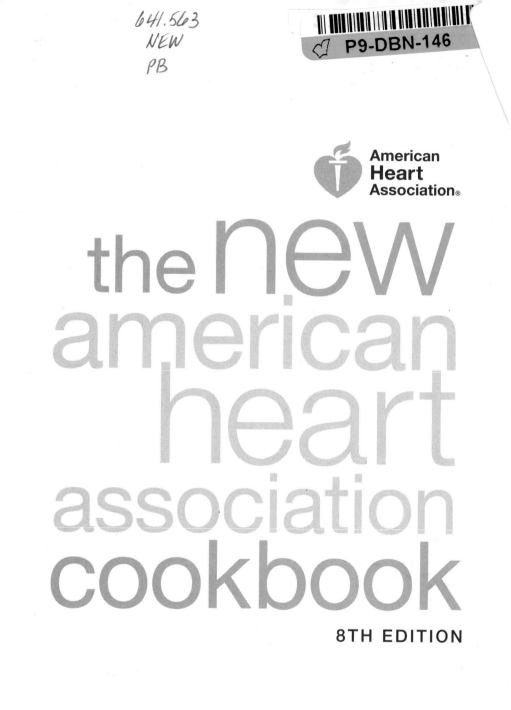

American
Heart
Association®

the new american heart association cookbook

8TH EDITION

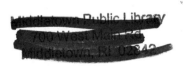

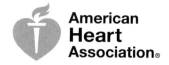
American Heart Association®

the new american heart association cookbook

8TH EDITION

CLARKSON POTTER/PUBLISHERS

NEW YORK

Copyright © 1973, 1975, 1979, 1984, 1991, 1998, 2004, 2010 by
American Heart Association
Illustrations copyright © 1998 by Paul Hoffman

Published in the United States by Clarkson Potter/Publishers, an imprint of
the Crown Publishing Group, a division of Random House, Inc., New York.
www.crownpublishing.com
www.clarksonpotter.com

CLARKSON POTTER is a trademark and POTTER with colophon is a registered
trademark of Random House, Inc.

Prior editions of this work were published in 1973, 1975, 1979, 1984, 1991, 1998,
and 2004

Your contributions to the American Heart Association support research that helps
make publications like this possible. For more information, call 1-800-AHA-USA1
(1-800-242-8721) or contact us online at www.americanheart.org.

Library of Congress Cataloging-in-Publication Data
American Heart Association new American cookbook / American Heart Association
—8th ed.
    p.   cm.
    Includes index.
    1. Heart—Disease—Diet therapy—Recipes.   2. Low-cholesterol diet—Recipes.
American Heart Association.   II. Title: New American cookbook.
    RC684.D5A44 2010
    641.5·6311—dc22   2009044692

ISBN 978-0-307-58757-2
eISBN 978-0-7704-3299-7

Printed in the United States of America

Book design by Stephanie Huntwork

Eighth Edition

CONTENTS

ACKNOWLEDGMENTS

American Heart Association Consumer Publications
Director: Linda S. Ball
Managing Editor: Deborah A. Renza
Senior Editor: Janice Roth Moss
Science Editor/Writer: Jacqueline F. Haigney
Assistant Editor: Roberta Westcott Sullivan

Recipe Developers for This and Previous Editions
Ellen C. Boeke
Claire Criscuolo
Sarah Fritschner
FRP
Nancy S. Hughes
Ruth Mossok Johnston
Jackie Mills, M.S., R.D.
Carol Ritchie
Julie Shapiro, R.D., L.D.
Marjorie Steenson
Linda Foley Woodrum

Nutrition Analyst
Tammi Hancock, R.D.

Today more than ever, the scientific community agrees that a healthy diet and lifestyle translate to a healthy body. Because food choices play such an important role in overall heart health, the American Heart Association has been publishing cookbooks for nearly four decades to help Americans eat well. Like the science behind it, this cookbook has undergone many transitions since the first edition was published in 1973. Our understanding of nutrition science has grown, new food products have emerged, and the cooking and eating habits of American families have changed. To keep up with these ongoing shifts, *The New American Heart Association Cookbook* is continuously revised to reflect the latest developments in cardiovascular science as well as new trends in taste and food preparation.

As the nation's leading authority on heart health, the American Heart Association creates our cookbooks and recipes to move our nutrition message from words into action. Eating good-for-you food does not have to come at the expense of good taste. To accomplish this goal, we work with a team of experts from both the health and culinary fields to ensure that each and every recipe delivers on all fronts. As a result, in these pages you'll find more than 600 dishes that meet not only our high standards for good heart health but also your expectations for exceptional flavor.

For the eighth edition of this practical and comprehensive cookbook, we have also updated the information on our dietary guidelines according to the most current scientific consensus. To help you adhere to those recommendations, we've made sure our recipes provide you with opportunities to incorporate more whole grains, vegetables, and fruits into your diet in delicious ways.

Having sold more than 3 million copies of this, our flagship cookbook, known over the years simply as "Big Red," we at the American Heart Association take great pleasure in knowing that our efforts have been helping individuals and families eat well and enjoy delicious meals together—while safeguarding their hearts—for more than 35 years. We are thrilled to carry on this tradition by offering you and your family this latest edition of Big Red for good eating and good health for years to come.

Rose Marie Robertson, M.D.
Chief Science Officer
American Heart Association/American Stroke Association

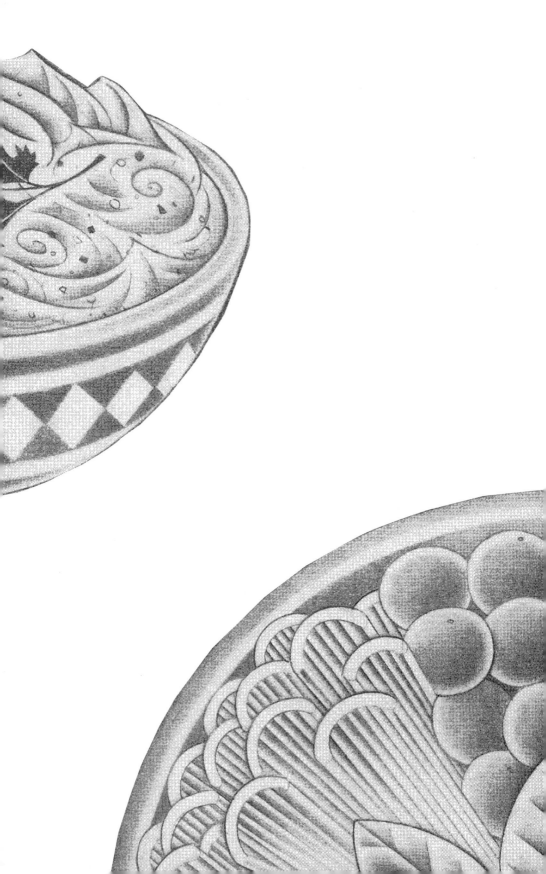

eat well to stay well

The cornerstone of good health is eating well. If you eat a balanced and nutritious diet, you have a much greater chance of achieving both long-term heart health and greater vitality. Cooking at home is one of the most effective ways to adopt healthy eating habits and to control which foods and how much you eat. With *The New American Heart Association Cookbook* in your kitchen, you can put healthy—and delicious—meals on your table night after night.

This eighth edition offers more than 600 nutritious and flavorful recipes—including 150 new dishes. You'll find favorite standards from previous editions, such as Chicken with Apricot Glaze and Grilled Stuffed Flank Steak. You'll also be intrigued by new recipes that showcase contemporary flavors and cooking trends, such as Pomegranate Walnut Chicken and Slow-Cooker Cioppino, and that let you experiment with foods you may not have tried but that provide big nutritional benefits. You'll find a broadened range of diverse flavors inspired by ethnic cuisines, including dishes such as Asian-Style Barbecue Pork, Chicken Gyros with Tzatziki Sauce, and Slow-Cooker Chile Verde Pork Chops. With literally hundreds of recipes to choose from, you're sure to find whatever you need, from make-it-in-a-hurry dishes to slow-cooker meals, from weeknight dinners to weekend entertaining, and from after-school snacks to special-occasion menus.

So whether you're an expert cook or just starting to find your way around the kitchen, this classic cookbook lets you celebrate the flavor and freshness of good food while nourishing your body with a variety of healthy ingredients. You can trust that each of the recipes is not only delicious but also follows the dietary guidelines of the American Heart Association.

We invite you to explore and experiment with the recipes in the pages that follow. We encourage you to let this cookbook be your guide to eating well as you work toward good heart health.

MAKING HEALTHY FOOD CHOICES

In 2006, the American Heart Association revised its dietary guidelines to emphasize how important good lifestyle choices are in achieving optimal health. The new guidelines also reflect how several long-held beliefs about diet and heart health have evolved as a result of ongoing research. For example, we now know that it's the type of fat, more than the quantity, that affects the development of cardiovascular disease. (For more information, see Appendix A, "How Your Diet Affects Your Heart," page 640.) We also know that changing how you eat and live can improve many of the factors—your "health factors"—that can delay or prevent heart disease. These factors include having a normal body mass index, being a nonsmoker, having normal blood pressure and cholesterol levels, and being physically active. No matter what your age or health status, you can eat well and enjoy a healthier lifestyle by following some simple, basic principles. You don't have to be perfect all the time, but every good choice you make counts toward better long-term health. The key is eating the right balance from a variety of food types and making smart, healthy choices most of the time.

EAT A WIDE VARIETY OF NUTRITIOUS FOODS

Each food group contributes to your overall health by providing a unique combination of nutrients. Your body requires the full spectrum, including fiber, vitamins, minerals, and other essentials, to stay healthy. That's why it's important to include vegetables, fruits, fat-free or low-fat (1%) dairy products, whole grains and other high-fiber foods, fish rich in omega-3 fatty acids, lean meats and poultry, and heart-healthy unsaturated oils and fats in your diet.

As you decide what to eat each day, focus on the foods that give you the best nutritional payback and limit foods and beverages that are high in calories but don't provide much nourishment. (To help you choose foods wisely as you sort through the array of choices in the supermarket, see Appendix B, "Shopping with Your Heart in Mind," page 642.)

Load Up on Vegetables and Fruits

Nutrition studies continue to demonstrate the many health benefits that come from eating a wide variety of vegetables and fruits. Eating more vegetables and fruits each day can help lower blood pressure and cholesterol, as well as keep your weight under control. Select produce in a wide variety of colors to be sure you get a broad range of nutrients. Don't get in a rut: Experiment with vegetables and fruits you haven't tried. For example, if you eat about 2,000 calories daily, you should aim for five servings of vegetables and four servings of fruits each day, including about 3 cups of dark green vegetables and 2 cups of different-colored vegetables and fruits in each week's total. This isn't as hard as it seems: Remember that one serving can be your choice of 1 cup raw leafy greens, ½ cup cut-up raw or cooked vegetables or fruit, ½ cup vegetable or fruit juice, 1 medium piece of fruit, or ¼ cup dried fruit.

> good-health tip Most frozen and canned vegetables and fruits have about the same nutritional value as fresh, but be sure to look for products that have no fat, salt, or sugar added during processing.

Choose Fat-Free and Low-Fat Dairy Products

Fat-free and low-fat (1%) dairy products, such as milk, cheeses, and yogurt, are an essential part of a well-rounded diet. They provide calcium, protein, and other vital nutrients with less artery-clogging saturated fat than their whole-milk or full-fat counterparts. If you are eating about 2,000 calories a day, aim for two to three servings of dairy each day, and choose fat-free products when possible. Examples of one serving include 1 cup of fat-free or low-fat milk and 1½ ounces of fat-free or natural (not processed) low-fat cheese.

> good-health tip If you drink whole milk, transition gradually to 2% fat, then 1%, then ½% (if available), and finally fat-free milk for the fewest calories, the least fat and cholesterol, and the greatest health benefit. Although 2% milk is considered "reduced-fat," it still contains almost half the fat of whole milk, which has 3½% fat.

	Whole Milk, 1 cup	Fat-Free Milk, 1 cup
Calories	146	83
Total Fat, g	8	0
Saturated Fat, g	5	0
Cholesterol, mg	24	5

Opt for Whole Grains

Unrefined whole grains contain important vitamins, minerals, and both soluble and insoluble fiber. Including enough soluble fiber in your diet has been shown to help lower blood levels of harmful LDL cholesterol. Insoluble fiber is digested slowly, so it also may help stabilize blood glucose levels and make you feel full, which helps prevent overeating and weight gain. A balanced 2,000-calorie diet should include about six servings of grain-based foods a day, and at least half those servings should come from whole-grain foods. Examples of one serving include one slice of whole-grain bread, ½ cup of whole-grain pasta, ½ cup of oatmeal, and ½ cup of brown rice.

good-health tip Be sure to check the labels on grain products. Look for breads, cereals, pastas, and other foods that list a whole grain as the first ingredient.

Eat Fish at Least Twice a Week

To help protect your heart, make fish a regular part of your diet. Because research suggests that eating fish that contain omega-3 fatty acids reduces the risk of heart disease, the American Heart Association recommends eating at least two servings of fish, preferably fatty fish, each week (one serving equals 3 ounces cooked weight, or 4 ounces raw). If you are concerned about the mercury in fish and shellfish, remember that the health risks from mercury exposure depend on the amount of seafood eaten and the level of mercury in the individual fish. In most cases, the benefits of fish far outweigh the risks.

good-health tip Examples of fish rich in heart-healthy fatty acids include salmon, trout, halibut, tuna, and mackerel.

Select Lean Meats and Poultry

Eating too much of the fats present in animal foods can put your heart health at risk. Lean and extra-lean cuts of meat and skinless poultry, however, are relatively low in these fats and are excellent sources of protein. The body uses protein for growth and tissue repair, but many American adults eat more than their bodies need. To avoid adding

good-health tip When planning a meal, imagine a plate divided into four parts: two for vegetables and fruits, one for grains, and the fourth for a serving of meat, poultry, or other protein source, such as beans. Try considering meat and poultry as a side dish instead of a main course.

unnecessary saturated fat and cholesterol to your diet, choose the leanest cuts and limit portion size. A healthy serving of cooked meat or poultry is about the size of a computer mouse or deck of playing cards, and about two servings (a total of 6 ounces cooked weight, 8 ounces raw) each day is plenty for most adults.

Incorporate Legumes, Nuts, and Seeds into Your Meal Planning

To help cut back on the saturated fat and cholesterol you eat each week, make vegetarian meals a regular part of your eating plan. Use legumes in entrées and side dishes as a great source of meatless protein and a terrific source of fiber. Try to serve these nutritional powerhouses three or four times a week. Examples include beans such as kidney beans and chickpeas, lentils, edamame (green soybeans), peas, and even peanuts. Walnuts, almonds, and most other nuts and seeds are nutrient dense, providing protein as well as heart-healthy unsaturated oils. They are also high in calories, however, so eat them in moderation and without added salt. Aim for a handful of nuts (about 1½ ounces, or one serving) three or four times a week.

> good-health tip Dry-roasting nuts and seeds intensifies their flavor without adding calories or salt. See "Cook's Tip on Dry-Roasting Nuts," page 87, for more information.

Use Unsaturated Fats

Including fats in your diet is essential: They provide energy, support cell growth, and help your body absorb nutrients and produce hormones. Of the four major types of dietary fat, the unsaturated fats found in vegetable oils such as olive and canola offer the most health benefits. Instead of butter or stick margarine, use fat-free spray margarines or the light tub spreads that are lowest in saturated and trans fats. Remember too that all fats are high in calories, so it's important to be aware of how much you use.

> good-health tip To help distinguish between the types of fat, remember that unsaturated fats stay liquid at room temperature, while saturated fats stay solid.

LIMIT NUTRIENT-POOR FOODS

If you concentrate first on choosing nutrient-rich foods and eating enough from the food groups described on the previous pages, you will meet your body's needs and feel satisfied, with little room left for foods that don't offer much benefit. On the other hand, nutrient-poor foods such as sugary sodas and French fries offer little or no nutritional value while adding the extra calories and dietary villains—saturated and trans fats, cholesterol, and sodium—that can jeopardize your health. Reducing your intake of these less-healthy foods will help you manage your weight and protect your heart.

Make Your Calories Count

Foods and beverages that are high in calories but low in nutrients may appease your hunger but do not contribute to your overall well-being, and they take the place of more nutritious foods that promote good health. When you do choose a high-calorie soda or snack, for example, make it an occasional treat rather than a habit. Also be mindful of portion sizes to keep your calorie intake in check. A steady diet of large portions of high-calorie food will increase your chance of becoming overweight or obese, a major risk factor for heart disease and stroke.

good-health tip Think before you drink that can of soda: A 12-ounce can of regular soda contains about 8 teaspoons of added sugar! No more than half of your daily discretionary calories should come from added sugars, which for most women means no more than 100 calories a day (about 6 teaspoons or 25 grams of added sugars), and for most men no more than 150 calories (about 9 teaspoons or 38 grams).

Limit Foods That Contain Saturated Fat, Trans Fat, and Cholesterol

We know that a steady diet of foods rich in saturated and trans fats raises the level of LDL ("bad") cholesterol in your blood and decreases HDL ("good") cholesterol. These changes in the cholesterol present in your bloodstream contribute to the gradual buildup of plaque in your arteries, which in turn can lead to heart disease, heart attack, or stroke. On the other hand, polyunsaturated and monounsaturated fats, such as those found in healthful oils and nuts and seeds, tend to lower the level of harmful LDL cholesterol and may help increase helpful HDL.

That's why we recommend that you limit saturated and trans fats while using more of the healthy unsaturated oils and fats. (For information on heart-healthy shopping, see Appendix B, "Shopping with Your Heart in Mind," page 642, and for cooking techniques, see Appendix C, "Cooking for a Healthy Heart," page 652.)

Saturated fats are found in foods from animal sources, such as meat, poultry, whole-milk dairy products (such as cream, butter, and cheese), and lard. They also occur in tropical vegetable oils, such as coconut, palm, and palm kernel oils. Check nutrition facts panels to keep your intake of saturated fats to less than 7 percent of your total daily calories.

> **good-health tip** To reduce saturated fat, choose the leanest cuts of meat and skinless poultry and prepare them without adding fats. Replace whole-fat dairy products with fat-free and low-fat (1%) alternatives. Use healthy cooking techniques and healthy unsaturated oils in limited amounts.

Trans fats (or *trans* fatty acids) are created in an industrial process that adds hydrogen to liquid vegetable oils to make them more solid; these altered oils are called "partially hydrogenated." Trans fat is especially common in commercial products, but many manufacturers and restaurants are reformulating their products to reduce or eliminate levels of trans fat. Check nutrition facts panels for trans fat, and aim to keep your intake of trans fat to less than 1 percent of your total daily calories. (Watch too for products that use unhealthy saturated fat to replace trans fat.)

> **good-health tip** Use liquid vegetable oils and soft margarine to replace stick margarine and shortening. Avoid foods that contain or are cooked in partially hydrogenated oils. These include commercial fried foods and many baked goods, such as doughnuts, cookies, and crackers.

Although high blood cholesterol levels are closely tied to consumption of saturated and trans fats, *dietary cholesterol* also may contribute to your body's production of LDL cholesterol. Aim for less than 300 milligrams of dietary cholesterol each day. If you are trying to lower your blood cholesterol, it makes sense to be aware of the foods that contain the most cholesterol, such as egg yolks, whole milk and full-fat cheese, animal fats, organ meats, and many shellfish. For example, one large egg has about 215 milligrams, and one 3-ounce serving of cooked shrimp has about 170 milligrams.

good-health tip Remember that dietary cholesterol comes only from animal products; vegetable-based foods do not contain cholesterol.

Limit Foods That Are High in Sodium

Sodium is vital in maintaining the complicated balance of fluids and electrolytes in your body, but most Americans consume much more of it than they need. Ideally, most people should limit their intake of sodium to less than 1,500 milligrams each day for significant health benefits. A reduced sodium intake can lower blood pressure, prevent and control high blood pressure, and help prevent cardiovascular disease. To transition to lower levels of sodium in your diet, begin by aiming to eat less than 2,300 milligrams of sodium per day. Limit prepared and packaged foods that contain high levels of sodium, and use less salt in cooking and at the table. (See page 656 for easy tips on adding flavor while reducing sodium.)

good-health tip Because most of the sodium in our food supply comes from processed foods, it's easy to eat more than you realize. To keep track, get in the habit of checking the nutrition information for foods you buy or eat away from home.

APPLY THE SAME NUTRITIONAL PRINCIPLES WHEN EATING OUT

Whether for work or pleasure, today most of us eat away from home more than ever. Although the typical menu offerings in most restaurants and fast-food eateries may not be as heart-healthy as they could be, you can still make healthy choices when you eat out. Just follow the same basic principles outlined here and—especially important—watch your portions. To keep to reasonable serving sizes, plan to take half your food home or share with a dining partner.

MAKING HEALTHY LIFESTYLE CHOICES

Good overall health comes from making positive lifestyle choices over time—as well as following the principles of a healthy diet. Choosing and maintaining habits that benefit your physical well-being can boost your energy, promote better overall health, and reduce your risk of cardiovascular disease.

BE PHYSICALLY ACTIVE

A regular routine of physical activity is an essential part of a healthy lifestyle. Exercise protects against heart disease in many ways: It strengthens the heart's pumping power, lowers blood pressure, and improves cholesterol levels. In general, it makes you feel better and more energized. You don't have to run marathons—any activity of enough intensity to increase your heart rate offers health benefits. For the most part, people succeed in making physical activity a consistent part of their lives when they like what they are doing. If going to the gym is not for you, try other types of physical activity, such as walking, playing basketball, biking, or dancing, until you find something you can stick with. When you get bored with one type of activity, switch to something different, or mix it up by alternating activities. If you haven't been active for a while, set reasonable goals, and as you achieve them, reward yourself.

You should aim for at least 150 minutes (2 hours and 30 minutes) of moderate-intensity or 75 minutes (1 hour and 15 minutes) of vigorous-intensity aerobic exercise each week. Moderate-intensity activities increase your heart rate to the point that you are able to talk but not sing while you are exercising. At vigorous intensity, you should not be able to say more than a few words without needing to catch your breath. You can combine activities at different intensities, and you can even break your workout time into sessions of 10 minutes or more, spread out through the week, to reach an equivalent total. Twice a week or more, you should also include moderate- or high-intensity muscle-strengthening activities that involve all the major muscle groups.

> **good-health tip** Wear a pedometer to count your steps for a week to gauge your typical activity level. Experts recommend aiming for 10,000 steps a day. If you aren't averaging that amount, slowly work your way up by adding about 250 steps each day.

MAINTAIN A HEALTHY WEIGHT

Extra pounds put extra stress on your heart and entire circulatory system, increasing your risk of heart disease, stroke, and diabetes. That's why the balance between the calories you eat and the calories you burn is critical to maintaining overall good health and a healthy weight. Calories measure energy—the energy your body uses and the energy in the foods you eat. If you eat more calories than your body uses, you gain weight; if you eat fewer, you lose weight. The right number of calories for you will vary based on your age and physical activity level. Your healthcare provider can help you determine your ideal weight and whether you should reduce, increase, or maintain your calorie intake. You can also find online information on weight management at www.americanheart.org.

good-health tip To lose about one pound a week, reduce your calorie intake by 500 calories a day. Reduce your calorie intake by 1,000 calories a day to lose about two pounds. Don't try to lose more than two pounds a week without the guidance of a healthcare professional.

BE MODERATE IN YOUR ALCOHOL USE

Alcohol adds calories yet has no nutritional value. Although current studies indicate that drinking moderate amounts of alcohol may help protect against heart disease, it's also clear that too much alcohol can lead to serious problems, including high blood pressure and an increased risk of stroke. If you do drink alcohol, do so in moderation. If you don't drink, don't start.

good-health tip Drinking in moderate amounts means one drink per day for a woman and two drinks per day for a man. One drink is equivalent to 12 ounces of beer, 4 ounces of wine, or 1½ ounces of 80-proof spirits.

ABOUT THE RECIPES

You will get the most from this cookbook if you know how to use the recipes and the information they include. We have provided a nutrition analysis for each recipe so you can plan your meals using the dishes that best meet your needs and be confident that the recipes you prepare reflect dietary principles that promote good heart health.

HOW THE RECIPES ARE ANALYZED

We make every effort to provide accurate nutrition information. Because of the many variables involved in analyzing foods, however, the values provided should be considered approximate. Also, food manufacturers continue to reformulate their products in response to changing trends, so check the nutrition facts panels on commercial products for the most up-to-date information.

- Each analysis is based on a single serving, unless otherwise indicated.
- When ingredient options are listed, the first one is analyzed.
- When a range of amounts is given, the average is analyzed.
- Optional ingredients and garnishes are not included in the nutrition analysis.
- The specific ingredients listed in each recipe are analyzed. If you make ingredient substitutions, remember that the nutrition values will change. In most cases, using similar foods (for example, bottled lemon juice for fresh or white onions instead of yellow) won't change the values enough to matter; if you use a low-fat cheese instead of fat-free, however, the fat values will be significantly different.
- We use the lowest-sodium products that are widely available for analysis, and we encourage you to compare nutrition facts labels and shop for low-sodium products whenever possible. If you have to substitute a high-sodium ingredient, remember to adjust the nutrition values for that recipe.
- Because product labeling in the marketplace can vary and change quickly, we use the generic terms "fat-free" and "low-fat" throughout to avoid confusion.
- We specify canola, corn, and olive oils in these recipes, but you can also use other heart-healthy unsaturated oils, such as safflower, soybean, and sunflower.

- Nutrient values except for fats are rounded to the nearest whole number. Values for saturated, trans, monounsaturated, and polyunsaturated fats are rounded to the nearest half gram; because of the rounding, they may not add up to the amount listed for total fat.
- Analyses of meat are based on cooked lean meat with all visible fat discarded.
- For ground beef, we use 95 percent fat-free meat.
- When meat, poultry, or seafood is marinated and the marinade is discarded, we calculate only the amount of marinade absorbed.
- In recipes that call for broth, we use our homemade broths (pages 42–44) in the analyses. We encourage you to make your own broth to keep sodium low and flavor high. If you do use commercial broths, be sure to choose the products lowest in sodium and fat.
- When alcohol is used in a dish that is cooked, we estimate that most of the alcohol calories evaporate during cooking.
- When no quantity is listed for an ingredient in a recipe (for example, the small amount of flour used to prepare a surface for kneading dough), that ingredient is not included in the analysis.
- We use the abbreviations "g" for gram and "mg" for milligram.

WHY CERTAIN INGREDIENTS ARE USED

We strive for the best ingredient choices that will produce the most delicious results while still following our nutrition guidelines. For example, to keep the level of sodium in our recipes low, we call for unprocessed foods or no-salt-added and low-sodium products when possible and add table salt sparingly for flavor. That might mean a recipe uses a can of no-salt-added tomatoes and ¼ teaspoon of table salt instead of a regular can of tomatoes and no table salt. In the same vein, to keep the cholesterol within reasonable limits, we often use egg substitute instead of whole eggs. Sometimes, though, especially with baked goods, for optimal taste and texture, we call for whole eggs or a combination of eggs and egg substitute.

We hope you will enjoy using this cookbook and that many of these recipes will become long-standing favorites. We encourage you to try all kinds of healthy foods, herbs and spices, varied healthy cooking techniques, and unusual ingredient combinations. Good food is more than the sum of its physical ingredients: A truly satisfying meal is also a social and emotional experience that encompasses good nutrition, creativity in the kitchen, and enjoyment at the table. Choosing to eat well for good health is an ongoing adventure—and a positive lifestyle move that will bring you lasting benefits for a lifetime.

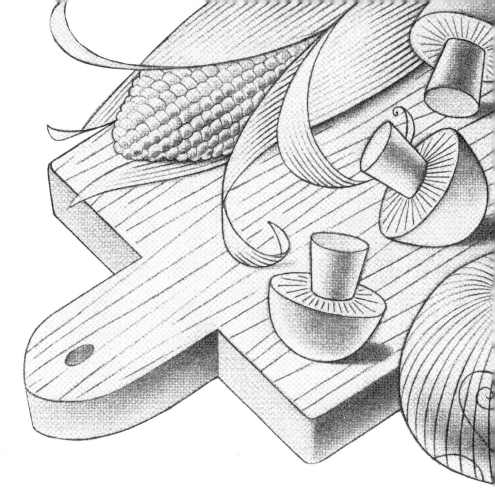

recipes

appetizers, snacks, and beverages

Mexican Bean Dip

Lots of Layers Dip

Cucumber and Yogurt Dip

Spinach Dip

Artichoke Dip

Ranch Dip

Apricot Dip

Luscious Berry Dip

Cinnamon-Sugar Pita Chips with Fruit Salsa

Fire-and-Ice Cream Cheese Spread

Roasted-Pepper Hummus

Torta with Chèvre and Sun-Dried Tomatoes

Plum Tomatoes with Blue Cheese

Plum Tomatoes with Feta Cheese

Red Potatoes with Feta Cheese and Basil

Orange Chicken Lettuce Wraps

Crumb-Crusted Mushrooms with Lemon

Crumb-Crusted Tomato Slices

Sweet-and-Sour Spring Rolls

Jalapeño Poppers

Mexican Potato Skins

Tortilla Pinwheels

Pepper-Topped Whole-Grain Tortilla Pizzas

Stuffed Mushrooms

Coconut Halibut Bites

Skewered Chicken Strips with Soy-Peanut Marinade

Meatballs in Beer Sauce

Spinach and Cheese Mini Quiches

mexican bean dip

SERVES 8; ¼ CUP PER SERVING

A colorful array of garnishes, such as cilantro, radishes, tomatoes, green and red onions, and jalapeños, would be the perfect finishing touches for this creamy dip, which is equally good hot or cold.

¼ cup hot water
2 teaspoons very low sodium beef bouillon granules
1 15.5-ounce can no-salt-added kidney beans, rinsed and drained
½ cup no-salt-added tomato sauce
½ cup chopped onion

¼ cup chopped green bell pepper
2½ tablespoons fresh lime juice
2 medium garlic cloves, minced
¼ teaspoon cayenne, or to taste
¼ teaspoon ground cumin (optional)
1 tablespoon olive oil (extra virgin preferred)

Put the water and bouillon granules in a food processor or blender. Pulse several times to dissolve the granules.

Add the remaining ingredients except the oil. Process until smooth.

To serve at room temperature, stir in the oil (don't process it). To serve warm, heat the dip in a small saucepan over medium heat for 5 to 6 minutes, stirring frequently. Remove from the heat. Stir in the oil.

COOK'S TIP on decorative veggie bowls

When entertaining, halve butternut and acorn squash lengthwise and discard the strings and seeds. Put a different garnish in each squash half. For the dip, cut the top off a large acorn squash and discard the strings and seeds. Cut a thin slice from the bottom side so the squash doesn't rock. Arrange the garnish-filled squash halves around the dip, and let each person choose the ones he or she prefers.

PER SERVING

CALORIES 78
TOTAL FAT 2.0 g
  Saturated Fat 0.0 g
  Trans Fat 0.0 g
  Polyunsaturated Fat 0.0 g
  Monounsaturated Fat 1.0 g
CHOLESTEROL 0 mg
SODIUM 6 mg
CARBOHYDRATES 13 g
  Fiber 3 g
  Sugars 3 g
PROTEIN 4 g
DIETARY EXCHANGES
  1 starch

lots of layers dip

SERVES 16; TWO 2-INCH SQUARES PER SERVING

A classic for football parties, this traditionally high-calorie, fat-laden dip goes light with fat-free dairy products and quick tomato salsa. Heating the chili powder for just a few minutes gives this dip an extra punch of flavor.

⅓ cup chopped avocado

¼ teaspoon fresh lime juice

1 15.5-ounce can no-salt-added pinto beans or no-salt-added black beans, rinsed and drained

2 tablespoons canned diced green chiles, drained

½ teaspoon canola or corn oil

¼ teaspoon garlic powder

1 14.5-ounce can no-salt-added diced tomatoes, drained

1 teaspoon ground cumin

1 teaspoon cider vinegar

¾ cup sliced green onions

1½ teaspoons chili powder

¾ cup fat-free sour cream

½ cup shredded fat-free Cheddar cheese

3 tablespoons sliced black olives, chopped

In a small bowl, gently stir together the avocado and lime juice. Set aside.

In an 8-inch square glass baking dish, mash the beans until broken into medium-size chunks. (A potato masher works well for this.) Stir in the chiles, oil, and garlic powder. Spread to cover the bottom of the dish.

In a medium bowl, stir together the tomatoes, cumin, and vinegar. Spread over the beans. Sprinkle with the green onions.

In a small nonstick skillet, heat the chili powder over low heat for 5 minutes, or until fragrant, stirring frequently.

Put the sour cream in a small bowl. Stir in the chili powder. Spread over the green onions.

Sprinkle with the Cheddar, then with the olives. Sprinkle the reserved avocado on top.

COOK'S TIP

If you have leftovers, you may want to remove the avocado because it will turn brown. For a quick lunch, warm the dip and some corn tortillas separately in the microwave, spread the dip over the tortillas, top with shredded lettuce, and roll up the tortillas.

PER SERVING

CALORIES 57
TOTAL FAT 1.0 g
  Saturated Fat 0.0 g
  Trans Fat 0.0 g
  Polyunsaturated Fat 0.0 g
  Monounsaturated Fat 0.5 g
CHOLESTEROL 3 mg
SODIUM 80 mg
CARBOHYDRATES 9 g
  Fiber 2 g
  Sugars 3 g
PROTEIN 4 g
DIETARY EXCHANGES
  ½ starch,
  ½ very lean meat

cucumber and yogurt dip

SERVES 8; SCANT 3 TABLESPOONS PER SERVING

Tasty as a dip, this recipe also makes an excellent sauce for poached or grilled salmon that has been chilled.

1 medium unpeeled cucumber, seeded and diced

4 to 5 medium green onions, finely chopped

½ cup fat-free plain yogurt

⅓ cup light mayonnaise

¼ cup shredded or grated Parmesan cheese

2 medium garlic cloves, minced

1 teaspoon white wine Worcestershire sauce

In a medium bowl, stir together the ingredients. Cover and refrigerate for at least 1 hour.

PER SERVING

CALORIES 50
TOTAL FAT 3.0 g
  Saturated Fat 0.5 g
  Trans Fat 0.0 g
  Polyunsaturated Fat 1.5 g
  Monounsaturated Fat 0.5 g
CHOLESTEROL 6 mg
SODIUM 145 mg
CARBOHYDRATES 3 g
  Fiber 1 g
  Sugars 2 g
PROTEIN 3 g
DIETARY EXCHANGES
  ½ fat

spinach dip

SERVES 6; ¼ CUP PER SERVING

Watercress adds a peppery bite and avocado provides a lush richness to this appetizer.

1 10-ounce package frozen chopped spinach	1 medium avocado, chopped
5 medium green onions, coarsely chopped	1¼ teaspoons salt-free garlic and herb seasoning blend
½ cup watercress leaves or baby arugula	⅛ teaspoon pepper
¼ cup fresh parsley, stems discarded	⅛ teaspoon salt
8 ounces fat-free plain yogurt	⅛ teaspoon red hot-pepper sauce, or to taste

Prepare the spinach using the package directions, omitting the salt and margarine. Drain well in a colander. Squeeze dry.

In a food processor or blender, process the spinach, green onions, watercress, and parsley until just blended. The mixture should be coarse. Transfer to a colander to drain well.

Process the remaining ingredients until smooth. Transfer to a medium bowl.

Stir the spinach mixture into the yogurt mixture. Cover and refrigerate for at least 1 hour.

COOK'S TIP

For chunkier avocado in this dip, mash it with a fork instead of processing it. Stir the avocado into the spinach and yogurt mixture.

PER SERVING
CALORIES 93
TOTAL FAT 5.5 g
Saturated Fat 1.0 g
Trans Fat 0.0 g
Polyunsaturated Fat 0.5 g
Monounsaturated Fat 3.5 g
CHOLESTEROL 1 mg
SODIUM 120 mg
CARBOHYDRATES 9 g
Fiber 4 g
Sugars 4 g
PROTEIN 5 g
DIETARY EXCHANGES
½ carbohydrate,
1 fat

artichoke dip

SERVES 8; SCANT ¼ CUP PER SERVING

Surround a bowl of this dip with whole-grain crackers or baked chips.

½ cup fat-free plain yogurt
4 ounces light tub cream cheese, at room temperature
2 medium green onions (green part only), thinly sliced
1½ teaspoons cream sherry
1 teaspoon dried Italian seasoning, crumbled
⅛ teaspoon garlic powder
⅛ teaspoon salt
1 9-ounce package frozen artichoke hearts, thawed, patted dry, and finely chopped

In a medium bowl, whisk together all the ingredients except the artichokes.

Stir in the artichokes. Cover and refrigerate for at least 1 hour. Stir before serving.

PER SERVING

CALORIES 57
TOTAL FAT 2.5 g
  Saturated Fat 1.5 g
  Trans Fat 0.0 g
  Polyunsaturated Fat 0.0 g
  Monounsaturated Fat 0.5 g
CHOLESTEROL 10 mg
SODIUM 130 mg
CARBOHYDRATES 5 g
  Fiber 2 g
  Sugars 2 g
PROTEIN 3 g
DIETARY EXCHANGES
  1 vegetable, ½ fat

ranch dip

SERVES 4; ¼ CUP PER SERVING

This old friend is low in fat and makes a great appetizer or snack when served with a variety of fresh vegetables, such as cucumber rounds, celery sticks, and jícama spears. The fresh parsley really perks up the flavor.

2 ounces light tub cream cheese	½ teaspoon onion powder
¾ cup low-fat buttermilk	¼ teaspoon dried oregano, crumbled
2 tablespoons snipped fresh parsley	⅛ teaspoon pepper
½ teaspoon garlic powder	

In a medium bowl, using an electric mixer on medium speed, beat the cream cheese for 1 minute, or until fluffy.

Using the mixer on medium low, gradually beat in the buttermilk for 1 to 2 minutes, or until smooth.

Add the remaining ingredients. Beat for about 30 seconds, or until combined. Serve or cover and refrigerate for up to four days for a more pronounced flavor.

PER SERVING

CALORIES 54
TOTAL FAT 2.5 g
  Saturated Fat 1.5 g
  Trans Fat 0.0 g
  Polyunsaturated Fat 0.0 g
  Monounsaturated Fat 1.0 g
CHOLESTEROL 11 mg
SODIUM 114 mg
CARBOHYDRATES 4 g
  Fiber 0 g
  Sugars 3 g
PROTEIN 3 g
DIETARY EXCHANGES
  ½ fat

apricot dip

SERVES 8; ¼ CUP PER SERVING

This recipe makes a fabulous dip for fresh fruits, such as strawberries, bananas, and apple slices.

1 cup fresh orange juice
½ cup finely chopped dried apricots
   (3 to 4 ounces)
½ cup unsweetened applesauce

¼ teaspoon ground cinnamon
2 dashes ground nutmeg
8 ounces fat-free vanilla yogurt

In a small nonreactive saucepan, stir together the orange juice and apricots. Bring to a boil over medium-high heat. Reduce the heat and bring to a simmer, stirring frequently. As the apricots become tender, mash them with the back of a spoon. Simmer for about 20 minutes, or until all the liquid is absorbed. Transfer to a medium bowl.

Stir in the applesauce, cinnamon, and nutmeg. Cover and let cool.

Stir the yogurt into the cooled mixture. Cover and refrigerate for at least 1 hour.

COOK'S TIP on cutting sticky foods

To cut dried apricots or other sticky foods easily, use kitchen shears lightly sprayed with cooking spray.

PER SERVING

CALORIES 76
TOTAL FAT 0.0 g
  Saturated Fat 0.0 g
  Trans Fat 0.0 g
  Polyunsaturated Fat 0.0 g
  Monounsaturated Fat 0.0 g
CHOLESTEROL 1 mg
SODIUM 21 mg
CARBOHYDRATES 18 g
  Fiber 1 g
  Sugars 16 g
PROTEIN 2 g
DIETARY EXCHANGES
  1 fruit

luscious berry dip

SERVES 8; ¼ CUP PER SERVING

This rich-tasting fruit dip is the perfect complement to just about every fruit imaginable.

1 cup fat-free ricotta cheese
¾ cup halved fresh or frozen strawberries, hulled if fresh, thawed if frozen
½ cup fresh or ¾ cup frozen unsweetened raspberries, thawed if frozen, undrained

¼ cup fat-free vanilla yogurt
1 tablespoon firmly packed light brown sugar
½ teaspoon ground cinnamon

In a food processor or blender, process all the ingredients until smooth. Transfer to a small serving bowl. Cover and refrigerate until ready to serve.

COOK'S TIP

Frozen raspberries lose quite a bit of volume when they thaw, which is why the recipe calls for a larger amount of frozen raspberries than of fresh.

PER SERVING

CALORIES 45
TOTAL FAT 0.0 g
    Saturated Fat 0.0 g
    Trans Fat 0.0 g
    Polyunsaturated Fat 0.0 g
    Monounsaturated Fat 0.0 g
CHOLESTEROL 3 mg
SODIUM 66 mg
CARBOHYDRATES 6 g
    Fiber 1 g
    Sugars 5 g
PROTEIN 5 g
DIETARY EXCHANGES
    ½ carbohydrate,
    ½ lean meat

cinnamon-sugar pita chips with fruit salsa

SERVES 8; 4 PITA CHIPS AND ¼ CUP SALSA PER SERVING

Depending on which fruits are favorites at your house, experiment with the salsa. Two cups of just about any fruit combination would work well. You can make the sweet, crisp pita chips up to four days ahead and store them in an airtight container at room temperature.

CINNAMON-SUGAR PITA CHIPS
2 6-inch whole-grain pita pockets
2 tablespoons sugar
¼ teaspoon ground cinnamon

FRUIT SALSA
2 medium kiwifruit, peeled and diced
1 medium banana, diced
1 8-ounce can pineapple chunks in their own juice, drained and diced
2 teaspoons fresh lime juice

Preheat the oven to 350°F.

Cut each pita into 8 wedges. Split each wedge in half (you will have 32 pieces). Line a large baking sheet with cooking parchment. Place the wedges in a single layer on the parchment.

In a small bowl, stir together the sugar and cinnamon. Sprinkle over the pita wedges.

Bake for 10 to 12 minutes, or until crisp. Transfer the baking sheet to a cooling rack and let the pita chips cool completely.

Meanwhile, in a medium bowl, stir together the salsa ingredients. Serve the salsa with the pita chips.

PER SERVING
CALORIES 91
TOTAL FAT 0.5 g
  Saturated Fat 0.0 g
  Trans Fat 0.0 g
  Polyunsaturated Fat 0.0 g
  Monounsaturated Fat 0.0 g
CHOLESTEROL 0 mg
SODIUM 82 mg
CARBOHYDRATES 21 g
  Fiber 2 g
  Sugars 10 g
PROTEIN 2 g
DIETARY EXCHANGES
  1 starch, ½ fruit

fire-and-ice cream cheese spread

SERVES 4; 3 TABLESPOONS PER SERVING

Easy but elegant, this cream cheese spread is spiced with hot red pepper and cooled with the sweetness of apricots. Serve with pear slices or heart-healthy crackers.

¼ cup light tub cream cheese
¼ cup fat-free sour cream
¼ cup all-fruit apricot spread

¼ teaspoon crushed red pepper flakes
2 tablespoons finely chopped red bell pepper

In a small mixing bowl, with an electric mixer on medium speed, beat the cream cheese and sour cream until well blended.

Line a small bowl with plastic wrap. Spoon the cream cheese mixture into the bowl. Press the mixture lightly to get rid of any air pockets. Smooth the surface with a rubber scraper. Cover with plastic wrap and refrigerate for at least 30 minutes to firm slightly.

Meanwhile, in a small saucepan, cook the apricot spread and red pepper flakes over medium heat for 3 minutes, or until the spread just begins to melt, stirring occasionally. Remove from the heat.

Stir in the bell pepper. Let cool to room temperature.

Uncover and invert the cream cheese mixture onto a small serving plate. Discard the plastic wrap that lined the bowl. Top the cream cheese mixture with the apricot mixture.

PER SERVING

CALORIES 89
TOTAL FAT 2.5 g
   Saturated Fat 1.5 g
   Trans Fat 0.0 g
   Polyunsaturated Fat 0.0 g
   Monounsaturated Fat 0.5 g
CHOLESTEROL 12 mg
SODIUM 77 mg
CARBOHYDRATES 14 g
   Fiber 0 g
   Sugars 10 g
PROTEIN 2 g
DIETARY EXCHANGES
   1 fruit, ½ fat

roasted-pepper hummus

SERVES 8; ¼ CUP PER SERVING

Roasted bell pepper not only boosts the flavor of this creamy chickpea spread but adds color as well. Serve with Pita Crisps (page 30), heart-healthy crackers, or vegetable dippers.

2 tablespoons sesame seeds, dry-roasted

1 15.5-ounce can no-salt-added chickpeas, rinsed and drained

½ cup diced roasted red bell pepper, drained if bottled

¼ cup water

2 tablespoons fresh lime juice

1 medium garlic clove, minced

¼ teaspoon salt

⅛ teaspoon pepper

In a food processor or blender, process the sesame seeds for 30 seconds.

Add the remaining ingredients. Process until smooth. Serve at room temperature or refrigerate in an airtight container to serve chilled.

PER SERVING

CALORIES 69
TOTAL FAT 1.5 g
  Saturated Fat 0.0 g
  Trans Fat 0.0 g
  Polyunsaturated Fat 0.5 g
  Monounsaturated Fat 0.5 g
CHOLESTEROL 0 mg
SODIUM 94 mg
CARBOHYDRATES 11 g
  Fiber 3 g
  Sugars 1 g
PROTEIN 3 g
DIETARY EXCHANGES
  ½ starch,
  ½ lean meat

torta with chèvre and sun-dried tomatoes

SERVES 12; 2 TABLESPOONS PER SERVING

Chèvre (SHEHV-ruh), or goat cheese, lends its unique flavor to this attractive layered spread. Serve with veggie dippers or heart-healthy crackers.

3 ounces fat-free block cream cheese, softened
2 ounces light tub cream cheese
3 ounces soft goat cheese
1 cup water and 1 to 2 teaspoons water (optional), divided use
½ cup dry-packed sun-dried tomatoes (about 1 ounce)

1 teaspoon dried oregano, crumbled
1 medium garlic clove, minced
¼ teaspoon dried basil, crumbled
⅛ teaspoon pepper
¼ cup finely snipped fresh parsley
¼ teaspoon paprika
1 tablespoon pine nuts

In a medium mixing bowl, with an electric mixer on medium speed, beat the cheeses for 1 to 2 minutes, or until smooth. Cover and refrigerate for 30 minutes.

Meanwhile, in a small saucepan, bring 1 cup water to a boil over high heat. Stir in the tomatoes. Turn off the heat. Let soak for 10 to 15 minutes. Using a slotted spoon, transfer the tomatoes to a small bowl. Discard the soaking liquid. Let the tomatoes cool for 5 minutes. Coarsely chop. Squeeze out the excess liquid.

In a food processor or blender, process the tomatoes, oregano, garlic, basil, and pepper for 20 to 30 seconds, or until the desired consistency. For a smoother texture, add the remaining 1 to 2 teaspoons water. Cover and refrigerate for 30 minutes.

Line a 1½-cup bowl or other round container with plastic wrap. Spread one-third of the cheese mixture in the container. Press the mixture lightly to get rid of any air pockets. Smooth the surface with a rubber scraper. Top with half the tomato mixture. Repeat the layers. Top with the remaining cheese mixture. Cover and refrigerate for at least 30 minutes.

Uncover and invert the torta onto a small serving plate. Discard the plastic wrap. Press the parsley onto the sides of the torta. Sprinkle with the paprika and pine nuts.

PER SERVING

CALORIES 49
TOTAL FAT 2.5 g
  Saturated Fat 1.5 g
  Trans Fat 0.0 g
  Polyunsaturated Fat 0.0 g
  Monounsaturated Fat 0.5 g
CHOLESTEROL 7 mg
SODIUM 100 mg
CARBOHYDRATES 3 g
  Fiber 0 g
  Sugars 1 g
PROTEIN 3 g
DIETARY EXCHANGES
  ½ very lean meat,
  ½ fat

plum tomatoes with blue cheese

SERVES 8; 3 PIECES PER SERVING

This colorful appetizer features tomatoes topped with a spicy blue cheese mixture and chopped green onions.

1½ ounces blue cheese	12 medium Italian plum (Roma)
1 tablespoon plus 2 teaspoons	tomatoes
fat-free milk	2 tablespoons finely chopped green
¼ teaspoon red hot-pepper sauce	onions

In a medium mixing bowl, with an electric mixer on low speed, beat the blue cheese, milk, and hot-pepper sauce until completely blended, scraping the side of the bowl with a rubber scraper. Transfer to a small container. Cover and refrigerate for 30 minutes to 24 hours.

Cut the tomatoes in half lengthwise. Top each half with the cheese mixture. Sprinkle with the green onions. Serve or cover and refrigerate for up to 1 hour.

PLUM TOMATOES WITH FETA CHEESE

Substitute 2 ounces low-fat feta cheese for the blue cheese. Substitute fat-free plain yogurt for the milk.

RED POTATOES WITH FETA CHEESE AND BASIL

Replace the tomatoes with eight small red potatoes, cut in half lengthwise. Steam for 10 minutes. Plunge the potatoes into a bowl of ice water for 2 minutes. Drain well. Pat dry. Top each piece with the cheese mixture in Plum Tomatoes with Feta Cheese. Sprinkle with 2 tablespoons chopped fresh basil or green onions.

PER SERVING	PER SERVING PLUM TOMATOES WITH FETA CHEESE	PER SERVING RED POTATOES WITH FETA CHEESE AND BASIL
CALORIES 37	CALORIES 32	CALORIES 44
TOTAL FAT 1.5 g	TOTAL FAT 1.0 g	TOTAL FAT 1.0 g
Saturated Fat 1.0 g	Saturated Fat 0.5 g	Saturated Fat 0.5 g
Trans Fat 0.0 g	Trans Fat 0.0 g	Trans Fat 0.0 g
Polyunsaturated Fat 0.0 g	Polyunsaturated Fat 0.0 g	Polyunsaturated Fat 0.0 g
Monounsaturated Fat 0.5 g	Monounsaturated Fat 0.0 g	Monounsaturated Fat 0.0 g
CHOLESTEROL 4 mg	CHOLESTEROL 3 mg	CHOLESTEROL 3 mg
SODIUM 82 mg	SODIUM 102 mg	SODIUM 100 mg
CARBOHYDRATES 4 g	CARBOHYDRATES 4 g	CARBOHYDRATES 7 g
Fiber 1 g	Fiber 1 g	Fiber 1 g
Sugars 3 g	Sugars 3 g	Sugars 1 g
PROTEIN 2 g	PROTEIN 2 g	PROTEIN 2 g
DIETARY EXCHANGES	DIETARY EXCHANGES	DIETARY EXCHANGES
1 vegetable, ½ fat	1 vegetable	½ starch

orange chicken lettuce wraps

SERVES 8; 2 LETTUCE WRAPS PER SERVING

Delight your guests with these cool and crisp appetizers or use this dish as an entrée for four.

2 heads iceberg lettuce
1 teaspoon grated orange zest
¼ cup fresh orange juice
¼ cup fat-free, low-sodium chicken broth, such as on page 43
1 tablespoon plain rice vinegar
2 teaspoons soy sauce (lowest sodium available)
1½ teaspoons cornstarch
½ teaspoon toasted sesame oil
1 teaspoon canola or corn oil

1 pound boneless, skinless chicken breasts, all visible fat discarded, cut into ½-inch cubes
1 medium bell pepper (yellow preferred), diced
1 cup packaged broccoli slaw or 1 cup chopped broccoli florets
½ cup sliced canned water chestnuts, drained
2 medium green onions, thinly sliced

Cut each head of lettuce in half vertically. Discard the cores. Carefully remove 4 outside leaves from each half. Set aside.

In a small bowl, whisk together the orange zest, orange juice, broth, vinegar, soy sauce, cornstarch, and sesame oil. Set aside.

In a large nonstick skillet, heat the canola oil over medium-high heat, swirling to coat the bottom. Cook the chicken for 3 to 4 minutes, or until lightly browned on the outside and no longer pink in the center, stirring constantly.

Stir in the bell pepper. Cook for 1 to 2 minutes, or until tender-crisp, stirring constantly.

Stir in the broccoli slaw, water chestnuts, and green onions. Cook for 1 to 2 minutes, or until the broccoli is tender-crisp and the water chestnuts are heated through.

Stir in the reserved orange juice mixture. Reduce the heat and simmer for 2 to 3 minutes, or until the sauce is thickened, stirring occasionally. Transfer to a serving bowl.

Place the bowl of chicken filling in the center of a platter. Arrange the lettuce leaves around the bowl. Let each person spoon some chicken mixture onto lettuce leaves and gently roll to enclose the filling.

PER SERVING

CALORIES 104
TOTAL FAT 1.5 g
  Saturated Fat 0.5 g
  Trans Fat 0.0 g
  Polyunsaturated Fat 0.5 g
  Monounsaturated Fat 0.5 g
CHOLESTEROL 33 mg
SODIUM 90 mg
CARBOHYDRATES 9 g
  Fiber 3 g
  Sugars 4 g
PROTEIN 15 g
DIETARY EXCHANGES
  2 vegetable,
  2 very lean meat

crumb-crusted mushrooms with lemon

SERVES 4; 2 MUSHROOMS PER SERVING

Coat whole mushrooms with yogurt and a crust of seasoned bread crumbs, bake them for a few minutes, and watch them disappear!

1½ teaspoons light tub margarine
 2 slices whole-grain bread (lowest sodium available), processed into crumbs
 4 medium garlic cloves, minced
 1 teaspoon dried Italian seasoning, crumbled
 ⅛ teaspoon salt-free lemon pepper

 1 tablespoon grated lemon zest
   Cooking spray
 8 medium button mushrooms (about 1 ounce each), stems discarded
 ⅓ cup fat-free plain yogurt
 ¼ teaspoon paprika
 1 medium lemon, quartered

In a large nonstick skillet, melt the margarine over medium-high heat, swirling to coat the bottom. Add the bread crumbs, garlic, Italian seasoning, and lemon pepper, stirring to combine. Cook for 6 minutes, or until golden brown, stirring frequently. Remove from the heat.

Stir in the lemon zest.

Preheat the oven to 450°F. Lightly spray a baking sheet with cooking spray.

In a large bowl, gently stir together the mushrooms and yogurt to coat. Place the mushrooms in a single layer about ¼ inch apart on the baking sheet. Sprinkle with the bread crumb mixture, then with the paprika.

Bake for 5 minutes, or until heated through.

Gently transfer the mushrooms to a serving plate. Sprinkle with any bread crumbs remaining on the baking sheet. Garnish with the lemon wedges.

CRUMB-CRUSTED TOMATO SLICES

Lightly spray a 9-inch square baking pan with cooking spray. Substitute 2 large tomatoes (about 8 ounces each) for the mushrooms. Cut the tomatoes into 4 slices each. Place the tomatoes in the pan. Spoon the yogurt over each slice. Top with the crumb topping. Bake at 450°F for 20 minutes, or until soft. Garnish with the lemon wedges.

PER SERVING

CALORIES 69
TOTAL FAT 1.5 g
  Saturated Fat 0.0 g
  Trans Fat 0.0 g
  Polyunsaturated Fat 0.5 g
  Monounsaturated Fat 0.5 g
CHOLESTEROL 1 mg
SODIUM 97 mg
CARBOHYDRATES 11 g
  Fiber 2 g
  Sugars 3 g
PROTEIN 5 g
DIETARY EXCHANGES
  ½ starch

PER SERVING

CRUMB-CRUSTED TOMATO SLICES
CALORIES 77
TOTAL FAT 1.5 g
  Saturated Fat 0.0 g
  Trans Fat 0.0 g
  Polyunsaturated Fat 0.5 g
  Monounsaturated Fat 0.5 g
CHOLESTEROL 0 mg
SODIUM 100 mg
CARBOHYDRATES 13 g
  Fiber 3 g
  Sugars 6 g
PROTEIN 4 g
DIETARY EXCHANGES
  ½ starch, 1 vegetable

sweet-and-sour spring rolls

SERVES 4; 3 SPRING ROLLS PER SERVING

These vegetarian spring rolls are pan-fried, then glazed with sweet-and-sour sauce.

1 teaspoon canola or corn oil and
1 teaspoon canola or corn oil,
divided use
1½ cups shredded cabbage
4 medium garlic cloves, minced
4 medium green onions, chopped
1 8-ounce can bamboo shoots,
drained

2 teaspoons soy sauce (lowest
sodium available)
⅛ teaspoon pepper
3 18 x 14-inch sheets frozen phyllo
dough, thawed in refrigerator
Cooking spray
1 tablespoon plus 1 teaspoon bottled
sweet-and-sour sauce (lowest
sodium available)

In a large nonstick skillet, heat 1 teaspoon oil over medium-high heat for 1 minute, swirling to coat the bottom. Cook the cabbage and garlic for 3 minutes, stirring constantly.

Stir in the green onions and bamboo shoots. Cook for 30 seconds, stirring constantly. Remove from the heat.

Stir in the soy sauce and pepper.

Keeping the unused phyllo covered with a damp cloth or damp paper towels to prevent drying, lightly spray one sheet of dough with cooking spray. Working quickly, cut that sheet into four 9 x 7-inch pieces. Put three of the quarter-sheets under the cloth. On the remaining quarter, put 1 rounded tablespoon cabbage mixture 2 to 3 inches from one short end. Fold that end over the filling, then fold in the sides. Roll tightly. Set aside with the seam side down. Repeat with the remaining phyllo and filling.

Wipe the skillet with paper towels. Heat the remaining 1 teaspoon oil over medium-high heat for 1 minute, swirling to coat the bottom. Cook the spring rolls for 6 minutes, turning occasionally, until they are brown on all sides. Transfer to a serving plate. Brush with the sweet-and-sour sauce.

PER SERVING

CALORIES 105
TOTAL FAT 3.0 g
Saturated Fat 0.0 g
Trans Fat 0.0 g
Polyunsaturated Fat 1.0 g
Monounsaturated Fat 1.5 g
CHOLESTEROL 0 mg
SODIUM 145 mg
CARBOHYDRATES 18 g
Fiber 2 g
Sugars 3 g
PROTEIN 3 g
DIETARY EXCHANGES
1 starch, 1 vegetable,
½ fat

jalapeño poppers

SERVES 12; 2 PIECES PER SERVING

Charring fresh jalapeños imparts a smoky flavor and makes the coating adhere better to the surface.

Cooking spray
12 large fresh jalapeños (about 1 pound), halved lengthwise, seeds and ribs discarded
8 ounces fat-free block cream cheese, softened
½ cup shredded low-fat Cheddar cheese
1 teaspoon ground cumin
¼ cup all-purpose flour
½ cup egg substitute
⅓ cup plain dry bread crumbs (lowest sodium available)
1 teaspoon salt-free all-purpose seasoning blend

Preheat the broiler. Lightly spray a broiler pan and rack and a large baking sheet with cooking spray.

Place the jalapeños with the cut side down on the broiler rack.

Broil about 2 inches from the heat for 3 to 4 minutes, or until slightly charred. Using tongs, turn the jalapeños over. Broil for 2 to 3 minutes, or until tender-crisp. Transfer the broiler pan and rack to a cooling rack.

Preheat the oven to 400°F.

In a small mixing bowl, with an electric mixer on low speed, beat the cream cheese until smooth. Stir in the Cheddar and cumin. Spoon into the jalapeños.

Put the flour and egg substitute in separate shallow dishes. In a third shallow dish, stir together the bread crumbs and seasoning blend. Set the dishes and baking sheet in a row, assembly-line fashion. Lightly coat each jalapeño in the flour, then in the egg substitute, and finally in the bread crumbs. Place with the stuffed side up on the baking sheet.

Bake for 8 to 10 minutes, or until golden brown and heated through. Put the baking sheet on a cooling rack. Let cool for 3 to 4 minutes.

PER SERVING

CALORIES 60
TOTAL FAT 0.5 g
　Saturated Fat 0.5 g
　Trans Fat 0.0 g
　Polyunsaturated Fat 0.0 g
　Monounsaturated Fat 0.0 g
CHOLESTEROL 4 mg
SODIUM 208 mg
CARBOHYDRATES 7 g
　Fiber 1 g
　Sugars 2 g
PROTEIN 6 g
DIETARY EXCHANGES
　½ starch

COOK'S TIP

You can grill the jalapeños (whole) before stuffing them. Using the tip of a knife, make a small hole in the stem ends of the jalapeños to keep them from bursting as they cook. Grill over medium-high heat for 4 to 5 minutes, or until the skins are slightly charred, turning after each minute of cooking time. When cool enough to handle, cut the jalapeños in half lengthwise, discarding the stems, seeds, and ribs, and stuff and bake as directed on page 20.

COOK'S TIP on handling hot chile peppers

Hot chile peppers contain oils that can burn your skin, lips, and eyes. Wear disposable gloves or wash your hands thoroughly with warm, soapy water immediately after handling hot peppers. Examples of hot peppers are Anaheim, ancho, cascabel, cayenne, cherry, chipotle, habanero, Hungarian wax, jalapeño, poblano, Scotch bonnet, serrano, and Thai. A rule of thumb is that the smaller the pepper, the hotter it is.

mexican potato skins

SERVES 4; 2 PIECES PER SERVING

For after-school snacking or casual entertaining, these tasty appetizers satisfy the need for something with a hint of heat. Use the reserved potato skins from Baked Potato Soup (page 80), or bake your own (see Cook's Tip below).

---

8 potato skin quarters from Baked Potato Soup, or 2 8-ounce baked potato skins
2 tablespoons plus 2 teaspoons fat-free sour cream

8 fresh cilantro leaves, finely snipped
¼ cup salsa (lowest sodium available), such as Salsa Cruda (page 508)
1 small fresh jalapeño, seeded and thinly sliced (optional)

Preheat the oven or toaster oven to 400°F.

Place the potato skins with the skin side down on a baking sheet.

Bake for 8 to 10 minutes, or until hot and crisp. For extra-crisp skins, use a toaster oven (the time is the same as for the full-size oven). Transfer to a plate.

Meanwhile, in a small bowl, stir together the sour cream and cilantro.

Spoon the salsa onto each potato skin. Top with the sour cream mixture and jalapeño.

COOK'S TIP on baked potato skins

Preheat the oven to 425°F. Bake the potatoes on the oven rack for 1 hour 15 minutes, or until slightly overdone (the skins will be crisp and will crackle slightly when you gently squeeze the potatoes, using an oven mitt or tongs). Transfer to a cooling rack. Let stand for 15 to 20 minutes, or until cool enough to handle. Halve the potatoes lengthwise, then halve crosswise (to make 4 quarters each). Using a spoon, scoop out the flesh, leaving about a ⅛-inch shell.

PER SERVING

CALORIES 38
TOTAL FAT 0.0 g
  Saturated Fat 0.0 g
  Trans Fat 0.0 g
  Polyunsaturated Fat 0.0 g
  Monounsaturated Fat 0.0 g
CHOLESTEROL 2 mg
SODIUM 68 mg
CARBOHYDRATES 8 g
  Fiber 0 g
  Sugars 1 g
PROTEIN 1 g
DIETARY EXCHANGES
  ½ starch

tortilla pinwheels

SERVES 10; 2 PIECES PER SERVING

You can vary the heat of this Tex-Mex finger food with the type of salsa you choose.

4 ounces light tub cream cheese

½ 15.5-ounce can no-salt-added black beans, rinsed, drained, and mashed

½ medium red bell pepper, finely chopped

¼ cup salsa (lowest sodium available), such as Salsa Cruda (page 508)

1 medium green onion, thinly sliced

¼ teaspoon ground cumin

⅛ teaspoon salt

5 6-inch corn tortillas

Preheat the oven to 350°F.

In a medium bowl, using an electric mixer on medium speed, beat the cream cheese until smooth. Stir in the remaining ingredients except the tortillas.

Wrap the tortillas in aluminum foil. Bake for 5 minutes, or until heated through. Remove the tortillas from the oven.

Put one tortilla on a cutting board, leaving the others wrapped. Spread ¼ cup bean mixture over the entire top of the tortilla. Roll up jelly-roll style and place with the seam side down on the cutting board. Insert four toothpicks about 1 inch apart into the tortilla roll. Using a sharp knife, slice between the toothpicks to make 4 pieces. Leaving the toothpicks in place, arrange the pieces on a serving plate. Repeat with the remaining filling and tortillas.

PER SERVING

CALORIES 69
TOTAL FAT 2.0 g
    Saturated Fat 1.0 g
    Trans Fat 0.0 g
    Polyunsaturated Fat 0.0 g
    Monounsaturated Fat 0.5 g
CHOLESTEROL 7 mg
SODIUM 108 mg
CARBOHYDRATES 9 g
    Fiber 2 g
    Sugars 2 g
PROTEIN 3 g
DIETARY EXCHANGES
    ½ starch, ½ fat

pepper-topped whole-grain tortilla pizzas

SERVES 8; 3 PIECES PER SERVING

Colorful and cheesy, these pizzas can satisfy even the most intense pizza craving in less than 20 minutes. Serve them as a snack for eight or as lunch or a light dinner for four.

1 teaspoon olive oil
1 medium red bell pepper, diced
1 medium orange bell pepper, diced
4 6-inch low-fat whole-grain tortillas (lowest sodium available)
¼ to ½ cup no-salt-added canned tomato sauce

½ cup shredded low-fat mozzarella cheese
¼ cup shredded or grated Parmesan cheese
¼ teaspoon pepper, or to taste
¼ teaspoon crushed red pepper flakes (optional)
4 fresh basil leaves, thinly sliced

Preheat the oven to 450°F.

In a medium skillet, heat the oil over medium-high heat, swirling to coat the bottom. Cook the bell peppers for 7 to 9 minutes, or until tender and nicely browned, stirring occasionally. Remove the skillet from the heat.

Heat the tortillas using the package directions.

Lay 2 tortillas on each of 2 baking sheets. Spoon 1 to 2 tablespoons tomato sauce onto each tortilla, spreading with the back of the spoon and leaving a ½-inch border. Spoon the bell peppers over the sauce. Sprinkle with the mozzarella and Parmesan, then with the pepper and red pepper flakes.

Bake for 5 minutes, or until the cheeses melt and begin to turn golden brown.

Sprinkle the basil over the pizzas. Cut each pizza into 6 pieces. Put 3 pieces on each plate. Serve immediately for the best texture.

COOK'S TIP on heating tortillas

If you have a gas burner, you can heat tortillas, one at a time, directly over the flame. It will take about 10 seconds on each side. Tongs work well for flipping the tortillas so you don't burn your fingers.

PER SERVING

CALORIES 80
TOTAL FAT 2.0 g
  Saturated Fat 1.0 g
  Trans Fat 0.0 g
  Polyunsaturated Fat 0.0 g
  Monounsaturated Fat 1.0 g
CHOLESTEROL 4 mg
SODIUM 181 mg
CARBOHYDRATES 13 g
  Fiber 2 g
  Sugars 2 g
PROTEIN 5 g
DIETARY EXCHANGES
  1 starch, ½ lean meat

stuffed mushrooms

SERVES 6; 3 MUSHROOMS PER SERVING

Savor these plump mushrooms as an appetizer or jazz up your next spaghetti dinner by placing them on the pasta and sauce.

18 medium button mushrooms (about 1 pound), stems minced
2 teaspoons olive oil
3 medium garlic cloves, minced
¼ medium red bell pepper, diced
¼ medium yellow bell pepper, diced
2 medium green onions, sliced

¾ cup fresh soft whole-grain bread crumbs (lowest sodium available)
¼ cup egg substitute
2 tablespoons shredded or grated Parmesan cheese
½ teaspoon salt-free Italian seasoning, crumbled

Preheat the oven to 425°F.

Place the mushroom caps with the smooth side down in a 13 x 9 x 2-inch baking pan. Set aside.

In a medium nonstick skillet, heat the oil over medium heat, swirling to coat the bottom. Cook the mushroom stems and garlic for 5 minutes, stirring occasionally.

Stir in the bell peppers. Cook for 2 to 3 minutes, or until tender.

Stir in the green onions. Cook for 2 minutes. Remove from the heat.

Stir in the remaining ingredients. Spoon the filling into the mushroom caps, packing the mixture lightly.

Bake for 25 minutes, or until heated through.

PER SERVING

CALORIES 67
TOTAL FAT 2.0 g
  Saturated Fat 0.5 g
  Trans Fat 0.0 g
  Polyunsaturated Fat 0.0 g
  Monounsaturated Fat 1.5 g
CHOLESTEROL 1 mg
SODIUM 97 mg
CARBOHYDRATES 7 g
  Fiber 2 g
  Sugars 1 g
PROTEIN 6 g
DIETARY EXCHANGES
  ½ carbohydrate, ½ fat

coconut halibut bites

SERVES 12; 2 PIECES PER SERVING

You'll be delighted with these tempting morsels of halibut, served with a triple-citrus sweet-and-sour dipping sauce.

Cooking spray
¼ cup all-purpose flour
¼ cup sweetened shredded coconut
¼ cup egg substitute
½ teaspoon dried dillweed, crumbled
⅛ teaspoon pepper
1 pound halibut fillets, rinsed and patted dry, cut into 1-inch cubes

CITRUS DIPPING SAUCE
½ cup sweet orange marmalade
1 teaspoon grated lime zest
1 tablespoon fresh lime juice
1 tablespoon fresh lemon juice

Preheat the oven to 400°F. Lightly spray a baking sheet with cooking spray.

In a small shallow dish, stir together the flour and coconut. In another small shallow dish, whisk together the egg substitute, dillweed, and pepper. Set the dishes and baking sheet in a row, assembly-line fashion. Working in batches, put the fish in the egg mixture, turning to coat. Using a slotted spoon, transfer the fish to the flour mixture, turning to coat and gently shaking off any excess. Place the fish on the baking sheet, spacing the cubes slightly apart so they brown evenly.

Bake for 7 to 8 minutes, or until the fish flakes easily when tested with a fork.

Meanwhile, in a small serving bowl, stir together the sauce ingredients. Place in the center of a platter. Arrange the fish cubes around the dipping sauce.

PER SERVING

CALORIES 94
TOTAL FAT 1.5 g
  Saturated Fat 0.5 g
  Trans Fat 0.0 g
  Polyunsaturated Fat 0.5 g
  Monounsaturated Fat 0.5 g
CHOLESTEROL 12 mg
SODIUM 39 mg
CARBOHYDRATES 12 g
  Fiber 0 g
  Sugars 9 g
PROTEIN 9 g
DIETARY EXCHANGES
  1 carbohydrate,
  1 very lean meat

skewered chicken strips with soy-peanut marinade

SERVES 16; 2 SKEWERS PER SERVING

This flavorful chicken strip appetizer will be the talk of your next party. (See the Cook's Tip on Skewered Food on page 249 for how to make a festive presentation.) Or try this recipe as an entrée for four, keeping the chicken breasts whole and serving them with brown rice and snow peas.

SOY-PEANUT MARINADE
- 2 tablespoons fresh lime juice
- 1 tablespoon peanut butter
- 1 tablespoon soy sauce (lowest sodium available)
- 1 tablespoon plain rice vinegar
- 2 medium garlic cloves, minced
- ½ teaspoon ground cumin
- ½ teaspoon toasted sesame oil

- ¼ teaspoon pepper

- 4 boneless, skinless chicken breast halves (about 4 ounces each), all visible fat discarded, flattened to ¼- to ½-inch thickness and each cut lengthwise into 8 strips
- Cooking spray

In a large shallow glass dish, whisk together the marinade ingredients. Add the chicken, turning to coat. Cover and refrigerate for 30 minutes to 8 hours, turning occasionally.

Soak 32 wooden skewers in cold water for at least 10 minutes to prevent charring, or use metal skewers.

Lightly spray the grill rack with cooking spray. Preheat the grill on medium high.

Thread one strip of chicken onto each skewer.

Grill for 2 to 3 minutes on each side (6 to 8 minutes on each side for unsliced chicken), or until no longer pink in the center. Serve or cover and refrigerate to serve chilled.

PER SERVING

CALORIES 28
TOTAL FAT 1.0 g
  Saturated Fat 0.0 g
  Trans Fat 0.0 g
  Polyunsaturated Fat 0.0 g
  Monounsaturated Fat 0.5 g
CHOLESTEROL 11 mg
SODIUM 39 mg
CARBOHYDRATES 0 g
  Fiber 0 g
  Sugars 0 g
PROTEIN 4 g
DIETARY EXCHANGES
  ½ lean meat

meatballs in beer sauce

SERVES 16; 2 MEATBALLS PER SERVING

You can make the sauce while these easy-to-prepare meatballs bake.

Cooking spray

MEATBALLS

2 slices whole-grain bread (lowest sodium available), cut into cubes
4 ounces beer (light or nonalcoholic)
1 pound extra-lean ground beef
½ cup shredded low-fat mozzarella cheese
½ teaspoon pepper, or to taste

SAUCE

1 teaspoon light tub margarine
½ cup chopped onion
1 tablespoon all-purpose flour
8 ounces beer (light or nonalcoholic)
2 tablespoons light brown sugar
2 tablespoons cider vinegar
2 tablespoons fat-free, no-salt-added beef broth, such as on page 42

Preheat the oven to 350°F. Lightly spray a baking sheet with cooking spray.

In a medium bowl, soak the bread cubes in 4 ounces beer for 2 to 3 minutes.

Add the beef, mozzarella, and pepper. With your hands or a spoon, combine the ingredients. Shape into 32 meatballs. Transfer to the baking sheet.

Bake for 15 minutes. Drain on paper towels to remove any fat.

Meanwhile, in a medium skillet, melt the margarine over medium-high heat, swirling to coat the bottom. Cook the onion for 3 minutes, or until soft, stirring occasionally.

Stir in the flour. Cook for 1 to 2 minutes, stirring constantly.

Stir in the remaining sauce ingredients. Reduce the heat and simmer for 10 minutes.

Add the meatballs to the sauce, stirring gently to coat. Simmer for 20 minutes, stirring occasionally.

PER SERVING

CALORIES 71
TOTAL FAT 2.0 g
  Saturated Fat 0.5 g
  Trans Fat 0.0 g
  Polyunsaturated Fat 0.0 g
  Monounsaturated Fat 1.0 g
CHOLESTEROL 17 mg
SODIUM 67 mg
CARBOHYDRATES 5 g
  Fiber 0 g
  Sugars 2 g
PROTEIN 8 g
DIETARY EXCHANGES
  ½ carbohydrate,
  1 lean meat

spinach and cheese mini quiches

SERVES 24; 2 PER SERVING

For occasions from bridal showers to brunch parties, these delicious mini quiches are the perfect size. They freeze well, so you can make them in advance.

Cooking spray
16 ounces fat-free cottage cheese
1 10-ounce package frozen chopped spinach, thawed, well drained, and squeezed dry
1 cup shredded low-fat Swiss cheese
¾ cup egg substitute
½ cup low-fat all-purpose baking mix (lowest sodium available)

2 medium green onions, thinly sliced
2 tablespoons shredded or grated Parmesan cheese
2 tablespoons fat-free half-and-half
1 tablespoon olive oil
1 tablespoon snipped fresh dillweed or 1 teaspoon dried, crumbled
¼ teaspoon pepper

Preheat the oven to 350°F. Lightly spray two 24-cup mini muffin pans with cooking spray.

In a large bowl, stir together the remaining ingredients until the baking mix is just moistened. Don't overmix. Spoon 1 heaping tablespoon batter into each muffin cup.

With the pans on separate oven racks, bake for 15 minutes. Switch the pans from top to bottom. Bake for 10 to 15 minutes, or until a wooden toothpick inserted in the center comes out clean. Transfer the pans to a cooling rack. Let cool for 5 minutes. Using a thin spatula, loosen the quiches. Transfer to a serving platter.

PER SERVING

CALORIES 44
TOTAL FAT 1.0 g
  Saturated Fat 0.5 g
  Trans Fat 0.0 g
  Polyunsaturated Fat 0.0 g
  Monounsaturated Fat 0.5 g
CHOLESTEROL 3 mg
SODIUM 138 mg
CARBOHYDRATES 4 g
  Fiber 1 g
  Sugars 2 g
PROTEIN 5 g
DIETARY EXCHANGES
  1 very lean meat

pita crisps

SERVES 12; 3 WEDGES PER SERVING

Excellent as snacks, these herb-flecked pita wedges also complement soups and salads.

¼ cup very finely snipped fresh parsley
2 medium green onions, finely chopped
1 teaspoon olive oil
¾ teaspoon dried basil, crumbled
½ teaspoon dried rosemary, crushed

1 medium garlic clove, minced
3 6-inch whole-grain pita pockets, split open into rounds
Olive oil spray
2 tablespoons shredded or grated Parmesan cheese

Preheat the oven to 350°F.

In a small bowl, stir together the parsley, green onions, oil, basil, rosemary, and garlic. Spread the mixture on the pita rounds.

Lightly spray the tops with olive oil spray. Sprinkle with the Parmesan. Cut each pita round into 6 wedges. Put the wedges on a baking sheet.

Bake for 12 minutes, or until crisp. Serve warm or let cool completely and store in an airtight container for up to one week.

PER SERVING

CALORIES 32
TOTAL FAT 0.5 g
 Saturated Fat 0.0 g
 Trans Fat 0.0 g
 Polyunsaturated Fat 0.0 g
 Monounsaturated Fat 0.5 g
CHOLESTEROL 1 mg
SODIUM 63 mg
CARBOHYDRATES 6 g
 Fiber 1 g
 Sugars 0 g
PROTEIN 1 g
DIETARY EXCHANGES
 ½ starch

peanutty caramel apple "gramwiches"

The protein in this after-school snack will keep the kids satisfied until dinner.

¼ cup peanut butter
2 tablespoons fat-free caramel
   topping
3 low-fat graham crackers
   (3 rectangular flats), each broken
   into 2 squares

1 large apple

In a small bowl, stir together the peanut butter and caramel topping. Spread on the graham crackers.

Holding the apple upright, cut 6 lengthwise slices, each ¼ to ½ inch wide, from the sides. (Discard the core and reserve any remaining apple for munching.) Place one apple slice on each graham cracker square.

PER SERVING

CALORIES 131
TOTAL FAT 6.0 g
   Saturated Fat 1.0 g
   Trans Fat 0.0 g
   Polyunsaturated Fat 1.5 g
   Monounsaturated Fat 2.5 g
CHOLESTEROL 0 mg
SODIUM 97 mg
CARBOHYDRATES 18 g
   Fiber 2 g
   Sugars 10 g
PROTEIN 3 g
DIETARY EXCHANGES
   1 carbohydrate, 1 fat

nibbles

SERVES 16; ½ CUP PER SERVING

By varying the cereal and nuts, you can create lots of different snack mixtures.

---

5 cups dry cereal (such as rice
    squares, wheat squares, oat circles,
    or puffed corn, or a combination)
2 cups unsalted pretzel sticks, broken
    in half
¼ cup light tub margarine
2 teaspoons Worcestershire sauce
    (lowest sodium available)

1 teaspoon celery flakes
1 teaspoon onion powder
½ teaspoon garlic powder
½ cup unsalted raw peanuts or other
    unsalted raw nuts

Preheat the oven to 275°F.

In a large bowl, stir together the cereal and pretzel sticks.

In a small saucepan, melt the margarine over low heat. Stir in the remaining ingredients except the nuts. Stir into the cereal mixture.

Stir in the nuts. Transfer the mixture to a shallow roasting pan.

Bake for 1 hour, stirring every 10 minutes. Serve warm or let cool completely and store in an airtight container for up to seven days.

SOUTHWESTERN NIBBLES
Add ½ teaspoon ground cumin, ½ teaspoon chili powder, and ⅛ teaspoon red hot-pepper sauce to the melted margarine with the other seasonings.

PER SERVING

CALORIES 92
TOTAL FAT 3.5 g
  Saturated Fat 0.5 g
  Trans Fat 0.0 g
  Polyunsaturated Fat 1.0 g
  Monounsaturated Fat 2.0 g
CHOLESTEROL 0 mg
SODIUM 105 mg
CARBOHYDRATES 13 g
  Fiber 1 g
  Sugars 1 g
PROTEIN 2 g
DIETARY EXCHANGES
  1 starch, ½ fat

animal crackers in my fruit

SERVES 16; ¼ CUP PER SERVING

The classic song "Animal Crackers in My Soup" inspired this snack. Kids of all ages will enjoy the stirring action when making this stovetop recipe.

⅔ cup walnut halves
2¼ cups animal crackers (about
    50 pieces)
    Cooking spray

½ teaspoon ground cinnamon
⅛ teaspoon ground nutmeg
12 ounces mixed dried fruit (any
    combination)

In a large nonstick saucepan or skillet over medium heat, dry-roast the walnuts for 3 to 4 minutes, or until golden brown, stirring occasionally.

Stir in the animal crackers. Remove from the heat. Lightly spray the mixture with cooking spray. Return to the heat.

Sprinkle the mixture with the cinnamon and nutmeg. Dry-roast for 1 minute, or until the cookies are slightly warmed, stirring constantly.

Stir in the dried fruit. Remove from the heat. Spread the mixture on a baking sheet or large platter to cool. Serve or refrigerate in an airtight container for up to five days.

PER SERVING

CALORIES 114
TOTAL FAT 4.0 g
    Saturated Fat 0.5 g
    Trans Fat 0.0 g
    Polyunsaturated Fat 2.0 g
    Monounsaturated Fat 1.0 g
CHOLESTEROL 0 mg
SODIUM 62 mg
CARBOHYDRATES 20 g
    Fiber 2 g
    Sugars 9 g
PROTEIN 2 g
DIETARY EXCHANGES
    ½ starch, 1 fruit,
    ½ fat

summer slush

SERVES 4

With its fruit, fruit juice, and yogurt, this drink is a fine way to start your morning or an easy way to enjoy fruit during the day.

2 cups frozen unsweetened strawberries or unsweetened sliced peaches

1½ cups pineapple-orange juice

1 large banana, sliced

6 ounces fat-free vanilla or fruit-flavored yogurt

2 tablespoons sugar

¼ to ½ teaspoon coconut extract

In a food processor or blender, process the ingredients until smooth.

COOK'S TIP

For an even colder treat, place the serving glasses in the freezer at least 30 minutes before serving.

creamy orange fizz

SERVES 4

Similar to a float, this fruity, low-fat drink sparkles!

---

2 cups orange sherbet
1 cup pineapple juice
1 cup club soda

½ cup frozen fat-free whipped topping,
thawed in refrigerator

Spoon ½ cup sherbet into each of 4 tall glasses or wine-glasses.

Pour ¼ cup pineapple juice and ¼ cup club soda into each glass.

Top each serving with 2 tablespoons whipped topping.

berry good smoothie

SERVES 2

This delicious combination will help you get three types of fruit into your diet at any time of day.

1 cup strawberries, hulled and halved, or raspberries
1 medium banana, cut into large pieces

1 cup fresh orange juice

In a food processor or blender, process the ingredients until smooth.

COOK'S TIP

Turn these smoothies into a sherbetlike dessert by adding ½ to 2 cups crushed ice.

PER SERVING

CALORIES 133
TOTAL FAT 0.5 g
  Saturated Fat 0.0 g
  Trans Fat 0.0 g
  Polyunsaturated Fat 0.0 g
  Monounsaturated Fat 0.0 g
CHOLESTEROL 0 mg
SODIUM 3 mg
CARBOHYDRATES 32 g
  Fiber 3 g
  Sugars 21 g
PROTEIN 2 g
DIETARY EXCHANGES
  2 fruit

sparkling cranberry cooler

SERVES 4

Chill your most festive glasses for serving this refreshing drink.

1½ cups unsweetened cranberry juice	2 teaspoons fresh lime juice
1 cup purple grape juice	1½ cups sugar-free lemon-lime soda
½ cup burgundy or other dry red wine (regular or nonalcoholic)	

In a glass pitcher, stir together all the ingredients except the soda. Refrigerate for at least 1 hour, or until well chilled.

To serve, stir in the soda. Add ice, if desired. Serve immediately.

SPARKLING ORANGE JUICE COOLER
Replace the cranberry juice with orange juice, the purple grape juice with white grape juice, and the burgundy with dry white wine (regular or nonalcoholic).

PER SERVING

CALORIES 103
TOTAL FAT 0.0 g
  Saturated Fat 0.0 g
  Trans Fat 0.0 g
  Polyunsaturated Fat 0.0 g
  Monounsaturated Fat 0.0 g
CHOLESTEROL 0 mg
SODIUM 21 mg
CARBOHYDRATES 22 g
  Fiber 0 g
  Sugars 21 g
PROTEIN 1 g
DIETARY EXCHANGES
  1½ fruit

PER SERVING

SPARKLING ORANGE JUICE COOLER
CALORIES 104
TOTAL FAT 0.0 g
  Saturated Fat 0.0 g
  Trans Fat 0.0 g
  Polyunsaturated Fat 0.0 g
  Monounsaturated Fat 0.0 g
CHOLESTEROL 0 mg
SODIUM 19 mg
CARBOHYDRATES 20 g
  Fiber 0 g
  Sugars 18 g
PROTEIN 1 g
DIETARY EXCHANGES
  1½ fruit

peppermint coffee chiller

SERVES 4

If you love gourmet coffees but want to cut the calories, the fat, and the cost, enjoy this delicious treat instead.

2 cups fat-free chocolate ice cream	1 tablespoon instant coffee granules
1 cup water	1 teaspoon vanilla extract
1 cup fat-free milk	¼ teaspoon peppermint extract
2 tablespoons sugar	

In a food processor or blender, process the ingredients until smooth. Serve over ice cubes.

PER SERVING

CALORIES 151
TOTAL FAT 0.0 g
  Saturated Fat 0.0 g
  Trans Fat 0.0 g
  Polyunsaturated Fat 0.0 g
  Monounsaturated Fat 0.0 g
CHOLESTEROL 1 mg
SODIUM 93 mg
CARBOHYDRATES 33 g
  Fiber 0 g
  Sugars 25 g
PROTEIN 6 g
DIETARY EXCHANGES
  2 carbohydrate

mexican hot chocolate

SERVES 4

With its hint of cinnamon, this supergood hot chocolate is supertasty without any of the superbad fats!

½ cup confectioners' sugar
⅓ cup unsweetened cocoa powder (dark preferred)
¼ teaspoon ground cinnamon and ¼ teaspoon ground cinnamon, divided use
½ cup fat-free milk and 3½ cups fat-free milk, divided use

¾ teaspoon vanilla extract
2 cinnamon sticks (each about 3 inches long)
¼ cup frozen fat-free whipped topping, thawed in refrigerator

In a small bowl, stir together the confectioners' sugar, cocoa powder, and ¼ teaspoon ground cinnamon.

Stir in ½ cup milk and the vanilla.

In a medium saucepan over medium-high heat, heat the remaining 3½ cups milk and cinnamon sticks for 5 to 7 minutes, or until the mixture begins to simmer. Remove from the heat. Discard the cinnamon sticks. Measure ½ cup of the heated milk and pour into the confectioners' sugar mixture, whisking until combined. (This helps prevent clumping.)

Pour the confectioners' sugar mixture into the milk remaining in the pan. Heat over medium heat for 5 minutes, or until hot, stirring occasionally. Pour into mugs. Garnish each with a dollop of the whipped topping and dust with the remaining ¼ teaspoon ground cinnamon.

soups

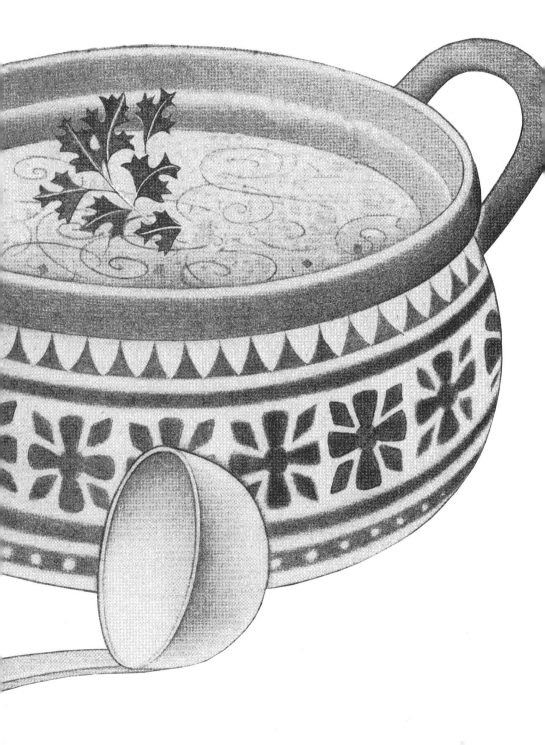

Beef Broth

Chicken Broth

Vegetable Broth

Vegetable Bouillon

Greek Egg and Lemon Soup

Peppery Cream of Carrot Soup

Creamy Asparagus Soup

Cream of Mushroom Soup

Fresh Mushroom Soup

Broccoli-Parmesan Soup

Onion Soup

Roasted Corn Soup

Spinach Pasta Soup

Hot-and-Sour Soup with Tofu

Thai-Style Lemon and Spinach Soup

Winter Squash Soup

Minestrone

Quick Vegetable Soup

Five-Minute Soup

Chilled Cucumber Watercress Soup

Creamy Basil-Tomato Soup

Flavorful Tomato Bouillon

Gazpacho

Yogurt-Fruit Soup

Minted Cantaloupe Soup with Fresh Lime

Tropical Minted Cantaloupe Soup with Fresh Lime

Southwestern Cod Soup

Sweet Corn Soup with Crab and Asparagus

Sweet Corn Soup with Chicken and Asparagus

Shrimp Gumbo

Shrimp and Tomato Soup with Chipotle Peppers

Chicken and Vegetable Soup

Chicken, Greens, and Potato Soup

Chile-Chicken Tortilla Soup

Turkey and Rice Soup

Vietnamese Beef and Rice Noodle Soup

Beef Barley Soup

White Bean Soup with Tarragon

Lentil Chili Soup

Curried Pumpkin Soup

Split Pea Soup

Baked Potato Soup

beef broth

MAKES 3½ QUARTS

Roasting the bones is the key to making this beef broth so flavorful. You'll need plenty of time to make this recipe, but the investment will be worth it—a heart-healthy broth that can be used in many, many dishes. And it freezes well!

Cooking spray
6 pounds beef bones
1 teaspoon canola or corn oil
2 large carrots, sliced
2 large leeks (green and white parts), sliced
2 medium ribs of celery with leaves, coarsely chopped

1 large onion, quartered
5 quarts water
8 whole peppercorns
6 to 8 sprigs of fresh parsley
3 sprigs of fresh thyme

Preheat the oven to 400°F. Lightly spray a large baking pan with cooking spray. Put the beef bones in the pan.

Roast for 40 minutes to 1 hour, or until browned.

Meanwhile, in a stockpot, heat the oil over medium-high heat, swirling to coat the bottom. Cook the carrots, leeks, celery, and onion for 5 minutes, stirring occasionally. Reduce the heat to medium. Cook, covered, for 15 to 20 minutes, or until the leeks are limp.

Stir in the browned bones and remaining ingredients. Increase the heat to high and bring to a boil. Reduce the heat and simmer, covered, for 4 to 5 hours. Strain the broth and discard the solids. Cover and refrigerate for at least 8 hours so the flavors blend and the fat rises to the surface. Discard the fat before reheating the broth.

COOK'S TIP on freezing broth

Freeze broth in airtight plastic containers for future use. For smaller amounts, freeze broth in a muffin pan or ice cube trays. Remove the frozen portions and store them in a resealable plastic freezer bag. Thaw the broth for several hours in the refrigerator or by heating in the microwave.

1 CUP OF BROTH

CALORIES 10
TOTAL FAT 0.0 g
  Saturated Fat 0.0 g
  Trans Fat 0.0 g
  Polyunsaturated Fat 0.0 g
  Monounsaturated Fat 0.0 g
CHOLESTEROL 0 mg
SODIUM 30 mg
CARBOHYDRATES 1 g
  Fiber 0 g
  Sugars 0 g
PROTEIN 2 g
DIETARY EXCHANGES
  Free

chicken broth

MAKES 4 QUARTS

Homemade broth is so flavorful that it really is worth taking the time to make your own. You can skip roasting the bones, but the roasting step definitely intensifies the flavor. (See the Cook's Tip on Freezing Broth, page 42, for how to ensure that you always have a supply of homemade broth on hand.)

Cooking spray
4 pounds chicken bones
1 teaspoon canola or corn oil
2 medium carrots, sliced
2 medium leeks (green and white parts), sliced
1 medium rib of celery with leaves, coarsely chopped

1 large onion, quartered
2 cups dry white wine (regular or nonalcoholic)
5 quarts water
6 to 8 sprigs of fresh parsley
3 sprigs of fresh thyme
8 whole peppercorns
1 medium dried bay leaf

Preheat the oven to 400°F. Lightly spray a large baking pan with cooking spray. Put the chicken bones in the pan.

Roast for 1 hour, or until browned. (If you prefer a lighter-colored broth, roast the bones for only 30 to 40 minutes.)

Meanwhile, in a stockpot, heat the oil over medium-high heat, swirling to coat the bottom. Cook the carrots, leeks, celery, and onion for 5 minutes, stirring occasionally. Reduce the heat to medium. Cook, covered, for 15 to 20 minutes, or until the leeks are limp.

Stir in the wine. Increase the heat to high and bring to a boil. Boil for 5 to 10 minutes, or until the wine has evaporated.

Stir in the browned bones and remaining ingredients. Bring to a boil. Reduce the heat and simmer, covered, for 4 to 5 hours. Strain the broth and discard the solids. Cover and refrigerate for at least 8 hours so the flavors blend and the fat rises to the surface. Discard the fat before reheating the broth.

1 CUP OF BROTH

CALORIES 10
TOTAL FAT 0.0 g
  Saturated Fat 0.0 g
  Trans Fat 0.0 g
  Polyunsaturated Fat 0.0 g
  Monounsaturated Fat 0.0 g
CHOLESTEROL 0 mg
SODIUM 25 mg
CARBOHYDRATES 1 g
  Fiber 0 g
  Sugars 0 g
PROTEIN 2 g
DIETARY EXCHANGES
  Free

vegetable broth

MAKES 1¾ QUARTS

This versatile broth has so many uses—try it as the base for other soups and vegetarian dishes and use it to replace water when you cook rice and other grains. (See the Cook's Tip on Freezing Broth, page 42, for how to ensure that you always have a supply of homemade broth on hand.)

1 teaspoon canola or corn oil	3 medium ribs of celery with leaves, coarsely chopped
2 medium onions, quartered	3 or 4 sprigs of fresh thyme
2 large leeks (green and white parts), sliced	3 large sprigs of fresh parsley
9 cups water	12 whole peppercorns
2 medium carrots, sliced	1 medium dried bay leaf

In a stockpot, heat the oil over medium-high heat, swirling to coat the bottom. Cook the onions and leeks for 4 to 5 minutes, stirring occasionally.

Stir in the remaining ingredients. Increase the heat to high and bring to a boil. Reduce the heat and simmer for 1 hour 15 minutes to 1 hour 30 minutes, or until reduced to about 8 cups. Strain the broth and discard the solids. Cover and refrigerate for at least 8 hours so the flavors blend.

VEGETABLE BOUILLON

Simmer the cooked broth for 20 to 30 minutes, or until reduced by half. Use the reduction when a recipe calls for canned bouillon.

---

1 CUP OF BROTH

CALORIES 5
TOTAL FAT 0.0 g
  Saturated Fat 0.0 g
  Trans Fat 0.0 g
  Polyunsaturated Fat 0.0 g
  Monounsaturated Fat 0.0 g
CHOLESTEROL 0 mg
SODIUM 10 mg
CARBOHYDRATES 1 g
  Fiber 0 g
  Sugars 0 g
PROTEIN 0 g
DIETARY EXCHANGES
  Free

---

1 CUP OF BROTH

VEGETABLE BOUILLON
CALORIES 10
TOTAL FAT 0.0 g
  Saturated Fat 0.0 g
  Trans Fat 0.0 g
  Polyunsaturated Fat 0.0 g
  Monounsaturated Fat 0.0 g
CHOLESTEROL 0 mg
SODIUM 20 mg
CARBOHYDRATES 1 g
  Fiber 0 g
  Sugars 0 g
PROTEIN 1 g
DIETARY EXCHANGES
  Free

greek egg and lemon soup

SERVES 4

Avgolemono (ahv-goh-LEH-moh-noh) is the Greek name for this simply delicious soup. Watch the egg-lemon mixture create an interesting texture and appearance as you stir it into the soup.

4 cups fat-free, low-sodium chicken broth, such as on page 43	¾ cup egg substitute, at room temperature
¼ cup uncooked rice	¼ cup fresh lemon juice

In a medium saucepan, bring the broth to a boil over medium-high heat.

Stir in the rice. Reduce the heat and simmer, covered, for 15 to 20 minutes, or until the rice is tender. Remove from the heat.

In a medium bowl, whisk together the egg substitute and lemon juice. Gradually whisk about half the broth into the egg substitute mixture. Pour the egg substitute mixture back into the remaining broth, whisking well. Return the pan to the heat.

Cook over low heat for 4 to 5 minutes, or just until the soup has thickened, whisking constantly, but lightly. Don't let the soup boil.

PER SERVING

CALORIES 79
TOTAL FAT 0.0 g
  Saturated Fat 0.0 g
  Trans Fat 0.0 g
  Polyunsaturated Fat 0.0 g
  Monounsaturated Fat 0.0 g
CHOLESTEROL 0 mg
SODIUM 120 mg
CARBOHYDRATES 12 g
  Fiber 0 g
  Sugars 1 g
PROTEIN 7 g
DIETARY EXCHANGES
  1 starch,
  ½ very lean meat

peppery cream of carrot soup

SERVES 4

Using part broth and part fat-free half-and-half results in a soup that is creamy without being overwhelmingly rich.

1 teaspoon olive oil
1 pound carrots, cut into 2 x ½-inch pieces
¾ cup chopped onion
2 medium garlic cloves, minced
¾ teaspoon grated peeled gingerroot
¼ teaspoon pepper

⅛ to ¼ teaspoon cayenne
⅛ teaspoon ground nutmeg
⅛ teaspoon salt
2 cups fat-free, low-sodium chicken broth, such as on page 43
1 cup fat-free half-and-half

In a large heavy saucepan, heat the oil over medium-high heat, swirling to coat the bottom. Cook the carrots and onion for 10 minutes, stirring frequently.

Stir in the garlic, gingerroot, pepper, cayenne, nutmeg, and salt. Cook for 30 seconds, stirring frequently.

Pour in the broth. Bring to a simmer, stirring frequently. Reduce the heat and simmer, covered, for 30 to 40 minutes, or until the carrots are tender, stirring occasionally.

Using a food processor or blender, process the soup in batches until smooth. Carefully return the soup to the pan.

Pour in the half-and-half. Cook over medium heat for 1 to 2 minutes, or until heated through, stirring constantly.

COOK'S TIP on whole nutmeg

We call for ground nutmeg in our recipes because that is what most home cooks use. However, freshly grated nutmeg is more fragrant and flavorful. If you keep whole nutmeg in a tightly sealed container in a cool, dark place, it will last indefinitely. Then use a grater or rasp zester to grate only the amount needed for your recipe. Give it a try and see what you've been missing!

PER SERVING

CALORIES 114
TOTAL FAT 2.0 g
  Saturated Fat 0.5 g
  Trans Fat 0.0 g
  Polyunsaturated Fat 0.5 g
  Monounsaturated Fat 1.0 g
CHOLESTEROL 0 mg
SODIUM 187 mg
CARBOHYDRATES 21 g
  Fiber 3 g
  Sugars 11 g
PROTEIN 6 g
DIETARY EXCHANGES
  ½ fat-free milk,
  2 vegetable

creamy asparagus soup

SERVES 4

Pureed rice provides creaminess, and adding the asparagus tips at the end of the cooking process gives the soup texture.

2 teaspoons canola or corn oil	1 10-ounce package frozen asparagus
1 small onion, chopped	spears, thawed
1 medium rib of celery, chopped	¼ cup uncooked rice
4 cups fat-free, low-sodium chicken	Dash of pepper (white preferred)
broth, such as on page 43	Dash of ground nutmeg

In a large saucepan, heat the oil over medium-high heat, swirling to coat the bottom. Cook the onion and celery for about 3 minutes, or until the onion is soft, stirring frequently.

Pour in the broth. Increase the heat to high and bring to a boil.

Meanwhile, cut the tips off the asparagus and set aside. Cut the stalks into 1-inch pieces.

When the broth is boiling, stir in the asparagus pieces (not the tips) and rice. Reduce the heat and simmer, covered, for 15 minutes, or until the rice is tender.

In a food processor or blender, process the broth mixture in batches until smooth. Carefully return the soup to the pan.

Gently stir in the asparagus tips, pepper, and nutmeg. Cook for about 5 minutes, or until heated through.

COOK'S TIP on immersion blenders

Also called a hand blender, this wand-shaped gadget with a blender blade at the bottom has become a staple in many kitchens. If you have one, you'll find that it is especially useful when you want to make creamy soup, because you blend the soup directly in the saucepan. No more burning yourself or spilling part of the soup when you transfer it from the pan to a blender or processor and back to the pan again.

PER SERVING

CALORIES 103
TOTAL FAT 2.5 g
  Saturated Fat 0.0 g
  Trans Fat 0.0 g
  Polyunsaturated Fat 1.0 g
  Monounsaturated Fat 1.5 g
CHOLESTEROL 0 mg
SODIUM 40 mg
CARBOHYDRATES 16 g
  Fiber 2 g
  Sugars 2 g
PROTEIN 6 g
DIETARY EXCHANGES
  ½ starch, 1 vegetable,
  ½ fat

cream of mushroom soup

SERVES 4

Rich-tasting, creamy mushroom soup is the perfect beginning to any meal.

1 teaspoon olive oil
1 cup chopped onion
1 large rib of celery, chopped
8 ounces button mushrooms, sliced
8 ounces baby bella mushrooms, sliced
⅛ teaspoon dried thyme, crumbled

2 medium garlic cloves, minced
2 tablespoons all-purpose flour
1½ cups fat-free, low-sodium chicken broth, such as on page 43
½ cup fat-free half-and-half
¼ cup shredded or grated Parmesan cheese

In a large heavy saucepan, heat the oil over medium-high heat, swirling to coat the bottom. Add the onion, celery, mushrooms, and thyme, stirring to combine. Cook for 8 to 10 minutes, or until the onion and mushrooms are soft and the celery is tender, stirring frequently.

Stir in the garlic. Cook for 30 seconds, stirring frequently.

Sprinkle the flour over the mixture. Cook for 1 minute, stirring frequently.

Stir in the broth. Bring to a simmer, stirring frequently. Reduce the heat and simmer, covered, for about 10 minutes, stirring occasionally.

In a food processor or blender, process the soup in batches, leaving some mushrooms chunky. Carefully return the soup to the pan.

Stir in the half-and-half and Parmesan. Cook over medium heat for 1 to 2 minutes, or until heated through, stirring constantly.

PER SERVING

CALORIES 116
TOTAL FAT 3.0 g
    Saturated Fat 1.0 g
    Trans Fat 0.0 g
    Polyunsaturated Fat 0.5 g
    Monounsaturated Fat 1.5 g
CHOLESTEROL 4 mg
SODIUM 144 mg
CARBOHYDRATES 17 g
    Fiber 3 g
    Sugars 6 g
PROTEIN 9 g
DIETARY EXCHANGES
    ½ starch, 2 vegetable,
    ½ fat

fresh mushroom soup

SERVES 4

Try a variety of mushrooms to make your soup exotic. Among the choices are shiitake, portobello, oyster, golden Italian, and, of course, button.

1 teaspoon light tub margarine
8 ounces fresh mushrooms, any variety, 4 ounces finely chopped and 4 ounces sliced
1 large onion, chopped
2 medium garlic cloves, minced
3½ cups fat-free, low-sodium chicken broth, such as on page 43
1 5-ounce can fat-free evaporated milk

⅓ cup all-purpose flour
1½ tablespoons finely snipped fresh parsley
1 tablespoon dry sherry
½ teaspoon grated lemon zest
1 teaspoon fresh lemon juice
⅛ teaspoon salt
⅛ teaspoon pepper (white preferred)

In a large saucepan, melt the margarine over medium heat, swirling to coat the bottom. Cook the mushrooms, onion, and garlic, covered, for 8 minutes, stirring occasionally. Increase the heat to high and cook, uncovered, for 2 to 3 minutes, or until the moisture evaporates.

In a medium bowl, whisk together the broth, milk, and flour. Immediately whisk into the mushroom mixture. Increase the heat to medium high and bring to a boil, stirring occasionally. Cook for 3 to 5 minutes, or until thickened, stirring occasionally.

Stir in the remaining ingredients.

COOK'S TIP

If you can't immediately add the broth mixture to the mushroom mixture, whisk the broth mixture again when you are ready to combine the mixtures. This will disperse the flour.

PER SERVING
CALORIES 121
TOTAL FAT 1.0 g
    Saturated Fat 0.0 g
    Trans Fat 0.0 g
    Polyunsaturated Fat 0.0 g
    Monounsaturated Fat 0.0 g
CHOLESTEROL 2 mg
SODIUM 154 mg
CARBOHYDRATES 21 g
    Fiber 2 g
    Sugars 9 g
PROTEIN 8 g
DIETARY EXCHANGES
    ½ starch, 1 vegetable,
    ½ fat-free milk

broccoli-parmesan soup

SERVES 6

Parmesan, parsley, and ginger set this recipe apart from the usual versions of broccoli-cheese soup.

1 teaspoon olive oil	1 tablespoon snipped fresh parsley
1 cup chopped onion	2 cups fat-free milk
¼ cup chopped celery	¼ cup all-purpose flour
2 medium garlic cloves, minced	¼ cup shredded or grated Parmesan
12 ounces broccoli florets	cheese
3 cups fat-free, low-sodium chicken	¼ teaspoon pepper
broth, such as on page 43	¼ teaspoon ground ginger

In a large heavy saucepan, heat the oil over medium-high heat, swirling to coat the bottom. Cook the onion and celery for 3 to 4 minutes, or until the onion is soft, stirring frequently.

Stir in the garlic. Cook for 30 seconds, stirring frequently.

Stir in the broccoli, broth, and parsley. Bring to a boil. Reduce the heat and simmer, covered, for 8 to 10 minutes, or until the broccoli is tender, stirring occasionally.

In a small bowl, whisk together the milk and flour. Stir into the soup. Increase the heat to medium high and bring to a boil, stirring frequently. Reduce the heat and simmer for 1 to 2 minutes, or until slightly thickened, stirring occasionally.

In a food processor or blender, process the soup in batches until slightly chunky. Carefully return the soup to the pan.

Stir in the Parmesan, pepper, and ginger.

COOK'S TIP

For a change of flavor, replace the ground ginger with curry powder to taste.

onion soup

SERVES 6

Caramelized onions give this soup its rich flavor. Once you master the necessary technique, you can use the onions to enhance the flavor of other dishes. For starters, try them in casseroles, in quiches, and on pizzas.

6 slices French bread, baguette-style (about 2 ounces total) (lowest sodium available)

2 tablespoons shredded or grated Parmesan cheese

1 teaspoon canola or corn oil

1 teaspoon light tub margarine

3 cups thinly sliced onions

½ teaspoon sugar

¼ teaspoon salt

6 cups fat-free, no-salt-added beef broth, such as on page 42

½ cup dry white wine (regular or nonalcoholic)

1 medium dried bay leaf

¼ teaspoon dried thyme, crumbled

¼ teaspoon pepper, or to taste

⅛ teaspoon ground nutmeg

Preheat the oven to 350°F.

Put the bread slices on a baking sheet.

Bake for 10 minutes, or until toasted. Sprinkle with the Parmesan. Bake for 1 to 2 minutes, or until the cheese melts. Set aside.

In a large saucepan, heat the oil and margarine over medium-high heat, swirling to coat the bottom. Cook the onions for 2 minutes, stirring occasionally. Reduce the heat to low. Cook, covered, until the onions are soft, about 5 minutes.

Stir in the sugar and salt. Increase the heat to medium high and cook, uncovered, for 15 to 20 minutes, or until the onions are golden brown, stirring occasionally. After the first 10 minutes, stir more often to keep the onions from sticking and burning.

Stir in the remaining ingredients. Bring to a boil. Reduce the heat and simmer, partially covered, for 15 minutes. Discard the bay leaf. Serve the soup topped with the toasted bread slices.

PER SERVING

CALORIES 92
TOTAL FAT 1.5 g
  Saturated Fat 0.5 g
  Trans Fat 0.0 g
  Polyunsaturated Fat 0.5 g
  Monounsaturated Fat 1.0 g
CHOLESTEROL 1 mg
SODIUM 225 mg
CARBOHYDRATES 12 g
  Fiber 1 g
  Sugars 3 g
PROTEIN 4 g
DIETARY EXCHANGES
  ½ starch, 1 vegetable

roasted corn soup

SERVES 4

Roasting the corn intensifies its sweetness, making this satisfying low-calorie soup a real standout.

Cooking spray
1 cup frozen whole-kernel corn, partially thawed
1 cup fat-free, no-salt-added beef broth, such as on page 42
1 cup chopped onion
1 medium garlic clove, minced
1¾ cups water

1 cup low-sodium mixed-vegetable juice
2 medium carrots, chopped
¼ large red bell pepper, chopped
¼ small green bell pepper, chopped
1 teaspoon chili powder
½ teaspoon ground cumin
2 tablespoons snipped fresh cilantro

Preheat the oven to 425°F.

Lightly spray a baking sheet with cooking spray. Spread the corn in a single layer on the baking sheet. Lightly spray the corn with cooking spray.

Roast for 12 to 14 minutes, or until lightly browned, stirring once halfway through. Remove from the oven.

About the time you stir the corn, combine the broth, onion, and garlic in a medium saucepan. Cook over medium-high heat for 4 minutes.

Stir in the corn and the remaining ingredients except the cilantro. Reduce the heat to medium and cook for 15 minutes, stirring occasionally. Just before serving, stir in the cilantro.

COOK'S TIP

Serving a broth-based vegetable soup such as this one with lunch or before dinner is a great way to take the edge off appetites and keep servings of higher-calorie dishes in proportion.

PER SERVING

CALORIES 95
TOTAL FAT 0.5 g
 Saturated Fat 0.0 g
 Trans Fat 0.0 g
 Polyunsaturated Fat 0.5 g
 Monounsaturated Fat 0.0 g
CHOLESTEROL 0 mg
SODIUM 112 mg
CARBOHYDRATES 21 g
 Fiber 4 g
 Sugars 8 g
PROTEIN 3 g
DIETARY EXCHANGES
 ½ starch, 2 vegetable

spinach pasta soup

SERVES 4

Very easy to make and attractive as well, this soup will become a fast favorite.

---

4 cups fat-free, low-sodium chicken
  broth, such as on page 43
½ cup water
¼ cup plus 1 tablespoon no-salt-
  added tomato paste
½ teaspoon grated lemon zest
¼ cup dried orzo or pastina

8 ounces fresh spinach, chopped,
  or ½ 10-ounce package frozen
  chopped spinach, thawed and well
  drained
2 medium green onions, sliced
¼ teaspoon pepper
⅛ teaspoon salt

In a medium saucepan, whisk together the broth, water, and tomato paste until smooth. Add the lemon zest. Bring to a boil over medium-high heat.

Stir in the pasta. Reduce the heat to medium and cook for 5 to 7 minutes, or until the pasta is tender.

Stir in the spinach and green onions. Cook for 2 to 3 minutes.

Stir in the pepper and salt.

COOK'S TIP on orzo

Orzo looks like, and is a good substitute for, rice, although it actually is very small pasta.

COOK'S TIP on pastina

Pastina, or "tiny pasta," is frequently used in soups. If you cannot find pastina, crush any type of macaroni.

PER SERVING

CALORIES 84
TOTAL FAT 0.5 g
  Saturated Fat 0.0 g
  Trans Fat 0.0 g
  Polyunsaturated Fat 0.0 g
  Monounsaturated Fat 0.0 g
CHOLESTEROL 0 mg
SODIUM 167 mg
CARBOHYDRATES 15 g
  Fiber 3 g
  Sugars 4 g
PROTEIN 6 g
DIETARY EXCHANGES
  ½ starch, 1 vegetable

hot-and-sour soup with tofu

SERVES 4

Although the list of ingredients is fairly long, this soup is easy to make.

2 cups water
2 cups low-sodium vegetable broth, such as on page 44, or fat-free, low-sodium chicken broth, such as on page 43
½ teaspoon sugar
½ teaspoon grated peeled gingerroot
2 cups thinly sliced button mushrooms
8 ounces light firm tofu, well drained and cut into ¼-inch cubes
2 ounces spinach, chopped, or whole baby spinach leaves

1 teaspoon cornstarch
3 tablespoons soy sauce (lowest sodium available)
3 tablespoons plain rice vinegar
1 teaspoon chili garlic paste or chili garlic sauce or ⅛ teaspoon crushed red pepper flakes
½ teaspoon toasted sesame oil
¼ cup thinly sliced green onions
2 tablespoons snipped fresh cilantro

In a large saucepan, stir together the water, broth, sugar, and gingerroot. Bring to a boil over medium-high heat.

Stir in the mushrooms. Reduce the heat and simmer, covered, for 10 minutes, or until soft.

Stir in the tofu and spinach. Cook for 2 minutes, or just until the spinach is wilted.

Meanwhile, put the cornstarch in a small bowl. Add the soy sauce and vinegar, stirring to dissolve. Stir into the soup. Cook for 1 minute, or until the soup slightly thickens. Remove from the heat.

Stir in the chili garlic paste and oil. Serve sprinkled with the green onions and cilantro.

COOK'S TIP on chili garlic paste and chili garlic sauce

Two staples of Asian cooking, spicy chili garlic paste and chili garlic sauce differ a bit but are almost always interchangeable. In addition to chopped chiles and garlic, the paste includes vinegar. Look for both products in the Asian section of the grocery store and in Asian markets when you want to heighten the flavor of soups, stir-fries, and dipping sauces.

PER SERVING

CALORIES 65
TOTAL FAT 1.5 g
  Saturated Fat 0.0 g
  Trans Fat 0.0 g
  Polyunsaturated Fat 0.5 g
  Monounsaturated Fat 0.5 g
CHOLESTEROL 0 mg
SODIUM 390 mg
CARBOHYDRATES 5 g
  Fiber 1 g
  Sugars 2 g
PROTEIN 7 g
DIETARY EXCHANGES
  ½ carbohydrate,
  1 lean meat

thai-style lemon and spinach soup

SERVES 4

So quick, so easy, so versatile! This soup is great as a starter and as a side dish, especially to accompany grilled chicken or fish.

3 cups fat-free, low-sodium chicken broth, such as on page 43
2 ounces dried whole-grain vermicelli, broken into thirds
1 ounce spinach, coarsely chopped
½ cup finely chopped green onions
½ cup finely snipped cilantro
4 lemon slices
½ teaspoon grated peeled gingerroot
⅛ teaspoon crushed red pepper flakes
⅛ teaspoon salt

In a large saucepan over high heat, bring the broth to a boil. Stir in the pasta. Return to a boil. Reduce the heat and simmer, covered, for 8 minutes, or until the pasta is tender.

Stir in the remaining ingredients. Increase the heat to high and bring just to a boil. Remove from the heat.

PER SERVING

CALORIES 66
TOTAL FAT 0.5 g
  Saturated Fat 0.0 g
  Trans Fat 0.0 g
  Polyunsaturated Fat 0.0 g
  Monounsaturated Fat 0.0 g
CHOLESTEROL 0 mg
SODIUM 176 mg
CARBOHYDRATES 12 g
  Fiber 2 g
  Sugars 1 g
PROTEIN 4 g
DIETARY EXCHANGES
  1 starch

winter squash soup

SERVES 6

It's very easy to transform leftover cooked winter squash or sweet potatoes into this creamy dish.

3 cups fat-free, low-sodium chicken broth, such as on page 43
2 cups mashed cooked winter squash (any variety) or sweet potatoes, thawed if frozen or well drained if canned

1 teaspoon onion powder
½ teaspoon garlic powder
½ teaspoon ground cumin
¼ teaspoon salt
¼ teaspoon pepper
1 cup fat-free half-and-half

In a medium saucepan, stir together all the ingredients except the half-and-half. Bring to a simmer over medium-high heat, stirring occasionally. Reduce the heat and simmer, covered, for 6 to 8 minutes.

Stir in the half-and-half. Cook for 2 to 3 minutes, or until heated through, stirring occasionally.

COOK'S TIP

For 2 cups mashed roasted acorn squash, cut a 2-pound squash in half lengthwise. Discard the seeds and strings. Lightly spray the squash with cooking spray. Place the squash on a nonstick baking sheet with the cut side up. Bake at 400°F for 50 to 60 minutes, or until tender when tested with the tip of a sharp knife or a fork. Scoop out the flesh and mash. For 2 cups mashed sweet potatoes, cook 1½ pounds sweet potatoes in boiling water for 30 minutes, or until tender. Discard the skins and mash the flesh.

COOK'S TIP on cutting winter squash

Some winter squash, such as butternut, are difficult to cut when raw. To make the job easy, pierce the squash several times with a fork and place the squash on a microwaveable plate. Microwave on 100 percent power (high) for 1 to 2 minutes. Let the squash stand for 5 minutes before cutting. Using a large, sturdy knife, cut off the stem end, then cut lengthwise from the stem end through the root end. With a spoon, discard the seeds and strings.

minestrone

SERVES 8

One of the best things about a recipe like this is that almost anything works in it. The combination of vegetables can be different each time you make the soup.

2 teaspoons olive oil

1 medium onion, chopped

2 medium carrots, chopped

2 medium ribs of celery with leaves, chopped

2 medium garlic cloves, chopped, and 1 medium garlic clove, whole, divided use

4 cups low-sodium vegetable broth, such as on page 44, or fat-free, no-salt-added beef broth, such as on page 42

1 15.5-ounce can no-salt-added navy beans, rinsed and drained

1 14.5-ounce can no-salt-added diced tomatoes, undrained

1 large potato, peeled and cubed

8 ounces fresh green beans, trimmed and cut into 1-inch pieces

1 small zucchini, cubed

½ cup dried whole-grain elbow macaroni or medium shell pasta

1 tablespoon dried basil, crumbled

1 teaspoon dried oregano, crumbled

1 teaspoon pepper, or to taste

¼ teaspoon salt

1 to 2 cups water, as needed

2 tablespoons shredded or grated Parmesan cheese

In a stockpot, heat the oil over medium-high heat, swirling to coat the bottom. Cook the onion, carrots, celery, and chopped garlic for about 3 minutes, or until the onion is soft, stirring frequently.

Stir in the broth, navy beans, tomatoes with liquid, potato, green beans, zucchini, pasta, basil, oregano, pepper, salt, and remaining whole garlic clove. Reduce the heat and simmer for 45 minutes.

Gradually stir in 1 cup water. Slightly mash the soup ingredients with a potato masher. Stir in more water as needed for the desired consistency. Serve sprinkled with the Parmesan.

COOK'S TIP on potato skins

Don't throw away potato skins—they're rich in vitamins and other nutrients. You can even use them to make a vegetable broth: Combine water and the peels of 6 to 7 raw potatoes with garlic, parsley, and coarsely chopped onion, carrot, and celery to taste; then gently simmer, covered, for about 1 hour 30 minutes. Either strain the broth or, for a thicker consistency, process it in a blender or food processor until smooth.

PER SERVING

CALORIES 155
TOTAL FAT 2.0 g
  Saturated Fat 0.5 g
  Trans Fat 0.0 g
  Polyunsaturated Fat 0.5 g
  Monounsaturated Fat 1.0 g
CHOLESTEROL 1 mg
SODIUM 151 mg
CARBOHYDRATES 29 g
  Fiber 6 g
  Sugars 7 g
PROTEIN 7 g
DIETARY EXCHANGES
  1½ starch, 2 vegetable

quick vegetable soup

SERVES 24; 1 CUP PER SERVING

This filling, fresh-tasting soup is sure to satisfy. It deliberately uses packaged vegetables, but you can certainly prep your own when saving money is more important than saving time. Leftovers keep for up to four days.

Cooking spray
1 pound packaged shredded carrots
14 to 16 ounces packaged ready-to-use celery sticks, chopped into ½-inch pieces
¾ cup frozen chopped onion
1 tablespoon dried Italian seasoning, crumbled, or other salt-free seasoning blend
1 to 1½ teaspoons crushed red pepper flakes
¾ teaspoon salt
8 single-serving packets sodium-free instant beef broth

12 cups water
1 12-ounce bag ready-to-use trimmed green beans, halved if desired
1 16-ounce bag frozen corn
1 10-ounce package frozen green peas
1 28-ounce can no-salt-added tomatoes, crushed, undrained
1 6-ounce can no-salt-added tomato paste
1 cup shredded or grated Parmesan cheese
24 fresh basil leaves

Lightly spray a stockpot with cooking spray. Cook the carrots, celery, onion, Italian seasoning, red pepper flakes, and salt, covered, over high heat for 4 minutes.

Stir in the instant broth, water, green beans, corn, and peas. Cook, covered, for 14 minutes.

Stir in the tomatoes with liquid and the tomato paste. Cook, covered, for 2 minutes. Serve topped with the Parmesan and basil.

PER SERVING

CALORIES 77
TOTAL FAT 1.5 g
  Saturated Fat 0.5 g
  Trans Fat 0.0 g
  Polyunsaturated Fat 0.0 g
  Monounsaturated Fat 0.5 g
CHOLESTEROL 2 mg
SODIUM 183 mg
CARBOHYDRATES 14 g
  Fiber 3 g
  Sugars 5 g
PROTEIN 4 g
DIETARY EXCHANGES
  ½ starch, 1 vegetable

five-minute soup

SERVES 6

Serve this quick-cooking soup immediately after preparing it, while the vegetables are fresh and colorful.

4 cups fat-free, low-sodium chicken broth, such as on page 43, heated

2 cups shredded fresh spinach, cabbage, or lettuce

1 medium zucchini, very thinly sliced

½ cup shredded skinless chicken breast or shredded lean meat, cooked without salt, all visible fat discarded

4 medium button mushrooms, sliced

1 medium tomato, cubed

In a large saucepan, stir together all the ingredients. Bring to a boil over medium-high heat. Reduce the heat and simmer for 5 minutes.

PER SERVING

CALORIES 41
TOTAL FAT 0.5 g
  Saturated Fat 0.0 g
  Trans Fat 0.0 g
  Polyunsaturated Fat 0.0 g
  Monounsaturated Fat 0.0 g
CHOLESTEROL 10 mg
SODIUM 40 mg
CARBOHYDRATES 3 g
  Fiber 1 g
  Sugars 1 g
PROTEIN 6 g
DIETARY EXCHANGES
  1 very lean meat

chilled cucumber watercress soup

SERVES 4

Dainty cucumber-and-watercress sandwiches are popular at high tea, and this soup combines the same mellow cucumber and peppery watercress. Serve it chilled at everything from tea to brunches.

2 teaspoons canola or corn oil
1 large onion, finely chopped
4 cups fat-free, low-sodium chicken broth, such as on page 43
1 large cucumber, cut in half lengthwise, seeded, and diced
2 large bunches watercress, stems discarded (about 2 cups packed leaves)

2 tablespoons uncooked rice
¼ teaspoon pepper (white preferred)
1 tablespoon finely snipped fresh dillweed or 1 teaspoon dried, crumbled
¼ cup fat-free plain yogurt
1 Italian plum (Roma) tomato, thinly sliced (optional)

In a large saucepan, heat the oil over medium-high heat, swirling to coat the bottom. Cook the onion for 3 to 4 minutes, or until soft, stirring frequently.

Reduce the heat to medium. Stir in the broth, cucumber, watercress, rice, and pepper. Cook for 15 to 20 minutes, or until the rice is tender.

Stir in the dillweed. Cook for 2 minutes.

In a food processor or blender, process the soup in batches until smooth. Cover and refrigerate until chilled.

Just before serving, whisk in the yogurt. Serve topped with the tomato slices.

PER SERVING

CALORIES 91
TOTAL FAT 2.5 g
  Saturated Fat 0.0 g
  Trans Fat 0.0 g
  Polyunsaturated Fat 0.5 g
  Monounsaturated Fat 1.5 g
CHOLESTEROL 0 mg
SODIUM 47 mg
CARBOHYDRATES 13 g
  Fiber 2 g
  Sugars 5 g
PROTEIN 5 g
DIETARY EXCHANGES
  ½ starch, 1 vegetable,
  ½ fat

creamy basil-tomato soup

SERVES 6

Fresh basil adds a flavor boost to traditional tomato soup.

1 teaspoon olive oil
¾ cup chopped onion
⅓ cup chopped celery
⅓ cup finely chopped carrots
2 medium garlic cloves, minced
½ teaspoon dried oregano, crumbled
⅛ teaspoon pepper
1 14.5-ounce can no-salt-added diced tomatoes, undrained
1 14.5-ounce can no-salt-added stewed tomatoes, undrained

1 cup fat-free, low-sodium chicken broth, such as on page 43
1 teaspoon sugar
¼ cup chopped fresh basil (about ½ ounce)
3 tablespoons fat-free sour cream
3 tablespoons shredded or grated Parmesan cheese

In a large saucepan, heat the oil over medium-high heat, swirling to coat the bottom. Cook the onion, celery, and carrots for 3 to 4 minutes, or until the onion is soft, stirring frequently.

Stir in the garlic, oregano, and pepper. Cook for 30 seconds, stirring constantly.

Stir in the diced tomatoes with liquid, stewed tomatoes with liquid, broth, and sugar. Bring to a simmer, stirring frequently. Reduce the heat and simmer, covered, for 15 to 20 minutes, stirring occasionally.

Stir in the basil.

In a food processor or blender, process the soup in batches until almost smooth. Carefully return the soup to the pan.

Stir in the sour cream and Parmesan. Cook over medium heat for 1 to 2 minutes, or until heated through, stirring constantly.

PER SERVING

CALORIES 79
TOTAL FAT 1.5 g
    Saturated Fat 0.5 g
    Trans Fat 0.0 g
    Polyunsaturated Fat 0.0 g
    Monounsaturated Fat 1.0 g
CHOLESTEROL 3 mg
SODIUM 80 mg
CARBOHYDRATES 12 g
    Fiber 2 g
    Sugars 7 g
PROTEIN 3 g
DIETARY EXCHANGES
    2 vegetable, ½ fat

flavorful tomato bouillon

SERVES 8

A variety of herbs and spices transforms basic tomato juice and beef broth into a soothing bouillon. Serve some today and freeze the rest for other uses, such as flavoring vegetables, poached fish, and pasta.

46 ounces no-salt-added tomato juice

2 cups fat-free, no-salt-added beef broth, such as on page 42

2 to 3 tablespoons snipped fresh dillweed or 2 teaspoons dried, crumbled

6 whole cloves

2 medium dried bay leaves

½ teaspoon dried basil, crumbled

½ teaspoon dried marjoram, crumbled

½ teaspoon dried oregano, crumbled

½ teaspoon sugar

½ teaspoon salt

¼ to ½ teaspoon pepper

8 thin slices lemon (optional)

In a medium saucepan, stir together all the ingredients except the lemon. Bring to a boil over medium-high heat. Reduce the heat and simmer for 30 minutes. Discard the cloves and bay leaves. Serve with a slice of lemon in each bowl.

PER SERVING

CALORIES 34
TOTAL FAT 0.0 g
  Saturated Fat 0.0 g
  Trans Fat 0.0 g
  Polyunsaturated Fat 0.0 g
  Monounsaturated Fat 0.0 g
CHOLESTEROL 0 mg
SODIUM 171 mg
CARBOHYDRATES 8 g
  Fiber 1 g
  Sugars 7 g
PROTEIN 2 g
DIETARY EXCHANGES
  2 vegetable

gazpacho

SERVES 6

This cold soup is versatile as well as refreshing. Make it part of a late-night supper with a sandwich or fat-free cheese and crackers, use it as a salsa for dipping baked chips, or spoon it over grilled chicken or fish.

SOUP

6 cups chopped tomatoes (peeled if desired) or canned no-salt-added Italian plum (Roma) tomatoes
1 medium garlic clove, minced
1 medium onion, coarsely chopped
½ medium green bell pepper, coarsely chopped
½ cup coarsely chopped cucumber
2 cups no-salt-added tomato juice
¼ cup red wine vinegar
½ teaspoon sugar
½ teaspoon ground cumin (optional)
¼ teaspoon salt
⅛ to ¼ teaspoon pepper

GARNISHES

1 cup finely chopped tomato
1 small to medium onion, finely chopped
½ medium green bell pepper, finely chopped
½ cup finely chopped cucumber

In a food processor or blender, process the 6 cups tomatoes, garlic, coarsely chopped onion, bell pepper, and cucumber in batches until smooth. Pour each batch into a large bowl.

Stir in the remaining soup ingredients. Cover and refrigerate for at least 30 minutes.

Meanwhile, put the garnishes in individual dishes. Serve with the soup.

PER SERVING
CALORIES 76
TOTAL FAT 0.5 g
Saturated Fat 0.0 g
Trans Fat 0.0 g
Polyunsaturated Fat 0.0 g
Monounsaturated Fat 0.0 g
CHOLESTEROL 0 mg
SODIUM 108 mg
CARBOHYDRATES 17 g
Fiber 4 g
Sugars 12 g
PROTEIN 3 g
DIETARY EXCHANGES
3 vegetable

yogurt-fruit soup

SERVES 4

Chilled soup is a wonderful way to begin a brunch or luncheon.

2 cups peeled and cubed peaches (about 4 medium)	½ cup fresh orange juice
	½ cup water
16 ounces fat-free plain yogurt	1 tablespoon honey
1 cup strawberries, hulled	4 sprigs of fresh mint (optional)

In a food processor or blender, process all the ingredients except the mint sprigs until smooth. Pour into a large glass bowl. Cover and refrigerate for at least 3 hours. Garnish with the mint.

COOK'S TIP

Try a wide variety of fruits in place of the fresh peaches and strawberries. For example, substitute unsweetened frozen peaches, blueberries, or mixed fruit for the fresh peaches, or use 1 to 2 medium bananas instead of the strawberries.

PER SERVING

CALORIES 135
TOTAL FAT 0.5 g
  Saturated Fat 0.0 g
  Trans Fat 0.0 g
  Polyunsaturated Fat 0.0 g
  Monounsaturated Fat 0.0 g
CHOLESTEROL 2 mg
SODIUM 89 mg
CARBOHYDRATES 26 g
  Fiber 2 g
  Sugars 24 g
PROTEIN 8 g
DIETARY EXCHANGES
  1 fruit, 1 fat-free milk

minted cantaloupe soup with fresh lime

SERVES 4

Delicately sweetened melon blended with vanilla, mint, and lime—what a refreshing treat on a hot summer day!

8 ounces fat-free vanilla yogurt	¼ cup chopped fresh mint
4 cups diced cantaloupe	1½ to 2 tablespoons fresh lime juice
1 tablespoon plus 1 teaspoon sugar	4 sprigs of fresh mint (optional)

Put the yogurt, cantaloupe, sugar, and ¼ cup mint in a food processor or blender. Process until smooth. Pour into a large glass bowl. Cover and refrigerate for at least 1 hour, or until well chilled.

Immediately before serving, stir in the lime juice. Garnish with the mint.

TROPICAL MINTED CANTALOUPE SOUP WITH FRESH LIME

Add 1 teaspoon grated peeled gingerroot and 3 tablespoons frozen orange-pineapple concentrate and process with the yogurt mixture.

TIME-SAVER

To chill the soup quickly, put it in the freezer for 20 to 25 minutes, or until very cold, occasionally stirring at the edges with a rubber scraper. Chill the soup bowls at the same time.

PER SERVING

CALORIES 127
TOTAL FAT 0.5 g
　Saturated Fat 0.0 g
　Trans Fat 0.0 g
　Polyunsaturated Fat 0.0 g
　Monounsaturated Fat 0.0 g
CHOLESTEROL 1 mg
SODIUM 68 mg
CARBOHYDRATES 28 g
　Fiber 2 g
　Sugars 26 g
PROTEIN 5 g
DIETARY EXCHANGES
　1 fruit, 1 carbohydrate

southwestern cod soup

SERVES 4

The mild flavor of cod marries well with the intense flavors of the Southwest, including green chiles, cumin, and cilantro. This dish is great any time of year, but it's especially comforting as the weather turns colder.

2 cups fat-free, low-sodium chicken broth, such as on page 43
1 14.5-ounce can no-salt-added diced tomatoes, undrained
6 small red potatoes, halved (about 6 ounces total)
1 medium carrot, sliced
1 4-ounce can chopped green chiles, drained

1 teaspoon ground cumin
2 medium garlic cloves, minced
¼ teaspoon salt
8 ounces cod fillets, rinsed, cut into ¾-inch cubes
2 tablespoons snipped fresh cilantro
1 teaspoon grated lime zest
1 teaspoon fresh lime juice

In a large saucepan, stir together the broth, tomatoes with liquid, potatoes, carrot, green chiles, cumin, garlic, and salt. Bring to a simmer over medium-high heat, stirring occasionally. Reduce the heat and simmer, covered, for 15 minutes, or until the potatoes are tender.

Stir in the remaining ingredients. Simmer, covered, for 5 minutes, or until the fish flakes easily when tested with a fork.

PER SERVING

CALORIES 119
TOTAL FAT 0.5 g
  Saturated Fat 0.0 g
  Trans Fat 0.0 g
  Polyunsaturated Fat 0.0 g
  Monounsaturated Fat 0.0 g
CHOLESTEROL 24 mg
SODIUM 350 mg
CARBOHYDRATES 16 g
  Fiber 4 g
  Sugars 5 g
PROTEIN 13 g
DIETARY EXCHANGES
  ½ starch, 2 vegetable,
  1½ very lean meat

sweet corn soup with crab and asparagus

SERVES 8

This Cantonese-style soup is practically a meal in itself. Round out your dinner with Easy Refrigerator Rolls (page 538) and Baked Ginger Pears (page 623),

1½ pounds fresh asparagus spears, trimmed, cut into 1-inch pieces
¼ cup water and 2 tablespoons water, divided use
2 tablespoons cornstarch
4 cups fat-free, low-sodium chicken broth, such as on page 43
1 15-ounce can no-salt-added cream-style corn
½ teaspoon salt

2 teaspoons soy sauce (lowest sodium available)
¾ cup egg substitute
2 6-ounce cans crabmeat, rinsed and drained, shells and cartilage discarded
½ teaspoon toasted sesame oil
6 medium green onions (green part only), finely chopped
Chili garlic sauce to taste (optional)

Put the asparagus and ¼ cup water in a medium microwaveable dish. Microwave, covered, on 100 percent power (high) for 5 minutes, or until tender-crisp. Don't overcook. Drain in a colander.

Meanwhile, put the cornstarch in a cup. Add the remaining 2 tablespoons water, whisking to dissolve.

In a large saucepan, bring the broth to a boil over high heat. Stir in the corn, salt, and soy sauce. Return to a boil.

Pour the cornstarch mixture into the broth mixture, stirring constantly.

Pour the egg substitute in a thin stream into the boiling soup. Remove from the heat.

Spoon the asparagus into soup bowls. Ladle the broth mixture over the asparagus. Top with the crabmeat, sesame oil, and green onions. Serve with the chili garlic sauce.

SWEET CORN SOUP WITH CHICKEN AND ASPARAGUS

Substitute 2 cups chopped cooked skinless chicken breasts, cooked without salt, for the crabmeat.

PER SERVING

CALORIES 133
TOTAL FAT 1.0 g
  Saturated Fat 0.0 g
  Trans Fat 0.0 g
  Polyunsaturated Fat 0.5 g
  Monounsaturated Fat 0.0 g
CHOLESTEROL 38 mg
SODIUM 387 mg
CARBOHYDRATES 16 g
  Fiber 3 g
  Sugars 5 g
PROTEIN 15 g
DIETARY EXCHANGES
  ½ starch, 1 vegetable,
  1½ very lean meat

PER SERVING

WITH CHICKEN AND ASPARAGUS
CALORIES 152
TOTAL FAT 2.5 g
  Saturated Fat 0.5 g
  Trans Fat 0.0 g
  Polyunsaturated Fat 0.5 g
  Monounsaturated Fat 0.5 g
CHOLESTEROL 30 mg
SODIUM 273 mg
CARBOHYDRATES 16 g
  Fiber 3 g
  Sugars 5 g
PROTEIN 17 g
DIETARY EXCHANGES
  ½ starch, 1 vegetable,
  1½ very lean meat

shrimp gumbo

SERVES 6

For a great winter meal, try this thick gumbo with a touch of hot-pepper sauce to warm up your taste buds.

1 teaspoon canola or corn oil
1 pound fresh okra, trimmed and sliced, or 1 10-ounce package frozen sliced okra
1 large onion, chopped
½ medium green bell pepper, chopped
1 medium rib of celery, chopped
3 medium garlic cloves, minced
½ teaspoon pepper, or to taste
2 cups fat-free, low-sodium chicken broth, such as on page 43
1 14.5-ounce can no-salt-added diced tomatoes, undrained

2 medium dried bay leaves
1 cup uncooked brown rice
1 tablespoon cornstarch
2 tablespoons water
1 pound raw medium shrimp, peeled, rinsed, and patted dry
1 tablespoon gumbo filé powder (optional)
¼ teaspoon salt
⅛ teaspoon red hot-pepper sauce, or to taste

In a stockpot, heat the oil over medium-high heat, swirling to coat the bottom. Cook the okra, onion, bell pepper, celery, garlic, and pepper for 5 minutes, stirring frequently.

Stir in the broth, tomatoes with liquid, and bay leaves. Increase the heat to high and bring to a boil. Reduce the heat and simmer, covered, for 45 minutes.

Meanwhile, prepare the rice using the package directions, omitting the salt and margarine. Set aside.

Put the cornstarch in a cup. Add the water, stirring to dissolve. Stir into the gumbo. Cook for 1 minute, or until thickened, stirring constantly.

Stir in the shrimp. Increase the heat to high and bring to a low boil. Reduce the heat and simmer, covered, for 3 to 5 minutes, or until the shrimp turn pink. Don't overcook, or the shrimp will become rubbery.

Discard the bay leaves. Stir in the filé powder, salt, and hot-pepper sauce. Serve over the rice.

PER SERVING

CALORIES 232
TOTAL FAT 2.5 g
  Saturated Fat 0.5 g
  Trans Fat 0.0 g
  Polyunsaturated Fat 1.0 g
  Monounsaturated Fat 1.0 g
CHOLESTEROL 112 mg
SODIUM 274 mg
CARBOHYDRATES 36 g
  Fiber 4 g
  Sugars 5 g
PROTEIN 17 g
DIETARY EXCHANGES
  2 starch, 2 vegetable,
  2 very lean meat

shrimp and tomato soup with chipotle peppers

SERVES 4

The mild, smoky heat of chipotle peppers nicely balances the mild sweetness of the tomatoes in this soup.

Cooking spray
1 large onion, finely chopped
1 medium green bell pepper, chopped
1¾ cups fat-free, low-sodium chicken broth, such as on page 43
1 14.5-ounce can no-salt-added stewed tomatoes, diced, undrained
1 medium fresh chipotle pepper, seeds and ribs discarded, finely chopped

1 pound raw medium shrimp, peeled, rinsed, and patted dry
1 tablespoon olive oil (extra virgin preferred)
1 medium lime, quartered
¼ cup fat-free sour cream
¼ cup snipped fresh cilantro

Lightly spray a Dutch oven with cooking spray. Cook the onion and bell pepper over medium-high heat for 3 to 4 minutes, or until the onion is soft, stirring frequently.

Stir in the broth, tomatoes with liquid, and chipotle pepper. Increase the heat to high and bring to a boil. Reduce the heat and simmer, covered, for 20 minutes, or until the bell pepper is tender.

Stir in the shrimp. Simmer, covered, for 5 minutes, or until the shrimp turn pink, stirring frequently. Remove from the heat. Stir in the oil.

Ladle into bowls. Squeeze a lime wedge over each serving. Top with the sour cream. Sprinkle with the cilantro.

PER SERVING

CALORIES 197
TOTAL FAT 4.5 g
    Saturated Fat 0.5 g
    Trans Fat 0.0 g
    Polyunsaturated Fat 1.0 g
    Monounsaturated Fat 2.5 g
CHOLESTEROL 171 mg
SODIUM 280 mg
CARBOHYDRATES 16 g
    Fiber 3 g
    Sugars 9 g
PROTEIN 22 g
DIETARY EXCHANGES
    3 vegetable, 3 lean meat

chicken and vegetable soup

SERVES 4

Although the amount of Parmesan used is small, the cheese adds just the right touch to make this soup complete.

Cooking spray
1 pound boneless, skinless chicken breasts, all visible fat discarded, cut into bite-size pieces
1 medium zucchini, thinly sliced
1 medium red bell pepper, chopped
1¾ cups fat-free, low-sodium chicken broth, such as on page 43
2 ounces dried no-yolk noodles
½ cup frozen whole-kernel corn

½ cup water
½ teaspoon dried thyme, crumbled
4 or 5 medium green onions, finely chopped
¼ cup finely snipped fresh parsley
1 tablespoon olive oil
½ teaspoon salt
¼ teaspoon pepper
2 tablespoons shredded or grated Parmesan cheese

Lightly spray a Dutch oven with cooking spray. Cook the chicken over medium-high heat for 2 to 3 minutes, or until no longer pink on the outside, stirring constantly. Transfer to a plate.

Lightly spray the Dutch oven again with cooking spray. Cook the zucchini and bell pepper for 2 minutes, or until just beginning to brown lightly on the edges, stirring constantly.

Stir in the broth, noodles, corn, water, and thyme. Increase the heat to high and bring to a boil. Reduce the heat and simmer, covered, for 10 minutes.

Stir in the chicken and any accumulated juices. Cook for 3 minutes, or until the chicken is no longer pink in the center. Remove from the heat.

Stir in the remaining ingredients except the Parmesan. Serve sprinkled with the Parmesan.

PER SERVING

CALORIES 273
TOTAL FAT 6.0 g
  Saturated Fat 1.5 g
  Trans Fat 0.0 g
  Polyunsaturated Fat 1.0 g
  Monounsaturated Fat 3.0 g
CHOLESTEROL 68 mg
SODIUM 441 mg
CARBOHYDRATES 22 g
  Fiber 4 g
  Sugars 5 g
PROTEIN 31 g
DIETARY EXCHANGES
  1 starch, 1 vegetable,
  3 lean meat

chicken, greens, and potato soup

SERVES 4

Adding chicken and mustard greens turns this potato soup into a main dish. Leeks, dillweed, and thyme make a good thing even better.

3 medium potatoes, peeled and cut into ½-inch pieces

2½ cups fat-free, low-sodium chicken broth, such as on page 43

2 teaspoons canola or corn oil

1 medium leek, sliced (white part only), or 9 medium green onions, sliced

4 medium garlic cloves, minced

10 ounces boneless, skinless chicken breasts, cut into bite-size pieces

1 12-ounce can fat-free evaporated milk

½ 10-ounce package frozen mustard greens, thawed and well drained

1 teaspoon snipped fresh dillweed or ¼ teaspoon dried, crumbled

1 teaspoon chopped fresh thyme or ¼ teaspoon dried, crumbled

¼ teaspoon salt

⅛ teaspoon pepper

In a Dutch oven, bring the potatoes and broth to a boil over medium-high heat. Reduce the heat and simmer, covered, for 20 minutes, or until the potatoes are tender. Don't drain. Remove from the heat and let cool slightly.

In a food processor or blender, process the potato mixture (in batches if necessary) until smooth. Set aside.

Wipe the Dutch oven with paper towels. Pour in the oil and heat over medium heat. Cook the leek for 5 minutes, stirring occasionally.

Stir in the garlic. Cook for 1 minute, stirring occasionally.

Stir in the chicken. Cook for 5 minutes, or until the chicken is no longer pink in the center, stirring frequently.

Stir in the potato mixture and the remaining ingredients. Reduce the heat to low and cook for about 3 minutes, or until heated through, stirring occasionally.

PER SERVING

CALORIES 271
TOTAL FAT 1.5 g
  Saturated Fat 0.5 g
  Trans Fat 0.0 g
  Polyunsaturated Fat 0.5 g
  Monounsaturated Fat 0.5 g
CHOLESTEROL 45 mg
SODIUM 339 mg
CARBOHYDRATES 36 g
  Fiber 4 g
  Sugars 13 g
PROTEIN 29 g
DIETARY EXCHANGES
  1½ starch, 1 fat-free milk, 1 vegetable

chile-chicken tortilla soup

SERVES 8

This is a terrific soup for using up leftover chicken.

1 teaspoon canola or corn oil
½ cup chopped onion
2 medium garlic cloves, minced
4 cups fat-free, low-sodium chicken broth, such as on page 43
1 15.5-ounce can no-salt-added pinto beans, rinsed and drained
1 14.5-ounce can no-salt-added crushed tomatoes, undrained
1 cup cubed cooked skinless chicken breast, cooked without salt
2 fresh Anaheim or poblano peppers, diced

1 teaspoon ground cumin
1 teaspoon chili powder and ½ teaspoon chili powder, divided use
½ teaspoon dried oregano, crumbled
¼ teaspoon salt
⅛ teaspoon pepper
Cooking spray
8 6-inch corn tortillas, halved and cut into ¼-inch strips
2 medium green onions, thinly sliced

In a large nonstick saucepan, heat the oil over medium-high heat, swirling to coat the bottom. Cook the onion and garlic for about 3 minutes, or until the onion is soft, stirring frequently.

Stir in the broth, beans, tomatoes with liquid, chicken, Anaheim peppers, cumin, 1 teaspoon chili powder, oregano, salt, and pepper. Bring to a boil. Reduce the heat and simmer, covered, for 20 to 25 minutes, stirring occasionally.

Meanwhile, preheat the oven to 350°F. Lightly spray a baking sheet with cooking spray.

Place the tortilla strips in a single layer on the baking sheet. Lightly spray with cooking spray. Sprinkle with the remaining ½ teaspoon chili powder.

Bake for 10 minutes, or until crisp.

Just before serving, sprinkle the tortilla strips and green onions over the soup.

PER SERVING

CALORIES 142
TOTAL FAT 2.0 g
  Saturated Fat 0.5 g
  Trans Fat 0.0 g
  Polyunsaturated Fat 0.5 g
  Monounsaturated Fat 1.0 g
CHOLESTEROL 15 mg
SODIUM 134 mg
CARBOHYDRATES 20 g
  Fiber 4 g
  Sugars 4 g
PROTEIN 11 g
DIETARY EXCHANGES
  1 starch, 1 vegetable,
  1 very lean meat

turkey and rice soup

SERVES 6

This soup gives you twice the rice—wild and brown—and is a good way to use leftover holiday turkey. Stir in sour cream at the end for a creamy treat.

2 cups chopped cooked turkey breast, cooked without salt (about 8 ounces), all visible fat discarded
1 cup chopped peeled butternut squash or carrots
1 cup sliced button mushrooms
1 medium rib of celery, sliced
½ cup uncooked wild rice
1½ teaspoons dried savory, crumbled, or 1 teaspoon dried thyme, crumbled, and ½ teaspoon dried sage

½ teaspoon pepper
4 cups water
2 cups fat-free, low-sodium chicken broth, such as on page 43
1 cup uncooked instant brown rice
¼ cup plus 2 tablespoons fat-free sour cream

In a 3½- or 4-quart slow cooker, stir together the turkey, squash, mushrooms, celery, wild rice, savory, and pepper. Stir in the water and broth. Cook, covered, on high for 3 to 4 hours or on low for 6 to 7 hours, or until the squash and wild rice are tender.

If using the low setting, turn to high. Stir in the brown rice. Cook for 30 minutes, or until the rice is tender. Stir a dollop of sour cream into each serving.

PER SERVING

CALORIES 217
TOTAL FAT 3.0 g
 Saturated Fat 1.0 g
 Trans Fat 0.0 g
 Polyunsaturated Fat 1.0 g
 Monounsaturated Fat 0.5 g
CHOLESTEROL 38 mg
SODIUM 70 mg
CARBOHYDRATES 28 g
 Fiber 2 g
 Sugars 2 g
PROTEIN 19 g
DIETARY EXCHANGES
 2 starch, 2 very lean meat

vietnamese beef and rice noodle soup

SERVES 6

Tender beef in a flavorful broth and a spike of lime just before serving characterize this classic Vietnamese soup. You can dress it up with bonus garnish ingredients, such as matchstick-size strips of fresh snow peas and shredded carrots.

4 cups water (if using rice noodles)
4 ounces dried rice noodles or dried whole-grain angel hair pasta
3 cups fat-free, no-salt-added beef broth, such as on page 42
2 cups fat-free, low-sodium chicken broth, such as on page 43
2 ¼-inch-thick slices unpeeled gingerroot

1 teaspoon grated lime zest
¼ teaspoon sugar
⅛ teaspoon ground allspice
1 pound boneless sirloin steak, all visible fat discarded, cut into slivers
1 teaspoon toasted sesame oil
⅓ cup loosely packed coarsely snipped fresh cilantro or mint
1 large lime, cut into 6 wedges

PER SERVING

WITH RICE NOODLES
CALORIES 184
TOTAL FAT 4.0 g
  Saturated Fat 1.5 g
  Trans Fat 0.0 g
  Polyunsaturated Fat 0.5 g
  Monounsaturated Fat 2.0 g
CHOLESTEROL 40 mg
SODIUM 71 mg
CARBOHYDRATES 16 g
  Fiber 0 g
  Sugars 0 g
PROTEIN 20 g
DIETARY EXCHANGES
  1 starch,
  2½ very lean meat

PER SERVING

WITH ANGEL HAIR PASTA
CALORIES 183
TOTAL FAT 4.5 g
  Saturated Fat 1.5 g
  Trans Fat 0.0 g
  Polyunsaturated Fat 0.5 g
  Monounsaturated Fat 2.0 g
CHOLESTEROL 40 mg
SODIUM 69 mg
CARBOHYDRATES 15 g
  Fiber 2 g
  Sugars 1 g
PROTEIN 21 g
DIETARY EXCHANGES
  1 starch,
  2½ very lean meat

If using the rice noodles, in a medium saucepan, bring the water to a boil over high heat. Stir in the noodles. Remove from the heat and let the noodles soak in the hot water for 3 to 4 minutes, or until tender. If using the angel hair pasta, prepare using the package directions, omitting the salt. Drain in a colander.

Rinse the pan. Put the broths, gingerroot, lime zest, sugar, and allspice in the pan, stirring to combine. Bring to a simmer over medium-high heat. Reduce the heat and simmer for 2 to 3 minutes, or until the broth is infused with ginger flavor, stirring occasionally.

Stir in the meat and oil. Bring to a simmer and simmer for 2 to 4 minutes, or until the meat is the desired doneness. Discard the gingerroot slices.

Put the noodles in bowls. Ladle the broth mixture over the noodles. Sprinkle with the cilantro. Squeeze the lime into the soup, or serve the lime wedges on the side.

COOK'S TIP

Because the gingerroot is removed before the soup is served, there is no need to peel it; the thin skin will not affect the flavor.

beef barley soup

SERVES 6

Served with a crisp salad topped with Zesty Tomato Dressing (page 136) and Whole-Wheat Muffins (page 542), this filling soup makes a meal that will help drive away the winter chill.

2 teaspoons canola or corn oil	1 medium dried bay leaf
1 pound bottom round steak, all visible fat discarded, cut into bite-size pieces	½ teaspoon salt and ½ teaspoon salt, divided use
1 medium onion, chopped	¼ teaspoon pepper
4 cups fat-free, no-salt-added beef broth, such as on page 42	2 medium potatoes, peeled and diced
	3 medium carrots, sliced
4 cups water	2 medium ribs of celery, thickly sliced on the diagonal
½ cup uncooked pearl barley	2 teaspoons dried thyme, crumbled

In a Dutch oven, heat the oil over medium heat, swirling to coat the bottom. Cook the beef for 10 minutes, or until brown, stirring occasionally.

Stir in the onion. Cook for 4 minutes, stirring occasionally.

Stir in the broth, water, barley, bay leaf, ½ teaspoon salt, and pepper. Increase the heat to high and bring to a boil. Reduce the heat and simmer, covered, for 1 hour, or until the beef is tender.

Stir in the potatoes, carrots, celery, thyme, and remaining ½ teaspoon salt. Increase the heat to medium high and bring to a boil. Reduce the heat and simmer, partially covered, for 20 to 25 minutes, or until the vegetables are tender. Discard the bay leaf.

PER SERVING

CALORIES 273
TOTAL FAT 5.5 g
   Saturated Fat 1.5 g
   Trans Fat 0.0 g
   Polyunsaturated Fat 1.0 g
   Monounsaturated Fat 3.0 g
CHOLESTEROL 45 mg
SODIUM 509 mg
CARBOHYDRATES 33 g
   Fiber 6 g
   Sugars 4 g
PROTEIN 22 g
DIETARY EXCHANGES
   2 starch, 1 vegetable, 2½ lean meat

white bean soup with tarragon

SERVES 4

Add tarragon to this traditionally mild comfort soup for a touch of sophistication.

Cooking spray
1 large onion, chopped
2 medium ribs of celery, thinly sliced
2 medium carrots, finely chopped
2 medium garlic cloves, minced
1 15.5-ounce can no-salt-added navy beans, rinsed and drained
1¾ cups fat-free, low-sodium chicken broth, such as on page 43
½ cup water
1 teaspoon ground cumin
½ teaspoon dried tarragon, crumbled
½ cup finely chopped green onions
¼ cup finely snipped fresh parsley
2 teaspoons olive oil (extra virgin preferred)

Lightly spray a Dutch oven with cooking spray. Put the onion, celery, carrots, and garlic in the Dutch oven. Lightly spray the vegetables and garlic with cooking spray. Cook over medium-high heat for 3 to 4 minutes, or until the onion is soft, stirring frequently.

Stir in the beans, broth, water, cumin, and tarragon. Increase the heat to high and bring to a boil. Reduce the heat and simmer, covered, for 15 minutes, or until the carrots are tender. Remove from the heat.

Stir in the green onions, parsley, and oil.

PER SERVING

CALORIES 167
TOTAL FAT 2.5 g
  Saturated Fat 0.5 g
  Trans Fat 0.0 g
  Polyunsaturated Fat 0.5 g
  Monounsaturated Fat 1.5 g
CHOLESTEROL 0 mg
SODIUM 67 mg
CARBOHYDRATES 28 g
  Fiber 7 g
  Sugars 9 g
PROTEIN 8 g
DIETARY EXCHANGES
  1 starch, 3 vegetable,
  ½ fat

lentil chili soup

SERVES 6

This robust soup gets its full-bodied flavor from beer and a variety of seasonings.

1 teaspoon canola or corn oil

2 medium onions, chopped

1 medium green bell pepper, finely chopped

3 medium garlic cloves, minced

3½ cups fat-free, low-sodium chicken broth, such as on page 43

12 ounces beer (light or nonalcoholic)

1¼ cups water and ½ to 1 cup water, as needed, divided use

1½ cups dried lentils, sorted for stones and shriveled lentils and rinsed (12 ounces)

1 6-ounce can no-salt-added tomato paste

2½ to 3 tablespoons chili powder

1½ teaspoons ground cumin

1 teaspoon salt-free all-purpose seasoning blend

1 teaspoon sugar

¼ teaspoon cayenne

½ cup grated fat-free Cheddar cheese

3 or 4 medium green onions, thinly sliced

In a stockpot, heat the oil over medium-high heat, swirling to coat the bottom. Cook the onions, bell pepper, and garlic for 10 minutes, stirring frequently.

Stir in the broth, beer, 1¼ cups water, lentils, tomato paste, chili powder, cumin, seasoning blend, sugar, and cayenne. Increase the heat to high and bring to a boil. Reduce the heat and simmer, partially covered, for 35 to 40 minutes, or until the lentils are tender, stirring occasionally. Gradually stir in the remaining ½ to 1 cup water as needed for the desired consistency. Serve sprinkled with the Cheddar and green onions.

PER SERVING

CALORIES 288
TOTAL FAT 1.5 g
    Saturated Fat 0.0 g
    Trans Fat 0.0 g
    Polyunsaturated Fat 0.5 g
    Monounsaturated Fat 0.5 g
CHOLESTEROL 2 mg
SODIUM 154 mg
CARBOHYDRATES 49 g
    Fiber 11 g
    Sugars 12 g
PROTEIN 21 g
DIETARY EXCHANGES
    2½ starch, 3 vegetable,
    2 very lean meat

curried pumpkin soup

SERVES 6

If you have been reluctant to try tofu, wait no more—this savory soup is a fine introduction. In addition to providing nutrients, tofu contributes to the creaminess of this versatile soup. Serve the soup as an entrée at home, tote it to work in a thermos for a satisfying lunch, or serve small portions as a first course at dinner.

1 teaspoon olive oil	2 tablespoons maple syrup
¼ cup chopped shallots	2 teaspoons curry powder
2 15-ounce cans solid-pack pumpkin (not pie filling)	¼ teaspoon salt
	⅛ teaspoon cayenne (optional)
2 cups low-sodium vegetable broth, such as on page 44	¼ cup unsalted pepitas (pumpkin seeds), dry-roasted
1 12-ounce can fat-free evaporated milk	2 tablespoons snipped fresh cilantro
12 ounces light firm tofu, drained and chopped	

In a large saucepan, heat the oil over medium-low heat, swirling to coat the bottom. Cook the shallots for 2 to 3 minutes, or until soft, stirring occasionally.

Stir in the pumpkin, broth, milk, tofu, maple syrup, curry powder, salt, and cayenne.

In a food processor or blender, process the soup in batches until smooth. Carefully return the soup to the pan.

Cook over medium-low heat for 15 to 20 minutes, or until the soup is heated through and the flavors have blended, stirring occasionally. Serve topped with the pumpkin seeds and cilantro.

COOK'S TIP on pepitas

Popular in Mexican cooking, pepitas are small green pumpkin seeds without the hull. Look for them in the Mexican or health food section of the supermarket.

PER SERVING

CALORIES 211
TOTAL FAT 6.5 g
  Saturated Fat 1.0 g
  Trans Fat 0.0 g
  Polyunsaturated Fat 2.0 g
  Monounsaturated Fat 2.0 g
CHOLESTEROL 3 mg
SODIUM 203 mg
CARBOHYDRATES 26 g
  Fiber 7 g
  Sugars 17 g
PROTEIN 15 g
DIETARY EXCHANGES
  2 vegetable,
  1 carbohydrate,
  2 lean meat

split pea soup

SERVES 4

Easy to prepare, homemade split pea soup is much lower in sodium than its canned cousin. Our version is flavorful even without the usual ham.

1 cup dried split peas, sorted for stones and shriveled peas and rinsed
1 teaspoon canola or corn oil
1 small onion, chopped
4 cups water
3 medium ribs of celery with leaves, chopped
1 medium carrot, chopped

½ cup snipped fresh parsley
1 teaspoon pepper, or to taste
½ teaspoon dried marjoram, crumbled
½ teaspoon dried thyme, crumbled
½ teaspoon dried basil, crumbled
½ teaspoon celery seeds
¼ teaspoon salt
1 medium dried bay leaf

Soak the split peas using the package directions.

In a large saucepan, heat the oil over medium-high heat, swirling to coat the bottom. Cook the onion for 5 minutes, or until lightly browned, stirring frequently.

Stir in the peas and remaining ingredients. Bring to a simmer. Reduce the heat and simmer, covered, for 1 hour to 1 hour 30 minutes, or until the peas are tender, stirring occasionally. Discard the bay leaf.

COOK'S TIP

If you like soup with lots of texture, serve as is. For a little less texture, use a potato masher to blend the ingredients. For an even smoother texture, process the soup in batches in a food processor or blender until it reaches the desired consistency.

PER SERVING

CALORIES 208
TOTAL FAT 2.0 g
    Saturated Fat 0.0 g
    Trans Fat 0.0 g
    Polyunsaturated Fat 0.5 g
    Monounsaturated Fat 1.0 g
CHOLESTEROL 0 mg
SODIUM 202 mg
CARBOHYDRATES 36 g
    Fiber 15 g
    Sugars 7 g
PROTEIN 13 g
DIETARY EXCHANGES
    2 starch, 1 vegetable,
    1 very lean meat

baked potato soup

SERVES 4 (PLUS 8 POTATO SKIN QUARTERS RESERVED)

Finished with a sprinkling of Cheddar and turkey bacon crumbles, this creamy but low-fat soup is comfort in a bowl. Use the leftover potato skins for Mexican Potato Skins (page 22).

2 8-ounce baking potatoes (russet preferred), pierced in several places
2 slices turkey bacon
1½ tablespoons canola or corn oil
1 medium bunch green onions, white and pale green parts chopped and ¼ cup chopped dark green parts (keep dark green parts separate), divided use

2½ tablespoons all-purpose flour
1¾ cups fat-free, low-sodium chicken broth, such as on page 43
1½ cups fat-free milk
½ cup fat-free sour cream
2 tablespoons low-fat Cheddar cheese

Preheat the oven to 425°F.

Bake the potatoes on the oven rack for 1 hour 15 minutes, or until slightly overdone (the skins will be crisp and will crackle slightly when you gently squeeze the potatoes, using an oven mitt or tongs). Transfer to a cooling rack. Let stand for 15 to 20 minutes, or until cool enough to handle. Halve the potatoes lengthwise, then halve crosswise (to make 4 quarters each). Using a spoon, scoop out the flesh, leaving about a ⅛-inch shell. Reserve the skins for use in Mexican Potato Skins. Cut the scooped-out flesh into bite-size pieces. Set aside.

In a Dutch oven or large skillet, cook the turkey bacon over medium heat for 8 minutes, or until lightly browned, turning frequently. Transfer to a small plate. When cool enough to handle, crumble onto the plate. Set aside.

Put the oil in the same skillet, swirling to coat the bottom. Cook the white and pale green parts of the green onions over medium-low heat for 3 to 4 minutes, or until beginning to soften, stirring occasionally.

Sprinkle the flour over the green onions. Cook for 1 minute, stirring frequently.

Slowly whisk in the broth until the flour is dissolved. Whisk in the milk. Increase the heat to medium high and bring to a boil. Reduce the heat and simmer for 5 minutes, stirring occasionally.

PER SERVING

CALORIES 231
TOTAL FAT 7.5 g
  Saturated Fat 1.0 g
  Trans Fat 0.0 g
  Polyunsaturated Fat 2.0 g
  Monounsaturated Fat 4.0 g
CHOLESTEROL 13 mg
SODIUM 230 mg
CARBOHYDRATES 31 g
  Fiber 2 g
  Sugars 8 g
PROTEIN 11 g
DIETARY EXCHANGES
  2 starch, ½ very lean meat, 1 fat

Stir in the potato pieces. Return to a simmer and simmer for 2 to 3 minutes.

Whisk in the sour cream by spoonfuls. Stir in the remaining ¼ cup chopped dark green onions. Cook for 2 to 3 minutes to heat through, but do not boil. Serve sprinkled with the Cheddar and turkey bacon.

COOK'S TIP

Potatoes are a great source of potassium and other important nutrients. The baked potato has gotten a bad reputation because of the company it keeps—the usual toppings of full-fat cheese and sour cream, butter, and regular bacon add calories and heart-stopping fats.

salads
and salad
dressings

Greek Village Salad (Horiatiki)

Hot and Spicy Watercress and Romaine Salad

Super Salad

Salad Greens with Oranges and Strawberries

Spinach Salad with Kiwifruit and Raspberries

Wilted Baby Spinach with Pear and Goat Cheese

Spinach-Chayote Salad with Orange Vinaigrette

Tex-Mex Cucumber Salad

Marinated Fresh Asparagus, Tomato, and Hearts of Palm Salad

Green Bean and Tomato Toss

Tomato, Basil, and Mozzarella Salad

Brussels Sprouts Caesar-Style

Spinach Salad with Roasted Beets and Pomegranate Vinaigrette

Dijon-Marinated Vegetable Medley

Asian Coleslaw

Confetti Coleslaw

Carrot Salad with Jícama and Pineapple

Cucumber and Mango Salad with Lime Dressing

Berry Explosion Salad

Ginger-Infused Watermelon and Mixed Berries

Fresh Fruit Salad Romanoff

Winter Fruit Salad with Spinach and Gorgonzola

Parsley Potato Salad

Mustard Potato Salad

Zesty Corn Relish

Mediterranean Veggie Couscous Salad

Tabbouleh

Wild Rice Salad with Cranberry Vinaigrette

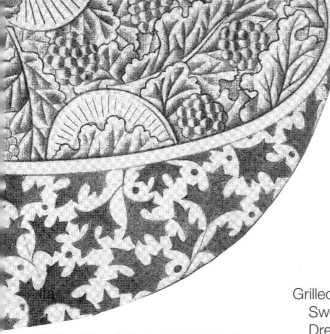

Italian Rice Salad with Artichokes

Sixteen-Bean Salad

Greek Pasta Salad

Sesame-Ginger Pasta Salad with Edamame

Salmon and Orzo Salad

Salmon and Spring Greens with Tangy-Sweet Dressing

Fresh Salmon Salad

Salade Niçoise

Curried Tuna Salad

Curried Chicken Salad

Six-Layer Salad with Chicken

Chicken Vegetable Salad

Tuna Vegetable Salad

Cajun Chicken Salad

Asian Chicken and Rice Salad

Island Chicken Salad with Fresh Mint

Grilled Flank Steak Salad with Sweet-and-Sour Sesame Dressing

Layered Taco Salad with Tortilla Chips

Southwestern Pork Salad

Warm Orzo Salad with Black Beans and Ham

Succotash Pasta Salad, California-Style

Double Spinach Tortellini Salad

Curried Quinoa Salad with Cranberries and Almonds

Barley and Asparagus Salad with Feta Cheese

Couscous Salad

Zesty Tomato Dressing

Poppy Seed Dressing with Kiwifruit

Chunky Cucumber and Garlic Dressing

Lemon Dressing

greek village salad (horiatiki)

SERVES 4

This chunky, veggie-filled salad has lots of color, texture, and flavor. The optional lemon wedges are for those who like a little extra tang.

DRESSING

- 1 tablespoon olive oil (extra virgin preferred)
- 1 tablespoon fresh lemon juice
- ¼ teaspoon Greek seasoning
- ¼ teaspoon pepper

SALAD

- 3 cups coarsely chopped romaine
- 1 small cucumber, peeled, halved lengthwise, and sliced
- 1 medium red or green bell pepper, coarsely chopped
- 1 cup halved cherry tomatoes or grape tomatoes
- ½ cup slivered red onion
- ¼ cup crumbled fat-free feta cheese
- ¼ cup kalamata olives, chopped

- 1 medium lemon, quartered (optional)

In a small bowl, whisk together the dressing ingredients.

In a large bowl, toss the salad ingredients. Pour in the dressing. Toss to coat. Serve with the lemon wedges to squeeze over the salad.

COOK'S TIP on olive oil

Use the best-quality olive oil you can for salads and other uncooked dishes. Since the oil is not heated, its flavor components don't break down; therefore, the deep, fruity flavors of a really good oil come through.

PER SERVING

CALORIES 99
TOTAL FAT 6.0 g
  Saturated Fat 1.0 g
  Trans Fat 0.0 g
  Polyunsaturated Fat 1.0 g
  Monounsaturated Fat 4.5 g
CHOLESTEROL 0 mg
SODIUM 276 mg
CARBOHYDRATES 9 g
  Fiber 3 g
  Sugars 4 g
PROTEIN 3 g
DIETARY EXCHANGES
  2 vegetable, 1 fat

hot and spicy watercress and romaine salad

SERVES 4

This salad combines jícama, also called Mexican potato, with peppery watercress, crunchy romaine, and several staples of Asian cooking. The result? Greens with an attitude.

SALAD
- 1 head romaine, torn into pieces
- 2 bunches watercress, stems discarded, leaves torn into pieces
- 6 medium radishes, thinly sliced
- ½ cup matchstick-size jícama strips
- 4 medium green onions, thinly sliced

DRESSING
- 1½ tablespoons soy sauce (lowest sodium available)
- 1 tablespoon white wine vinegar
- 2½ teaspoons toasted sesame oil
- 1½ teaspoons sugar
- 1 teaspoon hot-pepper oil

In a large bowl, toss the salad ingredients.

In a small bowl, whisk together the dressing ingredients until the sugar is dissolved. Pour over the salad, tossing gently to coat. Serve immediately for the best texture.

PER SERVING

CALORIES 93
TOTAL FAT 4.5 g
   Saturated Fat 0.5 g
   Trans Fat 0.0 g
   Polyunsaturated Fat 2.0 g
   Monounsaturated Fat 2.0 g
CHOLESTEROL 0 mg
SODIUM 179 mg
CARBOHYDRATES 12 g
   Fiber 5 g
   Sugars 5 g
PROTEIN 3 g
DIETARY EXCHANGES
   2 vegetable, 1 fat

super salad

SERVES 4

The creamy, slightly sweet dressing that coats this refreshing layered combo will appeal to even the choosy ones in the family.

DRESSING	SALAD
3 tablespoons light mayonnaise	½ medium unpeeled cucumber
3 tablespoons fat-free sour cream	4 ounces baby spinach
2 tablespoons sugar	2 cups bite-size pieces torn romaine
2 tablespoons water	1 medium carrot, peeled into thin
1½ tablespoons fresh lemon juice	ribbons
1 teaspoon yellow mustard	3 medium radishes, thinly sliced

In a small bowl, whisk together the dressing ingredients until smooth. Set aside.

Pressing firmly, run the tines of a fork down the cucumber to create small decorative grooves in the skin. Cut the cucumber crosswise into ⅛-inch slices.

In a glass trifle bowl or 11 x 7 x 2-inch glass baking dish, make one layer each of half the spinach, half the romaine, and half the carrot ribbons. Repeat. Arrange the cucumber and radish slices around the edge of the salad. Spoon the dressing over all. Serve or cover with plastic wrap and refrigerate for up to 4 hours.

COOK'S TIP on carrot ribbons

Make thin strips of carrot (carrot ribbons) by running a vegetable peeler down the length of the carrot, letting the ribbons fall into a small bowl. Turn the carrot frequently as you work. Repeat until the carrot is too small to use.

PER SERVING

CALORIES 86
TOTAL FAT 3.0 g
  Saturated Fat 0.0 g
  Trans Fat 0.0 g
  Polyunsaturated Fat 2.0 g
  Monounsaturated Fat 0.5 g
CHOLESTEROL 6 mg
SODIUM 161 mg
CARBOHYDRATES 14 g
  Fiber 2 g
  Sugars 9 g
PROTEIN 2 g
DIETARY EXCHANGES
  1 vegetable,
  ½ carbohydrate, ½ fat

salad greens with oranges and strawberries

SERVES 4

When it's sizzling outside, this salad is a must—cool and refreshing!

SALAD
- 6 cups mixed salad greens (spring greens preferred)
- 1 cup fresh strawberries, hulled and quartered
- 2 medium oranges, sectioned
- ½ cup thinly sliced red onion

DRESSING
- ⅓ cup fresh orange juice
- 3 tablespoons sugar
- 2 tablespoons cider vinegar
- 1½ tablespoons soy sauce (lowest sodium available)
- 1½ teaspoons grated orange zest
- 1¼ teaspoons ground cumin
- ¼ teaspoon crushed red pepper flakes

3 tablespoons slivered almonds, dry-roasted

In a large bowl, toss together the salad ingredients.

In a small bowl, whisk together the dressing ingredients until the sugar is dissolved.

At serving time, pour the dressing over the salad, tossing gently to coat. Sprinkle with the almonds.

COOK'S TIP on dry-roasting nuts

One way to dry-roast nuts is to heat them in an ungreased skillet over medium heat for 3 to 4 minutes, stirring occasionally. If you prefer, put them in a shallow baking pan and roast them in a 350°F oven for 10 to 15 minutes, stirring occasionally. For dry-roasted nuts ready at a moment's notice, prepare extras for storing in an airtight container in the freezer. You don't even need to thaw the nuts before using them.

PER SERVING

CALORIES 155
TOTAL FAT 3.0 g
    Saturated Fat 0.0 g
    Trans Fat 0.0 g
    Polyunsaturated Fat 1.0 g
    Monounsaturated Fat 1.5 g
CHOLESTEROL 0 mg
SODIUM 170 mg
CARBOHYDRATES 30 g
    Fiber 5 g
    Sugars 22 g
PROTEIN 4 g
DIETARY EXCHANGES
    1 fruit, 1 carbohydrate, ½ fat

spinach salad with kiwifruit and raspberries

SERVES 4

The raspberries contrast beautifully with the dark green spinach leaves in this easy, festive salad.

1½ tablespoons white wine vinegar
1 tablespoon all-fruit seedless raspberry spread
1½ tablespoons canola or corn oil

4 ounces spinach, torn into bite-size pieces
2 medium kiwifruit, peeled and sliced
½ cup fresh raspberries

Put the vinegar and raspberry spread in a blender or mini food processor. Add the oil in a stream, processing constantly until blended.

In a salad bowl, combine the spinach, half the kiwifruit, and half the raspberries.

Just before serving, add the vinegar mixture. Toss well. Top with the remaining kiwifruit and raspberries.

PER SERVING
CALORIES 96
TOTAL FAT 5.5 g
Saturated Fat 5.0 g
Trans Fat 0.0 g
Polyunsaturated Fat 1.5 g
Monounsaturated Fat 3.5 g
CHOLESTEROL 0 mg
SODIUM 24 mg
CARBOHYDRATES 11 g
Fiber 3 g
Sugars 6 g
PROTEIN 1 g
DIETARY EXCHANGES
1 fruit, 1 fat

wilted baby spinach with pear and goat cheese

SERVES 6

A warm, fruity dressing slightly wilts tender baby spinach, which is topped with pear slices and goat cheese. This dish is perfect for "fussy" entertaining without the fuss!

4 to 6 ounces baby spinach
½ cup thinly sliced red onion
DRESSING
3 tablespoons dry white wine (regular or nonalcoholic)
2 tablespoons red wine vinegar
2 tablespoons all-fruit seedless raspberry spread

2 teaspoons sugar
2 teaspoons toasted sesame oil
¼ teaspoon salt
——
1 small pear, thinly sliced
1½ ounces soft goat cheese, cut into small pieces

In a large bowl, toss together the spinach and onion.

In a small saucepan, stir together the dressing ingredients. Bring to a boil over high heat, stirring constantly. Remove from the heat. Immediately pour over the spinach mixture. Toss gently to coat. Transfer to plates.

Arrange the pear slices and goat cheese on the salad.

COOK'S TIP on goat cheese

If the goat cheese is too soft to cut easily, put it in the freezer for a few minutes to chill slightly.

PER SERVING

CALORIES 84
TOTAL FAT 3.0 g
   Saturated Fat 1.5 g
   Trans Fat 0.0 g
   Polyunsaturated Fat 0.5 g
   Monounsaturated Fat 1.0 g
CHOLESTEROL 3 mg
SODIUM 163 mg
CARBOHYDRATES 12 g
   Fiber 2 g
   Sugars 7 g
PROTEIN 2 g
DIETARY EXCHANGES
   1 carbohydrate, ½ fat

spinach-chayote salad with orange vinaigrette

SERVES 10

If you've wondered how to use the pale-green, pear-shaped chayote, this no-cook salad is one answer. Chayote, a member of the gourd family, is a good source of potassium and has a mild taste that combines the flavors of cucumber and zucchini.

DRESSING
- ½ teaspoon grated orange zest
- ½ cup fresh orange juice
- 2 tablespoons canola or corn oil
- 2 tablespoons sugar
- 1½ tablespoons white wine vinegar
- 1 tablespoon fresh lemon juice

SALAD
- 1 chayote (about 8 ounces), peeled, seeded, and thinly sliced
- 6 to 8 ounces spinach or other salad greens, torn into bite-size pieces
- 1 11-ounce can mandarin oranges in juice, well drained
- 1 small cucumber, thinly sliced
- 2 tablespoons sliced green onions

In a small bowl, whisk together the dressing ingredients until the sugar is dissolved.

In a large bowl, stir together the chayote and 2 tablespoons dressing. Let stand for 5 to 10 minutes.

Add the remaining salad ingredients to the chayote, tossing well.

Pour the remaining dressing over the salad, tossing to coat.

COOK'S TIP on chayote

The chayote (chy-OH-tay or ky-OH-tay), also called mirliton and christophene, is a mild-flavored summer squash. A vegetable peeler works well to remove the skin except at the puckered end, which requires a sharp knife. After peeling the squash, cut it in half lengthwise to remove its one seed. Use chayote raw in salads, cook it like other summer squash, or stuff and bake it like acorn squash.

PER SERVING
CALORIES 64
TOTAL FAT 3.0 g
  Saturated Fat 0.0 g
  Trans Fat 0.0 g
  Polyunsaturated Fat 1.0 g
  Monounsaturated Fat 2.0 g
CHOLESTEROL 0 mg
SODIUM 19 mg
CARBOHYDRATES 9 g
  Fiber 1 g
  Sugars 7 g
PROTEIN 1 g
DIETARY EXCHANGES
  ½ carbohydrate, ½ fat

tex-mex cucumber salad

SERVES 4

A delicious, easy way to serve fresh vegetables, this salad is a great companion to grilled fish, poultry, or meats and adds some bright color to your plate.

1 medium cucumber, peeled, seeded, and diced

1 medium tomato, seeded and diced

⅓ cup picante sauce (lowest sodium available)

2 medium green onions, finely chopped

2 tablespoons snipped fresh cilantro

1 tablespoon fresh lime juice

1 tablespoon olive oil (extra virgin preferred)

1 medium garlic clove, minced

Put the ingredients in a small bowl, tossing to combine. Serve immediately for peak flavor.

COOK'S TIP on seeding cucumbers

To seed cucumbers easily, cut them in half lengthwise and run the tip of a teaspoon down the center.

PER SERVING

CALORIES 55
TOTAL FAT 3.5 g
  Saturated Fat 0.5 g
  Trans Fat 0.0 g
  Polyunsaturated Fat 0.5 g
  Monounsaturated Fat 2.5 g
CHOLESTEROL 0 mg
SODIUM 94 mg
CARBOHYDRATES 5 g
  Fiber 1 g
  Sugars 3 g
PROTEIN 1 g
DIETARY EXCHANGES
  1 vegetable, 1 fat

marinated fresh asparagus, tomato, and hearts of palm salad

SERVES 6

This colorful and inviting salad is popular at any dinner party or buffet.

SALAD

- 8 ounces asparagus spears, trimmed and cut into 2-inch pieces
- 1 pound Italian plum (Roma) tomatoes, cut into ¼-inch slices
- 1 14-ounce can hearts of palm, well drained
- ¼ cup thinly sliced onion (yellow preferred)

DRESSING

- ¼ cup red wine vinegar
- 2 tablespoons dry red wine (regular or nonalcoholic)
- 2 teaspoons sugar
- ¼ teaspoon pepper

In a medium saucepan, steam the asparagus for 3 minutes, or until tender-crisp. Immediately transfer to a shallow glass casserole dish.

Gently stir in the tomatoes, hearts of palm, and onion.

In a small bowl, whisk together the dressing ingredients until the sugar is dissolved. Pour over the asparagus mixture. Cover and refrigerate for 30 minutes, stirring occasionally.

COOK'S TIP

You can make this salad up to 24 hours in advance, but don't add the hearts of palm until about 30 minutes before serving. They become discolored from the wine if added sooner.

COOK'S TIP on hearts of palm

Hearts of palm, which really do come from palm trees, taste somewhat like artichokes. Sometimes the outer stem of the larger pieces is a bit tough. Make a small slit in the tough layer and peel it off before using the tender part.

PER SERVING

CALORIES 44
TOTAL FAT 1.0 g
  Saturated Fat 0.0 g
  Trans Fat 0.0 g
  Polyunsaturated Fat 0.0 g
  Monounsaturated Fat 0.0 g
CHOLESTEROL 0 mg
SODIUM 165 mg
CARBOHYDRATES 8 g
  Fiber 3 g
  Sugars 4 g
PROTEIN 3 g
DIETARY EXCHANGES
  2 vegetable

green bean and tomato toss

SERVES 4

Fresh and pretty, this heart-friendly salad can go anywhere—from the kitchen table to an elegant buffet.

8 ounces green beans, trimmed	1 tablespoon Dijon mustard
4 ounces grape tomatoes	¼ teaspoon pepper
3 tablespoons fresh lemon juice	⅛ teaspoon salt
2 tablespoons olive oil (extra virgin preferred)	

In a medium saucepan, steam the beans for 5 minutes, or until just tender-crisp.

Meanwhile, fill a medium bowl with ice water.

When the beans are cooked, using a slotted spoon, immediately plunge them into the ice water to stop the cooking (this technique is called "shocking," and it helps preserve the beans' bright color). Drain well in a colander. Transfer to an 8-inch square glass baking dish or other glass dish large enough to hold the beans in a single layer.

Sprinkle the tomatoes over the beans.

In a small glass bowl, whisk together the remaining ingredients. Pour over the green bean mixture, tossing to coat. Cover the dish and refrigerate for 1 to 2 hours, or until well chilled, tossing occasionally. Drain, discarding the marinade.

PER SERVING

CALORIES 57
TOTAL FAT 3.5 g
    Saturated Fat 0.5 g
    Trans Fat 0.0 g
    Polyunsaturated Fat 0.5 g
    Monounsaturated Fat 2.5 g
CHOLESTEROL 0 mg
SODIUM 117 mg
CARBOHYDRATES 6 g
    Fiber 2 g
    Sugars 2 g
PROTEIN 1 g
DIETARY EXCHANGES
    1 vegetable, 1 fat

tomato, basil, and mozzarella salad

SERVES 4

Decoratively arranged bright red tomatoes, deep-green basil, and creamy white mozzarella, drizzled with zesty balsamic vinaigrette, make a vibrant and visually appealing salad. The apple juice and Dijon mustard give this recipe, based on the popular Caprese salad, an interesting flavor twist.

DRESSING
- 2 tablespoons balsamic vinegar
- 2 tablespoons frozen unsweetened apple juice concentrate, thawed
- 2 teaspoons Dijon mustard
- 1 teaspoon olive oil (extra virgin preferred)
- 1 medium garlic clove, minced

SALAD
- 4 medium Italian plum (Roma) tomatoes, cored, each cut into 8 slices
- 2 ounces fat-free mozzarella cheese, cut into 16 small, thin slices
- 16 medium fresh basil leaves (as uniform in size as possible)
- ¼ teaspoon pepper

In a small bowl, whisk together the dressing ingredients.

On each salad plate, make a circle of 8 overlapping tomato slices. Tuck 4 mozzarella slices and 4 basil leaves between the tomato slices on each plate, as follows: tomato slice, mozzarella slice, tomato slice, basil leaf, repeating the pattern until all are used. Drizzle with the vinaigrette. Sprinkle with the pepper. Serve immediately for the best texture.

COOK'S TIP on vinegar

Balsamic vinegar is used in this recipe for its robust and slightly sweet flavor. If you prefer a less pungent flavor, try mild unseasoned rice vinegar (seasoned rice vinegar is high in sodium), which is made from fermented rice. It can be found near the vinegars or in the Asian section of the grocery store.

PER SERVING

CALORIES 70
TOTAL FAT 1.5 g
  Saturated Fat 0.0 g
  Trans Fat 0.0 g
  Polyunsaturated Fat 0.0 g
  Monounsaturated Fat 1.0 g
CHOLESTEROL 2 mg
SODIUM 153 mg
CARBOHYDRATES 10 g
  Fiber 1 g
  Sugars 7 g
PROTEIN 5 g
DIETARY EXCHANGES
  ½ carbohydrate,
  1 lean meat

brussels sprouts caesar-style

SERVES 4

Vitamin-rich brussels sprouts are teamed with a Caesar-style dressing, crisp homemade croutons, and juicy tomato slices. This twist on a classic might convince even the most finicky eaters to eat their brussels sprouts!

4 ounces fresh or frozen brussels sprouts (about 10)
1 slice whole-grain bread (lowest sodium available), cut into ¾-inch cubes
Olive oil spray
¼ teaspoon garlic powder

DRESSING
1 tablespoon shredded or grated Parmesan cheese
1½ teaspoons Dijon mustard

1½ teaspoons fresh lemon juice
1½ teaspoons Worcestershire sauce (lowest sodium available)
1½ teaspoons white wine vinegar
1 teaspoon olive oil
½ teaspoon sugar
⅛ teaspoon pepper

———

2 medium Italian plum (Roma) tomatoes, thinly sliced

Preheat the oven to 350°F.

If using fresh brussels sprouts, trim the ends. Remove the outer leaves if necessary. Fill a medium saucepan half-full of water. Bring to a boil over high heat. Add the brussels sprouts. Reduce the heat and simmer for 10 to 12 minutes, or until tender. If using frozen brussels sprouts, prepare using the package directions, omitting the salt and margarine. For fresh or frozen brussels sprouts, drain well. Let cool slightly. Cut in half lengthwise.

Meanwhile, put the bread cubes on a nonstick baking sheet. Lightly spray with olive oil spray. Sprinkle with the garlic powder.

Bake for 5 minutes, or until golden brown. Transfer the baking sheet to a cooling rack and let cool.

In a small bowl, whisk together the dressing ingredients.

Arrange the tomatoes in one layer on plates. Arrange the brussels sprouts on top. Drizzle with the dressing. Sprinkle with the toasted bread cubes.

PER SERVING

CALORIES 50
TOTAL FAT 2.0 g
  Saturated Fat 0.5 g
  Trans Fat 0.0 g
  Polyunsaturated Fat 0.0 g
  Monounsaturated Fat 1.0 g
CHOLESTEROL 1 mg
SODIUM 100 mg
CARBOHYDRATES 8 g
  Fiber 2 g
  Sugars 3 g
PROTEIN 2 g
DIETARY EXCHANGES
  ½ carbohydrate, ½ fat

spinach salad with roasted beets and pomegranate vinaigrette

SERVES 4

This sweet and colorful salad brims with nutrients, flavor, and texture. Beets, orange segments, and spinach provide everything from folic acid to fiber, and pomegranate juice adds antioxidants and a pleasant sweetness to the dressing.

2 medium beets, stems trimmed to about 1 inch
Cooking spray
2 teaspoons cumin seeds
4 ounces baby spinach
1 8-ounce red onion, halved lengthwise, each half cut crosswise into ¼-inch slices

DRESSING
2 tablespoons frozen orange juice concentrate
1 tablespoon balsamic vinegar

2 medium garlic cloves, finely chopped
2 teaspoons olive oil (extra virgin preferred)
1 teaspoon honey
⅓ cup pure pomegranate juice (not a blend)

————

1 large seedless orange, peeled and segmented
1 tablespoon sliced almonds, dry-roasted

Preheat the oven to 375°F.

Place each beet on a separate piece of aluminum foil large enough to enclose the beet. Lightly spray the beets with cooking spray. Sprinkle with the cumin seeds. Wrap tightly. Put on a baking sheet.

Bake for 40 to 45 minutes, or until tender when pierced with a fork. Carefully unwrap the beets to avoid steam burns. Let stand for 5 to 10 minutes, or just until cool enough to handle. Wearing disposable plastic gloves (to keep from staining your fingers), peel the skins using your fingers or a paring knife. Discard the skins, including any cumin seeds that stick to them. Cut each beet crosswise into ¼-inch slices. Set aside.

Meanwhile, in a medium bowl, toss together the spinach and onion.

In a small bowl, whisk together the dressing ingredients except the pomegranate juice. Whisk in the pomegranate juice.

When the beets are ready, drizzle half the dressing over the spinach mixture. Toss gently to coat. Mound the spinach mixture on salad plates. Arrange the beet slices and orange segments on top. Drizzle with the remaining dressing. Sprinkle with the almonds. Serve immediately for the best texture.

COOK'S TIP

When you buy fresh beets, don't throw away the beet greens. They're packed with vitamins. Use them as you would spinach, either cut into slivers and steamed or cooked quickly in a small amount of olive oil. You can even toss them with your favorite whole-grain pasta.

TIME-SAVER

Fresh roasted beets give this salad a delicious concentrated beet flavor. However, if you don't have time to roast fresh beets, you can use a 16-ounce can of no-salt-added diced beets, rinsed and drained.

dijon-marinated vegetable medley

SERVES 4

This salad offers a rainbow of color to brighten any lunch or dinner, whether at home, at the park, or by the lake.

SALAD
- ¾ cup frozen whole-kernel corn, thawed
- ¾ cup frozen cut green beans, thawed
- ¾ cup no-salt-added canned black beans, rinsed and drained
- 2 cups chopped tomatoes
- ½ cup chopped red onion

DRESSING
- ¼ to ½ cup balsamic vinegar plus water to make ¾ cup
- 2 tablespoons Dijon mustard
- 2 tablespoons chopped fresh basil or 2 teaspoons dried, crumbled
- 1 tablespoon chopped fresh thyme or 1 teaspoon dried, crumbled
- 1 tablespoon olive oil (extra virgin preferred)
- 1 teaspoon sugar
- 2 medium garlic cloves, minced
- ¼ teaspoon pepper (white preferred)

4 large lettuce leaves

In a large bowl, gently toss together the salad ingredients.

In a medium bowl, whisk together the dressing ingredients. Pour over the salad, gently tossing to coat. Cover and refrigerate for 4 to 8 hours, tossing occasionally. Drain, discarding the dressing. Spoon onto the lettuce.

PER SERVING

CALORIES 173
TOTAL FAT 4.5 g
    Saturated Fat 0.5 g
    Trans Fat 0.0 g
    Polyunsaturated Fat 0.5 g
    Monounsaturated Fat 2.5 g
CHOLESTEROL 0 mg
SODIUM 195 mg
CARBOHYDRATES 30 g
    Fiber 5 g
    Sugars 13 g
PROTEIN 6 g
DIETARY EXCHANGES
    1 starch, 3 vegetable,
    ½ fat

asian coleslaw

SERVES 10

You can make this salad a day ahead, and there's no mayonnaise to worry about—perfect picnic or potluck fare.

SLAW

- 1 small napa cabbage (about 2 pounds), thinly sliced
- 2 medium carrots, coarsely grated
- 1 medium red bell pepper, thinly sliced
- 2 medium green onions, thinly sliced on the diagonal

DRESSING

- 2 tablespoons soy sauce (lowest sodium available)
- 2 tablespoons plain rice vinegar
- 1 tablespoon finely grated peeled gingerroot or 1 teaspoon ground ginger
- 2 teaspoons toasted sesame oil
- 1 medium garlic clove, finely chopped
- ¼ teaspoon crushed red pepper flakes

In a large bowl, toss together the slaw ingredients.

In a small bowl, stir together the dressing ingredients. Pour over the slaw. Toss well. Serve at room temperature or cover and refrigerate until needed, tossing again just before serving.

COOK'S TIP on napa cabbage

Napa, or Chinese, cabbage has long, crinkly, cream-colored leaves with pale green tips. It's delicious in salads, soups, and stir-fries. You can store napa cabbage in the vegetable bin of your refrigerator for up to five days.

TIME-SAVER

Use a food processor for the slicing and grating. The salad won't be as pretty, but the preparation will be fast.

PER SERVING

CALORIES 41
TOTAL FAT 1.0 g
  Saturated Fat 0.0 g
  Trans Fat 0.0 g
  Polyunsaturated Fat 0.5 g
  Monounsaturated Fat 0.5 g
CHOLESTEROL 0 mg
SODIUM 102 mg
CARBOHYDRATES 5 g
  Fiber 2 g
  Sugars 3 g
PROTEIN 2 g
DIETARY EXCHANGES
  1 vegetable

confetti coleslaw

SERVES 12

Bursting with color and flavor, this tangy coleslaw is excellent with barbecued chicken or beef.

DRESSING
- ⅓ cup white wine vinegar
- ¼ cup sugar
- 1 tablespoon canola or corn oil
- 1 tablespoon honey
- ¼ teaspoon salt
- ¼ teaspoon pepper (coarsely ground preferred)

SLAW
- 12 ounces green cabbage, shredded (about 4 cups)
- 8 ounces red cabbage, shredded (about 3 cups)
- 4 medium green onions, thinly sliced
- ½ medium red bell pepper, diced
- ½ medium green bell pepper, diced

In a large bowl, whisk together the dressing ingredients until the sugar is dissolved.

Add the slaw ingredients, tossing to coat. Cover and refrigerate for at least 30 minutes.

PER SERVING

CALORIES 53
TOTAL FAT 1.0 g
  Saturated Fat 0.0 g
  Trans Fat 0.0 g
  Polyunsaturated Fat 0.5 g
  Monounsaturated Fat 0.5 g
CHOLESTEROL 0 mg
SODIUM 61 mg
CARBOHYDRATES 11 g
  Fiber 2 g
  Sugars 8 g
PROTEIN 1 g
DIETARY EXCHANGES
  1 vegetable,
  ½ carbohydrate

carrot salad with jícama and pineapple

SERVES 6

A longtime favorite gets an update with the refreshing crunch of jícama.

DRESSING
- ¼ cup fat-free plain yogurt
- 2 tablespoons light mayonnaise
- 2 tablespoons fresh lemon juice
- 1 teaspoon sugar

SALAD
- 2 cups shredded carrots
- ½ cup diced jícama
- ½ cup drained pineapple tidbits canned in their own juice
- ¼ cup golden raisins

In a large bowl, whisk together the dressing ingredients.

Add the salad ingredients, tossing well.

COOK's TIP on jícama

A Mexican vegetable, jícama (HEE-kah-mah) looks like a fat turnip in a potato skin. Peeled and sliced or diced, it looks and tastes somewhat like apple, although not as sweet, and somewhat like potato, although not as bland, and even somewhat like cucumber. Either raw or cooked, jícama adds a nice crunchy texture. For an easy appetizer, cut jícama into sticks and sprinkle with fresh lime juice and cayenne.

PER SERVING

CALORIES 70
TOTAL FAT 1.5 g
  Saturated Fat 0.0 g
  Trans Fat 0.0 g
  Polyunsaturated Fat 1.0 g
  Monounsaturated Fat 0.5 g
CHOLESTEROL 2 mg
SODIUM 80 mg
CARBOHYDRATES 15 g
  Fiber 2 g
  Sugars 10 g
PROTEIN 1 g
DIETARY EXCHANGES
  ½ fruit, 1 vegetable

cucumber and mango salad with lime dressing

SERVES 6

Cucumber and mango combine to make a crunchy, sweet salad with an unusual mix of flavors. Serve this refreshing salad with grilled salmon or shrimp.

SALAD
- 1 large mango, thinly sliced
- 1 large cucumber (English, or hothouse, preferred), halved lengthwise and crosswise, seeded, and cut into thin strips
- 1 medium red bell pepper, thinly sliced
- ¼ cup snipped fresh cilantro
- 1 teaspoon seeded and minced fresh jalapeño

DRESSING
- 1 teaspoon grated lime zest
- 2 tablespoons fresh lime juice
- 1 tablespoon olive oil (extra virgin preferred)
- 1 teaspoon honey
- ½ teaspoon ground cumin
- ¼ teaspoon salt

In a large bowl, toss the salad ingredients.

In a small bowl, whisk together the dressing ingredients. Pour over the salad. Toss to coat.

COOK'S TIP

For the prettiest salad, cut the mango, cucumber, and bell pepper into slices that are about the same size.

PER SERVING

CALORIES 62
TOTAL FAT 2.5 g
  Saturated Fat 0.5 g
  Trans Fat 0.0 g
  Polyunsaturated Fat 0.5 g
  Monounsaturated Fat 1.5 g
CHOLESTEROL 0 mg
SODIUM 100 mg
CARBOHYDRATES 11 g
  Fiber 1 g
  Sugars 8 g
PROTEIN 1 g
DIETARY EXCHANGES
  ½ fruit, ½ fat

berry explosion salad

SERVES 4

Big, bold flavors are infused in this salad, every bite of which "explodes" with freshness.

2 cups berries, such as blueberries, raspberries, blackberries, or sliced hulled strawberries, or a combination	1 tablespoon light brown sugar
	½ medium kiwifruit, peeled and halved
	½ cup fat-free vanilla yogurt
	½ teaspoon grated lemon zest
½ medium mango, cubed	2 tablespoons sliced almonds, dry-roasted
4 fresh mint leaves, finely chopped	

Put the berries and mango in a large bowl.

In a small bowl, stir together the mint and brown sugar, mashing the mixture with the back of the spoon. Add to the berry mixture. Using two spoons, toss gently.

In another small bowl, mash the kiwifruit with a fork. Stir in the yogurt and lemon zest.

Sprinkle the berry mixture with the almonds. Top with the yogurt dressing, or serve the dressing on the side.

COOK'S TIP

Mashing the mint "bruises" it, bringing out its full flavor. You can use a mortar and pestle for this step if you have one.

PER SERVING

CALORIES 115
TOTAL FAT 2.0 g
  Saturated Fat 0.0 g
  Trans Fat 0.0 g
  Polyunsaturated Fat 0.5 g
  Monounsaturated Fat 1.0 g
CHOLESTEROL 1 mg
SODIUM 24 mg
CARBOHYDRATES 24 g
  Fiber 3 g
  Sugars 19 g
PROTEIN 3 g
DIETARY EXCHANGES
  1 fruit, ½ carbohydrate, ½ fat

ginger-infused watermelon and mixed berries

SERVES 4

The watermelon absorbs the sweet and tart flavors of the liquid mixture in this salad.

2 cups bite-size watermelon cubes
1 cup strawberries, hulled and quartered
½ cup blueberries, thawed and patted dry if frozen
¼ cup white grape juice

2 tablespoons fresh lemon juice
1 tablespoon sugar
2 teaspoons grated peeled gingerroot
4 ounces spring greens, torn into bite-size pieces, or 4 whole Bibb lettuce leaves (optional)

In a medium bowl, stir together all the ingredients except the spring greens or Bibb lettuce "cups." Spoon over the greens or into the cups. Serve immediately for peak flavors and texture.

COOK'S TIP

Omit the spring greens or lettuce leaves and spoon the fruit mixture into wine goblets or dessert dishes for a refreshing, light dessert.

PER SERVING

CALORIES 72
TOTAL FAT 0.5 g
 Saturated Fat 0.0 g
 Trans Fat 0.0 g
 Polyunsaturated Fat 0.0 g
 Monounsaturated Fat 0.0 g
CHOLESTEROL 0 mg
SODIUM 3 mg
CARBOHYDRATES 18 g
 Fiber 2 g
 Sugars 14 g
PROTEIN 1 g
DIETARY EXCHANGES
 1 fruit

fresh fruit salad romanoff

SERVES 4

The sour cream and brown sugar topping served over this delectable five-fruit salad is reminiscent of a style of cuisine favored by old-world Russian royalty, the Romanoffs. Serve as a side dish or for dessert.

SALAD
- 2 medium peaches, peeled and chopped
- 1 cup honeydew melon cubes or balls
- ½ cup blueberries
- ½ cup hulled and sliced strawberries
- 20 red grapes, halved

- 3 tablespoons fresh orange juice
- 2 tablespoons light brown sugar and 2 tablespoons light brown sugar, divided use
- ½ cup light sour cream

In a large bowl, gently stir together the salad ingredients.

In a small bowl, stir together the orange juice and 2 tablespoons brown sugar until the sugar is dissolved. Sprinkle over the fruit salad. Toss gently. Cover and refrigerate for about 2 hours, or until thoroughly chilled.

At serving time, in a small bowl, stir together the sour cream and remaining 2 tablespoons brown sugar until the sugar is dissolved. Spoon over the fruit salad.

PER SERVING

CALORIES 171
TOTAL FAT 2.5 g
   Saturated Fat 1.5 g
   Trans Fat 0.0 g
   Polyunsaturated Fat 0.0 g
   Monounsaturated Fat 0.5 g
CHOLESTEROL 10 mg
SODIUM 43 mg
CARBOHYDRATES 39 g
   Fiber 3 g
   Sugars 33 g
PROTEIN 3 g
DIETARY EXCHANGES
   1½ fruit, 1 carbohydrate, ½ fat

winter fruit salad with spinach and gorgonzola

SERVES 6

The beauty of this salad lies not only in the presentation but also in the fact that you can prepare the fruit mixture ahead, then assemble the salad quickly at the last minute. The juices of the cooked fruit mingle with the raspberry vinegar for a simple yet sensational dressing.

2 medium Granny Smith or Gala apples, peeled and thinly sliced

2 medium Bosc or Bartlett pears, peeled and thinly sliced

¼ cup unsweetened cranberry juice

2 tablespoons light brown sugar

4 ounces baby spinach

2 tablespoons crumbled Gorgonzola cheese

3 tablespoons walnut halves, dry-roasted

3 tablespoons raspberry vinegar or red wine vinegar

¼ teaspoon pepper

In a medium saucepan, bring the apples, pears, cranberry juice, and brown sugar to a simmer over medium-high heat. Reduce the heat and simmer, covered, for 5 to 6 minutes, or until the fruit is tender. Transfer the fruit with juices to a medium bowl. Let cool for 5 to 10 minutes.

Put the spinach in a large bowl or on a platter. Spoon the fruit mixture with juices over the spinach. Sprinkle with the remaining ingredients.

PER SERVING

CALORIES 118
TOTAL FAT 3.0 g
  Saturated Fat 0.5 g
  Trans Fat 0.0 g
  Polyunsaturated Fat 1.5 g
  Monounsaturated Fat 0.5 g
CHOLESTEROL 2 mg
SODIUM 60 mg
CARBOHYDRATES 24 g
  Fiber 4 g
  Sugars 17 g
PROTEIN 2 g
DIETARY EXCHANGES
  1 fruit, ½ carbohydrate, ½ fat

parsley potato salad

SERVES 6

Great flavor, crunch, and color—this salad has it all!

2 cups diced cooked red potatoes
(about 3 medium)
1 medium rib of celery, chopped
2 tablespoons snipped fresh parsley
1 tablespoon chopped onion
1 tablespoon chopped red bell pepper
1½ teaspoons cider vinegar
1 teaspoon dry mustard

½ teaspoon celery seeds
⅛ teaspoon salt
⅛ teaspoon pepper
¼ cup light mayonnaise
1 red bell pepper, cut into 12 strips,
or 1 to 2 tablespoons pimiento
(optional)

In a large bowl, lightly toss together the potatoes, celery, parsley, onion, bell pepper, vinegar, mustard, celery seeds, salt, and pepper.

Stir in the mayonnaise. Arrange the bell pepper strips on top of the salad. Cover and refrigerate for several hours.

MUSTARD POTATO SALAD

Reduce the mayonnaise to 2 tablespoons. Replace the dry mustard with 2 tablespoons yellow mustard, adding it with the mayonnaise.

PER SERVING

CALORIES 75
TOTAL FAT 2.5 g
  Saturated Fat 0.0 g
  Trans Fat 0.0 g
  Polyunsaturated Fat 1.5 g
  Monounsaturated Fat 0.5 g
CHOLESTEROL 3 mg
SODIUM 144 mg
CARBOHYDRATES 12 g
  Fiber 1 g
  Sugars 1 g
PROTEIN 1 g
DIETARY EXCHANGES
  1 starch, ½ fat

PER SERVING

MUSTARD POTATO SALAD
CALORIES 66
TOTAL FAT 1.5 g
  Saturated Fat 0.0 g
  Trans Fat 0.0 g
  Polyunsaturated Fat 1.0 g
  Monounsaturated Fat 0.5 g
CHOLESTEROL 2 mg
SODIUM 158 mg
CARBOHYDRATES 12 g
  Fiber 1 g
  Sugars 1 g
PROTEIN 1 g
DIETARY EXCHANGES
  1 starch

zesty corn relish

SERVES 8

Serve this corn and bell pepper combination on leaf lettuce as a salad, or use small portions as a condiment with ham or turkey.

1 tablespoon olive oil

3 cups frozen corn kernels, thawed

1 medium red bell pepper, finely diced

¼ cup minced red onion

½ medium fresh jalapeño, seeds and ribs discarded, minced

2 tablespoons dry white wine (regular or nonalcoholic) (optional)

6 medium fresh basil leaves, finely chopped, or ½ teaspoon dried, crumbled

3 or 4 sprigs of cilantro, coarsely snipped, or ⅛ teaspoon dried coriander seeds, crushed

3 sprigs of fresh thyme, stems discarded, or ½ to 1 teaspoon dried thyme, crumbled

2 teaspoons fresh lime juice

1 small garlic clove, crushed

¼ teaspoon salt

¼ teaspoon pepper, or to taste

In a large skillet, heat the oil over medium heat, swirling to coat the bottom. Cook the corn, bell pepper, onion, and jalapeño for about 3 minutes, or until tender. Remove the skillet from the heat. Let the mixture cool for about 10 minutes.

Stir in the remaining ingredients. Transfer to a glass dish. Cover and refrigerate for 30 minutes to two days.

PER SERVING

CALORIES 73

TOTAL FAT 2.5 g

  Saturated Fat 0.5 g

  Trans Fat 0.0 g

  Polyunsaturated Fat 0.5 g

  Monounsaturated Fat 1.5 g

CHOLESTEROL 0 mg

SODIUM 83 mg

CARBOHYDRATES 13 g

  Fiber 2 g

  Sugars 3 g

PROTEIN 2 g

DIETARY EXCHANGES

  1 starch, ½ fat

mediterranean veggie couscous salad

SERVES 8

Fresh basil and colorful vegetables team with couscous in a refreshing Mediterranean-inspired side dish.

¾ cup water
⅔ cup uncooked whole-wheat couscous
½ cup diced zucchini
½ cup quartered grape tomatoes
⅓ cup diced red bell pepper
¼ cup finely chopped red onion
3 to 4 tablespoons chopped fresh basil

1 6-ounce jar marinated quartered artichoke hearts, rinsed, drained, and chopped
2 tablespoons low-fat creamy balsamic dressing (lowest sodium available)
1 ounce fat-free feta cheese, crumbled

In a small saucepan, bring the water to a boil over high heat. Remove from the heat. Stir in the couscous. Let stand, covered, for 5 minutes, or until the water is absorbed. Pour into a medium bowl. Fluff lightly with a fork.

Stir in the remaining ingredients. Serve or cover and refrigerate for several hours so the flavors blend more.

PER SERVING

CALORIES 108
TOTAL FAT 2.5 g
   Saturated Fat 0.0 g
   Trans Fat 0.0 g
   Polyunsaturated Fat 1.0 g
   Monounsaturated Fat 1.0 g
CHOLESTEROL 0 mg
SODIUM 136 mg
CARBOHYDRATES 19 g
   Fiber 4 g
   Sugars 1 g
PROTEIN 4 g
DIETARY EXCHANGES
   1½ starch

tabbouleh

SERVES 10

Tabbouleh, a fresh-tasting salad made with bulgur, parsley, and vegetables and seasoned with lemon juice and mint, originated in Lebanon. It is particularly good with lean cuts of roasted lamb or grilled meats.

SALAD
- ½ cup uncooked fine or medium bulgur
- 2 cups snipped fresh parsley
- 1 medium red bell pepper, diced
- 1 medium cucumber, peeled, seeded, and cubed
- 4 medium green onions, finely chopped
- ⅓ cup chopped fresh mint

- ½ teaspoon pepper
- ¼ teaspoon salt

- ¼ cup plus 2 tablespoons fresh lemon juice
- 2 tablespoons olive oil (extra virgin preferred)
- 1 to 2 medium garlic cloves, crushed or minced
- 20 cherry tomatoes, quartered

Put the bulgur in a large bowl. Add hot water to cover. Let stand for 15 to 30 minutes, or until softened. Drain in a fine sieve, pressing to remove all the liquid. Return the bulgur to the bowl and fluff with a fork.

Stir the remaining salad ingredients into the bulgur.

In a small bowl, whisk together the lemon juice, olive oil, and garlic. Pour over the salad and toss. Cover and refrigerate for 3 to 4 hours.

Just before serving, stir in the tomatoes.

COOK'S TIP on bulgur

Bulgur, which lends a nutty flavor and texture to food, is wheat kernels that have been steamed, dried, and coarsely broken or ground into grain. Supermarkets usually stock medium, or #2, bulgur; you may need to go to Middle Eastern markets or health food stores for fine, or #1, bulgur. Neither of these requires cooking.

PER SERVING

CALORIES 73
TOTAL FAT 3.0 g
  Saturated Fat 0.5 g
  Trans Fat 0.0 g
  Polyunsaturated Fat 0.5 g
  Monounsaturated Fat 2.0 g
CHOLESTEROL 0 mg
SODIUM 73 mg
CARBOHYDRATES 11 g
  Fiber 3 g
  Sugars 2 g
PROTEIN 2 g
DIETARY EXCHANGES
  ½ starch, 1 vegetable,
  ½ fat

wild rice salad
with cranberry vinaigrette

SERVES 4

Although this salad is elegant and unusual, it is a snap to prepare.

⅓ cup uncooked wild rice
⅓ cup chopped mixed dried fruit
2 tablespoons finely chopped pecans, dry-roasted
3 tablespoons finely chopped red onion

¼ cup thinly sliced celery
¼ cup sweetened cranberry juice
2 teaspoons red wine vinegar
½ teaspoon grated peeled gingerroot
½ teaspoon toasted sesame oil

Prepare the rice using the package directions, omitting the salt and margarine. Transfer to a medium bowl and let cool to room temperature.

Gently stir in the remaining ingredients.

TIME-SAVER

If you don't want to cook the wild rice yourself, you can buy precooked wild rice at health food stores.

PER SERVING

CALORIES 117
TOTAL FAT 3.0 g
    Saturated Fat 0.5 g
    Trans Fat 0.0 g
    Polyunsaturated Fat 1.0 g
    Monounsaturated Fat 1.5 g
CHOLESTEROL 0 mg
SODIUM 30 mg
CARBOHYDRATES 20 g
    Fiber 2 g
    Sugars 9 g
PROTEIN 3 g
DIETARY EXCHANGES
    ½ starch, 1 fruit, ½ fat

italian rice salad with artichokes

SERVES 6

This salad reflects the red, white, and green of the Italian flag.

SALAD

8 ounces uncooked arborio rice

1 9-ounce package frozen artichoke hearts, thawed, patted dry, and halved lengthwise

4 medium Italian plum (Roma) tomatoes, cut in half lengthwise and thinly sliced

1 cup frozen green peas, thawed

¼ cup diced red onion

DRESSING

2 tablespoons shredded or grated Parmesan cheese

2 tablespoons fresh lemon juice

1 tablespoon chopped fresh basil or 1 teaspoon dried, crumbled

1 tablespoon olive oil (extra virgin preferred)

1 medium garlic clove, minced

½ teaspoon sugar

¼ teaspoon salt

⅛ teaspoon pepper

Prepare the rice using the package directions, omitting the salt and margarine. Transfer to a large bowl and let cool to room temperature.

Gently stir in the remaining salad ingredients.

In a food processor or blender, process the dressing ingredients for about 20 seconds. Pour over the salad. Using a rubber scraper, stir gently. Cover and refrigerate for several hours.

COOK'S TIP on arborio rice

Arborio rice absorbs more flavor than other rice. It is also what gives this dish and risottos their creaminess.

PER SERVING

CALORIES 213
TOTAL FAT 3.0 g
  Saturated Fat 0.5 g
  Trans Fat 0.0 g
  Polyunsaturated Fat 0.5 g
  Monounsaturated Fat 2.0 g
CHOLESTEROL 1 mg
SODIUM 175 mg
CARBOHYDRATES 41 g
  Fiber 5 g
  Sugars 3 g
PROTEIN 6 g
DIETARY EXCHANGES
  2 starch, 2 vegetable

sixteen-bean salad

SERVES 4

Here's one way to eat your soup with a fork! Using soup mix provides real variety with a minimum of effort.

1 cup 16-bean soup mix, sorted for stones and shriveled beans and rinsed	3 medium green onions, thinly sliced
½ cup chopped tomato	¼ cup salsa (lowest sodium available), such as Salsa Cruda (page 508)
⅓ medium red bell pepper, chopped	1 tablespoon snipped fresh cilantro
⅓ medium yellow bell pepper, chopped	⅛ teaspoon pepper
	4 ounces mixed salad greens, torn into bite-size pieces

Cook the beans until just tender using the package directions, omitting the salt and seasoning packet. Drain and let cool for about 30 minutes, or until room temperature. Transfer to a large bowl.

Add the remaining ingredients except the salad greens, tossing gently. Cover and refrigerate for 4 hours, stirring occasionally. Spoon over the salad greens.

COOK'S TIP

For a really quick lunch, wrap some of the leftovers minus the salad greens in a fat-free flour tortilla (look for the lowest sodium available). Zap the wrap in the microwave until warm.

PER SERVING

CALORIES 193
TOTAL FAT 1.0 g
  Saturated Fat 0.0 g
  Trans Fat 0.0 g
  Polyunsaturated Fat 0.5 g
  Monounsaturated Fat 0.5 g
CHOLESTEROL 0 mg
SODIUM 87 mg
CARBOHYDRATES 34 g
  Fiber 6 g
  Sugars 4 g
PROTEIN 11 g
DIETARY EXCHANGES
  1 starch, 1 vegetable,
  1 very lean meat

greek pasta salad

SERVES 8

Feta cheese and fresh dillweed enhance this pasta-vegetable combination.

SALAD

12 ounces dried tricolor rotini

1¼ cups frozen petite green peas, thawed

1 medium red bell pepper, diced

⅔ cup unpeeled seeded and diced cucumber

4 medium green onions, thinly sliced

4 ounces fat-free feta cheese, crumbled

DRESSING

½ cup fat-fat cottage cheese

½ cup fat-free plain yogurt

¼ cup light mayonnaise

¼ cup thinly sliced green onions (green part only)

1 to 2 tablespoons finely snipped fresh dillweed

¼ teaspoon pepper

Prepare the pasta using the package directions, omitting the salt. Drain well in a colander. Transfer to a large bowl.

Stir in the remaining salad ingredients.

In a food processor or blender, process the cottage cheese, yogurt, mayonnaise, and ¼ cup green onions until smooth. Stir in the dillweed and pepper. Pour over the pasta mixture, tossing to coat. Cover and refrigerate for about 30 minutes, or until chilled.

PER SERVING

CALORIES 237
TOTAL FAT 2.5 g
  Saturated Fat 0.5 g
  Trans Fat 0.0 g
  Polyunsaturated Fat 1.5 g
  Monounsaturated Fat 0.5 g
CHOLESTEROL 3 mg
SODIUM 381 mg
CARBOHYDRATES 41 g
  Fiber 3 g
  Sugars 6 g
PROTEIN 12 g
DIETARY EXCHANGES
  2½ starch,
  ½ very lean meat

sesame-ginger pasta salad with edamame

SERVES 4

You can serve this entrée salad on its own or stretch it to serve more people by spooning it over a bed of mixed baby greens, arugula, or baby spinach.

SALAD

12 ounces dried whole-grain angel hair pasta

1 cup frozen shelled edamame (green soybeans)

1 large cucumber (English, or hothouse, preferred), halved lengthwise, seeded, and sliced crosswise

4 medium green onions, thinly sliced

1 medium red bell pepper, cut into short, thin strips

½ cup snipped fresh cilantro

DRESSING

3 tablespoons plain rice vinegar

2 tablespoons soy sauce (lowest sodium available)

1 tablespoon canola or corn oil

1½ teaspoons grated peeled gingerroot

½ teaspoon toasted sesame oil

⅛ teaspoon cayenne

Prepare the pasta using the package directions, omitting the salt and adding the edamame during the last 3 minutes of cooking. Drain in a colander. Rinse under cold water until cool. Drain well. Transfer to a large bowl.

Stir in the remaining salad ingredients.

In a small bowl, whisk together the dressing ingredients. Pour over the salad. Toss to coat.

PER SERVING

CALORIES 426
TOTAL FAT 8.5 g
    Saturated Fat 0.5 g
    Trans Fat 0.0 g
    Polyunsaturated Fat 2.0 g
    Monounsaturated Fat 3.0 g
CHOLESTEROL 0 mg
SODIUM 207 mg
CARBOHYDRATES 73 g
    Fiber 13 g
    Sugars 8 g
PROTEIN 17 g
DIETARY EXCHANGES
    4½ starch, 1 vegetable,
    ½ very lean meat, ½ fat

salmon and orzo salad

SERVES 4

Made with petite pasta, crunchy cucumbers, healthful salmon, and a burst of lemon, this dish gives you an enjoyable variation on tuna-pasta salad. Serve it with sliced kiwifruit on the side.

8 ounces dried orzo

1 7-ounce vacuum-sealed pouch pink salmon, flaked

¼ medium English, or hothouse, cucumber or ½ medium cucumber, diced

2 medium green onions, thinly sliced

½ cup light mayonnaise

1 teaspoon grated lemon zest

2 tablespoons fresh lemon juice

1 teaspoon dried dillweed, crumbled

½ teaspoon salt-free lemon pepper, or ¼ teaspoon pepper and ½ teaspoon grated lemon zest

Prepare the orzo using the package directions, omitting the salt. Drain in a colander. Rinse with cold water to cool. Drain well. Transfer to a medium bowl. Let cool for 10 minutes.

Gently stir in the remaining ingredients. Serve or cover and refrigerate for up to three days.

PER SERVING

CALORIES 291
TOTAL FAT 9.5 g
  Saturated Fat 1.5 g
  Trans Fat 0.0 g
  Polyunsaturated Fat 5.5 g
  Monounsaturated Fat 2.0 g
CHOLESTEROL 28 mg
SODIUM 514 mg
CARBOHYDRATES 36 g
  Fiber 2 g
  Sugars 3 g
PROTEIN 15 g
DIETARY EXCHANGES
  2½ starch, 1½ lean meat,
  ½ fat

salmon and spring greens with tangy-sweet dressing

SERVES 4

This full-bodied salad pops with flavor and texture.

¾ cup dried whole-grain rotini pasta (about 2 ounces)
¼ cup red wine vinegar
2 tablespoons sugar
2 tablespoons Dijon mustard (coarse grain preferred)
1 tablespoon canola or corn oil

5 ounces spring greens
¼ cup thinly sliced red onion
1 medium fresh Anaheim or poblano pepper, seeds and ribs discarded, cut in thin rounds
1 7-ounce vacuum-sealed pouch pink salmon, flaked

Prepare the pasta using the package directions, omitting the salt. Drain in a colander. Rinse under cold water. Drain well.

Meanwhile, in a small bowl, whisk together the vinegar, sugar, mustard, and oil until the sugar is dissolved.

Arrange the spring greens on plates. Top with the pasta, onion, and Anaheim pepper. Pour the dressing over the salad. Top with the salmon.

COOK'S TIP

A serrated knife is helpful when slicing the Anaheim pepper.

PER SERVING

CALORIES 184
TOTAL FAT 6.0 g
   Saturated Fat 1.0 g
   Trans Fat 0.0 g
   Polyunsaturated Fat 1.5 g
   Monounsaturated Fat 2.5 g
CHOLESTEROL 15 mg
SODIUM 382 mg
CARBOHYDRATES 23 g
   Fiber 4 g
   Sugars 10 g
PROTEIN 10 g
DIETARY EXCHANGES
   1 starch, 1 vegetable,
   1 lean meat, ½ fat

fresh salmon salad

SERVES 6

When served on dark, crisp greens, this salad is especially attractive. You can grill the salmon instead of baking it if you prefer.

Olive oil spray

2 tablespoons fresh lemon juice and 2 to 3 tablespoons fresh lemon juice, divided use

1 1½-pound salmon steak, ¾ to 1 inch thick, rinsed and patted dry

½ teaspoon dried thyme, crumbled

¼ teaspoon pepper, or to taste

2 medium ribs of celery, diced

½ medium red bell pepper, diced

½ cup finely diced onion

½ cup light mayonnaise

10 small black olives, thinly sliced (optional)

2 tablespoons finely snipped fresh parsley

¼ teaspoon red hot-pepper sauce, or to taste

Preheat the oven to 450°F. Lightly spray a 13 x 9 x 2-inch glass baking dish with olive oil spray.

Pour 2 tablespoons lemon juice over the fish. Lightly spray one side of the fish with olive oil spray. Sprinkle that side with the thyme and pepper. Place the fish in the baking dish, seasoned side up.

Bake for 10 minutes, or to the desired doneness. Discard the skin and bones.

In a medium bowl, flake the fish with a fork. Stir in the celery, bell pepper, onion, mayonnaise, olives, parsley, hot-pepper sauce, and remaining 2 to 3 tablespoons lemon juice. Cover and refrigerate for several hours before serving.

PER SERVING

CALORIES 187
TOTAL FAT 9.0 g
  Saturated Fat 1.0 g
  Trans Fat 0.0 g
  Polyunsaturated Fat 5.0 g
  Monounsaturated Fat 2.5 g
CHOLESTEROL 61 mg
SODIUM 303 mg
CARBOHYDRATES 5 g
  Fiber 1 g
  Sugars 2 g
PROTEIN 21 g
DIETARY EXCHANGES
  ½ carbohydrate,
  3 lean meat

salade niçoise

SERVES 12

The next time you're invited to a potluck or picnic dinner, forget taking the usual entrée. Instead, surprise everyone with this lovely French salad.

DRESSING
- ¼ cup white wine vinegar
- 3 tablespoons olive oil
- 2 tablespoons Dijon mustard
- 2 teaspoons chopped fresh thyme or 1 teaspoon dried, crumbled
- 3 medium garlic cloves, minced
- 1 teaspoon sugar
- ½ teaspoon pepper, or to taste

SALAD
- 2 pounds green beans, trimmed and cut into 1-inch pieces
- 3 5-ounce cans very low sodium albacore tuna, packed in water, drained and flaked
- 5 medium red potatoes, cooked and sliced
- 4 medium ribs of celery, sliced
- 1 pint cherry tomatoes
- 1 large red onion, sliced and separated into rings
- 1 medium green bell pepper, cut into rings
- 1 medium red bell pepper, cut into rings
- 10 large black olives, sliced
- 10 large pimiento-stuffed green olives, sliced
- ⅓ cup snipped fresh parsley
- 2 medium green onions, finely chopped
- 2 tablespoons chopped fresh basil or 2 teaspoons dried, crumbled

In a small bowl, whisk together the dressing ingredients. Cover and refrigerate.

In a medium saucepan, steam the green beans for 6 to 8 minutes, or until tender-crisp. Transfer to a large bowl.

Stir in the remaining salad ingredients.

Pour the dressing over the salad, tossing to coat.

PER SERVING

CALORIES 181
TOTAL FAT 5.5 g
   Saturated Fat 0.5 g
   Trans Fat 0.0 g
   Polyunsaturated Fat 0.5 g
   Monounsaturated Fat 3.0 g
CHOLESTEROL 15 mg
SODIUM 200 mg
CARBOHYDRATES 24 g
   Fiber 6 g
   Sugars 5 g
PROTEIN 13 g
DIETARY EXCHANGES
   1 starch, 2 vegetable, 1½ lean meat

curried tuna salad

SERVES 4

A quick lunch for four, this salad features a mild tuna mixture seasoned with a sweet curry mayonnaise and crunchy celery, water chestnuts, and red bell peppers. Clusters of seedless red grapes make an attractive accompaniment.

TUNA SALAD
- ½ cup light mayonnaise
- 1 tablespoon plus 1 teaspoon sugar
- 2 teaspoons curry powder
- ⅛ teaspoon cayenne
- 2 5-ounce cans very low sodium albacore tuna, packed in water, drained and flaked
- 1 8-ounce can sliced water chestnuts, drained

- 1 medium red bell pepper, chopped
- 1½ medium ribs of celery, chopped

- 8 large red-leaf lettuce leaves
- 4 slices pineapple, fresh or canned in their own juice
- 2 tablespoons finely chopped pecans, dry-roasted

In a medium bowl, whisk together the mayonnaise, sugar, curry powder, and cayenne.

Stir in the remaining tuna salad ingredients.

Arrange the lettuce leaves on plates. Place the pineapple slices in the center of the lettuce. Top with scoops of tuna salad. Sprinkle with the pecans.

PER SERVING

CALORIES 245
TOTAL FAT 11.0 g
  Saturated Fat 1.0 g
  Trans Fat 0.0 g
  Polyunsaturated Fat 6.0 g
  Monounsaturated Fat 3.0 g
CHOLESTEROL 41 mg
SODIUM 327 mg
CARBOHYDRATES 21 g
  Fiber 4 g
  Sugars 12 g
PROTEIN 20 g
DIETARY EXCHANGES
  ½ fruit, 1 vegetable,
  ½ carbohydrate,
  2½ lean meat, ½ fat

curried chicken salad

SERVES 6

Chill this salad and serve it on a bed of lettuce, or heat it gently and serve it over cooked rice or noodles.

½ cup light mayonnaise
1 tablespoon fresh lemon juice
2 teaspoons plain rice vinegar or white vinegar
½ teaspoon curry powder
¼ teaspoon salt
⅛ teaspoon pepper

⅛ teaspoon cayenne
4 cups cubed cooked skinless chicken breasts, cooked without salt, all visible fat discarded
4 medium ribs of celery, chopped
12 thin strips green bell pepper (optional)

In a large bowl, whisk together the mayonnaise, lemon juice, vinegar, curry powder, salt, pepper, and cayenne.

Stir in the chicken and celery. Cover and refrigerate for at least 30 minutes. Serve topped with the bell pepper.

COOK'S TIP on rice vinegar

Used in Chinese and Japanese cooking, rice vinegar is slightly milder than most North American vinegars. Unless a recipe specifies black rice vinegar, use white or red rice vinegar. The black has a distinctive, heavier flavor; the red and the white are interchangeable. We call for plain rice vinegar because the seasoned varieties are high in sodium.

PER SERVING

CALORIES 214
TOTAL FAT 9.0 g
  Saturated Fat 1.5 g
  Trans Fat 0.0 g
  Polyunsaturated Fat 4.5 g
  Monounsaturated Fat 2.5 g
CHOLESTEROL 86 mg
SODIUM 364 mg
CARBOHYDRATES 3 g
  Fiber 1 g
  Sugars 1 g
PROTEIN 29 g
DIETARY EXCHANGES
  4 lean meat

six-layer salad with chicken

SERVES 4

Layer this salad the night before you'll need it using the reserved chicken breasts from Country-Time Baked Chicken (page 215). Unlike most lettuce salads that have to be served immediately, this one is even better the next day!

DRESSING
- ⅓ cup fat-free sour cream
- 1 ounce low-fat blue cheese, crumbled
- 3 tablespoons light mayonnaise
- 2 tablespoons water
- 1½ teaspoons cider vinegar

SALAD
- 5 cups packed shredded romaine (about 5 ounces)
- 1 medium red bell pepper, chopped
- ½ cup frozen green peas, partially thawed
- ½ cup finely chopped white or yellow onion or green part of green onions
- 2 cooked chicken breast halves from Country-Time Baked Chicken, shredded or chopped
- ¼ cup plus 2 tablespoons shredded fat-free sharp Cheddar cheese

In a blender, process the dressing ingredients until smooth.

In a 13 x 9 x 2-inch glass baking dish, make one layer of each salad ingredient as follows: romaine, bell pepper, peas, and onion. Spoon the dressing evenly over the salad, spreading to cover. Sprinkle the chicken and Cheddar over all. Serve immediately, or for peak flavor, cover and refrigerate for up to 24 hours.

PER SERVING

CALORIES 216
TOTAL FAT 7.0 g
  Saturated Fat 1.5 g
  Trans Fat 0.0 g
  Polyunsaturated Fat 2.5 g
  Monounsaturated Fat 2.5 g
CHOLESTEROL 52 mg
SODIUM 435 mg
CARBOHYDRATES 13 g
  Fiber 3 g
  Sugars 5 g
PROTEIN 24 g
DIETARY EXCHANGES
  ½ starch, 1 vegetable,
  3 lean meat

chicken vegetable salad

SERVES 6

Serve this crunchy mixture over salad greens or in pita pockets.

2 cups diced cooked skinless chicken breast, cooked without salt	¼ medium green bell pepper, diced
½ medium cucumber, peeled and diced	2 medium green onions, sliced
	¼ cup chopped pimiento, patted dry
1 medium rib of celery, diced	¼ cup light mayonnaise
½ cup sliced water chestnuts, drained	2 tablespoons capers, drained
	¼ teaspoon paprika

In a large bowl, stir together the chicken, cucumber, celery, water chestnuts, bell pepper, green onions, pimiento, and mayonnaise.

Sprinkle with the capers and paprika.

TUNA VEGETABLE SALAD

Substitute two 5-ounce cans very low sodium albacore tuna, packed in water, drained and flaked, for the chicken.

PER SERVING

CALORIES 122
TOTAL FAT 4.5 g
  Saturated Fat 1.0 g
  Trans Fat 0.0 g
  Polyunsaturated Fat 2.0 g
  Monounsaturated Fat 1.0 g
CHOLESTEROL 43 mg
SODIUM 218 mg
CARBOHYDRATES 5 g
  Fiber 2 g
  Sugars 1 g
PROTEIN 15 g
DIETARY EXCHANGES
  1 vegetable, 2 lean meat

PER SERVING

TUNA VEGETABLE SALAD
CALORIES 90
TOTAL FAT 3.5 g
  Saturated Fat 0.0 g
  Trans Fat 0.0 g
  Polyunsaturated Fat 1.5 g
  Monounsaturated Fat 0.5 g
CHOLESTEROL 24 mg
SODIUM 211 mg
CARBOHYDRATES 5 g
  Fiber 2 g
  Sugars 1 g
PROTEIN 13 g
DIETARY EXCHANGES
  1 vegetable, 2 lean meat

cajun chicken salad

SERVES 4

Need a little spice in your life? Try this bed of mixed salad greens piled high with roasted red bell peppers, mushrooms, and strips of reserved chicken breasts from Triple-Pepper Chicken (page 242).

DRESSING
- ¼ cup plus 2 tablespoons cider vinegar
- 1 tablespoon olive oil (extra virgin preferred)
- 3 medium garlic cloves, minced
- 1½ teaspoons sugar
- ½ teaspoon red hot-pepper sauce

SALAD
- 8 ounces button mushrooms, sliced
- 1 7.2-ounce jar roasted red bell peppers, drained and thinly sliced, or 1 large red bell pepper, roasted and thinly sliced
- 3 medium green onions, chopped
- 4 cooked chicken breast halves from Triple-Pepper Chicken, cut into thin strips
- 6 ounces mixed salad greens, torn

In a small bowl, whisk together the dressing ingredients.

In a large glass bowl, stir together the mushrooms, bell peppers, and green onions. Pour the dressing over all, tossing to coat. Let stand for 20 minutes.

Stir the chicken into the mushroom mixture. Spoon over the salad greens.

COOK'S TIP

You can make the mushroom mixture up to 8 hours in advance. Cover and refrigerate it until serving time.

PER SERVING

CALORIES 244
TOTAL FAT 7.5 g
  Saturated Fat 1.0 g
  Trans Fat 0.0 g
  Polyunsaturated Fat 1.5 g
  Monounsaturated Fat 4.5 g
CHOLESTEROL 66 mg
SODIUM 220 mg
CARBOHYDRATES 13 g
  Fiber 4 g
  Sugars 4 g
PROTEIN 30 g
DIETARY EXCHANGES
  2 vegetable, 3 lean meat

asian chicken and rice salad

SERVES 8

Made in a ring mold, this salad is a worthy centerpiece for a luncheon.

SALAD
- ¾ cup uncooked rice
- 1½ pounds diced cooked skinless chicken breasts, cooked without salt, all visible fat discarded
- 1 10-ounce package frozen green peas, thawed
- 4 medium green onions, sliced
- 1 medium rib of celery, diced
- 2 tablespoons diced green bell pepper

DRESSING
- ¼ cup plain rice vinegar
- 2 tablespoons canola or corn oil
- 2 tablespoons dry sherry
- 1 tablespoon soy sauce (lowest sodium available)
- 1 tablespoon Dijon mustard
- ¼ teaspoon hot-pepper oil (optional)
- ⅛ teaspoon ground ginger

————

Cooking spray (if using ring mold)
Sprigs of fresh cilantro (optional)

Prepare the rice using the package directions, omitting the salt and margarine. Transfer to a large bowl and let cool to room temperature.

Gently stir in the remaining salad ingredients.

In a small bowl, whisk together the dressing ingredients. Pour over the salad, tossing to coat.

If using a ring mold, lightly spray with cooking spray. Spoon the salad into the mold, packing firmly. If you prefer, leave the salad in the large bowl. Cover the mold or the bowl with plastic wrap and refrigerate for at least 30 minutes. Turn the salad out onto the serving platter, garnishing it by placing the cilantro in the center. Or mound the salad on plates. Garnish with the cilantro.

COOK'S TIP

Another attractive way to serve this salad is to spoon it into hollowed tomatoes or bell pepper halves.

PER SERVING

CALORIES 242
TOTAL FAT 5.0 g
  Saturated Fat 0.5 g
  Trans Fat 0.0 g
  Polyunsaturated Fat 1.5 g
  Monounsaturated Fat 2.5 g
CHOLESTEROL 49 mg
SODIUM 189 mg
CARBOHYDRATES 23 g
  Fiber 3 g
  Sugars 3 g
PROTEIN 23 g
DIETARY EXCHANGES
  1½ starch, 2½ lean meat

island chicken salad with fresh mint

SERVES 4

Light and utterly refreshing, this salad begins with chicken left over from Sweet-Spice Glazed Chicken (page 239) on a bed of mixed salad greens. Mango and kiwifruit with a bit of jalapeño heat surround the salad, and a cooling sweet citrus dressing and fresh mint top it.

½ cup fresh lime juice
3 tablespoons sugar
2 teaspoons canola or corn oil
4 ounces mixed salad greens, torn into bite-size pieces
4 cooked chicken breast halves from Sweet-Spice Glazed Chicken, cut into thin strips

2 to 3 medium mangoes, diced
3 medium kiwifruit, peeled and diced
1 to 2 medium fresh jalapeños, seeds and ribs discarded, finely chopped (optional)
¼ cup chopped fresh mint

In a small bowl, whisk together the lime juice, sugar, and oil until the sugar is dissolved.

Just before serving, place the salad greens on plates. Top with the chicken. Arrange the mango and kiwifruit around the chicken. Sprinkle with the jalapeños. Drizzle with the lime mixture. Sprinkle with the mint.

COOK'S TIP on cutting mangoes

To cut a mango, lay it on its flattest side. Cutting horizontally, slice off the top half of the mango. (The large pit won't "let go" of the flesh, so you can't cut the fruit exactly in half.) Turn the mango so the pit side is down. Slice off the top part of the second side, near the pit. Trim and discard all the peel from the three pieces. Cut off the flesh still on the pit. Slice, chop, or dice all the flesh.

PER SERVING

CALORIES 367
TOTAL FAT 7.0 g
   Saturated Fat 1.0 g
   Trans Fat 0.0 g
   Polyunsaturated Fat 2.0 g
   Monounsaturated Fat 3.5 g
CHOLESTEROL 66 mg
SODIUM 109 mg
CARBOHYDRATES 45 g
   Fiber 5 g
   Sugars 35 g
PROTEIN 28 g
DIETARY EXCHANGES
   1½ fruit, 1½ carbohydrate,
   3 lean meat

grilled flank steak salad with sweet-and-sour sesame dressing

SERVES 4

Leftover steak is a rare occurrence. If you plan ahead, however, you'll have some reserved Grilled Lemongrass Flank Steak (page 296) to use in this salad of colorful vegetables and earthy wild rice. A sweet-and-sour dressing melds the varied flavors and textures.

⅔ cup uncooked wild rice

DRESSING
2 tablespoons fresh lemon juice
2 tablespoons plain rice vinegar
1 tablespoon Chinese plum sauce
1 tablespoon light brown sugar
1 tablespoon toasted sesame seeds
½ teaspoon grated lemon zest

4 cups shredded napa cabbage
(12 to 16 ounces)

4 medium asparagus spears, trimmed and cooked
8 cherry tomatoes (gold preferred)
½ medium cucumber, thinly sliced
½ medium red bell pepper, thinly sliced
½ medium red onion, thinly sliced
6 ounces grilled flank steak from Grilled Lemongrass Flank Steak, thinly sliced against the grain, warm or chilled

Prepare the rice using the package directions, omitting the salt and margarine. Transfer to a large bowl. Cover and refrigerate until chilled.

In a medium bowl, whisk together the dressing ingredients.

Spread the cabbage on a platter. Mound the rice in the center of the cabbage. Decoratively arrange the asparagus, tomatoes, cucumber, bell pepper, and onion on the cabbage. Lay the beef slices on the rice. Drizzle the dressing over all.

PER SERVING

CALORIES 239
TOTAL FAT 5.0 g
    Saturated Fat 1.5 g
    Trans Fat 0.0 g
    Polyunsaturated Fat 1.0 g
    Monounsaturated Fat 2.0 g
CHOLESTEROL 24 mg
SODIUM 92 mg
CARBOHYDRATES 30 g
    Fiber 4 g
    Sugars 9 g
PROTEIN 18 g
DIETARY EXCHANGES
    1½ starch, 1 vegetable,
    2 lean meat

layered taco salad with tortilla chips

SERVES 4

This is a fun dish to have for lunch or dinner—any day of the week!

1 teaspoon canola or corn oil
8 ounces extra-lean ground beef
¾ teaspoon ground cumin
8 ounces lettuce, shredded
½ 15.5-ounce can no-salt-added kidney beans, rinsed and well drained
½ medium green bell pepper, thinly sliced lengthwise and cut into 2-inch pieces

½ cup fat-free sour cream
⅓ cup medium or hot picante sauce (lowest sodium available)
1 cup grape tomatoes, quartered
1½ ounces shredded low-fat sharp Cheddar cheese
¼ cup snipped fresh cilantro
2 ounces baked tortilla chips, slightly crushed

In a large nonstick skillet, heat the oil over medium-high heat, swirling to coat the bottom. Cook the ground beef for 4 to 5 minutes, or until browned on the outside and no longer pink inside, stirring frequently to turn and break up the beef. Remove the skillet from the heat.

Stir in the cumin. Spoon the beef mixture in a thin layer on a large plate to cool quickly, about 8 minutes.

Meanwhile, spread the lettuce in an 11 x 7 x 2-inch glass baking dish. Sprinkle with the beans and bell pepper.

In a small bowl, stir together the sour cream and picante sauce. Spoon over the salad.

Sprinkle the beef mixture over the salad. If not serving immediately, cover and refrigerate for up to 2 hours. Just before serving, top with the remaining ingredients.

TIME-SAVER

Check the produce area for bagged shredded lettuce if you need to shave a few minutes from your prep time.

COOK'S TIP

For a change, use no-salt-added black beans instead of kidney beans and substitute salsa verde (lowest sodium available) for the picante sauce.

PER SERVING

CALORIES 277
TOTAL FAT 7.0 g
  Saturated Fat 2.0 g
  Trans Fat 0.0 g
  Polyunsaturated Fat 1.5 g
  Monounsaturated Fat 3.0 g
CHOLESTEROL 39 mg
SODIUM 378 mg
CARBOHYDRATES 31 g
  Fiber 4 g
  Sugars 7 g
PROTEIN 23 g
DIETARY EXCHANGES
  1½ starch, 1 vegetable,
  2 lean meat

southwestern pork salad

SERVES 6

This salad is especially delicious if you use Cuban Black Beans (page 385) instead of the canned variety. You'll get the flavors you love without the heaviness of some southwestern pork dishes.

2 cups cubed cooked pork tenderloin, cooked without salt
1 cup Cuban Black Beans or canned no-salt-added black beans (about ½ 15.5-ounce can), rinsed and drained
4 medium green onions, finely chopped
½ medium green or red bell pepper, chopped
1 small garlic clove, minced

DRESSING
¼ cup snipped fresh parsley
¼ cup cider vinegar
2 tablespoons canola or corn oil
1½ tablespoons sugar
2 teaspoons olive oil (extra virgin preferred)
½ teaspoon dried oregano, crumbled
½ teaspoon dry mustard

———

3 cups salad greens
1 cup cherry tomatoes, quartered
6 medium black olives, chopped
Orange slices (optional)
Green grapes (optional)

In a large bowl, stir together the pork, beans, green onions, bell pepper, and garlic.

In a small bowl, whisk together the dressing ingredients. Pour over the pork mixture, tossing to coat. Cover and refrigerate for at least 30 minutes, stirring occasionally.

To serve, spread the salad greens on plates. Gently stir the tomatoes and olives into the pork mixture. Spoon over the salad greens. Garnish with the orange slices and grapes.

PER SERVING

CALORIES 222
TOTAL FAT 8.5 g
  Saturated Fat 1.5 g
  Trans Fat 0.0 g
  Polyunsaturated Fat 1.0 g
  Monounsaturated Fat 5.5 g
CHOLESTEROL 35 mg
SODIUM 151 mg
CARBOHYDRATES 19 g
  Fiber 4 g
  Sugars 8 g
PROTEIN 17 g
DIETARY EXCHANGES
  1 starch, 1 vegetable,
  2 lean meat, ½ fat

warm orzo salad with black beans and ham

SERVES 4

Bright yellow pasta, dark black beans, and colorful bell peppers make this currylike salad beautiful. It's a great one-dish meal to take on a picnic or pack for brown bag lunches.

2 teaspoons olive oil and 2 teaspoons olive oil, divided use
1 medium onion, diced
1 medium garlic clove, minced
2 large red or yellow bell peppers or a combination, diced
½ cup dry white wine (regular or nonalcoholic)
½ to 1 cup frozen whole-kernel corn
1 cup dried orzo or dried pastina

2 tablespoons red wine vinegar
1 teaspoon ground cumin
½ teaspoon ground turmeric
⅛ to ¼ teaspoon crushed red pepper flakes
1 15.5-ounce can no-salt-added black beans, rinsed and drained
4 to 5 ounces lower-sodium, low-fat ham, minced (about 1 cup)

In a large nonstick skillet, heat 2 teaspoons oil, swirling to coat the bottom. Cook the onion and garlic over medium-high heat for 3 minutes, stirring occasionally.

Reduce the heat to medium. Stir in the bell peppers. Cook for 2 to 3 minutes.

Pour in the wine. Cook for 5 minutes, or until the peppers are very soft and most of the wine has evaporated.

Stir in the corn. Cook for 2 minutes, or just until heated through. Remove from the heat.

Prepare the orzo using the package directions, omitting the salt. Drain well in a colander.

In a large bowl, stir together the vinegar, remaining 2 teaspoons oil, cumin, turmeric, and red pepper flakes.

Stir in the beans, ham, bell pepper mixture, and orzo. Serve warm or at room temperature.

PER SERVING

CALORIES 413
TOTAL FAT 7.0 g
  Saturated Fat 1.0 g
  Trans Fat 0.0 g
  Polyunsaturated Fat 1.0 g
  Monounsaturated Fat 4.0 g
CHOLESTEROL 14 mg
SODIUM 277 mg
CARBOHYDRATES 65 g
  Fiber 9 g
  Sugars 12 g
PROTEIN 19 g
DIETARY EXCHANGES
  3½ starch, 2 vegetable,
  1½ very lean meat

succotash pasta salad, california-style

SERVES 4

Break away from traditional pasta salads with this colorful, crunchy garden-fresh version.

4 ounces dried whole-grain rotini
1 15.5-ounce can no-salt-added black beans, rinsed and well drained
1 small zucchini, diced
1 medium avocado, diced
½ cup frozen whole-kernel corn
1 medium rib of celery, thinly sliced

¼ cup finely snipped fresh parsley
3 tablespoons cider vinegar
2 tablespoons olive oil (extra virgin preferred)
1 teaspoon dried oregano, crumbled
½ teaspoon salt

Prepare the pasta using the package directions, omitting the salt. Pour into a colander and run under cold water to cool completely. Drain well.

Meanwhile, in a large bowl, gently toss the remaining ingredients.

Add the pasta, gently tossing to combine.

COOK'S TIP

If you're making the salad ahead of time, combine all the ingredients except the avocado. To prevent discoloration, add the avocado just before serving the salad.

PER SERVING

CALORIES 366
TOTAL FAT 15.0 g
  Saturated Fat 2.0 g
  Trans Fat 0.0 g
  Polyunsaturated Fat 2.0 g
  Monounsaturated Fat 10.0 g
CHOLESTEROL 0 mg
SODIUM 309 mg
CARBOHYDRATES 49 g
  Fiber 12 g
  Sugars 6 g
PROTEIN 12 g
DIETARY EXCHANGES
  3 starch, 1 lean meat, 2 fat

double spinach tortellini salad

SERVES 6

For double the flavor, combine spinach tortellini and frozen chopped spinach. Serve this hearty salad with colorful fresh fruit.

SALAD
- 1 9-ounce package fresh spinach-and-cheese tortellini
- 1 10-ounce package frozen chopped spinach
- 1 medium zucchini, thinly sliced
- 1 medium yellow summer squash, thinly sliced
- 1 large carrot, thinly sliced
- 1 large yellow or red tomato, diced

DRESSING
- ½ cup fat-free, low-sodium chicken broth, such as on page 43
- ⅓ cup white wine vinegar
- 1 tablespoon olive oil
- 2 teaspoons sugar
- 2 medium garlic cloves, minced
- 1 teaspoon dried oregano, crumbled
- 1 teaspoon dried basil, crumbled
- ¼ teaspoon pepper

Prepare the tortellini using the package directions, omitting the salt. Drain well in a colander. Transfer to a large bowl. Let cool for 10 minutes.

Meanwhile, prepare the spinach using the package directions, omitting the salt and margarine. Drain well and squeeze dry.

Add the spinach and remaining salad ingredients to the tortellini. Toss gently to combine.

In a small bowl, whisk together the dressing ingredients. Pour over the pasta mixture, tossing gently to coat. Serve or cover and refrigerate until needed, up to three days.

PER SERVING

CALORIES 161
TOTAL FAT 5.5 g
  Saturated Fat 2.0 g
  Trans Fat 0.0 g
  Polyunsaturated Fat 1.5 g
  Monounsaturated Fat 2.5 g
CHOLESTEROL 10 mg
SODIUM 157 mg
CARBOHYDRATES 23 g
  Fiber 4 g
  Sugars 5 g
PROTEIN 8 g
DIETARY EXCHANGES
  1 starch, 1 vegetable, 1 fat

curried quinoa salad with cranberries and almonds

SERVES 4

Toss quinoa (KEEN-wah) with a sweet soy and curry sauce, then top it with toasted almonds for this entrée salad.

2 cups water

1 cup uncooked quinoa, rinsed and drained

2 tablespoons soy sauce (lowest sodium available)

1 tablespoon cider vinegar

1 tablespoon honey

½ teaspoon curry powder

¼ teaspoon crushed red pepper flakes, or to taste

1 8-ounce can sliced water chestnuts, drained

½ medium green bell pepper, chopped

1 medium rib of celery, finely chopped

½ cup sweetened dried cranberries or dried mixed fruit

½ teaspoon grated orange zest

½ cup sliced almonds, dry-roasted

In a medium saucepan, bring the water to a boil over high heat. Stir in the quinoa. Reduce the heat and simmer for 15 minutes, or until the water is absorbed. Remove from the heat and let cool.

Meanwhile, in a small bowl, whisk together the soy sauce, vinegar, honey, curry powder, and red pepper flakes.

In a large bowl, stir together the remaining ingredients except the almonds.

Gently stir in the cooled quinoa, then the soy sauce mixture. Sprinkle with the almonds.

COOK'S TIP on quinoa

Serve quinoa hot or cold, press it into molds to serve as timbales, make it into a curry, or vary the vegetables and herbs to give it a Mediterranean or all-American flavor. Try it for breakfast as a hot cereal topped with fruit and fat-free milk.

TIME-SAVER

A quick way to cool cooked quinoa is to spread it in a thin layer on a baking sheet or large piece of aluminum foil on a cooling rack and let stand for 5 to 10 minutes.

PER SERVING

CALORIES 317
TOTAL FAT 8.5 g
  Saturated Fat 0.5 g
  Trans Fat 0.0 g
  Polyunsaturated Fat 3.0 g
  Monounsaturated Fat 4.5 g
CHOLESTEROL 0 mg
SODIUM 214 mg
CARBOHYDRATES 53 g
  Fiber 7 g
  Sugars 18 g
PROTEIN 10 g
DIETARY EXCHANGES
  2 starch, 1 fruit,
  1 vegetable, 1½ fat

barley and asparagus salad with feta cheese

SERVES 4

Barley replaces the pasta you might expect in this highly flavored dish, which gets an added pop from feta cheese.

2 cups water
½ cup uncooked quick-cooking barley
4 ounces asparagus spears, trimmed and cut into 2-inch pieces
2 ounces spring greens, coarsely chopped
2 tablespoons cider vinegar
1 tablespoon capers, drained

1 tablespoon olive oil (extra virgin preferred)
2 teaspoons dried basil, crumbled
½ teaspoon dried rosemary, crushed
1 cup grape tomatoes, quartered
4 ounces fat-free feta cheese, crumbled

In a medium saucepan, bring the water to a boil over high heat. Stir in the barley. Reduce the heat and simmer, covered, for 8 minutes.

Stir in the asparagus. Cook for 2 minutes. Pour the barley mixture into a colander and run under cold water to cool completely. Shake off any excess liquid.

Meanwhile, in a medium bowl, toss together the spring greens, vinegar, capers, oil, basil, and rosemary.

Add the tomatoes, feta, and barley mixture, tossing gently.

COOK'S TIP

Try using a rubber scraper to toss ingredients. It will keep them from bruising.

COOK'S TIP on asparagus

An asparagus spear has a natural bending point where the tough stem ends. Holding a spear of asparagus at the top and the bottom, bend the spear; snap at the bending point. Discard the tough part, or save it to use in making broths and other soups.

PER SERVING

CALORIES 175
TOTAL FAT 4.0 g
  Saturated Fat 0.5 g
  Trans Fat 0.0 g
  Polyunsaturated Fat 0.5 g
  Monounsaturated Fat 2.5 g
CHOLESTEROL 0 mg
SODIUM 522 mg
CARBOHYDRATES 27 g
  Fiber 6 g
  Sugars 4 g
PROTEIN 10 g
DIETARY EXCHANGES
  1½ starch, 1 vegetable, 1 lean meat

couscous salad

SERVES 4

Couscous rehydrates so quickly that it makes short work of preparing this lemon-enhanced entrée salad.

1 cup water
¾ cup uncooked couscous
1 cup shredded fat-free mozzarella
  cheese
1 cup diced tomatoes
½ cup finely snipped fresh parsley
12 kalamata olives, finely chopped

1 teaspoon grated lemon zest
2 tablespoons fresh lemon juice
½ medium garlic clove, minced
⅛ teaspoon salt
¼ teaspoon crushed red pepper flakes
2 cups coarsely chopped fresh
  spinach

In a small saucepan, bring the water to a boil over high heat. Remove from the heat. Stir in the couscous. Let stand, covered, for 5 minutes, or until the liquid is absorbed. Fluff with a fork. Spread the couscous in a thin layer on a baking sheet or large piece of aluminum foil on a cooling rack. Let stand for 5 to 10 minutes, or until cooled.

Meanwhile, in a large bowl, stir together the remaining ingredients except the spinach. Add the couscous, tossing gently. Add the spinach, tossing gently.

PER SERVING

CALORIES 216
TOTAL FAT 3.5 g
  Saturated Fat 0.5 g
  Trans Fat 0.0 g
  Polyunsaturated Fat 0.5 g
  Monounsaturated Fat 2.5 g
CHOLESTEROL 5 mg
SODIUM 480 mg
CARBOHYDRATES 32 g
  Fiber 3 g
  Sugars 2 g
PROTEIN 14 g
DIETARY EXCHANGES
  2 starch,
  1½ very lean meat

zesty tomato dressing

SERVES 10; 2 TABLESPOONS PER SERVING

Fresh lemon juice and dry mustard make this dressing sparkle.

1 cup no-salt-added tomato juice
2 medium green onions, thinly sliced
2 tablespoons fresh lemon juice
2 tablespoons red wine vinegar
1 teaspoon dried parsley, crumbled
1 teaspoon sugar
½ teaspoon dried oregano, crumbled
½ teaspoon dry mustard
½ teaspoon soy sauce (lowest sodium available)
¼ teaspoon pepper

In a medium bowl, whisk together the ingredients. Cover and refrigerate for up to three days.

PER SERVING

CALORIES 10
TOTAL FAT 0.0 g
  Saturated Fat 0.0 g
  Trans Fat 0.0 g
  Polyunsaturated Fat 0.0 g
  Monounsaturated Fat 0.0 g
CHOLESTEROL 0 mg
SODIUM 10 mg
CARBOHYDRATES 2 g
  Fiber 0 g
  Sugars 2 g
PROTEIN 0 g
DIETARY EXCHANGES
  Free

poppy seed dressing with kiwifruit

SERVES 8; 2 TABLESPOONS PER SERVING

Serve this delicately sweet dressing over a crisp lettuce and jícama salad, seasonal fresh fruit, or fat-free cottage cheese or fat-free frozen yogurt.

¾ cup pineapple juice	2 tablespoons honey
1 tablespoon cornstarch	1 tablespoon fresh lime juice
2 medium kiwifruit, peeled and coarsely diced	1 teaspoon poppy seeds

In a small saucepan, whisk together the pineapple juice and cornstarch. Bring to a boil over medium-high heat, whisking occasionally. Reduce the heat and simmer for 3 to 4 minutes, or until the mixture thickens, whisking occasionally. Spoon into a small bowl. Let cool at room temperature for 5 minutes. Cover and refrigerate until chilled, at least 15 minutes.

In a food processor or blender, process the pineapple mixture, kiwifruit, honey, and lime juice until smooth. Pour into a bowl.

Stir in the poppy seeds. Serve or cover and refrigerate for up to five days.

COOK'S TIP on kiwifruit

Choose kiwifruit that yields to gentle pressure (it should not be soft or mushy). If the kiwifruit is extremely firm, let it sit on the counter for a few days to ripen. Although the fuzzy skin is almost always removed, it is edible, as are the tiny black seeds.

PER SERVING

CALORIES 46
TOTAL FAT 0.0 g
  Saturated Fat 0.0 g
  Trans Fat 0.0 g
  Polyunsaturated Fat 0.0 g
  Monounsaturated Fat 0.0 g
CHOLESTEROL 0 mg
SODIUM 2 mg
CARBOHYDRATES 11 g
  Fiber 1 g
  Sugars 8 g
PROTEIN 0 g
DIETARY EXCHANGES
  ½ carbohydrate

chunky cucumber and garlic dressing

SERVES 6; 2 TABLESPOONS PER SERVING

Be as cool as a cucumber on a hot summer day and serve this dressing on your favorite salad or on a grilled chicken, pork, or beef pita sandwich.

½ cup fat-free plain yogurt
½ medium cucumber, peeled, seeded, and chopped
1 tablespoon sugar
1 tablespoon canola or corn oil

½ teaspoon dried onion flakes
¼ teaspoon garlic powder
¼ teaspoon pepper
1 tablespoon red wine vinegar

In a small bowl, whisk the yogurt until smooth.

Whisk in the remaining ingredients except the vinegar.

Gradually whisk in the vinegar until combined. Cover and refrigerate for at least 4 hours.

PER SERVING

CALORIES 43
TOTAL FAT 2.5 g
  Saturated Fat 0.0 g
  Trans Fat 0.0 g
  Polyunsaturated Fat 0.5 g
  Monounsaturated Fat 1.5 g
CHOLESTEROL 0 mg
SODIUM 16 mg
CARBOHYDRATES 4 g
  Fiber 0 g
  Sugars 4 g
PROTEIN 1 g
DIETARY EXCHANGES
  ½ fat

lemon dressing

SERVES 8; 2 TABLESPOONS PER SERVING

Tangy and flavorful, this dressing is a rousing accompaniment for salads and other fresh vegetables.

½ cup fresh lemon juice	1 tablespoon honey
2 tablespoons water	1 tablespoon Dijon mustard
1 tablespoon snipped fresh parsley	2 medium garlic cloves, minced
1 tablespoon snipped fresh oregano	½ teaspoon fennel seeds, crushed
1 tablespoon olive oil (extra virgin preferred)	

In a small bowl, whisk together all the ingredients.

COOK'S TIP on fennel

Known primarily as an Italian spice and herb, fennel has a delicate anise flavor. The two main kinds of fennel both have feathery leaves and celerylike stems. Garden, or common, fennel produces the fennel seed that is used as a spice. Fennel seeds resemble caraway seeds and are usually ground before using. Florence fennel, or finocchio, is prized for the thickened leaf stalks that form a bulb at the base. The bulb and stems of both kinds can be used as a vegetable, raw or cooked, much as celery is used. The leaves can be snipped and used for flavoring. Add to cooked dishes at the last minute so the flavor doesn't dissipate.

PER SERVING

CALORIES 31
TOTAL FAT 2.0 g
  Saturated Fat 0.0 g
  Trans Fat 0.0 g
  Polyunsaturated Fat 0.0 g
  Monounsaturated Fat 1.0 g
CHOLESTEROL 0 mg
SODIUM 39 mg
CARBOHYDRATES 4 g
  Fiber 0 g
  Sugars 3 g
PROTEIN 0 g
DIETARY EXCHANGES
  ½ fat

seafood

Bronzed Catfish with Remoulade Sauce

Baked Catfish

Crispy Cajun Catfish Nibbles with Red Sauce

Catfish with Zesty Slaw Topping

Cod Baked with Vegetables

Seared Fish with Rosemary Aïoli

Fish Fillets with Zesty Rosemary Oil

So Simple, So Fast, So Good Fillets

Haddock with Tomatoes and Ginger

Mediterranean Fish

Fish in Crazy Water

Fish Tacos with Pico de Gallo

Coconut-Rum Baked Fish

Teriyaki Halibut

Orange Roughy with Tomatoes and Spinach

Dilled Orange Roughy with Lemon-Caper Sauce

Ginger-Walnut Salmon and Asparagus

Baked Salmon with Cucumber Relish

Salmon Fillets with Mango-Strawberry Salsa

Broiled Salmon with Citrus Salsa

Grilled Pineapple-Lime Salmon

Grilled Salmon with Cilantro Sauce

Salmon Alfredo

Sesame-Orange Salmon

Salmon Cakes with Creole Aïoli

Snapper with Fresh Tomatoes and Capers

Mushroom-Stuffed Fish Roll-Ups

Fish Fillets in Foil

Fish Fillets with Lemon and Spinach

Fish Fillets with Basil, Tomato, and Green Onion

Fish Fillets with Dill and Cucumber

Fish Fillets with Thyme and Celery

Fish Fillets with Curried Vegetables

Crispy Baked Fillet of Sole

Bay-Style Fillets

Sole with Walnuts and White Wine

Sole with Parsley and Mint

Sole Parmesan

Stovetop Fish with Vegetable Rice, Mexican Style

Tex-Mex Tilapia

Baked Tilapia with Sausage-Flecked Rice

Tilapia Amandine

Greek Fish Fillets

Grilled Fish with Mediterranean Salsa

Almond-Topped Baked Trout

Baked Trout with Tartar Sauce

Crisp Pan-Seared Trout with Green Onions

Braised Tuna Steaks with Orange-Cranberry Glaze

Grilled Tuna with Pineapple-Nectarine Salsa

Sesame Tuna with Pineapple Sauce

Stuffed Shells with Albacore Tuna and Vegetables

Spicy Tuna Pitas

Tuna Chili

Linguine with White Clam Sauce

Crabmeat Maryland

Crab Primavera Alfredo

Scallops and Asparagus in Wine Sauce

Oven-Fried Scallops with Cilantro and Lime

Shrimp and Okra Étouffée

Fiery Shrimp Dijon

Curried Shrimp Risotto

Little Shrimp Cakes

Slow-Cooker Cioppino

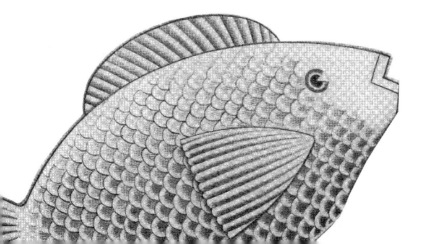

bronzed catfish with remoulade sauce

SERVES 4

The bronzing technique used in this recipe is similar to the blackening used for dishes such as blackened redfish. To get that bronzed look, however, the fish is cooked at a more moderate temperature so the seasonings do not burn.

REMOULADE SAUCE
- 2 medium green onions, thinly sliced
- 1 small rib of celery, finely chopped
- 2 tablespoons snipped fresh parsley
- 2 tablespoons no-salt-added ketchup
- 1 tablespoon Creole mustard or coarse-grain Dijon mustard
- 1 tablespoon red wine vinegar
- 2 teaspoons Worcestershire sauce (lowest sodium available)
- 2 teaspoons olive oil (extra virgin preferred)

- 1 medium garlic clove, minced
- ½ teaspoon paprika
- ¼ teaspoon salt

- 4 catfish fillets (about 4 ounces each), rinsed and patted dry
- Cooking spray
- 2 teaspoons salt-free Creole or Cajun seasoning blend and 2 teaspoons salt-free Creole or Cajun seasoning blend (such as on page 463), divided use

In a medium glass bowl, stir together the remoulade sauce ingredients. Cover and refrigerate for up to three days.

Lightly spray both sides of the fish with cooking spray. Sprinkle 2 teaspoons seasoning blend over one side of the fish.

Heat a nonstick skillet over medium-high heat. Put the fish with the seasoned side down in the skillet. Cook for 5 minutes, or until golden brown. Sprinkle the unseasoned side with the remaining 2 teaspoons seasoning blend. Turn over. Cook for 4 to 5 minutes, or until the bottom side is browned and the fish flakes easily when tested with a fork. Serve topped with the sauce.

PER SERVING

CALORIES 142
TOTAL FAT 5.5 g
  Saturated Fat 1.0 g
  Trans Fat 0.0 g
  Polyunsaturated Fat 1.0 g
  Monounsaturated Fat 2.5 g
CHOLESTEROL 66 mg
SODIUM 271 mg
CARBOHYDRATES 3 g
  Fiber 1 g
  Sugars 2 g
PROTEIN 19 g
DIETARY EXCHANGES
  3 lean meat

baked catfish

SERVES 6

Crisp on the outside and moist on the inside, these fish fillets go well with mashed potatoes, such as Mashed Potatoes with Parmesan and Green Onions (page 462).

Cooking spray
¾ cup low-fat buttermilk
¼ teaspoon salt
¼ teaspoon red hot-pepper sauce
3 ounces fat-free, low-sodium whole-grain crackers, crushed (about 30)

6 catfish fillets (about 4 ounces each), rinsed and patted dry
1 tablespoon light tub margarine, melted
2 tablespoons snipped fresh parsley
1 large lemon, cut into 6 wedges (optional)

Preheat the oven to 400°F. Lightly spray a 13 x 9 x 2-inch baking pan with cooking spray.

In a small shallow dish, stir together the buttermilk, salt, and hot-pepper sauce. Put the cracker crumbs on a plate. Set the dish, plate, and baking pan in a row, assembly-line fashion. Dip one fillet in the buttermilk mixture, turning to coat and letting the excess drip off. Dip in the crumbs, turning to coat and gently shaking off the excess. Transfer to the baking pan. Repeat with the remaining fillets, placing them in a single layer. Drizzle with the margarine and lightly spray with cooking spray.

Bake for 15 to 20 minutes, or until the fish flakes easily when tested with a fork. Sprinkle with the parsley. Serve with the lemon wedges to squeeze over the fish.

PER SERVING

CALORIES 188
TOTAL FAT 5.5 g
  Saturated Fat 1.0 g
  Trans Fat 0.0 g
  Polyunsaturated Fat 1.0 g
  Monounsaturated Fat 1.5 g
CHOLESTEROL 67 mg
SODIUM 235 mg
CARBOHYDRATES 12 g
  Fiber 1 g
  Sugars 3 g
PROTEIN 22 g
DIETARY EXCHANGES
  1 starch, 3 lean meat

crispy cajun catfish nibbles with red sauce

SERVES 4

If you like fried popcorn shrimp, you'll love these crisp bites of catfish. They're served with a zesty sauce similar to cocktail sauce.

Cooking spray

FISH
- 3 tablespoons yellow cornmeal
- ½ teaspoon chili powder
- ½ teaspoon ground cumin
- ¼ teaspoon salt
- ¼ teaspoon garlic powder
- ⅛ teaspoon pepper
- 1 pound catfish fillets, rinsed and patted dry, cut into ½-inch cubes

- ¼ cup egg substitute
- ½ cup cornflake crumbs

RED SAUCE
- ¼ cup no-salt-added ketchup
- 2 tablespoons white wine vinegar
- 2 tablespoons fresh lemon juice
- 1 tablespoon honey
- 1 tablespoon bottled white horseradish

Preheat the oven to 400°F. Lightly spray a baking sheet with cooking spray.

In a large dish, stir together the cornmeal, chili powder, cumin, salt, garlic powder, and pepper. Add the fish, turning gently to coat.

Put the egg substitute and cornflake crumbs in two separate shallow dishes. Set the dishes and a large baking sheet in a row, assembly-line fashion. Dip the fish in batches in the egg substitute, turning to coat and letting the excess drip off. Dip in the cornflake crumbs to coat lightly, gently shaking off any excess. Transfer the fish to the baking sheet in a single layer. Repeat with the remaining fish. Lightly spray the tops with cooking spray.

Bake for 7 to 8 minutes, or until the fish flakes easily when tested with a fork.

Meanwhile, in a small bowl, whisk together the sauce ingredients. Serve with the fish.

PER SERVING

CALORIES 213
TOTAL FAT 3.5 g
  Saturated Fat 1.0 g
  Trans Fat 0.0 g
  Polyunsaturated Fat 1.0 g
  Monounsaturated Fat 1.0 g
CHOLESTEROL 66 mg
SODIUM 326 mg
CARBOHYDRATES 25 g
  Fiber 1 g
  Sugars 8 g
PROTEIN 22 g
DIETARY EXCHANGES
  1 starch, ½ carbohydrate, 3 very lean meat

catfish with zesty slaw topping

SERVES 4

A New Orleans favorite gets a lean update with crispy baked catfish and a broccoli-slaw topping, kicked up with Cajun or Creole seasoning and horseradish. Serve with melon wedges on the side.

Cooking spray
¼ cup whole-wheat flour or all-purpose flour
1 teaspoon salt-free spicy all-purpose seasoning blend
¼ cup egg substitute, lightly beaten
¾ cup cornflake crumbs
1 pound catfish fillets, rinsed and patted dry, cut into 1-inch cubes

SLAW TOPPING
4 cups packaged broccoli slaw or shredded green cabbage
1 medium carrot, shredded
2 medium green onions, thinly sliced
2 tablespoons light mayonnaise
1 teaspoon white wine vinegar
1 teaspoon bottled white horseradish
½ teaspoon salt-free Creole or Cajun seasoning blend, such as on page 463

Preheat the oven to 400°F. Lightly spray a large baking sheet with cooking spray.

In a shallow dish, stir together the flour and spicy seasoning blend. Put the egg substitute and cornflake crumbs in two separate shallow dishes. Set the dishes and the baking sheet in a row, assembly-line fashion. Dip the fish in batches in the flour mixture, turning to coat. Dip in the egg substitute, turning to coat and letting the excess drip off. Dip in the cornflake crumbs to coat lightly, gently shaking off any excess. Transfer to the baking sheet, spacing the cubes at least 1 inch apart. Repeat with the remaining fish. Lightly spray the tops with cooking spray.

Bake for 10 to 12 minutes, or until the fish flakes easily when tested with a fork. Transfer the baking sheet to a cooling rack. Let cool for 5 minutes.

Meanwhile, in a medium bowl, stir together the slaw topping ingredients. Serve over the fish.

PER SERVING

CALORIES 252
TOTAL FAT 5.0 g
  Saturated Fat 1.0 g
  Trans Fat 0.0 g
  Polyunsaturated Fat 2.5 g
  Monounsaturated Fat 1.5 g
CHOLESTEROL 68 mg
SODIUM 305 mg
CARBOHYDRATES 28 g
  Fiber 5 g
  Sugars 5 g
PROTEIN 24 g
DIETARY EXCHANGES
  1½ starch, 1 vegetable, 3 very lean meat

cod baked with vegetables

SERVES 6

This one-dish comfort meal preserves the mildness of cod yet is full of flavors.

Cooking spray

10 to 12 ounces red potatoes, cut into 1-inch cubes

2 medium carrots, cut into ¼-inch slices

2 tablespoons light tub margarine, melted

2 tablespoons fresh lemon juice

¼ teaspoon salt and ¼ teaspoon salt, divided use

¼ teaspoon pepper and ¼ teaspoon pepper, divided use

1½ pounds cod fillets, rinsed and patted dry, cut into 2-inch cubes

4 medium green onions, sliced

2 tablespoons snipped fresh parsley or 2 teaspoons dried, crumbled

1 tablespoon finely snipped fresh dillweed or 1 teaspoon dried, crumbled

Preheat the oven to 400°F. Lightly spray a 13 x 9 x 2-inch glass baking dish with cooking spray.

Put the potatoes and carrots in the baking dish.

In a small bowl, stir together the margarine, lemon juice, ¼ teaspoon salt, and ¼ teaspoon pepper. Pour over the potatoes and carrots.

Bake, covered, for 25 minutes.

Sprinkle the fish with the remaining ¼ teaspoon salt and ¼ teaspoon pepper, then the green onions. Gently stir into the potatoes and carrots. Sprinkle with the parsley and dillweed.

Bake, covered, for 15 to 20 minutes, or until the fish flakes easily when tested with a fork.

MICROWAVE METHOD

Prepare the potatoes, carrots, and margarine mixture as directed. Cover and microwave at 100 percent power (high) for 8 to 10 minutes. Add the remaining ingredients and microwave, covered and vented, at 100 percent power (high) for 5 to 7 minutes.

PER SERVING

CALORIES 151
TOTAL FAT 2.5 g
  Saturated Fat 0.0 g
  Trans Fat 0.0 g
  Polyunsaturated Fat 0.5 g
  Monounsaturated Fat 1.0 g
CHOLESTEROL 43 mg
SODIUM 309 mg
CARBOHYDRATES 13 g
  Fiber 2 g
  Sugars 3 g
PROTEIN 19 g
DIETARY EXCHANGES
  1 starch, 3 very lean meat

seared fish with rosemary aïoli

SERVES 4

Aïoli (ay-OH-lee or I-OH-lee) is basically mayonnaise with herbs and fresh garlic. The use of a particular herb is generally what makes the big difference. Rosemary is the choice for this assertive entrée!

ROSEMARY AÏOLI
- ¼ cup low-fat sour cream
- 2 tablespoons fat-free milk
- 2 tablespoons light mayonnaise
- 1 medium garlic clove, minced
- ¼ teaspoon dried rosemary, crushed
- ¼ teaspoon salt

- ½ teaspoon paprika
- ¼ teaspoon pepper
- ⅛ teaspoon salt

- 4 mild fish fillets, such as tilapia (about 4 ounces each), rinsed and patted dry

In small bowl, whisk together the aïoli ingredients.

Sprinkle both sides of the fish with the paprika, pepper, and remaining ⅛ teaspoon salt. Using your fingertips, gently press the seasoning so it adheres to the fish.

Heat a large nonstick skillet over medium-high heat. Cook the fish for 3 minutes on each side, or until it flakes easily when tested with a fork. Serve with the aïoli.

PER SERVING

CALORIES 149
TOTAL FAT 4.5 g
    Saturated Fat 1.5 g
    Trans Fat 0.0 g
    Polyunsaturated Fat 2.0 g
    Monounsaturated Fat 1.0 g
CHOLESTEROL 62 mg
SODIUM 358 mg
CARBOHYDRATES 3 g
    Fiber 0 g
    Sugars 1 g
PROTEIN 24 g
DIETARY EXCHANGES
    3 lean meat

fish fillets with zesty rosemary oil

SERVES 4

Just a hint of cider vinegar is added to heighten the flavor of this already-tasty fish dish. The sauce is very intense, so a little goes a very long way.

4 mild fish fillets, such as tilapia (about 4 ounces each), rinsed and patted dry
1 teaspoon grated lemon zest
1 tablespoon fresh lemon juice
1 tablespoon olive oil (extra virgin preferred)

½ teaspoon cider vinegar
½ medium garlic clove, minced
¼ teaspoon salt
⅛ teaspoon dried rosemary, crushed

Heat a large nonstick skillet over medium heat. Cook the fish for 3 minutes on each side, or until it flakes easily when tested with a fork.

Meanwhile, in a small bowl, stir together the remaining ingredients. Drizzle the sauce over the fish.

PER SERVING

CALORIES 141
TOTAL FAT 5.5 g
  Saturated Fat 1.0 g
  Trans Fat 0.0 g
  Polyunsaturated Fat 1.0 g
  Monounsaturated Fat 3.0 g
CHOLESTEROL 57 mg
SODIUM 205 mg
CARBOHYDRATES 1 g
  Fiber 0 g
  Sugars 0 g
PROTEIN 23 g
DIETARY EXCHANGES
  3 lean meat

so simple, so fast, so good fillets

SERVES 4

If you want something easy to prepare and easy to clean up, keep this recipe close at hand. You'll use it over and over and over again!

4 mild fish fillets, such as tilapia
  (about 4 ounces each), rinsed and
  patted dry
½ teaspoon dried thyme, crumbled
  (optional)
¼ teaspoon salt

¼ teaspoon pepper
2 tablespoons light tub margarine
2 tablespoons snipped fresh parsley
  (optional)
1 medium lemon, quartered

Sprinkle both sides of the fish with the thyme, salt, and pepper.

Heat a large nonstick skillet over medium heat. Cook the fish for 3 minutes on each side, or until it flakes easily when tested with a fork.

Spread the margarine over the fish. Sprinkle with the parsley. Squeeze the lemon over all.

PER SERVING

CALORIES 132
TOTAL FAT 4.0 g
  Saturated Fat 1.0 g
  Trans Fat 0.0 g
  Polyunsaturated Fat 1.0 g
  Monounsaturated Fat 2.0 g
CHOLESTEROL 57 mg
SODIUM 250 mg
CARBOHYDRATES 1 g
  Fiber 0 g
  Sugars 0 g
PROTEIN 23 g
DIETARY EXCHANGES
  3 lean meat

haddock with tomatoes and ginger

SERVES 6

A citrusy tomato sauce with an Asian flair tops mild haddock fillets.

Cooking spray
3 tablespoons all-purpose flour
Dash of pepper
6 haddock fillets (about 4 ounces each), rinsed and patted dry
1 tablespoon canola or corn oil
1 tablespoon grated peeled gingerroot
2 medium garlic cloves, minced
2 cups chopped tomatoes

2 or 3 medium green onions, sliced
1 cup fresh orange juice
½ cup dry white wine (regular or nonalcoholic)
1½ tablespoons cornstarch
1 tablespoon soy sauce (lowest sodium available)
1 tablespoon snipped fresh parsley

Preheat the oven to 350°F. Lightly spray a 13 x 9 x 2-inch glass baking dish with cooking spray.

In a shallow dish, stir together the flour and pepper. Dip one fillet in the flour mixture, turning to coat and gently shaking off any excess. Transfer the fish to a plate. Repeat with the remaining fish.

In a large nonstick skillet, heat the oil over medium-high heat, swirling to coat the bottom. Cook the fish for 1 minute on each side. Transfer to the baking dish, leaving any remaining oil in the skillet.

Bake for 10 to 15 minutes, or until the fish flakes easily when tested with a fork.

Meanwhile, in the same skillet, cook the gingerroot and garlic in the oil over medium heat for 2 to 3 minutes, stirring occasionally. Stir in the tomatoes and green onions. Bring to a simmer. Reduce the heat and simmer for 3 to 4 minutes.

In a small bowl, whisk together the remaining ingredients except the parsley. Stir into the tomato mixture. Increase the heat to medium high and cook for 2 to 3 minutes, or until thickened, whisking constantly. Stir in the parsley. Spoon the sauce over the fish.

PER SERVING

CALORIES 192
TOTAL FAT 3.5 g
  Saturated Fat 0.5 g
  Trans Fat 0.0 g
  Polyunsaturated Fat 1.0 g
  Monounsaturated Fat 1.5 g
CHOLESTEROL 65 mg
SODIUM 150 mg
CARBOHYDRATES 13 g
  Fiber 1 g
  Sugars 6 g
PROTEIN 23 g
DIETARY EXCHANGES
  1 carbohydrate,
  3 very lean meat

mediterranean fish

SERVES 6

You can use almost any fish fillets—thick or thin—in this dish.

Cooking spray
1 medium onion, thinly sliced
1½ pounds fish fillets (thin or thick), such as orange roughy, rinsed and patted dry, cut into serving pieces as necessary
2 large tomatoes, sliced
6 ounces button mushrooms, sliced
½ medium green bell pepper, sliced
¼ cup snipped fresh parsley

½ cup dry white wine (regular or nonalcoholic)
2 tablespoons fresh lemon juice
1 teaspoon snipped fresh dillweed or ¼ teaspoon dried, crumbled
Pepper to taste
½ cup plain dry bread crumbs (lowest sodium available)
1 tablespoon olive oil
½ teaspoon dried basil, crumbled

Preheat the oven to 350°F. Lightly spray a 13 x 9 x 2-inch glass baking dish with cooking spray.

Arrange the onion in the baking dish. Place the fish on the onion.

In a medium bowl, stir together the tomatoes, mushrooms, bell pepper, and parsley. Spoon over the fish.

In a small bowl, stir together the wine, lemon juice, dillweed, and pepper. Pour over the vegetable mixture.

Bake thinner fish, such as orange roughy, covered, for 15 minutes. If using thicker fish, such as halibut, add about 5 minutes.

Meanwhile, in a small bowl, stir together the bread crumbs, oil, and basil. Sprinkle over the fish mixture after the baking time given.

Bake, uncovered, for 5 to 10 minutes, or until the fish flakes easily when tested with a fork.

PER SERVING

CALORIES 184
TOTAL FAT 4.0 g
  Saturated Fat 0.5 g
  Trans Fat 0.0 g
  Polyunsaturated Fat 0.5 g
  Monounsaturated Fat 2.0 g
CHOLESTEROL 68 mg
SODIUM 156 mg
CARBOHYDRATES 13 g
  Fiber 2 g
  Sugars 5 g
PROTEIN 22 g
DIETARY EXCHANGES
  ½ starch, 1 vegetable,
  3 very lean meat

fish in crazy water

SERVES 4

Like some cooks in Italian coastal villages do when they prepare fish, we add vegetables and wine to the poaching liquid here. Serve the fish with brown rice along with the vegetables from this "crazy water."

4 mild fish steaks or fillets, such as halibut (about 4 ounces each), rinsed and patted dry
¼ teaspoon salt
1 cup white wine (regular or nonalcoholic)
1 cup fat-free, low-sodium chicken broth, such as on page 43
1 medium yellow bell pepper, chopped

2 Italian plum (Roma) tomatoes, chopped
1 tablespoon capers, drained and crushed
1 tablespoon olive oil
3 medium garlic cloves, minced
¼ teaspoon crushed red pepper flakes
¼ cup snipped fresh parsley

Sprinkle the fish with the salt.

In a large skillet, stir together the remaining ingredients except the parsley. Bring to a boil over high heat. Reduce the heat and simmer for 5 minutes, stirring occasionally.

Add the fish, turning to coat. Increase the heat to medium high and return to a simmer. Cook, covered, for 4 to 6 minutes per ½-inch thickness of fish, or until the fish flakes easily when tested with a fork.

Using a slotted spatula, transfer the fish to plates. Using a slotted spoon, spoon the vegetables and capers over the fish. Sprinkle with the parsley.

PER SERVING

CALORIES 216
TOTAL FAT 6.0 g
    Saturated Fat 1.0 g
    Trans Fat 0.0 g
    Polyunsaturated Fat 1.5 g
    Monounsaturated Fat 3.5 g
CHOLESTEROL 36 mg
SODIUM 284 mg
CARBOHYDRATES 5 g
    Fiber 1 g
    Sugars 2 g
PROTEIN 25 g
DIETARY EXCHANGES
    1 vegetable, 3 lean meat

fish tacos with pico de gallo

SERVES 4

Fish tacos are all the rage at many restaurants. Our version includes a margarita-style marinade and fresh pico de gallo enhanced with the delicate crunch of jícama.

PICO DE GALLO
1 cup diced jícama
2 medium Italian plum (Roma) tomatoes, diced
¼ small red onion, finely chopped
1 medium fresh jalapeño, seeds and ribs discarded, finely chopped
2 tablespoons coarsely chopped fresh cilantro
2 teaspoons fresh lime juice

1 tablespoon tequila or dry white wine (regular or nonalcoholic) (optional)

1 tablespoon fresh lime juice
1 teaspoon grated orange zest
1 teaspoon canola or corn oil
1 pound firm fish fillets, such as mahimahi, rinsed and patted dry, cut into ¾-inch cubes
8 6-inch corn tortillas

In a medium glass bowl, stir together the pico de gallo ingredients. Cover and refrigerate for up to two days.

In another medium glass bowl, stir together the tequila, remaining 1 tablespoon lime juice, orange zest, and oil. Add the fish, gently turning to coat. Cover and refrigerate for 10 to 30 minutes.

In a large nonstick skillet, cook the fish with the marinade over medium-high heat for 4 to 6 minutes, or until the fish flakes easily when tested with a fork and most of the liquid has evaporated. Transfer the fish to a large plate.

Meanwhile, using the package directions, warm the tortillas.

Spoon the fish down the center of each tortilla. Spoon the pico de gallo over the fish. Roll up the tortillas to enclose the filling. Serve with the seam side down.

PER SERVING

CALORIES 192
TOTAL FAT 3.0 g
  Saturated Fat 0.5 g
  Trans Fat 0.0 g
  Polyunsaturated Fat 1.0 g
  Monounsaturated Fat 1.0 g
CHOLESTEROL 83 mg
SODIUM 148 mg
CARBOHYDRATES 18 g
  Fiber 4 g
  Sugars 2 g
PROTEIN 23 g
DIETARY EXCHANGES
  1 starch, 1 vegetable,
  3 very lean meat

coconut-rum baked fish

SERVES 4

Take one bite of this incredible fish and you'll want to make reservations for a Caribbean cruise. Stir-fried sugar snap peas and wedges of fresh pineapple make terrific accompaniments.

2 tablespoons rum or ½ teaspoon rum extract
1 teaspoon grated lime zest
1 tablespoon fresh lime juice
½ teaspoon coconut extract
4 tilapia fillets (about 4 ounces each), rinsed and patted dry
Cooking spray

½ cup egg substitute
¼ cup all-purpose flour
⅓ cup plain dry bread crumbs (lowest sodium available)
2 tablespoons shredded sweetened coconut
2 tablespoons chopped macadamia nuts

In a medium glass dish, stir together the rum, lime zest, lime juice, and coconut extract. Add the fish, turning to coat. Cover and refrigerate for 10 minutes to 1 hour.

Preheat the oven to 400°F. Lightly spray a baking sheet with cooking spray.

Put the egg substitute and flour in separate shallow dishes. In a third shallow dish, stir together the bread crumbs, coconut, and macadamia nuts. Set the dishes and baking sheet in a row, assembly-line fashion. Drain the fish, discarding the marinade. Dip one piece of fish in the flour, turning to coat lightly. Dip in the egg substitute, turning to coat and letting the excess drip off. Dip in the bread crumb mixture, turning to coat and gently shaking off any excess. Transfer to the baking sheet. Repeat with the remaining fish. Lightly spray the tops with cooking spray.

Bake for 10 to 12 minutes, or until the fish is light golden brown and flakes easily when tested with a fork.

PER SERVING

CALORIES 231
TOTAL FAT 6.5 g
 Saturated Fat 2.0 g
 Trans Fat 0.0 g
 Polyunsaturated Fat 1.0 g
 Monounsaturated Fat 3.0 g
CHOLESTEROL 57 mg
SODIUM 197 mg
CARBOHYDRATES 15 g
 Fiber 1 g
 Sugars 2 g
PROTEIN 28 g
DIETARY EXCHANGES
 1 starch, 3 lean meat

teriyaki halibut

SERVES 8

Prepare some brown rice and steam bright-green sugar snap peas to complement this dish.

MARINADE
- ½ cup dry white wine (regular or nonalcoholic)
- 3 tablespoons soy sauce (lowest sodium available)
- 1 tablespoon light brown sugar
- 1 teaspoon all-purpose flour
- 1 teaspoon canola or corn oil
- ½ teaspoon dry mustard

- 2 pounds halibut fillets, rinsed and patted dry, cut into 8 servings
- Cooking spray
- 8 slices pineapple, canned in their own juice, drained

In a small saucepan, whisk together the marinade ingredients. Bring to a boil over medium-high heat. Reduce the heat and simmer for 3 minutes. Pour into a small bowl. Cover and refrigerate for 30 minutes to 1 hour.

In a large shallow glass dish, combine the fish and marinade, turning to coat. Refrigerate for 15 minutes.

Preheat the broiler. Lightly spray a broiler pan and rack with cooking spray.

Transfer the fish to the broiler rack. Pour the marinade into a small saucepan. Bring to a boil over medium-high heat. Boil for 5 minutes. Brush the fish with the hot marinade, discarding any that isn't used.

Broil the fish 5 to 6 inches from the heat for 5 minutes. Turn over. Top with the pineapple. Broil for about 5 minutes, or until the fish flakes easily when tested with a fork.

COOK'S TIP

Seafood doesn't need to marinate for long. Too much marinating time can cause it to become rubbery or mushy.

PER SERVING

CALORIES 182
TOTAL FAT 3.5 g
  Saturated Fat 0.5 g
  Trans Fat 0.0 g
  Polyunsaturated Fat 1.0 g
  Monounsaturated Fat 1.0 g
CHOLESTEROL 36 mg
SODIUM 214 mg
CARBOHYDRATES 11 g
  Fiber 1 g
  Sugars 9 g
PROTEIN 24 g
DIETARY EXCHANGES
  ½ fruit, 3 very lean meat

orange roughy with tomatoes and spinach

SERVES 6

While this aromatic dish bakes, slice some crusty whole-grain bread to serve with it. Juicy fresh strawberries would be nice for dessert.

Cooking spray
1 teaspoon olive oil
1 large onion, finely chopped
3 medium garlic cloves, minced
3 tablespoons water and
   2 tablespoons water (optional),
   divided use
1 28-ounce can no-salt-added Italian
   plum (Roma) tomatoes, undrained
½ cup dry white wine (regular or
   nonalcoholic)

10 ounces spinach, coarsely torn
2 tablespoons finely snipped fresh
   dillweed
2 tablespoons snipped fresh parsley
2 tablespoons fresh lemon juice
6 orange roughy fillets (about
   4 ounces each), rinsed and
   patted dry
½ teaspoon pepper
2 tablespoons cornstarch (optional)

Preheat the oven to 400°F. Lightly spray a 13 x 9 x 2-inch glass baking dish with cooking spray.

In a large nonstick skillet, heat the oil over medium-high heat, swirling to coat the bottom. Cook the onion and garlic for 2 minutes, stirring frequently. Pour in 3 tablespoons water. Cook until the water has evaporated, stirring constantly.

Stir in the tomatoes with liquid and the wine. Crush the tomatoes with a spoon. Cook for 7 to 8 minutes, or until the liquid is reduced slightly.

Stir in the spinach. Cook, covered, for 3 to 5 minutes, or until the spinach is wilted. Remove from the heat. Stir in the dillweed, parsley, and lemon juice.

Pour half the sauce into the baking dish. Place the fish on the sauce. Sprinkle with the pepper. Fold each fillet in half. Top with the remaining sauce.

Bake, covered, for 15 to 18 minutes, or until the fish flakes easily when tested with a fork. Transfer the fish to a small platter.

If the sauce is the consistency you like, spoon over the fish. If you prefer a thicker sauce, cover the fish to keep warm. Pour the sauce into a large nonstick skillet. Put the cornstarch in a small bowl. Add the remaining 2 tablespoons water, whisking to dissolve. Stir into the sauce. Bring to a boil over medium-high heat. Cook until the desired consistency, stirring constantly. Spoon the sauce over the fish.

COOK'S TIP on cooking wine

Avoid wine bottled and labeled as cooking wine. It's loaded with sodium. It won't do your dish—or your body—any good.

dilled orange roughy with lemon-caper sauce

SERVES 4

One skillet is all you need to cook this fish, enveloped in a creamy lemon sauce. Serve with steamed asparagus.

¼ cup all-purpose flour

1 tablespoon snipped fresh dillweed or 1 teaspoon dried, crumbled

¼ teaspoon pepper

4 orange roughy fillets (about 4 ounces each), rinsed and patted dry

2 teaspoons olive oil

½ cup fat-free, low-sodium chicken broth, such as on page 43

1 teaspoon grated lemon zest

1 tablespoon fresh lemon juice

1 tablespoon capers, drained

In a shallow dish, stir together the flour, dillweed, and pepper. Dip one fillet in the flour mixture, turning to coat and gently shaking off any excess. Transfer to a plate. Repeat with the remaining fish.

In a large nonstick skillet, heat the oil over medium-high heat, swirling to coat the bottom. Cook the fish for 1 minute on each side, or until lightly browned.

Add the remaining ingredients without stirring. Bring to a simmer. Reduce the heat and simmer, covered, for 7 to 8 minutes, or until the fish flakes easily when tested with a fork. Serve the fish topped with the sauce.

PER SERVING

CALORIES 138
TOTAL FAT 3.0 g
  Saturated Fat 0.5 g
  Trans Fat 0.0 g
  Polyunsaturated Fat 0.5 g
  Monounsaturated Fat 2.0 g
CHOLESTEROL 68 mg
SODIUM 149 mg
CARBOHYDRATES 7 g
  Fiber 1 g
  Sugars 0 g
PROTEIN 22 g
DIETARY EXCHANGES
  ½ starch,
  3 very lean meat

ginger-walnut salmon and asparagus

SERVES 4

Walnuts add a bit of crunch to this yummy salmon and asparagus dish. Preparation is fast, and because the fish cooks in aluminum foil packets, cleanup is easy.

Cooking spray
12 medium asparagus spears (about 1 pound), trimmed
4 salmon fillets with skin (about 5 ounces each), rinsed and patted dry
¼ cup firmly packed light brown sugar
3 tablespoons honey

1½ tablespoons Worcestershire sauce (lowest sodium available)
1 tablespoon cornstarch
1 teaspoon grated peeled gingerroot
¼ cup chopped walnuts
1 tablespoon plus 1 teaspoon chopped crystallized ginger (optional)

Preheat the oven to 450°F.

Lightly spray four 15 x 12-inch sheets of aluminum foil with cooking spray. Place 3 asparagus spears in the center of each. Top with the fish with the skin side down.

In a small bowl, whisk together the brown sugar, honey, Worcestershire sauce, cornstarch, and gingerroot until the sugar is dissolved. Spoon over the top and sides of the fish. Sprinkle with the walnuts and crystallized ginger. Wrap the foil loosely and seal tightly (this leaves room for the heat to circulate inside). Place the packets on a baking sheet.

Bake for 20 minutes. Being careful to avoid steam burns, slowly open a packet. Check to see whether the fish is cooked to the desired doneness. If it isn't quite ready, reseal the packet and bake a little longer. Open the packets carefully. Remove the skin if desired (tongs work well). Transfer the fish and asparagus to plates. Top with the sauce.

COOK'S TIP on crystallized ginger

The optional crystallized ginger (also known as candied ginger) provides an extra-special taste treat, so do add it if you can. Made from gingerroot that has been cooked in sugar syrup and coated with sugar, crystallized ginger has a spicy-sweet flavor. You can find sliced or chopped crystallized ginger in the spice section of most supermarkets. It is pricey, but you don't need to use much. Try some of what is left over in desserts, sweet breads, and glazes.

PER SERVING

CALORIES 357
TOTAL FAT 10.0 g
  Saturated Fat 1.5 g
  Trans Fat 0.0 g
  Polyunsaturated Fat 5.5 g
  Monounsaturated Fat 2.0 g
CHOLESTEROL 81 mg
SODIUM 118 mg
CARBOHYDRATES 34 g
  Fiber 3 g
  Sugars 29 g
PROTEIN 34 g
DIETARY EXCHANGES
  1 vegetable,
  2 carbohydrate,
  4 lean meat

baked salmon with cucumber relish

SERVES 4

This attractive salmon dish has two crisscrossed toppings, one a fiery cucumber-based relish and the other a tangy yogurt and lemon mixture.

Cooking spray
4 salmon fillets (about 4 ounces each), rinsed and patted dry
¼ teaspoon pepper
¼ teaspoon salt and ¼ teaspoon salt, divided use
½ cup fat-free plain yogurt

1 teaspoon grated lemon zest
1 tablespoon fresh lemon juice
½ medium cucumber, peeled, seeded, and chopped
¼ cup finely chopped red onion
1 medium fresh jalapeño, seeds and ribs discarded, finely chopped

Preheat the oven to 400°F. Line a baking sheet with aluminum foil. Lightly spray with cooking spray.

Put the fish on the baking sheet. Sprinkle with the pepper and ¼ teaspoon salt.

Bake for 20 minutes, or to the desired doneness.

Meanwhile, in a small bowl, stir together the yogurt, lemon zest, lemon juice, and remaining ¼ teaspoon salt.

In a medium bowl, stir together the cucumber, red onion, and jalapeño.

Transfer the fish to a small platter. Spoon the yogurt mixture diagonally over each piece of fish. Spoon the cucumber mixture diagonally in the other direction over the fish.

PER SERVING

CALORIES 158
TOTAL FAT 4.0 g
  Saturated Fat 0.5 g
  Trans Fat 0.0 g
  Polyunsaturated Fat 1.5 g
  Monounsaturated Fat 1.0 g
CHOLESTEROL 60 mg
SODIUM 391 mg
CARBOHYDRATES 5 g
  Fiber 1 g
  Sugars 3 g
PROTEIN 25 g
DIETARY EXCHANGES
  ½ carbohydrate,
  3 lean meat

salmon fillets with mango-strawberry salsa

SERVES 4

The very versatile salsa in this recipe is perfect not only over salmon but also over grilled chicken and pork, or as a "dip" for heart-healthy chips.

MANGO-STRAWBERRY SALSA
- ½ medium mango, finely chopped, or ½ cup frozen mango slices, thawed and finely chopped
- ½ cup strawberries, hulled and finely chopped
- ¼ medium fresh poblano pepper, seeds and ribs discarded, finely chopped
- 1 tablespoon fresh lime juice

- 1 teaspoon grated peeled gingerroot
　——
- 2 tablespoons fresh lime juice
- 1½ teaspoons salt-free jerk seasoning blend
- ¼ teaspoon salt
- 4 salmon fillets (about 4 ounces each), rinsed and patted dry
- 1 teaspoon canola or corn oil

In a small bowl, stir together the salsa ingredients. Set aside.

Sprinkle the remaining 2 tablespoons lime juice, seasoning blend, and salt over one side of the fish.

In a large nonstick skillet, heat the oil over medium-high heat, swirling to coat the bottom. Cook the fish with the seasoned side down for 3 minutes. Turn over and cook for 3 minutes, or to the desired doneness. Serve the fish with the seasoned side up and the salsa on the side.

COOK'S TIP

If you want to make your own salt-free jerk seasoning blend, combine ½ teaspoon ground allspice, ½ teaspoon ground cinnamon, ½ teaspoon garlic powder, and ¼ teaspoon dried thyme, crumbled. That mixture will give you exactly the amount you need for this recipe.

PER SERVING

CALORIES 170
TOTAL FAT 5.0 g
　Saturated Fat 0.5 g
　Trans Fat 0.0 g
　Polyunsaturated Fat 2.0 g
　Monounsaturated Fat 2.0 g
CHOLESTEROL 59 mg
SODIUM 223 mg
CARBOHYDRATES 7 g
　Fiber 1 g
　Sugars 5 g
PROTEIN 23 g
DIETARY EXCHANGES
　½ fruit, 3 lean meat

broiled salmon with citrus salsa

SERVES 4

A delightfully minty fruit salsa dresses up just-about-foolproof broiled salmon. This so-easy entrée is ideal when you're entertaining.

Cooking spray
4 salmon fillets (about 4 ounces each), rinsed and patted dry
¼ teaspoon salt
¼ teaspoon pepper

CITRUS SALSA
1½ cups grapefruit and orange sections, finely chopped

¼ cup finely chopped red onion
2 tablespoons chopped fresh mint
1 teaspoon sugar
¼ teaspoon crushed red pepper flakes

Preheat the broiler. Lightly spray a broiler pan and rack with cooking spray.

Put the fish in the pan. Sprinkle it with the salt and pepper.

Broil for 5 minutes on each side, or to the desired doneness.

Meanwhile, in a medium bowl, stir together the salsa ingredients. Serve with the fish.

PER SERVING

CALORIES 171
TOTAL FAT 4.0 g
  Saturated Fat 0.5 g
  Trans Fat 0.0 g
  Polyunsaturated Fat 1.5 g
  Monounsaturated Fat 1.0 g
CHOLESTEROL 59 mg
SODIUM 224 mg
CARBOHYDRATES 10 g
  Fiber 2 g
  Sugars 8 g
PROTEIN 23 g
DIETARY EXCHANGES
  ½ fruit, 3 lean meat

grilled pineapple-lime salmon

SERVES 6

It's summertime and the grilling is easy. Once the salmon soaks up the pineapple-lime marinade flavors, it's ready in almost no time.

MARINADE
 6 ounces pineapple juice
 ½ cup finely chopped onion
 ½ teaspoon grated lime zest
 2 tablespoons fresh lime juice
 1 tablespoon grated peeled gingerroot
 1 tablespoon soy sauce (lowest
   sodium available)

2 medium garlic cloves, minced
1 teaspoon hot-pepper oil (optional)
1 teaspoon canola or corn oil
———
6 salmon steaks or fillets (about
   4 ounces each), rinsed and
   patted dry
   Cooking spray

In a large shallow glass dish, stir together the marinade ingredients. Add the fish, turning to coat. Cover and refrigerate for 15 minutes to 1 hour, turning occasionally.

Lightly spray the grill rack or a broiler pan and rack with cooking spray. Preheat the grill on medium high or preheat the broiler.

Drain the fish, discarding the marinade. Grill or broil 4 to 5 inches from the heat for 5 to 7 minutes on each side, or to the desired doneness.

COOK'S TIP on hot-pepper oil

Also called chili oil, this is vegetable oil flavored with hot red chiles. Commonly used in Chinese cuisine, it can be very hot. You can make your own by steeping crushed red pepper flakes in canola or corn oil.

PER SERVING

CALORIES 133
TOTAL FAT 4.0 g
 Saturated Fat 0.5 g
 Trans Fat 0.0 g
 Polyunsaturated Fat 1.5 g
 Monounsaturated Fat 1.0 g
CHOLESTEROL 59 mg
SODIUM 141 mg
CARBOHYDRATES 0 g
 Fiber 0 g
 Sugars 0 g
PROTEIN 23 g
DIETARY EXCHANGES
 3 lean meat

grilled salmon with cilantro sauce

SERVES 4

With its fresh and slightly crunchy cilantro sauce, this grilled salmon pairs nicely with a cool and refreshing cucumber salad such as Cucumber and Mango Salad with Lime Dressing (page 102).

Cooking spray

CILANTRO SAUCE

1 cup packed fresh cilantro leaves

¼ cup sliced almonds, dry-roasted

¼ cup shredded or grated Parmesan cheese

¼ cup cold water

2 tablespoons thinly sliced green onions

1 tablespoon plus 2 teaspoons fresh lime juice

1 tablespoon olive oil (extra virgin preferred)

1 small garlic clove, chopped

½ medium fresh jalapeño, seeded and chopped

4 salmon fillets with skin (about 5 ounces each), rinsed and patted dry

½ teaspoon ground cumin

¼ teaspoon ground coriander

¼ teaspoon salt

Pinch of cayenne

Lightly spray the grill rack with cooking spray. Preheat the grill on medium high.

In a food processor or blender, process the sauce ingredients until chunky. Cover and refrigerate until ready to serve.

Sprinkle the flesh side of the fish with the remaining ingredients.

Grill the fish for 5 to 7 minutes on each side, or to the desired doneness. Remove the skin if desired (tongs work well). Serve with the sauce.

PER SERVING

CALORIES 252
TOTAL FAT 12.5 g
  Saturated Fat 2.5 g
  Trans Fat 0.0 g
  Polyunsaturated Fat 3.0 g
  Monounsaturated Fat 6.0 g
CHOLESTEROL 76 mg
SODIUM 328 mg
CARBOHYDRATES 3 g
  Fiber 1 g
  Sugars 1 g
PROTEIN 31 g
DIETARY EXCHANGES
  3½ lean meat, ½ fat

COOK'S TIP

Grill salmon with the skin still on so it doesn't fall apart when you turn it. The skin comes off easily once the fish is cooked.

salmon alfredo

SERVES 4

The sauce in this high-protein dish is as rich-tasting as conventional Alfredo but without all the unwanted fat. Tofu adds an unexpected and interesting new twist to this classic sauce.

8 ounces dried plain or spinach fettuccine or spaghetti
8 ounces salmon fillets with skin, rinsed and patted dry
12 ounces light firm tofu, drained
2/3 cup fat-free milk
Cooking spray
3 medium garlic cloves, minced

2 ounces light tub cream cheese
1/4 to 1/2 teaspoon pepper (white preferred)
1/8 teaspoon ground nutmeg
2/3 cup frozen green peas, thawed
1 tablespoon shredded or grated Parmesan cheese
1 tablespoon fresh lemon juice

Prepare the pasta using the package directions, omitting the salt. Drain well in a colander. Cover to keep warm.

Meanwhile, steam or poach the fish for 6 to 8 minutes, or to the desired doneness. Discard the skin. Set the fish aside.

In a food processor or blender, process the tofu and milk until smooth.

Lightly spray a large saucepan with cooking spray. Cook the garlic over medium-high heat for about 30 seconds. Remove from the heat.

Whisk in the tofu mixture, cream cheese, pepper, and nutmeg. Cook over medium-high heat for 2 to 3 minutes, or until the cream cheese is melted and the mixture is smooth, whisking constantly.

Stir in the peas, Parmesan, and lemon juice. Cook for 1 minute.

Flake the fish into the tofu mixture. Stir. Cook for about 1 minute, or until heated through. Serve over the pasta.

PER SERVING

CALORIES 396
TOTAL FAT 7.0 g
  Saturated Fat 2.5 g
  Trans Fat 0.0 g
  Polyunsaturated Fat 1.5 g
  Monounsaturated Fat 1.5 g
CHOLESTEROL 40 mg
SODIUM 198 mg
CARBOHYDRATES 51 g
  Fiber 3 g
  Sugars 6 g
PROTEIN 30 g
DIETARY EXCHANGES
  3½ starch, 3 lean meat

sesame-orange salmon

SERVES 4

A light crust of sesame seeds and an orange glaze dress up salmon so fast, you can serve it any weeknight.

Cooking spray

4 salmon fillets with skin (about 5 ounces each) or skinless salmon steaks (about 4 ounces each), rinsed and patted dry

2 tablespoons fresh orange juice and ½ cup fresh orange juice, divided use

3 tablespoons sesame seeds

1 tablespoon grated orange zest

¼ teaspoon salt-free lemon pepper

1 teaspoon soy sauce (lowest sodium available)

½ teaspoon toasted sesame oil

Preheat the oven to 425°F. Line a 13 x 9 x 2-inch baking pan with aluminum foil. Lightly spray the foil with cooking spray.

Place the fish in the pan (skin side down if using fillets). Brush the top side with 2 tablespoons orange juice.

In a small bowl, stir together the sesame seeds, orange zest, and lemon pepper. Sprinkle over the top of the fish. Using your fingertips, gently press the mixture so it adheres to the fish.

Bake for 10 to 12 minutes, or until the fish is cooked to the desired doneness. Remove the skin if desired (tongs work well).

Meanwhile, pour the remaining ½ cup orange juice into a small saucepan. Cook over medium-high heat for 4 minutes, or until reduced by about half. Remove from the heat.

Stir in the soy sauce and sesame oil. Drizzle over the fish.

COOK'S TIP on toasted sesame oil

Widely used in Asian and Indian cuisines, this polyunsaturated oil is also called Asian sesame oil and fragrant toasted sesame oil.

salmon cakes with creole aïoli

SERVES 4

Skip the tartar sauce and serve these salmon cakes with a spicy "upscale" sauce, which is perfect with grilled fish or chicken, too.

Cooking spray

SALMON CAKES

- 1 7-ounce vacuum-sealed pouch pink salmon, flaked
- ½ cup panko (Japanese bread crumbs)
- ½ cup finely chopped red bell pepper
- ¼ cup finely chopped green bell pepper
- 2 large egg whites
- 2 tablespoons fat-free milk
- 1 small fresh jalapeño, finely chopped (optional)

CREOLE AÏOLI

- ⅓ cup fat-free sour cream
- 2 tablespoons light mayonnaise
- 2 teaspoons Dijon mustard (coarse-grain preferred)
- 1 teaspoon Louisiana hot sauce, or to taste
- ½ medium garlic clove, minced
- ⅛ teaspoon salt

Preheat the oven to 375°F. Lightly spray a baking sheet with cooking spray.

In a medium bowl, stir together the salmon cake ingredients. Form into 8 patties, each about 2½ inches in diameter and ½ inch thick. Arrange the salmon cakes on the baking sheet. Lightly spray the tops with cooking spray.

Bake for about 22 minutes, or until the cakes are golden.

Meanwhile, in a small bowl, whisk together the aïoli ingredients. Serve the salmon cakes with the aïoli on the side.

PER SERVING

CALORIES 131
TOTAL FAT 3.5 g
  Saturated Fat 1.0 g
  Trans Fat 0.0 g
  Polyunsaturated Fat 1.5 g
  Monounsaturated Fat 0.5 g
CHOLESTEROL 21 mg
SODIUM 469 mg
CARBOHYDRATES 12 g
  Fiber 1 g
  Sugars 3 g
PROTEIN 12 g
DIETARY EXCHANGES
  1 starch, 1½ lean meat

snapper with fresh tomatoes and capers

SERVES 4

You get maximum flavor for minimal effort when you prepare this attractive dish. The brief amount of cooking turns the fresh vegetables into an assertive sauce.

4 snapper fillets (about 4 ounces each), rinsed and patted dry
4 medium green onions, chopped
½ medium tomato, finely chopped
2 tablespoons capers, drained
1 teaspoon grated lemon zest

2 tablespoons fresh lemon juice
1 tablespoon olive oil (extra virgin preferred)
1 medium garlic clove, minced
¾ teaspoon dried oregano, crumbled
¼ teaspoon salt

Heat a large nonstick skillet over medium-high heat. Cook the fish for 3 minutes. Turn the fish over.

Add the remaining ingredients. Cook for 3 minutes, or until the fish flakes easily when tested with a fork.

PER SERVING

CALORIES 157
TOTAL FAT 5.0 g
　Saturated Fat 1.0 g
　Trans Fat 0.0 g
　Polyunsaturated Fat 1.0 g
　Monounsaturated Fat 2.5 g
CHOLESTEROL 40 mg
SODIUM 327 mg
CARBOHYDRATES 4 g
　Fiber 2 g
　Sugars 2 g
PROTEIN 23 g
DIETARY EXCHANGES
　3 lean meat

mushroom-stuffed fish roll-ups

SERVES 6

Bits of fresh vegetables fill these baked fish rolls.

Cooking spray
1 teaspoon light tub margarine
12 ounces button mushrooms, finely diced
8 medium green onions, thinly sliced
½ medium red bell pepper, diced
2 tablespoons finely snipped fresh parsley and 2 tablespoons finely snipped fresh parsley, divided use
6 thin fish fillets, such as sole (about 4 ounces each), rinsed and patted dry

¼ teaspoon salt
¼ teaspoon pepper
2 to 3 tablespoons fresh lemon juice
½ cup dry white wine (regular or nonalcoholic)
2 tablespoons all-purpose flour
2 tablespoons water
¾ teaspoon paprika

Preheat the oven to 350°F. Lightly spray a 9-inch round or square baking pan with cooking spray.

In a large nonstick skillet, melt the margarine over medium heat, swirling to coat the bottom. Cook the mushrooms, green onions, bell pepper, and 2 table-spoons parsley for 3 to 5 minutes, or until the bell pep-per is tender, stirring occasionally.

Sprinkle the fish with the salt and pepper. Spoon the mushroom mixture evenly down the center of each fillet. Starting at a short side, roll up jelly-roll style and secure with wooden toothpicks. Place the fish in the baking pan. Sprinkle with the lemon juice. Pour the wine over all.

Bake, covered, for 25 to 35 minutes, or until the fish flakes easily when tested with a fork. Using a slotted spoon, transfer the fish to a platter. Remove the tooth-picks. Cover to keep warm. Pour the cooking liquid into a small saucepan.

In a small bowl, whisk together the flour, water, and paprika. Whisk into the cooking liquid. Cook over medium heat for 2 to 3 minutes, or until thickened, whisking constantly. Spoon over the fish. Sprinkle with the remaining 2 tablespoons parsley.

PER SERVING

CALORIES 149
TOTAL FAT 2.0 g
    Saturated Fat 0.5 g
    Trans Fat 0.0 g
    Polyunsaturated Fat 0.5 g
    Monounsaturated Fat 0.5 g
CHOLESTEROL 53 mg
SODIUM 197 mg
CARBOHYDRATES 8 g
    Fiber 2 g
    Sugars 3 g
PROTEIN 21 g
DIETARY EXCHANGES
    1 vegetable,
    3 very lean meat

fish fillets in foil

SERVES 4

Cooking fish in aluminum foil packets keeps the filling and the fillets moist. Custom-design your dinner by replacing the mushroom sauce with one of the variations on page 171.

Cooking spray
4 thin fish fillets, such as sole (about 4 ounces each), rinsed and patted dry
½ teaspoon pepper

MUSHROOM SAUCE
1 teaspoon light tub margarine
1 tablespoon chopped shallots or green onions

8 ounces button mushrooms, chopped
3 tablespoons dry white wine (regular or nonalcoholic)
1 tablespoon snipped fresh parsley
1 tablespoon fresh lemon juice

Preheat the oven to 400°F. Lightly spray four 8-inch-square pieces of heavy-duty aluminum foil with cooking spray.

Place a fish fillet on each piece of foil. Sprinkle with the pepper.

In a medium nonstick skillet, melt the margarine over medium-high heat, swirling to coat the bottom. Cook the shallots for 2 to 3 minutes, or until soft, stirring occasionally.

Stir in the mushrooms. Cook for 5 minutes, stirring occasionally.

Stir in the wine, parsley, and lemon juice. Cook for 2 to 3 minutes, or until most of the liquid has evaporated. Spoon over the fish. Wrap the foil loosely and seal tightly (this leaves room for the heat to circulate inside).

Bake with the smooth side of the packets down for 20 minutes. Being careful to avoid steam burns, open a foil packet to see if the fish flakes easily when tested with a fork. If not, reseal the packet and bake a little longer. Serve in the foil.

PER SERVING

CALORIES 119
TOTAL FAT 2.0 g
 Saturated Fat 0.5 g
 Trans Fat 0.0 g
 Polyunsaturated Fat 0.5 g
 Monounsaturated Fat 0.5 g
CHOLESTEROL 53 mg
SODIUM 94 mg
CARBOHYDRATES 3 g
 Fiber 1 g
 Sugars 1 g
PROTEIN 21 g
DIETARY EXCHANGES
 3 very lean meat

In place of the mushroom sauce, use any of the variations listed below. Amounts of all the ingredients except the margarine may be changed to suit individual taste. Use the margarine to dot each serving.

FISH FILLETS WITH LEMON AND SPINACH

Spinach, fresh or frozen, thawed and squeezed dry if frozen
Fresh lemon juice
Ground nutmeg
1 teaspoon light tub margarine

FISH FILLETS WITH BASIL, TOMATO, AND GREEN ONION

Tomato, thinly sliced or chopped
Green onions, thinly sliced
Basil, fresh and chopped or dried and crumbled
Fresh lemon juice
1 teaspoon light tub margarine

FISH FILLETS WITH DILL AND CUCUMBER

Fresh lemon juice
Fresh dillweed and/or parsley, snipped
1 teaspoon light tub margarine
Cucumber, thinly sliced (add after baking fish)

FISH FILLETS WITH THYME AND CELERY

Celery, thinly sliced
Fresh lemon juice
Thyme, fresh and chopped or dried and crumbled
1 teaspoon light tub margarine

FISH FILLETS WITH CURRIED VEGETABLES

Green onions, thinly sliced
Carrots, very thinly sliced
Curry powder
Green bell pepper, thinly sliced
1 teaspoon light tub margarine

crispy baked fillet of sole

SERVES 6

Fish fillets absorb Asian flavor from a soy sauce and gingerroot marinade and then are coated with an aromatic crumb coating and baked for crispness. Steamed carrots and Fresh Green Beans with Water Chestnuts (page 420) complete the meal.

MARINADE
¾ cup finely chopped onion
2 teaspoons grated lime zest
¼ cup fresh lime juice
1 tablespoon grated peeled gingerroot
1 tablespoon canola or corn oil
1 tablespoon soy sauce (lowest sodium available)
¼ teaspoon salt
¼ teaspoon pepper

6 thin fish fillets, such as sole (about 4 ounces each), rinsed

Cooking spray
1¼ cups plain dry bread crumbs (lowest sodium available)
2 tablespoons snipped fresh parsley
2 tablespoons finely chopped green onions

In a large shallow glass dish, stir together the marinade ingredients. Add the fish, turning to coat. Cover and refrigerate for 15 minutes to 1 hour.

Preheat the oven to 450°F. Lightly spray a 13 x 9 x 2-inch glass baking dish with cooking spray.

In a large shallow dish, stir together the bread crumbs, parsley, and green onions. Drain the fish, discarding the marinade. Dip one fillet into the bread crumb mixture, turning to coat and gently shaking off any excess. Transfer to the baking dish. Repeat with the remaining fillets.

Bake for 15 to 18 minutes, or until the fish flakes easily when tested with a fork.

PER SERVING
CALORIES 183
TOTAL FAT 2.5 g
  Saturated Fat 0.5 g
  Trans Fat 0.0 g
  Polyunsaturated Fat 1.0 g
  Monounsaturated Fat 0.5 g
CHOLESTEROL 53 mg
SODIUM 411 mg
CARBOHYDRATES 17 g
  Fiber 1 g
  Sugars 2 g
PROTEIN 22 g
DIETARY EXCHANGES
  1 starch, 3 very lean meat

bay-style fillets

SERVES 4

Here is the recipe for people who think cooking fish is daunting. All you do is bake fish with one ingredient sprinkled on top, then melt margarine right on the fish for a sauce that practically makes itself.

Cooking spray

4 thin fish fillets, such as sole (about 4 ounces each), rinsed and patted dry

1 teaspoon seafood seasoning blend

2 tablespoons light tub margarine

Preheat the oven to 350°F. Line a baking sheet with aluminum foil. Lightly spray with cooking spray.

Place the fish on the baking sheet. Sprinkle with the seasoning blend.

Bake for 10 minutes, or until the fish flakes easily when tested with a fork. Spread the margarine over the fish.

PER SERVING

CALORIES 112
TOTAL FAT 3.5 g
  Saturated Fat 0.5 g
  Trans Fat 0.0 g
  Polyunsaturated Fat 1.0 g
  Monounsaturated Fat 1.5 g
CHOLESTEROL 53 mg
SODIUM 277 mg
CARBOHYDRATES 0 g
  Fiber 0 g
  Sugars 0 g
PROTEIN 19 g
DIETARY EXCHANGES
  3 very lean meat

sole with walnuts and white wine

SERVES 4

White sauce with walnuts makes this dish something special. Serve with steamed broccoli and fresh peach slices.

Cooking spray

4 thin fish fillets, such as sole (about 4 ounces each), rinsed

½ cup dry white wine and ½ cup dry white wine (regular or nonalcoholic), divided use

½ cup fat-free, low-sodium chicken broth and ½ cup fat-free, low-sodium chicken broth, such as on page 43, divided use

Dash of cayenne

2 tablespoons light tub margarine

2 tablespoons all-purpose flour

¼ cup fat-free milk

Dash of pepper (white preferred)

2 tablespoons chopped walnuts, dry-roasted

Sprigs of fresh parsley (optional)

Preheat the oven to 325°F. Lightly spray a 9-inch square baking pan with cooking spray.

Put the fish in the baking pan. Pour in ½ cup wine and ½ cup broth. Sprinkle with the cayenne.

Bake, covered, for 20 minutes, or until the fish flakes easily when tested with a fork.

Meanwhile, in a small saucepan, melt the margarine over low heat, swirling to coat the bottom. Whisk in the flour. Cook for 1 minute, whisking occasionally. (Don't let the flour brown.) Increase the heat to medium high.

Whisk in the remaining ½ cup wine, remaining ½ cup broth, milk, and pepper. Cook for 3 to 4 minutes, or until thickened, whisking constantly.

Stir in the walnuts. Reduce the heat and simmer for 1 minute. Spoon over the fish. Garnish with the parsley.

PER SERVING

CALORIES 198
TOTAL FAT 6.0 g
  Saturated Fat 0.5 g
  Trans Fat 0.0 g
  Polyunsaturated Fat 2.5 g
  Monounsaturated Fat 2.0 g
CHOLESTEROL 54 mg
SODIUM 143 mg
CARBOHYDRATES 5 g
  Fiber 0 g
  Sugars 1 g
PROTEIN 21 g
DIETARY EXCHANGES
  ½ carbohydrate,
  3 lean meat

sole with parsley and mint

SERVES 4

Serve this dish with or without the sauce—either way is easy and unusual.

Cooking spray
2 tablespoons finely snipped fresh parsley
1 tablespoon snipped fresh mint
2 teaspoons canola or corn oil
1 medium garlic clove, chopped
¼ teaspoon salt
4 thin fish fillets, such as sole (about 4 ounces each), rinsed and patted dry

SAUCE (OPTIONAL)
1 teaspoon light tub margarine
1 medium green onion (green part only), chopped
½ cup dry white wine (regular or nonalcoholic)
¼ cup water
¼ teaspoon pepper (white preferred)

Preheat the broiler. Lightly spray the broiler pan and rack with cooking spray.

In a small bowl, stir together the parsley, mint, oil, garlic, and salt (the mixture will be pastelike). Rub over one side of the fish.

Broil the fish with the seasoned side up about 4 inches from the heat for 5 to 8 minutes, or until it flakes easily when tested with a fork.

Meanwhile, if serving with the sauce, in a medium nonstick skillet, melt the margarine over medium-high heat, swirling to coat the bottom. Cook the green onion for 1 to 2 minutes, stirring frequently. Stir in the wine, water, and pepper. Cook for 2 to 3 minutes, or until heated through. Spoon over the fish.

COOK'S TIP on white pepper

Milder in flavor than black pepper, white pepper is often used because its color blends in with a white or light-colored sauce. You can buy whole white peppercorns or ground white pepper.

PER SERVING

CALORIES 115
TOTAL FAT 3.5 g
  Saturated Fat 0.5 g
  Trans Fat 0.0 g
  Polyunsaturated Fat 1.0 g
  Monounsaturated Fat 1.5 g
CHOLESTEROL 53 mg
SODIUM 228 mg
CARBOHYDRATES 1 g
  Fiber 0 g
  Sugars 0 g
PROTEIN 19 g
DIETARY EXCHANGES
  3 lean meat

PER SERVING

WITH OPTIONAL SAUCE
CALORIES 141
TOTAL FAT 4.0 g
  Saturated Fat 0.5 g
  Trans Fat 0.0 g
  Polyunsaturated Fat 1.5 g
  Monounsaturated Fat 2.0 g
CHOLESTEROL 53 mg
SODIUM 239 mg
CARBOHYDRATES 1 g
  Fiber 0 g
  Sugars 0 g
PROTEIN 19 g
DIETARY EXCHANGES
  3 lean meat

sole parmesan

SERVES 4

Lots of Italian seasoning spices up mild sole fillets.

Cooking spray
¾ cup plain dry bread crumbs (lowest sodium available)
1 teaspoon dried oregano, crumbled
1 teaspoon garlic powder
¼ teaspoon pepper
¼ cup egg substitute
4 sole fillets (about 4 ounces each), rinsed and patted dry

½ cup shredded low-fat mozzarella cheese
¼ cup shredded or grated Parmesan cheese
1 teaspoon olive oil
1 small garlic clove, minced
½ cup no-salt-added tomato sauce
2 tablespoons chopped fresh basil

Preheat the oven to 400°F. Line a baking sheet with aluminum foil. Lightly spray with cooking spray.

In a shallow dish, stir together the bread crumbs, oregano, garlic powder, and pepper. Pour the egg substitute into another shallow dish. Set the dishes and baking sheet in a row, assembly-line fashion. Dip one piece of fish in the bread crumb mixture, turning to coat and gently shaking off any excess. Dip in the egg substitute, turning to coat and letting any excess drip off. Transfer to the baking sheet. Repeat with the remaining fish. Lightly spray the tops with cooking spray.

Bake for 10 minutes, or until the fish flakes easily when tested with a fork. Sprinkle with the mozzarella and Parmesan. Bake for 2 minutes, or until the cheese is melted.

Meanwhile, in a small saucepan, heat the oil over low heat, swirling to coat the bottom. Cook the garlic for 5 to 10 seconds, stirring occasionally.

Stir in the tomato sauce and basil. Increase the heat to medium high and bring to a simmer, stirring occasionally. Reduce the heat and simmer for about 5 minutes, stirring occasionally. Serve over the fish.

COOK'S TIP

Keep your pantry stocked with no-salt-added canned products such as tomato sauce, tomato paste, and diced and whole tomatoes. Regular tomato puree, however, is already low in sodium.

PER SERVING

CALORIES 256
TOTAL FAT 6.0 g
  Saturated Fat 2.0 g
  Trans Fat 0.0 g
  Polyunsaturated Fat 1.0 g
  Monounsaturated Fat 2.0 g
CHOLESTEROL 62 mg
SODIUM 451 mg
CARBOHYDRATES 19 g
  Fiber 2 g
  Sugars 4 g
PROTEIN 29 g
DIETARY EXCHANGES
  1½ starch,
  4 very lean meat

stovetop fish with vegetable rice, mexican style

SERVES 4

Cumin-seasoned fillets and turmeric rice tossed with fresh vegetables, cilantro, and lemon are a winning combination for nights when you don't want to use your oven.

½ cup uncooked instant brown rice
½ teaspoon ground turmeric (optional)
1½ teaspoons ground cumin
1 teaspoon paprika
¼ teaspoon salt and ¼ teaspoon salt, divided use
¼ teaspoon cayenne
4 tilapia or other mild fish fillets (about 4 ounces each), rinsed and patted dry

1 cup finely chopped green bell pepper or fresh poblano pepper, seeds and ribs discarded
2 medium Italian plum (Roma) tomatoes, chopped
⅓ cup snipped fresh cilantro
1 teaspoon grated lemon zest
3 tablespoons fresh lemon juice
1 tablespoon olive oil (extra virgin preferred)

Prepare the rice using the package directions, adding the turmeric and omitting the salt and margarine.

Meanwhile, in a small bowl, stir together the cumin, paprika, ¼ teaspoon salt, and cayenne. Sprinkle over one side of the fish. Using your fingertips, gently press the mixture so it adheres to the fish.

Heat a large nonstick skillet over high heat. Cook the fish for 1 minute on each side.

Reduce the heat to medium. Turn the fish over again. Cook for 2 minutes. Turn over and cook for 1 minute, or until the fish flakes easily when tested with a fork. Transfer to plates.

In a medium bowl, stir together the bell pepper, tomatoes, cilantro, lemon zest, lemon juice, oil, and remaining ¼ teaspoon salt.

Spoon the rice onto the plates. Top the rice with the bell pepper mixture.

PER SERVING

CALORIES 202
TOTAL FAT 6.0 g
  Saturated Fat 1.5 g
  Trans Fat 0.0 g
  Polyunsaturated Fat 1.0 g
  Monounsaturated Fat 3.5 g
CHOLESTEROL 57 mg
SODIUM 354 mg
CARBOHYDRATES 13 g
  Fiber 2 g
  Sugars 2 g
PROTEIN 25 g
DIETARY EXCHANGES
  1 starch, 3 lean meat

tex-mex tilapia

SERVES 4

Shredded zucchini, red onions, enchilada sauce, and green chiles perk up mild-flavored tilapia and keep it moist while it bakes. Serve with ice-cold wedges of juicy watermelon on the side.

4 tilapia fillets (about 4 ounces each), rinsed and patted dry
1 teaspoon ground cumin
1 medium zucchini, shredded
½ medium red onion, thinly sliced
2 tablespoons canned chopped green chiles, drained

2 tablespoons sliced black olives
1 10-ounce can enchilada sauce
½ cup fat-free shredded Cheddar cheese

Preheat the oven to 400°F.

Put the fish in a nonstick 8-inch square baking pan. Sprinkle with the cumin. Place the zucchini, onion, green chiles, and olives on the fish. Pour the enchilada sauce over all.

Bake, covered, for 35 to 40 minutes, or until the fish flakes easily when tested with a fork. Sprinkle with the Cheddar.

PER SERVING

CALORIES 183
TOTAL FAT 4.0 g
  Saturated Fat 1.0 g
  Trans Fat 0.0 g
  Polyunsaturated Fat 1.0 g
  Monounsaturated Fat 1.5 g
CHOLESTEROL 59 mg
SODIUM 588 mg
CARBOHYDRATES 8 g
  Fiber 1 g
  Sugars 3 g
PROTEIN 29 g
DIETARY EXCHANGES
  ½ carbohydrate,
  3½ very lean meat

baked tilapia with sausage-flecked rice

SERVES 4

It's amazing how such a small amount of low-fat sausage can have such a large impact on flavor. This dish is similar to what cooks in New Orleans fondly call "dirty rice."

⅓ cup uncooked brown rice Cooking spray 4 tilapia fillets (about 4 ounces each), rinsed and patted dry ¼ teaspoon dried thyme, crumbled ⅛ teaspoon salt and ¼ teaspoon salt, divided use Paprika to taste	3 ounces low-fat bulk breakfast sausage 1 medium red bell pepper, finely chopped ½ cup finely chopped green onions ¼ cup finely snipped fresh parsley ⅛ teaspoon cayenne (optional)

Prepare the rice using the package directions, omitting the salt and margarine.

Meanwhile, preheat the oven to 400°F. Line a baking sheet with aluminum foil. Lightly spray with cooking spray.

Put the fish on the baking sheet. Sprinkle with the thyme, ⅛ teaspoon salt, and paprika.

Bake for 12 minutes, or until the fish flakes easily when tested with a fork.

Meanwhile, in a medium nonstick skillet, cook the sausage over medium-high heat for 2 minutes, stirring to break up the larger pieces.

Stir in the bell pepper and green onions. Cook for 1 minute, or until the sausage begins to lightly brown, stirring constantly. Remove from the heat.

Stir in the rice, parsley, cayenne, and remaining ¼ teaspoon salt. Serve beside or on top of the fish.

COOK'S TIP on buying bulk sausage

Bulk sausage is ground meat that hasn't been stuffed into a casing. Look for sausage that is packaged in a cylinder-shaped roll rather than in individual casings.

PER SERVING

CALORIES 210
TOTAL FAT 3.0 g
  Saturated Fat 1.0 g
  Trans Fat 0.0 g
  Polyunsaturated Fat 0.5 g
  Monounsaturated Fat 1.0 g
CHOLESTEROL 67 mg
SODIUM 414 mg
CARBOHYDRATES 16 g
  Fiber 2 g
  Sugars 2 g
PROTEIN 28 g
DIETARY EXCHANGES
  1 starch,
  3½ very lean meat

tilapia amandine

SERVES 4

Worcestershire sauce and fresh lemon juice provide the flavor boost for this delicate dish.

¼ cup all-purpose flour
½ teaspoon paprika
⅛ teaspoon pepper
4 tilapia fillets (about 4 ounces each), rinsed and patted dry
¼ cup water

2 tablespoons fresh lemon juice
1 tablespoon light tub margarine
2 teaspoons Worcestershire sauce (lowest sodium available)
¼ teaspoon salt
¼ cup sliced almonds, dry-roasted

In a shallow dish, stir together the flour, paprika, and pepper. Dip one fillet in the mixture, turning to coat and gently shaking off any excess. Transfer to a plate. Repeat with the remaining fish.

In a large nonstick skillet, cook the fish over medium heat for 5 minutes on each side, or until it flakes easily when tested with a fork. Transfer to plates.

Meanwhile, in a small bowl, stir together the remaining ingredients except the almonds. Pour into the skillet, scraping the bottom and side with a rubber scraper to dislodge any browned bits. Cook for 2 minutes, or until the liquid is reduced to about ¼ cup. Spoon over the fish. Sprinkle with the almonds.

PER SERVING

CALORIES 184
TOTAL FAT 6.0 g
  Saturated Fat 1.0 g
  Trans Fat 0.0 g
  Polyunsaturated Fat 1.5 g
  Monounsaturated Fat 3.0 g
CHOLESTEROL 57 mg
SODIUM 231 mg
CARBOHYDRATES 8 g
  Fiber 1 g
  Sugars 1 g
PROTEIN 25 g
DIETARY EXCHANGES
  ½ starch, 3 lean meat

greek fish fillets

SERVES 4

It can't get much easier than this, from the simple seasonings to the simple cleanup.

1 teaspoon dried oregano, crumbled
1 teaspoon salt-free lemon pepper
¼ teaspoon paprika
¼ teaspoon salt
4 thin fish fillets, such as tilapia (about 4 ounces each), rinsed and patted dry

Cooking spray
1 tablespoon plus 1 teaspoon olive oil (extra virgin preferred)
1 medium lemon, quartered

Preheat the broiler.

In a small bowl, stir together the oregano, lemon pepper, paprika, and salt.

Put the fish on a nonstick baking sheet. Lightly spray the top side of the fish with cooking spray. Sprinkle with the oregano mixture.

Broil about 4 inches from the heat with the seasoned side up for 5 minutes, or until the fish flakes easily when tested with a fork. Transfer to plates.

Drizzle the fish with the oil. Squeeze a lemon quarter over each piece.

PER SERVING

CALORIES 154
TOTAL FAT 6.5 g
    Saturated Fat 1.5 g
    Trans Fat 0.0 g
    Polyunsaturated Fat 1.0 g
    Monounsaturated Fat 4.0 g
CHOLESTEROL 57 mg
SODIUM 205 mg
CARBOHYDRATES 1 g
    Fiber 0 g
    Sugars 0 g
PROTEIN 23 g
DIETARY EXCHANGES
    3 lean meat

grilled fish with mediterranean salsa

SERVES 4

Tilapia fillets are delicious grilled, especially when topped with this chilled sauce inspired by heart-healthy Mediterranean cuisine.

Cooking spray
1 small Italian plum (Roma) tomato, diced
1 medium green onion, thinly sliced
2 tablespoons crumbled fat-free feta cheese
1 tablespoon sliced black olives
1 teaspoon dried oregano, crumbled

1 teaspoon grated lemon zest
2 medium garlic cloves, minced
¼ teaspoon pepper
2 teaspoons olive oil
4 tilapia fillets (about 4 ounces each), rinsed and patted dry
1 small lemon, quartered (can use the one that is zested)

Lightly spray the grill rack with cooking spray. Preheat the grill on medium high.

Meanwhile, in a small bowl, stir together the tomato, green onion, feta, and black olives. Cover and refrigerate until ready to use.

Sprinkle the oregano, lemon zest, garlic, and pepper over a small platter. Drizzle the oil over the mixture. Put the fish on the platter, turning to coat. Using your fingertips, gently press the mixture so it adheres to the fish.

Grill for 4 to 5 minutes on each side, or until the fish flakes easily when tested with a fork. Transfer to plates. Squeeze the lemon over the fish. Serve topped with the tomato mixture.

COOK'S TIP

If you frequently grill fish, you may want to buy a grilling basket designed to use with fish. It is especially useful for thin, delicate fish fillets, such as tilapia. A perforated flat grilling pan would also work and is useful for grilling other types of food as well.

almond-topped baked trout

SERVES 4

Dinner will be ready in minutes when you prepare this simple fish dish.

Cooking spray
4 trout fillets with skin (about 5 ounces each), rinsed and patted dry
¼ cup panko (Japanese bread crumbs)
2 tablespoons shredded or grated Parmesan cheese

½ teaspoon dried basil, crumbled
½ teaspoon paprika
¼ teaspoon garlic powder
¼ teaspoon pepper
¼ cup sliced almonds, dry-roasted
4 lemon slices

Preheat the oven to 400°F. Lightly spray a large baking sheet with cooking spray.

Place the fish with the skin side down on the baking sheet.

In a small bowl, stir together the panko, Parmesan, basil, paprika, garlic powder, and pepper. Spoon over the fish. Using your fingertips, gently press the mixture so it adheres to the fish.

Spoon the almonds over the panko mixture, lightly pressing so they will adhere. Lightly spray with cooking spray.

Bake for 10 to 15 minutes, or until the fish flakes easily when tested with a fork.

Remove the skin if desired (tongs work well). Serve the fish with the crust side up and a lemon slice on top of each piece.

PER SERVING

CALORIES 210
TOTAL FAT 8.0 g
    Saturated Fat 1.5 g
    Trans Fat 0.0 g
    Polyunsaturated Fat 2.5 g
    Monounsaturated Fat 3.5 g
CHOLESTEROL 77 mg
SODIUM 88 mg
CARBOHYDRATES 4 g
    Fiber 1 g
    Sugars 0 g
PROTEIN 29 g
DIETARY EXCHANGES
    3½ lean meat

baked trout with tartar sauce

SERVES 4

Panko and nutritious wheat germ give this trout a tasty, crisp coating, which is brightened by lemon zest.

Olive oil spray
1 teaspoon onion powder
¼ teaspoon paprika
⅛ teaspoon salt
4 trout fillets with skin (about 5 ounces each), rinsed and patted dry
3 tablespoons all-purpose flour
¼ cup egg substitute
1 teaspoon fresh lemon juice

COATING

¾ cup panko (Japanese bread crumbs)
3 tablespoons toasted wheat germ
1 tablespoon snipped fresh dillweed
2 medium garlic cloves, minced
1 teaspoon grated lemon zest
⅛ teaspoon salt
⅛ teaspoon cayenne

TARTAR SAUCE

¼ cup light mayonnaise
1 tablespoon fat-free sour cream
1 tablespoon drained sweet pickle relish
1 tablespoon finely chopped red bell pepper
1 teaspoon fresh lemon juice
⅛ teaspoon paprika

1 medium lemon, quartered

Preheat the oven to 400°F. Line a baking sheet with aluminum foil. Lightly spray the foil with olive oil spray.

In a small bowl, stir together the onion powder, paprika, and salt. Sprinkle over the flesh side of the fish. Using your fingertips, gently press the mixture so it adheres to the fish.

Put the flour on a plate. In a shallow dish, stir together the egg substitute and lemon juice. Set the plate, dish, and baking sheet in a row, assembly-line fashion. Dip the flesh side of one piece of fish in the flour, gently shaking off any excess. Dip the flesh side in the egg substitute mixture, letting the excess drip off. Transfer the fish with the skin side down to the baking sheet. Repeat with the remaining fish.

On a shallow plate, stir together the coating ingredients. Sprinkle over the fish. Using your fingertips, gently press the coating so it adheres to the fish. Lightly spray the top of the fish with olive oil spray.

Bake for 10 minutes, or until the top is lightly browned and the fish flakes easily when tested with a fork.

Meanwhile, in a small bowl, stir together the tartar sauce ingredients.

Carefully place each piece of fish with the skin side up on a separate plate. Let cool for about 3 minutes. Using tongs, gently peel off and discard the skin. Turn the fish over so the coated side is up. Serve with the tartar sauce and lemon wedges.

COOK'S TIP on storing fresh dillweed

To store fresh dillweed, put it in a resealable plastic bag and refrigerate it in the refrigerator crisper. For longer storage, rinse the dillweed, pat it dry, and freeze it in an airtight container.

crisp pan-seared trout with green onions

SERVES 4

Rich in omega-3 fatty acids, trout gets dressed up for dinner with a crisp coat made of flour and Chinese five-spice seasoning. It's then topped with thinly sliced green onions and a drizzle of vinegar and soy sauce. Serve with soba noodles tossed with a small amount of toasted sesame oil.

3 tablespoons red wine vinegar
2 teaspoons soy sauce (lowest sodium available)
1 teaspoon toasted sesame oil
¼ cup all-purpose flour
1 teaspoon five-spice powder

4 trout fillets with skin (about 5 ounces each), rinsed and patted dry
2 teaspoons canola or corn oil
Cooking spray
8 medium green onions (green part only), thinly sliced

In a small bowl, stir together the vinegar, soy sauce, and sesame oil. Set aside.

In a shallow dish, stir together the flour and five-spice powder. Dip one fillet in the flour mixture to coat the flesh side of the fish, gently shaking off any excess. Transfer to a plate. Repeat with the remaining fillets.

In a large nonstick skillet, heat the canola oil over medium-high heat, swirling to coat the bottom. Cook the fish with the flesh side down for 3 to 4 minutes, or until browned. Remove from the heat.

Lightly spray the skin side of each fillet with cooking spray. Turn over. Cook with the skin side down for 3 to 4 minutes, or until the fish flakes easily when tested with a fork.

Transfer the fish with the skin side up to plates. Let cool for about 1 minute. Using tongs, gently peel off and discard the skin. Turn the fish over so the seasoned side is up. Sprinkle with the green onions. Pour the vinegar mixture over the fish.

PER SERVING

CALORIES 235
TOTAL FAT 8.0 g
  Saturated Fat 1.5 g
  Trans Fat 0.0 g
  Polyunsaturated Fat 2.5 g
  Monounsaturated Fat 3.5 g
CHOLESTEROL 75 mg
SODIUM 115 mg
CARBOHYDRATES 11 g
  Fiber 2 g
  Sugars 2 g
PROTEIN 27 g
DIETARY EXCHANGES
  ½ starch, 3 lean meat

braised tuna steaks with orange-cranberry glaze

SERVES 4

Simmering lightly browned tuna steaks keeps them moist, and the rosemary-infused glaze makes them delicious.

4 tuna steaks (about 4 ounces each), rinsed and patted dry
½ teaspoon ground pink peppercorns or ¼ teaspoon black pepper
1 teaspoon olive oil
1 teaspoon grated orange zest
½ cup fresh orange juice

½ cup unsweetened cranberry juice
2 tablespoons port (optional)
1 tablespoon coarsely chopped fresh rosemary or 1 teaspoon dried, crushed
2 teaspoons light brown sugar

Sprinkle both sides of the fish with the pepper.

In a large nonstick skillet, heat the oil over medium-high heat, swirling to coat the bottom. Cook the fish for 1 minute on each side, or until lightly browned.

Stir in the remaining ingredients. Bring to a simmer. Reduce the heat and simmer, covered, for 7 to 9 minutes for slightly pink centers, or until the fish is the desired doneness. Transfer to plates. Cover to keep warm.

Increase the heat to medium high. Cook the remaining liquid until reduced by half (about ½ cup). Pour over the fish.

grilled tuna with pineapple-nectarine salsa

SERVES 4

Citrus-marinated tuna sizzles on the grill, then is topped with a cool, refreshing fruit salsa.

MARINADE
- 1 teaspoon grated lime zest
- 2 tablespoons fresh lime juice
- 2 tablespoons fresh orange juice
- 1 tablespoon snipped fresh cilantro
- 1 teaspoon canola or corn oil
- ¼ teaspoon salt
- ⅛ teaspoon pepper

- 1 pound tuna or other firm-fleshed fish, rinsed and patted dry, cut into 4 pieces

PINEAPPLE-NECTARINE SALSA
- 1 8-ounce can pineapple tidbits in their own juice, drained
- 1 medium nectarine, diced
- 1 medium kiwifruit, peeled and diced
- 2 tablespoons diced red onion
- 1 tablespoon snipped fresh cilantro
- 1 teaspoon fresh lemon juice

In a large shallow glass dish, stir together the marinade ingredients. Add the fish, turning to coat. Cover and refrigerate for 15 minutes to 1 hour, turning occasionally.

Meanwhile, in a medium bowl, stir together the salsa ingredients. Cover and refrigerate.

Preheat the grill on medium high.

Grill the fish for 5 to 7 minutes on each side, or to the desired doneness. Transfer to plates. Serve topped with the salsa.

PER SERVING

CALORIES 173
TOTAL FAT 1.5 g
  Saturated Fat 0.5 g
  Trans Fat 0.0 g
  Polyunsaturated Fat 0.5 g
  Monounsaturated Fat 0.0 g
CHOLESTEROL 51 mg
SODIUM 192 mg
CARBOHYDRATES 12 g
  Fiber 2 g
  Sugars 9 g
PROTEIN 27 g
DIETARY EXCHANGES
  1 fruit, 3 very lean meat

sesame tuna with pineapple sauce

SERVES 4

Turmeric turns the rice a brilliant yellow, dressing up this dish so it's perfect for when you want to impress without a lot of effort.

1 cup uncooked instant brown rice
½ teaspoon ground turmeric
3 tablespoons dry-roasted sesame seeds
2 teaspoons all-purpose flour
¼ teaspoon salt
¼ teaspoon pepper
4 tuna steaks (about 4 ounces each), rinsed and patted dry
Cooking spray

½ cup pineapple juice
1 tablespoon sugar
1 tablespoon soy sauce (lowest sodium available)
2 teaspoons cornstarch
½ teaspoon grated peeled gingerroot
¼ teaspoon crushed red pepper flakes
¼ cup finely chopped green onions (optional)

Prepare the rice using the package directions, omitting the salt and margarine and adding the turmeric. Set aside.

Meanwhile, in a shallow dish, stir together the sesame seeds, flour, salt, and pepper. Dip one piece of fish in the mixture, turning to coat both sides. Don't shake off any excess. Transfer to a plate. Repeat with the remaining fish.

Lightly spray a large skillet with cooking spray. Heat over medium-high heat. Cook the fish for 2 minutes on each side for a very pink center, or until the desired doneness.

Meanwhile, in a small saucepan, stir together the pineapple juice, sugar, soy sauce, cornstarch, gingerroot, and red pepper flakes until the cornstarch is dissolved. Bring to a boil over medium-high heat. Boil for 1 minute, or until thickened, stirring frequently. Remove from the heat.

Stir the green onions into the rice. Spoon onto the center of a serving platter. Arrange the fish around the rice. Pour the sauce over the fish.

PER SERVING

CALORIES 294
TOTAL FAT 6.0 g
  Saturated Fat 1.0 g
  Trans Fat 0.0 g
  Polyunsaturated Fat 2.5 g
  Monounsaturated Fat 2.0 g
CHOLESTEROL 51 mg
SODIUM 295 mg
CARBOHYDRATES 28 g
  Fiber 2 g
  Sugars 6 g
PROTEIN 30 g
DIETARY EXCHANGES
  1½ starch, ½ fruit,
  3 lean meat

stuffed shells with albacore tuna and vegetables

SERVES 4

A tuna noodle casserole variation goes gourmet with an upscale white sauce enhanced with Dijon mustard.

12 jumbo dried pasta shells (about 4 ounces)
1 cup fat-free, low-sodium chicken broth, such as on page 43
3 tablespoons all-purpose flour
1 cup fat-free half-and-half
2 teaspoons Dijon mustard
1 teaspoon salt-free all-purpose seasoning blend

⅛ teaspoon salt
1 1-pound package frozen mixed vegetables (any combination), thawed
2 5-ounce cans very low sodium albacore tuna in water, drained and flaked
2 tablespoons shredded or grated Parmesan cheese

Prepare the pasta using the package directions, omitting the salt. Drain well in a colander. Set aside.

Preheat the oven to 350°F.

In a medium saucepan, whisk together the broth and flour. Bring to a simmer over medium-high heat, stirring occasionally. Reduce the heat and simmer for 1 to 2 minutes, or until thickened.

Whisk in the half-and-half, mustard, seasoning blend, and salt. Reduce the heat to medium low. Cook for 1 minute, or until heated through, whisking occasionally. Remove from the heat.

In a medium bowl, stir together ¼ cup sauce, the vegetables, and the tuna.

Gently spoon ¼ cup tuna mixture into each pasta shell. Place the shells with the open side up in a nonstick 13 x 9 x 2-inch baking pan. Pour the remaining sauce over all. Sprinkle with the Parmesan.

Bake, covered, for 25 to 30 minutes, or until heated through. Serve the stuffed shells topped with the sauce remaining in the pan.

PER SERVING

CALORIES 325
TOTAL FAT 3.0 g
  Saturated Fat 0.5 g
  Trans Fat 0.0 g
  Polyunsaturated Fat 0.5 g
  Monounsaturated Fat 0.5 g
CHOLESTEROL 32 mg
SODIUM 302 mg
CARBOHYDRATES 50 g
  Fiber 5 g
  Sugars 9 g
PROTEIN 31 g
DIETARY EXCHANGES
  3 starch, 1 vegetable,
  3 very lean meat

spicy tuna pitas

SERVES 4

The tang of lime juice combined with the distinctive flavor of cumin and the mildest kick from a bit of cayenne gives a unique twist to tuna salad.

2 5-ounce cans very low sodium albacore tuna in water, drained and flaked
½ medium rib of celery, chopped
2 medium green onions, chopped
¼ cup finely snipped fresh cilantro
⅓ cup light mayonnaise

1 tablespoon fresh lime juice
1 teaspoon ground cumin
⅛ teaspoon cayenne
2 7-inch whole-grain pita pockets, halved
4 medium lettuce leaves, such as red leaf

In a medium bowl, stir together the tuna, celery, green onions, and cilantro.

Stir in the mayonnaise, lime juice, cumin, and cayenne.

Line each pita half with lettuce. Spoon the tuna salad into the pitas.

PER SERVING

CALORIES 227
TOTAL FAT 6.5 g
  Saturated Fat 0.5 g
  Trans Fat 0.0 g
  Polyunsaturated Fat 4.0 g
  Monounsaturated Fat 1.0 g
CHOLESTEROL 28 mg
SODIUM 397 mg
CARBOHYDRATES 22 g
  Fiber 3 g
  Sugars 1 g
PROTEIN 22 g
DIETARY EXCHANGES
  1½ starch, 2½ lean meat

tuna chili

SERVES 4

Here's an easy way to work more seafood into your diet—a warming bowl of chili with tuna instead of beef.

2 teaspoons olive oil
1 medium onion, chopped
1 medium green bell pepper, chopped
2 medium garlic cloves, minced
4 medium tomatoes, chopped
1 15.5-ounce can no-salt-added pinto beans, rinsed and drained
2 5-ounce cans very low sodium albacore tuna in water, drained and flaked

⅔ cup salsa (lowest sodium available), such as Salsa Cruda (page 508)
1½ teaspoons chili powder
1 teaspoon ground cumin
1 tablespoon plus 1 teaspoon shredded fat-free Cheddar cheese
1 tablespoon plus 1 teaspoon sliced green onions

In a large saucepan, heat the oil over medium-high heat, swirling to coat the bottom. Cook the onion, bell pepper, and garlic for 4 to 5 minutes, or until the onion begins to brown, stirring occasionally.

Stir in the tomatoes, beans, tuna, salsa, chili powder, and cumin. Reduce the heat and simmer, covered, for 20 to 30 minutes, or until the onion is soft, the bell pepper is tender, and the mixture is heated through. Ladle into bowls.

Sprinkle with the Cheddar and green onions.

PER SERVING

CALORIES 251
TOTAL FAT 4.0 g
  Saturated Fat 0.5 g
  Trans Fat 0.0 g
  Polyunsaturated Fat 0.5 g
  Monounsaturated Fat 1.5 g
CHOLESTEROL 31 mg
SODIUM 240 mg
CARBOHYDRATES 30 g
  Fiber 8 g
  Sugars 11 g
PROTEIN 27 g
DIETARY EXCHANGES
  1 starch, 3 vegetable,
  3 very lean meat

linguine with white clam sauce

SERVES 4

We suggest fresh green beans and Tomato, Basil, and Mozzarella Salad (page 94) to go with this longtime favorite.

2 6.5-ounce cans minced clams, drained, liquid reserved (about 1 cup)
½ cup dry white wine (regular or nonalcoholic)
8 ounces dried linguine
1 teaspoon olive oil
½ cup finely chopped onion

4 medium garlic cloves, minced
2 tablespoons all-purpose flour
2 tablespoons finely snipped fresh parsley
2 tablespoons shredded or grated Parmesan cheese
Pepper to taste

In a small saucepan, stir together the clam liquid and wine. Bring to a boil over high heat. Boil for about 5 minutes, or until the mixture is reduced to 1¼ cups. Set aside.

Prepare the pasta using the package directions, omitting the salt. Drain well in a colander. Cover to keep warm.

Meanwhile, in a small nonstick skillet, heat the oil over medium-high heat, swirling to coat the bottom. Cook the onion for about 3 minutes, or until soft, stirring frequently.

Stir in the garlic. Cook for 2 minutes, stirring frequently.

Stir in the flour. Cook for 1 minute, stirring frequently.

Pour in the clam liquid mixture. Cook for 2 to 3 minutes, or until thickened, stirring constantly.

Stir in the clams and parsley. Cook for 2 minutes, or until heated through, stirring constantly. Spoon over the pasta. Sprinkle with the Parmesan and pepper.

PER SERVING
CALORIES 325
TOTAL FAT 3.0 g
    Saturated Fat 0.5 g
    Trans Fat 0.0 g
    Polyunsaturated Fat 0.5 g
    Monounsaturated Fat 1.0 g
CHOLESTEROL 33 mg
SODIUM 488 mg
CARBOHYDRATES 53 g
    Fiber 2 g
    Sugars 3 g
PROTEIN 17 g
DIETARY EXCHANGES
    3½ starch,
    1 very lean meat

crabmeat maryland

SERVES 8

Maryland's Chesapeake Bay is famous for crabs. Serve this decadent crab dish in individual casseroles for a special touch.

Cooking spray
2 tablespoons minced onion
2 cups fat-free milk
3 tablespoons all-purpose flour
1 medium rib of celery, finely chopped, or ¼ teaspoon celery seeds
1 2-ounce jar diced pimientos, drained
2 tablespoons minced green bell pepper
1 tablespoon snipped fresh parsley

Dash of red hot-pepper sauce
2 tablespoons dry sherry
¼ cup egg substitute
3 cups flaked crabmeat, thawed if frozen or rinsed and drained if canned, shells and cartilage discarded
¼ teaspoon pepper, or to taste
2 slices whole-grain bread (lowest sodium available), lightly toasted and crumbled

Preheat the oven to 350°F. Lightly spray eight individual casserole dishes with cooking spray.

In a large nonstick skillet, cook the onion over medium-high heat for about 3 minutes, or until soft, stirring frequently.

In a medium bowl, whisk together the milk and flour. Stir into the onion. Cook for 3 to 5 minutes, or until thickened, stirring occasionally.

Stir in the celery, pimientos, bell pepper, parsley, and hot-pepper sauce. Remove from the heat. Stir in the sherry.

Pour the egg substitute into a small bowl. Whisk in a little sauce. Slowly pour the mixture into the sauce in the skillet, whisking constantly.

Stir in the crabmeat and pepper. Spoon into the casserole dishes. Sprinkle with the bread crumbs. Lightly spray with cooking spray.

Bake for 15 to 20 minutes, or until lightly browned.

PER SERVING

CALORIES 118
TOTAL FAT 1.0 g
  Saturated Fat 0.0 g
  Trans Fat 0.0 g
  Polyunsaturated Fat 0.5 g
  Monounsaturated Fat 0.0 g
CHOLESTEROL 42 mg
SODIUM 276 mg
CARBOHYDRATES 10 g
  Fiber 1 g
  Sugars 4 g
PROTEIN 16 g
DIETARY EXCHANGES
  ½ starch, 2 very lean meat

crab primavera alfredo

SERVES 4

Lump crabmeat is simply irresistible, especially when you serve it in a creamy sauce with tender vegetables over pasta.

4 ounces whole-grain dried fettuccine
1 teaspoon olive oil
2 medium shallots, coarsely chopped
8 ounces broccoli florets, cut into bite-size pieces
½ cup halved matchstick-size carrot strips
1 medium yellow summer squash, thinly sliced
½ cup fat-free, low-sodium chicken broth, such as on page 43
½ cup fat-free half-and-half
1½ tablespoons all-purpose flour
½ teaspoon dried dillweed, crumbled
2 tablespoons shredded or grated Parmesan cheese
1 6-ounce can lump crabmeat, drained

Prepare the pasta using the package directions, omitting the salt. Drain well in a colander. Transfer to a medium bowl. Cover to keep warm.

Meanwhile, in a large skillet, heat the oil over medium-high heat, swirling to coat the bottom. Cook the shallots for about 3 minutes, or until soft, stirring frequently.

Stir in the broccoli and carrots. Cook for about 3 minutes, or until tender-crisp.

Stir in the squash. Cook for 2 to 3 minutes, or until the broccoli and carrots are tender.

In a small bowl, whisk together the broth, half-and-half, flour, and dillweed. Pour into the broccoli mixture. Bring to a simmer. Reduce the heat and simmer for 1 to 2 minutes, or until thickened, stirring occasionally.

Stir in the Parmesan. Carefully fold in the crabmeat so the lumps don't break up too much. Cook for 2 to 3 minutes, or until heated through, gently stirring occasionally. Spoon over the pasta.

PER SERVING

CALORIES 235
TOTAL FAT 3.5 g
　Saturated Fat 1.0 g
　Trans Fat 0.0 g
　Polyunsaturated Fat 0.5 g
　Monounsaturated Fat 1.5 g
CHOLESTEROL 40 mg
SODIUM 244 mg
CARBOHYDRATES 35 g
　Fiber 6 g
　Sugars 6 g
PROTEIN 18 g
DIETARY EXCHANGES
　2 starch, 1 vegetable,
　1½ very lean meat

scallops and asparagus in wine sauce

SERVES 4

A velvety sauce and tender asparagus complement the delicate flavor of scallops in this dish. Serve with your favorite pasta.

1 8-ounce bottle clam juice
½ cup dry white wine (regular or nonalcoholic)
3 tablespoons all-purpose flour
¼ teaspoon pepper
6 ounces asparagus, trimmed, or 4 ounces frozen asparagus, thawed; cut diagonally into 1-inch pieces

1 teaspoon light tub margarine
¼ cup minced shallots (about 4 large)
1 pound sea or bay scallops, rinsed and patted dry, quartered if large
3 tablespoons finely snipped fresh parsley
1 tablespoon fresh lemon juice

In a large saucepan, whisk together the clam juice, wine, flour, and pepper. Bring to a boil over medium-high heat. Boil for 4 to 5 minutes, or until thickened, stirring occasionally.

Meanwhile, in a medium saucepan, steam the fresh asparagus for 2 minutes, or until tender-crisp. (Don't cook the asparagus if using thawed frozen).

In a small nonstick skillet, melt the margarine over medium-high heat, swirling to coat the bottom. Cook the shallots for 2 to 3 minutes, or until soft, stirring frequently.

Stir the shallots and scallops into the sauce. Reduce the heat to medium and cook for 5 minutes, stirring frequently. Don't let the mixture come to a boil. Stir in the asparagus, parsley, and lemon juice. Cook for 2 to 3 minutes, or until the scallops are opaque and the mixture is heated through. Be careful not to overcook or the scallops will become rubbery.

PER SERVING

CALORIES 163
TOTAL FAT 1.5 g
  Saturated Fat 0.0 g
  Trans Fat 0.0 g
  Polyunsaturated Fat 0.5 g
  Monounsaturated Fat 0.5 g
CHOLESTEROL 37 mg
SODIUM 475 mg
CARBOHYDRATES 11 g
  Fiber 1 g
  Sugars 1 g
PROTEIN 21 g
DIETARY EXCHANGES
  1 carbohydrate,
  3 very lean meat

oven-fried scallops with cilantro and lime

SERVES 4

Tender, moist scallops soak in a cilantro-buttermilk marinade with the bright taste of lime before being coated in bread crumbs and baked.

Cooking spray
½ cup low-fat buttermilk
2 tablespoons snipped fresh cilantro
2 tablespoons fresh lime juice
¼ teaspoon pepper
⅛ teaspoon salt
1 pound sea scallops, rinsed and patted dry

½ cup plain dry bread crumbs (lowest sodium available)
Dash of paprika
4 sprigs of fresh cilantro, stems discarded (optional)
4 lime wedges (optional)

Preheat the oven to 400°F. Lightly spray a 9-inch round or square baking pan with cooking spray.

In a shallow glass bowl, whisk together the buttermilk, cilantro, lime juice, pepper, and salt.

Stir the scallops into the buttermilk mixture, turning to coat. Let soak for 10 minutes. Drain, discarding the buttermilk mixture.

Put the bread crumbs on a plate. Roll the scallops in the crumbs to coat, gently shaking off any excess. Place the scallops in a single layer in the baking dish.

Sprinkle the scallops with the paprika. Lightly spray with cooking spray.

Bake for 10 to 13 minutes, or until opaque. Be careful not to overcook or the scallops will become rubbery. Serve sprinkled with the cilantro leaves and garnished with the lime wedges.

PER SERVING

CALORIES 168
TOTAL FAT 2.0 g
  Saturated Fat 0.5 g
  Trans Fat 0.0 g
  Polyunsaturated Fat 0.5 g
  Monounsaturated Fat 0.5 g
CHOLESTEROL 39 mg
SODIUM 387 mg
CARBOHYDRATES 15 g
  Fiber 1 g
  Sugars 2 g
PROTEIN 22 g
DIETARY EXCHANGES
  1 starch, 3 very lean meat

shrimp and okra étouffée

SERVES 6

This heart-healthy version of étouffée (ay-too-FAY) is every bit as rich tasting as the classic Louisiana dish.

1½ cups uncooked instant brown rice
¼ cup all-purpose flour
1 teaspoon canola or corn oil
1 medium green bell pepper, finely chopped
1 medium onion, finely chopped
1 medium rib of celery, finely chopped
2 cups fresh or frozen sliced okra

2 cups fat-free, low-sodium chicken broth, such as on page 43
2 teaspoons salt-free Creole or Cajun seasoning blend, such as on page 463
1 pound raw medium shrimp, peeled, rinsed, and patted dry

Prepare the rice using the package directions, omitting the salt and margarine. Cover to keep warm.

Meanwhile, in a large nonstick skillet, cook the flour over medium heat for 8 to 10 minutes, or until browned, stirring occasionally. Transfer to a medium bowl. Let cool for 5 minutes. Wipe the skillet with paper towels.

In the same skillet, heat the oil over medium heat, swirling to coat the bottom. Cook the bell pepper, onion, and celery for 2 to 3 minutes, or until tender-crisp, stirring occasionally.

Stir in the okra. Cook for 2 to 3 minutes (4 to 5 minutes if using frozen), or until the okra is tender-crisp.

Whisk the broth into the flour (there may be a few lumps). Stir the broth mixture and seasoning blend into the bell pepper mixture. Increase the heat to medium high and bring to a simmer, stirring occasionally. Reduce the heat and simmer, covered, for 15 minutes.

Stir in the shrimp. Simmer, covered, for 2 to 3 minutes, or until the shrimp are pink on the outside. Spoon over the rice.

PER SERVING

CALORIES 194
TOTAL FAT 2.5 g
  Saturated Fat 0.5 g
  Trans Fat 0.0 g
  Polyunsaturated Fat 1.0 g
  Monounsaturated Fat 1.0 g
CHOLESTEROL 112 mg
SODIUM 152 mg
CARBOHYDRATES 27 g
  Fiber 3 g
  Sugars 3 g
PROTEIN 16 g
DIETARY EXCHANGES
  1½ starch, 1 vegetable,
  2 very lean meat

fiery shrimp dijon

SERVES 4

The addition of fresh lime juice makes the other intense ingredients in this dish explode with flavor. You'll hardly be able to believe that you can make such a tasty entrée in such a short time and with so little effort.

2 tablespoons light tub margarine	⅛ teaspoon salt
2 tablespoons Dijon mustard	Cooking spray
1½ teaspoons dried tarragon, crumbled	1 pound raw medium shrimp, peeled,
¼ teaspoon cayenne	rinsed, and patted dry
¼ teaspoon pepper	2 medium limes, quartered

In a small bowl, stir together the margarine, mustard, tarragon, cayenne, pepper, and salt.

Lightly spray a large skillet with cooking spray. Cook the shrimp over medium heat for 3 minutes, or until pink on the outside, stirring frequently.

Stir in the margarine mixture to coat the shrimp. Serve with the lime wedges.

PER SERVING

CALORIES 119
TOTAL FAT 4.0 g
  Saturated Fat 0.5 g
  Trans Fat 0.0 g
  Polyunsaturated Fat 1.0 g
  Monounsaturated Fat 1.5 g
CHOLESTEROL 168 mg
SODIUM 465 mg
CARBOHYDRATES 2 g
  Fiber 1 g
  Sugars 1 g
PROTEIN 19 g
DIETARY EXCHANGES
  3 lean meat

curried shrimp risotto

SERVES 4

Plump shrimp, curry powder, veggies, and brown rice come together beautifully in this no-stress risotto. The touch of fat-free half-and-half rounds out the curry flavor and adds the creaminess associated with risotto.

2½ cups fat-free, low-sodium chicken broth, such as on page 43
1 teaspoon olive oil and 1 teaspoon olive oil, divided use
1 medium green bell pepper, chopped
1 pound raw medium shrimp, peeled, rinsed, and patted dry
1 tablespoon plus 1 teaspoon curry powder
1 cup chopped onion

¾ cup thin carrot strips, coarsely chopped
1 cup uncooked instant brown rice
1 tablespoon grated peeled gingerroot
3 medium garlic cloves, minced
2 tablespoons fat-free half-and-half
½ teaspoon crushed red pepper flakes
⅛ teaspoon salt
¾ cup frozen green peas, thawed
2 medium green onions, thinly sliced

In a small saucepan, bring the broth to a boil, covered, over low heat. Remove from the heat. Keep covered.

Meanwhile, pour 1 teaspoon oil into a Dutch oven, swirling to coat the bottom. Cook the bell pepper over medium-high heat for 3 minutes, or until tender-crisp, stirring occasionally.

Stir in the shrimp and curry powder. Cook for 3 minutes, or until the shrimp turn pink on the outside, stirring frequently. Transfer the mixture to a plate. Cover and set aside.

Decrease the heat to medium. Pour the remaining 1 teaspoon oil into the Dutch oven, swirling to coat the bottom. Add the onion and carrots. Stir in 2 tablespoons of the heated broth, continuing to keep the remaining broth covered. Cook for 2 minutes, or until the onion and carrots just begin to soften, stirring frequently.

Stir the rice, gingerroot, and garlic into the pot. Cook for 2 minutes, stirring constantly.

Stir in the remaining broth. Bring to a simmer, still over medium heat. Reduce the heat and simmer, covered, for 10 minutes, or until the liquid is almost absorbed, stirring occasionally. Remove from the heat.

PER SERVING

CALORIES 267
TOTAL FAT 4.5 g
  Saturated Fat 0.5 g
  Trans Fat 0.0 g
  Polyunsaturated Fat 1.0 g
  Monounsaturated Fat 2.5 g
CHOLESTEROL 168 mg
SODIUM 336 mg
CARBOHYDRATES 32 g
  Fiber 5 g
  Sugars 6 g
PROTEIN 25 g
DIETARY EXCHANGES
  1½ starch, 2 vegetable, 3 very lean meat

In a small bowl, stir together the half-and-half, red pepper flakes, and salt. Add to the cooked rice mixture.

Stir in the peas and the shrimp mixture. Remove from the heat. Cover and let rest for 2 minutes. Serve sprinkled with the green onions.

little shrimp cakes

SERVES 4

Perfect for dinner, these shrimp cakes are also great for appetizers. The use of lots of lemon really sets them apart.

1 pound raw medium shrimp, peeled, rinsed, and patted dry
1 cup grated plain soft bread crumbs (lowest sodium available)
3 large egg whites
½ medium red bell pepper, finely chopped
1 medium green onion, finely chopped
2 tablespoons light mayonnaise

½ teaspoon Worcestershire sauce (lowest sodium available)
½ teaspoon seafood seasoning blend
⅛ to ¼ teaspoon cayenne
2 teaspoons canola or corn oil and 2 teaspoons canola or corn oil, divided use
2 medium lemons, quartered

In a large nonstick skillet, cook the shrimp over medium heat for 5 minutes, or until pink on the outside, stirring frequently. Transfer to a baking sheet or sheet of aluminum foil, spreading in a single layer to cool quickly.

Meanwhile, in a medium bowl, stir together the bread crumbs, egg whites, bell pepper, green onion, mayonnaise, Worcestershire sauce, seasoning blend, and cayenne.

Finely chop the shrimp. Stir into the bread-crumb mixture. Shape into 16 small patties.

In the same skillet, heat 2 teaspoons oil over medium heat, swirling to coat the bottom. Cook 8 patties for 3 minutes. Turn over. Cook for 2 to 3 minutes, or until golden. Transfer to a plate. Cover to keep warm. Repeat with the remaining oil and patties.

Serve with the lemon wedges.

PER SERVING

CALORIES 194
TOTAL FAT 8.0 g
  Saturated Fat 1.0 g
  Trans Fat 0.0 g
  Polyunsaturated Fat 3.0 g
  Monounsaturated Fat 3.5 g
CHOLESTEROL 171 mg
SODIUM 453 mg
CARBOHYDRATES 8 g
  Fiber 1 g
  Sugars 2 g
PROTEIN 22 g
DIETARY EXCHANGES
  ½ starch, 3 lean meat

slow-cooker cioppino

SERVES 4

Often made with shellfish and the catch of the day, cioppino (chuh-PEE-no) lends itself to just about any combination of seafood you like.

2 cups fat-free, low-sodium chicken broth, such as on page 43

1 14.5-ounce can no-salt-added diced tomatoes, undrained

2 medium potatoes, peeled and cut into ¾-inch cubes

½ medium onion, cut into ¾-inch cubes

½ medium yellow or green bell pepper, cut into ¾-inch squares

½ cup 1 x ½-inch carrot sticks

1 large rib of celery, cut into ½-inch slices

2 medium garlic cloves, minced

1 teaspoon olive oil

½ teaspoon dried basil, crumbled

½ teaspoon dried oregano, crumbled

½ teaspoon fennel seeds, crushed (optional)

¼ teaspoon salt

¼ teaspoon pepper

¼ teaspoon crushed red pepper flakes (optional)

8 ounces fish fillets, such as cod, red snapper, halibut, or a combination, rinsed, patted dry, and cut into 1-inch cubes

8 ounces raw medium shrimp, peeled, rinsed, and patted dry

2 tablespoons snipped fresh parsley

In a 3½- or 4-quart slow cooker, stir together the broth, tomatoes with liquid, potatoes, onion, bell pepper, carrots, celery, garlic, oil, basil, oregano, fennel seeds, salt, pepper, and red pepper flakes. Cook, covered, on low for 7 to 9 hours or on high for 3 to 4 hours, or until the vegetables are tender. About 10 minutes before the end of the cooking time if using high or 20 minutes before if using low, stir in the fish, shrimp, and parsley.

poultry

Pomegranate Walnut Chicken

Chicken with Apricot Glaze

Caribbean Grilled Chicken Breasts

Chicken, Barley, and Broccoli Bake

Sherry Chicken and Vegetables

Lemon-Basil Chicken with Mushrooms

Rosemary Chicken

Country-Time Baked Chicken

Mexican Chicken and Vegetables with Chipotle Peppers

Chicken Stew with Cornmeal Dumplings

Chicken Jambalaya

Crispy Baked Chicken

Szechuan Orange Chicken

Sesame Chicken

Slow-Cooker Dilled Chicken with Rice, Green Beans, and Carrots

Herbed Italian Chicken and Rice Casserole

Slow-Cooker Thyme-Garlic Chicken with Couscous

Chicken Scallops al Limone

Italian Chicken Roll-Ups

Sun-Dried Tomato and Kalamata Olive Chicken

Chicken Columbo

Chicken with One-Minute Tomato Sauce

Chicken with Bell Peppers and Mushrooms

Rosé Chicken with Artichoke Hearts and Mushrooms

Southwestern Chicken

Burgundy Chicken with Mushrooms

Stuffed Chicken with Blue Cheese

Grilled Lemon-Sage Chicken

Sweet-Spice Glazed Chicken

Maple-Glazed Chicken

Triple-Pepper Chicken

Lemon-Cayenne Chicken

Spicy Chicken and Grits

Sweet-and-Sour Baked Chicken

Chicken and Mushroom Stir-Fry

Beef-Vegetable Stir-Fry

Sesame Chicken and Vegetable Stir-Fry

Broiled Chicken with Hoisin-Barbecue Sauce

Curried Sweet-and-Sour Chicken

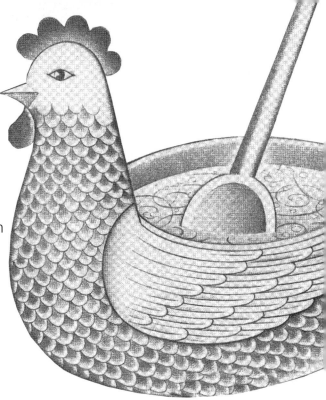

Italian Double Toss

Chicken Stufino

Baked Chicken Parmesan

Orange Microwave Chicken
  with Vegetables

Couscous Paella

Tandoori Ginger Chicken
  Strips

Chicken Gyros with
  Tzatziki Sauce

  Chicken Gyro Pitas

Boneless Buffalo Wings

Chicken and Barley Chili

  Bean and Barley Chili

Slow-Cooker White Chili

Chipotle Chicken Wraps

Chicken-Spinach Manicotti

Spaghetti with Grilled Chicken,
  Mixed Bell Peppers, and
  Zucchini

Linguine with Chicken and
  Artichokes

Chicken Curry in a Hurry

Cider-Glazed Turkey Tenderloin
  with Harvest Vegetables

Five-Spice Turkey Medallions

Turkey Rolls with Garden Pesto

Turkey Fillets with Fresh Herbs

Turkey Sausage Patties

Turkey Lasagna

Turkey Enchiladas

Turkey Loaf

Mediterranean Turkey Burgers

Southwestern Turkey Wraps

Turkey with Vegetables and
  Brown Rice

Stuffed Cornish Hens with
  Orange-Brandy Sauce

pomegranate walnut chicken

SERVES 4

Loaded with antioxidants, pomegranate juice adds its sweet tang to the deep mahogany sauce in this truly delicious dish. A garnish of oranges brings the flavors and colors to life.

2 teaspoons ground cumin
1 teaspoon poultry seasoning
1 teaspoon ground cinnamon
¼ teaspoon ground turmeric
¼ teaspoon ground nutmeg
4 boneless, skinless chicken breast halves (about 4 ounces each), all visible fat discarded
2 teaspoons olive oil and 1 teaspoon olive oil, divided use
1 large onion, halved lengthwise, then each half cut crosswise into ¼-inch half-circles
2 large garlic cloves, finely chopped
½ cup fat-free, low-sodium chicken broth, such as on page 43

1 tablespoon no-salt-added tomato paste
1 cup pure pomegranate juice (not a blend)
2 teaspoons frozen orange juice concentrate, thawed
2 teaspoons honey
¼ teaspoon salt
⅛ teaspoon cayenne
2 tablespoons chopped walnuts, dry-roasted
2 medium to large oranges, each cut crosswise into 6 slices

In a small bowl, stir together the cumin, poultry seasoning, cinnamon, turmeric, and nutmeg.

Put the chicken on a large plate. Using your fingers, rub the cumin mixture into the chicken.

Heat a large nonstick skillet over medium-high heat for 2 minutes. Add 2 teaspoons oil, swirling to coat the bottom. Cook the chicken with the smooth side down for 4 minutes, or until lightly browned. Turn over. Cook for 2 minutes, or until crusty and lightly browned (the chicken won't be done at this point). Transfer the chicken to a separate large plate. Cover to keep warm. Set aside.

In the same skillet, heat the remaining 1 teaspoon oil over medium heat, swirling to coat the bottom. Add the onion. Reduce the heat to low. Cook for 8 minutes, or until the onion begins to turn light brown, stirring frequently.

Stir in the garlic. Cook for 1 minute, stirring constantly.

Stir in the broth and tomato paste. Bring to a simmer, still on low heat, and simmer for 3 minutes, or until most of the broth has cooked away, stirring frequently.

Pour in the pomegranate juice. Increase the heat to medium and bring to a boil. Reduce the heat and simmer for 5 minutes, or until the sauce thickens and becomes syrupy.

Stir in the orange juice concentrate, honey, salt, and cayenne. Add the chicken with any accumulated juices. Spoon the sauce over the chicken. Return to a simmer. Simmer, covered, for 5 minutes, or until the chicken is no longer pink in the center. Serve the sauce over the chicken. Sprinkle with the walnuts. Garnish with the orange slices.

chicken with apricot glaze

SERVES 4

Serve steamed brown rice and a bright green vegetable to complement this palate-pleaser.

¼ cup all-purpose flour
⅛ teaspoon pepper (white preferred)
4 boneless, skinless chicken breast halves (about 4 ounces each), all visible fat discarded
Cooking spray
1 tablespoon canola or corn oil
½ cup all-fruit apricot spread
⅔ cup pineapple juice
1 tablespoon dry sherry

2 teaspoons soy sauce (lowest sodium available)
1 teaspoon dried marjoram, crumbled
1 teaspoon grated peeled gingerroot
1 teaspoon grated lemon zest
⅛ teaspoon red hot-pepper sauce
1 16-ounce can apricot halves in extra-light syrup, drained with liquid reserved, quartered
1 medium green bell pepper, diced

In a medium shallow dish, stir together the flour and pepper. Dip one piece of chicken in the mixture, turning to coat and gently shaking off any excess. Transfer the chicken with the smooth side up to a plate. Repeat with the remaining chicken. Lightly spray the tops with cooking spray.

In a large nonstick skillet, heat the oil over medium-high heat, swirling to coat the bottom. Cook the chicken with the smooth side down for 5 to 6 minutes, or until lightly browned. Remove from the heat. Lightly spray the side facing up with cooking spray. Turn over. Cover the browned side of the chicken with the apricot spread.

In a medium bowl, stir together the pineapple juice, sherry, soy sauce, marjoram, gingerroot, lemon zest, hot-pepper sauce, and reserved apricot liquid. Pour into the skillet. Bring to a simmer over medium-high heat. Reduce the heat and simmer, covered, for 10 minutes, or until the chicken is no longer pink in the center.

Stir in the bell pepper. Cook for 7 to 8 minutes. Serve the chicken topped with the apricots and sauce.

PER SERVING

CALORIES 353
TOTAL FAT 5.0 g
  Saturated Fat 0.5 g
  Trans Fat 0.0 g
  Polyunsaturated Fat 1.5 g
  Monounsaturated Fat 2.5 g
CHOLESTEROL 66 mg
SODIUM 145 mg
CARBOHYDRATES 47 g
  Fiber 3 g
  Sugars 32 g
PROTEIN 28 g
DIETARY EXCHANGES
  2 fruit, 1 carbohydrate,
  3 lean meat

caribbean grilled chicken breasts

SERVES 4

An important part of this delicious blend of flavors, bananas are easier to handle on the grill if they're slightly underripe.

MARINADE
- ⅔ cup pineapple juice
- 2 tablespoons minced onion
- 2 tablespoons fresh lime juice
- 1 tablespoon curry powder
- 1 tablespoon honey
- ¼ teaspoon salt
- ¼ teaspoon pepper
- ¼ teaspoon red hot-pepper sauce

- 4 boneless, skinless chicken breast halves (about 4 ounces each), all visible fat discarded
- 2 slightly underripe bananas, halved lengthwise and crosswise (8 pieces total)

In a large shallow glass dish, stir together the marinade ingredients. Add the chicken, turning to coat. Cover and refrigerate for 2 to 12 hours, turning occasionally.

Preheat the grill on medium.

Remove the chicken from the marinade. Pour the marinade into a small saucepan. Bring to a boil over high heat. Boil for 5 minutes.

Brush the bananas generously with the marinade. Grill the chicken and bananas for 10 to 15 minutes, or until the chicken is no longer pink in the center, turning over halfway through. Brush the chicken and bananas with the marinade before serving.

PER SERVING

CALORIES 224
TOTAL FAT 2.0 g
  Saturated Fat 0.5 g
  Trans Fat 0.0 g
  Polyunsaturated Fat 0.5 g
  Monounsaturated Fat 0.5 g
CHOLESTEROL 66 mg
SODIUM 225 mg
CARBOHYDRATES 25 g
  Fiber 2 g
  Sugars 16 g
PROTEIN 27 g
DIETARY EXCHANGES
  1½ fruit, 3 very lean meat

chicken, barley, and broccoli bake

SERVES 4

This homey one-dish meal tastes great and is packed with nutritious ingredients.

2 cups fat-free, low-sodium chicken broth, such as on page 43
1 cup fat-free milk
2 tablespoons all-purpose flour
1 teaspoon dried basil, crumbled
¼ teaspoon salt
Dash of pepper

⅔ cup uncooked pearl barley
4 boneless, skinless chicken breast halves (about 4 ounces each), all visible fat discarded
1 10-ounce package frozen chopped broccoli, partially thawed if needed to break into small pieces

Preheat the oven to 350°F.

In a medium saucepan, whisk together the broth, milk, flour, basil, salt, and pepper until smooth. Cook over medium heat for 7 to 10 minutes, or until the sauce just starts to boil, whisking frequently.

Meanwhile, spread the barley to cover the bottom of a 9-inch square metal pan. Top with the chicken. Pour the sauce over the chicken. Sprinkle the broccoli on top.

Bake for 1 hour 20 minutes, or until the barley is cooked and has absorbed the sauce and the chicken is no longer pink in the center.

PER SERVING

CALORIES 314
TOTAL FAT 2.0 g
  Saturated Fat 0.5 g
  Trans Fat 0.0 g
  Polyunsaturated Fat 0.5 g
  Monounsaturated Fat 0.5 g
CHOLESTEROL 67 mg
SODIUM 289 mg
CARBOHYDRATES 38 g
  Fiber 9 g
  Sugars 5 g
PROTEIN 36 g
DIETARY EXCHANGES
  2 starch, 2 vegetable,
  3 very lean meat

sherry chicken and vegetables

SERVES 4

The unusual combination of sherry and dill flavor this simple chicken dish.

Cooking spray
2 medium potatoes, peeled and chopped into ½-inch cubes
2 large carrots, cut into 1-inch pieces
2 medium onions, each cut into 8 wedges
4 whole medium garlic cloves

¼ teaspoon salt
4 boneless, skinless chicken breast halves (about 4 ounces each), all visible fat discarded
½ cup dry sherry
½ teaspoon pepper
½ teaspoon dried dillweed, crumbled

Preheat the oven to 350°F. Lightly spray a deep baking pan with cooking spray.

Put the potatoes, carrots, onions, and garlic in the baking pan. Sprinkle with the salt. Arrange the chicken on top. Pour the sherry over all. Sprinkle with the pepper and dillweed.

Bake, covered, for 30 minutes, or until the chicken is no longer pink in the center and the potatoes, carrots, and onions are tender.

PER SERVING

CALORIES 272
TOTAL FAT 1.5 g
  Saturated Fat 0.5 g
  Trans Fat 0.0 g
  Polyunsaturated Fat 0.5 g
  Monounsaturated Fat 0.5 g
CHOLESTEROL 66 mg
SODIUM 255 mg
CARBOHYDRATES 31 g
  Fiber 4 g
  Sugars 7 g
PROTEIN 30 g
DIETARY EXCHANGES
  1½ starch, 2 vegetable, 3 lean meat

lemon-basil chicken with mushrooms

SERVES 4

Lemon juice and basil team up to give this dish a lot of zing. Cooking the mushrooms separately and serving them as a bed for the chicken and sauce lets the mushroom flavor shine on its own.

4 boneless, skinless chicken breast halves (about 4 ounces each), all visible fat discarded
½ teaspoon pepper
¼ teaspoon salt
2 medium garlic cloves, finely chopped, and 1 medium garlic clove, finely chopped, divided use
1½ teaspoons grated lemon zest
1 teaspoon olive oil and 1 teaspoon olive oil, divided use

½ cup sliced onion, sliced about ¼ inch thick
8 ounces button mushrooms, sliced
1 teaspoon cornstarch
½ cup fat-free, low-sodium chicken broth, such as on page 43
⅓ cup chopped fresh basil
3 tablespoons fresh lemon juice

Sprinkle both sides of the chicken with the pepper and salt.

In a small bowl, stir together 2 chopped garlic cloves, lemon zest, and 1 teaspoon oil. Using your fingertips, rub the mixture into both sides of the chicken.

Heat a large nonstick skillet over medium-high heat for 2 minutes. Cook the chicken with the smooth side down for 4 minutes, or until lightly browned. Turn over. Cook for 2 minutes (the chicken won't be done at this point). Transfer to a plate. Cover to keep warm.

Discard any garlic in the skillet. Pour the remaining 1 teaspoon oil into the skillet, swirling to coat the bottom. Reduce the heat to low. Cook the onion and remaining 1 chopped garlic clove for 3 minutes, or until the onion begins to soften, stirring frequently.

Stir in the mushrooms. Increase the heat to medium-high. Cook for 6 minutes, or until the mushrooms soften and lightly brown, stirring frequently. Transfer to a small bowl. Cover to keep warm.

Meanwhile, put the cornstarch in a small bowl. Pour in the broth, whisking to dissolve.

PER SERVING

CALORIES 175
TOTAL FAT 4.0 g
  Saturated Fat 0.5 g
  Trans Fat 0.0 g
  Polyunsaturated Fat 0.5 g
  Monounsaturated Fat 2.0 g
CHOLESTEROL 66 mg
SODIUM 227 mg
CARBOHYDRATES 6 g
  Fiber 1 g
  Sugars 2 g
PROTEIN 29 g
DIETARY EXCHANGES
  1 vegetable, 3 lean meat

After you remove the mushrooms from the skillet, pour the cornstarch mixture into the skillet, whisking to combine. Return the chicken and any accumulated juices to the skillet. Spoon the broth mixture over the chicken. Bring to a simmer over medium-high heat. Reduce the heat and simmer, covered, for 8 minutes, or until the sauce thickens and the chicken is cooked through. Remove from the heat.

Spoon the mushroom mixture onto plates. Leaving the sauce in the skillet, place the chicken on the mushrooms. Stir the basil and lemon juice into the sauce. Spoon over the chicken and mushrooms.

COOK'S TIP on chicken

Skinless breast meat is the leanest part of a whole chicken, with half as much saturated fat as skinless dark meat.

rosemary chicken

SERVES 4

While the chicken bakes, make the sauce, cook some brown rice, and steam some broccoli. Then sit down and enjoy a fine dinner.

Cooking spray

4 boneless, skinless chicken breast halves (about 4 ounces each), all visible fat discarded

2 tablespoons chopped fresh rosemary or 2 teaspoons dried rosemary, crushed

2 ounces button mushrooms, thinly sliced

½ cup fat-free, low-sodium chicken broth, such as on page 43

¼ cup dry white wine (regular or nonalcoholic)

1 tablespoon fresh lemon juice
Pepper to taste

½ medium lemon, quartered (optional)

4 sprigs of parsley (optional)

Preheat the oven to 350°F. Lightly spray a 9-inch square baking pan with cooking spray.

Rub the chicken with the rosemary. Lightly spray with cooking spray. Place the chicken with the smooth side down in the pan.

Bake for 15 minutes.

Meanwhile, in a medium bowl, stir together the mushrooms, broth, wine, lemon juice, and pepper. Pour over the chicken.

Bake for 15 minutes, or until the chicken is no longer pink in the center. Garnish with the lemon, parsley, or both.

PER SERVING

CALORIES 142
TOTAL FAT 1.5 g
  Saturated Fat 0.5 g
  Trans Fat 0.0 g
  Polyunsaturated Fat 0.5 g
  Monounsaturated Fat 0.5 g
CHOLESTEROL 66 mg
SODIUM 79 mg
CARBOHYDRATES 1 g
  Fiber 0 g
  Sugars 0 g
PROTEIN 27 g
DIETARY EXCHANGES
  3 very lean meat

country-time baked chicken

SERVES 4 (PLUS 2 CHICKEN BREAST HALVES RESERVED)

As this nicely seasoned chicken bakes, it releases juices to reduce into a rich-tasting sauce. Reserve two of the cooked chicken breast halves to use in Six-Layer Salad with Chicken (page 122).

Cooking spray	½ teaspoon garlic powder
6 skinless chicken breast halves with bone (about 6 ounces each), all visible fat discarded	¼ teaspoon salt
	¼ teaspoon pepper
	1½ tablespoons olive oil
¾ teaspoon poultry seasoning	3 tablespoons snipped fresh parsley
½ teaspoon paprika	and 2 tablespoons snipped fresh
½ teaspoon onion powder	parsley, divided use

Preheat the oven to 325°F. Lightly spray a 13 x 9 x 2-inch glass baking dish with cooking spray.

Put the chicken with the smooth side up in the baking dish.

In a small bowl, stir together the poultry seasoning, paprika, onion powder, garlic powder, salt, and pepper. Sprinkle over the top of the chicken.

Drizzle the oil over the chicken. Sprinkle with 3 table-spoons parsley.

Bake, covered, for 40 minutes, or until the chicken is no longer pink in the center, turning several times to coat the chicken with the drippings. Transfer 4 pieces of chicken to plates. Put the remaining pieces in an air-tight storage container for use within two to three days in Six-Layer Salad with Chicken.

Pour the drippings from the baking dish into a small saucepan. Bring to a boil over high heat. Boil for 2 minutes, or until reduced to ¼ cup liquid. Spoon over the chicken. Sprinkle with the remaining 2 tablespoons parsley.

COOK'S TIP

Simple baked chicken is one of the most versatile foods to keep on hand. The extra chicken could alternatively be used in sandwiches, soups, or casseroles.

PER SERVING

CALORIES 184
TOTAL FAT 5.0 g
    Saturated Fat 1.0 g
    Trans Fat 0.0 g
    Polyunsaturated Fat 1.0 g
    Monounsaturated Fat 3.0 g
CHOLESTEROL 79 mg
SODIUM 188 mg
CARBOHYDRATES 1 g
    Fiber 0 g
    Sugars 0 g
PROTEIN 32 g
DIETARY EXCHANGES
    4 lean meat

mexican chicken and vegetables with chipotle peppers

SERVES 4 (PLUS 4 CHICKEN BREAST HALVES AND 1 CUP TOMATO MIXTURE RESERVED)

Chicken simmered with bell peppers and tomatoes, richly seasoned with chipotle peppers (smoked jalapeños), and served over yellow rice will satisfy the most demanding Mexican-food enthusiast. The extra chicken and sauce are ready for use in Chipotle Chicken Wraps (page 261) later in the week.

1½ cups water
4 dried chipotle peppers
Olive oil spray
8 boneless, skinless chicken breast halves (about 4 ounces each), all visible fat discarded
2 large onions, chopped
4 medium garlic cloves, minced
1 cup uncooked rice
½ teaspoon ground turmeric
1 medium fresh jalapeño, seeds and ribs discarded, minced (optional)

1 14.5-ounce can no-salt-added diced tomatoes, undrained
1 medium green bell pepper, chopped
2 teaspoons ground cumin
1½ teaspoons dried oregano, crumbled
1 teaspoon chili powder
½ teaspoon salt
1 to 2 teaspoons olive oil (extra virgin preferred)

In a small saucepan, bring the water to a boil over high heat. Remove from the heat. Add the chipotle peppers. Let stand for 30 minutes.

Meanwhile, lightly spray a Dutch oven with olive oil spray. Cook half the chicken with the smooth side down over medium-high heat for 6 minutes. Turn over. Cook for 4 to 6 minutes, or until no longer pink in the center. Transfer to a plate. Repeat with the remaining chicken.

Put the onions and garlic in the Dutch oven. Cook for 5 to 7 minutes, stirring frequently and scraping to dislodge any browned bits. Remove from the heat.

Drain the chipotle peppers, reserving the water. Discard the seeds, ribs, and stems from the peppers. In a food processor or blender, process the peppers and reserved water until smooth.

Prepare the rice using the package directions, omitting the salt and margarine and adding the turmeric. When the rice is done, stir in the jalapeño.

Meanwhile, chop or shred the chicken.

Stir the tomatoes with liquid, bell pepper, cumin, oregano, chili powder, chipotle pepper mixture, and chicken and any juices into the onion mixture. Bring to a boil over medium heat. Reduce the heat and simmer, covered, for 20 minutes. Remove from the heat. Transfer half the chicken and 1 cup tomato mixture to an airtight container. Refrigerate and reserve for use in Chipotle Chicken Wraps.

Before serving, stir the salt and oil into the remaining chicken mixture. Serve over the rice.

COOK'S TIP

This stew is even better if refrigerated overnight. It's a good dish to make on the weekend for a quick dinner. Just reheat the stew, add the salt and oil, and prepare the rice.

chicken stew with cornmeal dumplings

SERVES 6

Chicken and dumplings is a family-style dish found on many southern dinner tables. This creamy version is full of lean chicken and vegetables, topped with cornmeal dumplings.

STEW

- 2 teaspoons canola or corn oil
- 1 medium onion, chopped
- 1 medium garlic clove, minced
- 4 boneless, skinless chicken breast halves (about 4 ounces each), all visible fat discarded
- 4½ cups fat-free, low-sodium chicken broth, such as on page 43
- 2 medium ribs of celery, sliced
- 1 large carrot, sliced
- 1 medium dried bay leaf
- 1½ teaspoons dried basil, crumbled
- 1½ teaspoons dried oregano, crumbled
- ½ teaspoon salt
- ½ teaspoon pepper
- ¼ teaspoon dried sage
- 1 medium zucchini, halved lengthwise and sliced
- 1 medium yellow summer squash, halved lengthwise and sliced
- 1 cup fat-free milk
- ½ cup all-purpose flour

CORNMEAL DUMPLINGS

- ⅓ cup cornmeal
- ¼ cup snipped fresh parsley
- 1½ teaspoons baking powder
- ½ cup all-purpose flour
- ¼ teaspoon salt
- ⅛ teaspoon pepper
- ¼ cup egg substitute
- ¼ cup fat-free milk
- 1 tablespoon canola or corn oil

In a Dutch oven, heat the oil over medium-high heat, swirling to coat the bottom. Cook the onion and garlic for 3 to 4 minutes, or until the onion is soft, stirring frequently.

Add the chicken and cook for 2 to 3 minutes on each side, or until lightly browned (the chicken won't be done at this point).

Stir in the broth, celery, carrot, bay leaf, basil, oregano, ½ teaspoon salt, ½ teaspoon pepper, and sage. Bring to a low boil, still over medium-high heat. Reduce the heat and simmer, covered, for 10 minutes, or until the chicken is no longer pink except in the center. Transfer the chicken to a cutting board. Discard the bay leaf.

Stir the zucchini and yellow squash into the stew.

In a medium bowl, whisk together 1 cup milk and ½ cup flour. Stir into the stew. Bring to a boil over medium-high heat. Reduce the heat to medium and cook for 5 minutes, or until thickened and bubbly, stirring constantly.

When the chicken is cool enough to handle, cut into bite-size pieces. Stir into the stew. Bring to a simmer.

In a small bowl, stir together the remaining ½ cup flour, cornmeal, parsley, baking powder, remaining ¼ teaspoon salt, and remaining ⅛ teaspoon pepper.

In a separate small bowl, whisk together the remaining dumpling ingredients. Add to the flour mixture, whisking just until moistened.

Using a spoon, drop the dumpling batter in 6 mounds on the simmering stew. Reduce the heat and simmer, covered, for 10 to 12 minutes, or until a wooden toothpick inserted in one of the dumplings comes out clean. (Don't peek at the dumplings while they cook.)

chicken jambalaya

SERVES 4

Capture the flavors of Louisiana with this casserole. Your family will love the taste—and you'll love the simple preparation.

Cooking spray
1 cup fat-free, low-sodium chicken broth, such as on page 43
1 cup dry white wine (regular or nonalcoholic)
1 large onion, chopped
1 medium green bell pepper, chopped
2 medium ribs of celery, chopped
¼ cup snipped fresh parsley
½ teaspoon dried basil, crumbled
½ teaspoon dried thyme, crumbled

1 large dried bay leaf
¼ teaspoon red hot-pepper sauce
1 14.5-ounce can no-salt-added diced tomatoes, undrained
1 cup uncooked rice
½ cup cubed lower-sodium, low-fat ham
4 boneless, skinless chicken breast halves (about 4 ounces each), all visible fat discarded

Preheat the oven to 350°F. Lightly spray a 13 x 9 x 2-inch glass baking dish or 2-quart glass casserole dish with cooking spray.

In a medium saucepan, stir together the broth, wine, onion, bell pepper, celery, parsley, basil, thyme, bay leaf, and hot-pepper sauce. Bring to a boil over medium-high heat, stirring occasionally. Remove from the heat.

In the baking dish, stir together the tomatoes with liquid, rice, and ham. Place the chicken on top. Pour the hot broth mixture over all.

Bake, covered, for 45 to 55 minutes, or until the chicken is no longer pink in the center and the rice is tender. Discard the bay leaf.

PER SERVING

CALORIES 392
TOTAL FAT 2.0 g
  Saturated Fat 0.5 g
  Trans Fat 0.0 g
  Polyunsaturated Fat 0.5 g
  Monounsaturated Fat 0.5 g
CHOLESTEROL 74 mg
SODIUM 295 mg
CARBOHYDRATES 49 g
  Fiber 4 g
  Sugars 8 g
PROTEIN 35 g
DIETARY EXCHANGES
  2½ starch, 2 vegetable,
  3½ very lean meat

crispy baked chicken

SERVES 4

Remember when you didn't want to fry chicken because it was such a mess to clean up? Now you have two good reasons to cook this chicken—no pan to wash and the fact that it's really moist low-fat "fried" chicken!

Cooking spray
1 cup fat-free milk
1 cup cornflake crumbs
1 teaspoon dried rosemary, crushed

½ teaspoon pepper
4 boneless, skinless chicken breast halves (about 4 ounces each), all visible fat discarded

Preheat the oven to 400°F. Line a 13 x 9 x 2-inch baking pan with aluminum foil. Lightly spray with cooking spray.

Pour the milk into a shallow dish. In a separate shallow dish, stir together the cornflake crumbs, rosemary, and pepper. Set the dishes and baking pan in a row, assembly-line fashion. Dip one piece of chicken in the milk, turning to coat and letting the excess drip off. Dip in the crumb mixture, gently shaking off any excess. Transfer to the baking pan. Repeat with the remaining chicken, arranging so the pieces don't touch. Let stand for 5 to 10 minutes so the coating will adhere.

Bake for 30 minutes, or until the chicken is no longer pink in the center and the crumbs form a crisp "skin."

PER SERVING

CALORIES 212
TOTAL FAT 1.5 g
    Saturated Fat 0.5 g
    Trans Fat 0.0 g
    Polyunsaturated Fat 0.5 g
    Monounsaturated Fat 0.5 g
CHOLESTEROL 66 mg
SODIUM 241 mg
CARBOHYDRATES 21 g
    Fiber 0 g
    Sugars 3 g
PROTEIN 28 g
DIETARY EXCHANGES
    1½ starch,
    3 very lean meat

szechuan orange chicken

SERVES 4

When you want to give everyday ingredients an exotic touch, try this recipe. The spices, panko, and orange sauce add an Asian taste without the high fat and sodium content of takeout. By using the high heat of the broiler and the speed of microwave cooking, you'll have this healthy version of fast food on the table in no time!

Cooking spray
1 teaspoon garlic powder
1 teaspoon onion powder
1 teaspoon ground ginger/2 teaspoons ground ginger, divided use
½ teaspoon crushed red pepper flakes and ½ teaspoon crushed red pepper flakes, divided use
1 pound chicken breast tenders, all visible fat discarded, cut into 1-inch cubes
1 teaspoon plain rice vinegar

¼ cup egg substitute
1 cup panko (Japanese bread crumbs)
¼ cup plus 2 tablespoons frozen orange juice concentrate, thawed
¼ cup plus 2 tablespoons water
1 tablespoon plus 1 teaspoon honey
2 medium garlic cloves, finely chopped
2 teaspoons soy sauce (lowest sodium available)
1 teaspoon toasted sesame oil

Preheat the broiler. Line a baking sheet with aluminum foil. Lightly spray with cooking spray.

In a medium bowl, stir together the garlic powder, onion powder, 1 teaspoon ginger, and ½ teaspoon red pepper flakes. Add the chicken, turning to coat. Using your fingertips, gently press the mixture so it adheres to the chicken.

Drizzle with the vinegar, tossing to coat. Let stand for 5 minutes.

Meanwhile, pour the egg substitute into a shallow dish. Put the panko in a separate shallow dish. Set the dishes and baking sheet in a row, assembly-line fashion. Dip a few chicken cubes at a time in the egg substitute, turning to coat and letting the excess drip off. Dip in the panko, turning to coat and gently shaking off any excess. Using your fingertips, gently press the panko so it adheres to all sides of the chicken. Put the chicken on the baking sheet in a single layer, making sure the cubes don't touch. Lightly spray the tops and sides of the chicken with cooking spray.

Broil about 6 inches from the heat for 8 minutes, or until the chicken is no longer pink in the center and the coating is golden brown and crisp.

Meanwhile, in a small microwaveable bowl, stir together the orange juice concentrate, water, honey, remaining 2 teaspoons ginger, garlic, and soy sauce. Microwave, covered, on 100 percent power (high) for 3 minutes, or until hot and bubbly.

Stir in the sesame oil and remaining ½ teaspoon red pepper flakes. Drizzle over the chicken.

COOK'S TIP on panko

Panko, or Japanese bread crumbs, is made from the soft centers of bread rather than the crust. It has a pleasant crunchiness, is lighter than traditional bread crumbs, and contains considerably less sodium and fewer calories.

sesame chicken

SERVES 4

Lemon juice and wine flavor meaty chicken pieces, and a light crust of sesame seeds keeps them moist. Serve with a half recipe of Stir-Fried Bok Choy with Green Onion Sauce (page 428) and have Claret-Spiced Oranges (page 622) for dessert.

Cooking spray
⅓ cup all-purpose flour
¼ teaspoon pepper
4 boneless, skinless chicken breast halves (about 4 ounces each), all visible fat discarded

1 tablespoon fresh lemon juice
¼ cup sesame seeds
3 tablespoons minced green onions
½ cup dry white wine (regular or nonalcoholic) (plus more as needed)

Preheat the oven to 375°F. Lightly spray a 13 x 9 x 2-inch baking pan with cooking spray.

In a shallow dish, stir together the flour and pepper. Dip one piece of chicken in the mixture, turning to coat and gently shaking off any excess. Lightly spray the smooth side with cooking spray. Transfer with the sprayed side down to the baking pan. Repeat with the remaining chicken, arranging the pieces so they don't touch. Lightly spray the tops.

Sprinkle the lemon juice and half the sesame seeds over the chicken.

Bake for 30 minutes, or until lightly browned. Turn over. Sprinkle with the remaining sesame seeds and the green onions. Pour the wine around (not over) the chicken.

Bake for 30 to 45 minutes, or until the chicken is no longer pink in the center, basting occasionally.

PER SERVING

CALORIES 246
TOTAL FAT 7.5 g
  Saturated Fat 1.0 g
  Trans Fat 0.0 g
  Polyunsaturated Fat 3.0 g
  Monounsaturated Fat 2.5 g
CHOLESTEROL 66 mg
SODIUM 82 mg
CARBOHYDRATES 10 g
  Fiber 2 g
  Sugars 0 g
PROTEIN 29 g
DIETARY EXCHANGES
  ½ starch, 3 lean meat

slow-cooker dilled chicken with rice, green beans, and carrots

SERVES 4

There's no need to prepare the rice separately for this one-dish slow-cooker winner. Just add instant brown rice to the chicken and vegetables for the last half-hour of cooking.

2 medium carrots, chopped
1 cup frozen cut green beans
1 medium rib of celery, sliced
1 medium onion, chopped
1½ teaspoons dried dillweed, crumbled
⅛ teaspoon cayenne or ¼ teaspoon pepper

4 boneless, skinless chicken breast halves (about 4 ounces each), all visible fat discarded
1 10.75-ounce can low-fat condensed cream of chicken soup (lowest sodium available)
1 cup water
2 cups uncooked instant brown rice

In a 3½- or 4-quart slow cooker, stir together the carrots, green beans, celery, onion, dillweed, and cayenne. Put the chicken on top.

In a small bowl, whisk together the soup and water. Pour over the chicken. Cook, covered, on high for 2½ to 3 hours or on low for 5 to 6 hours, or until the chicken is no longer pink in the center and the vegetables are tender.

If using the low-heat setting, turn to high. Stir in the rice. Cook for 30 minutes, or until the rice is tender.

PER SERVING

CALORIES 383
TOTAL FAT 4.5 g
  Saturated Fat 1.0 g
  Trans Fat 0.0 g
  Polyunsaturated Fat 1.5 g
  Monounsaturated Fat 1.5 g
CHOLESTEROL 69 mg
SODIUM 441 mg
CARBOHYDRATES 50 g
  Fiber 5 g
  Sugars 6 g
PROTEIN 33 g
DIETARY EXCHANGES
  3 starch, 1 vegetable,
  3 very lean meat

herbed italian chicken and rice casserole

SERVES 4

Destined to become a family favorite, this casserole is an easy one-dish meal that combines classic flavors.

Cooking spray

1 14.5-ounce can no-salt-added stewed tomatoes, undrained

1 pound boneless, skinless chicken breasts, all visible fat discarded, cut into bite-size pieces

3 ounces button mushrooms, sliced

2 ounces baby spinach, chopped

¾ cup fat-free, low-sodium chicken broth, such as on page 43

¾ cup uncooked instant brown rice

½ cup chopped onion

¼ cup chopped fresh basil

2 medium garlic cloves, minced

½ teaspoon dried oregano, crumbled

½ teaspoon salt-free all-purpose seasoning blend

¼ teaspoon pepper

⅛ teaspoon salt

2 tablespoons shredded or grated Parmesan cheese

Preheat the oven to 375°F. With cooking spray, lightly spray an 11 x 7 x 1½-inch glass baking dish.

Pour the tomatoes with liquid into a large bowl. Break up any large pieces.

Stir in the remaining ingredients except the Parmesan. Pour into the baking dish.

Bake, covered, for 35 to 40 minutes, or until the chicken is no longer pink in the center and the rice is tender. Serve sprinkled with the Parmesan.

COOK'S TIP

Casseroles are a handy place to unobtrusively introduce more veggies and whole grains into your family's meals. The next time you prepare your usual rice or noodle bake, switch to brown rice or whole-grain pasta and add a colorful vegetable, such as spinach or kale.

PER SERVING

CALORIES 250
TOTAL FAT 3.0 g
  Saturated Fat 1.0 g
  Trans Fat 0.0 g
  Polyunsaturated Fat 0.5 g
  Monounsaturated Fat 1.0 g
CHOLESTEROL 68 mg
SODIUM 223 mg
CARBOHYDRATES 23 g
  Fiber 4 g
  Sugars 6 g
PROTEIN 31 g
DIETARY EXCHANGES
  1 starch, 2 vegetable,
  3 very lean meat

slow-cooker thyme-garlic chicken with couscous

SERVES 4

A colorful couscous mixture that includes fresh spinach and tomato is the bed for chicken breasts prepared in a slow cooker.

4 boneless, skinless chicken breast halves (about 4 ounces each), all visible fat discarded
1 teaspoon dried thyme, crumbled
¼ teaspoon salt
1 teaspoon grated orange zest
½ cup fresh orange juice
1 tablespoon balsamic vinegar

4 medium garlic cloves, minced
1 cup uncooked whole-wheat couscous
2 cups shredded spinach, stems discarded (about 2 ounces)
1 medium tomato, seeded and chopped

Sprinkle the chicken on both sides with the thyme and salt. Place in a 3½- or 4-quart slow cooker.

In a small bowl, stir together the orange zest, orange juice, vinegar, and garlic. Pour over the chicken. Cook, covered, on high for 2 to 2½ hours or on low for 4 to 5 hours, or until the chicken is no longer pink in the center.

Prepare the couscous using the package directions, omitting the salt and oil.

Add the spinach and tomato to the couscous, stirring until the spinach is wilted. Serve the chicken over the couscous. If desired, spoon a little of the cooking liquid on top.

PER SERVING

CALORIES 367
TOTAL FAT 2.5 g
   Saturated Fat 0.5 g
   Trans Fat 0.0 g
   Polyunsaturated Fat 1.0 g
   Monounsaturated Fat 0.5 g
CHOLESTEROL 66 mg
SODIUM 234 mg
CARBOHYDRATES 52 g
   Fiber 8 g
   Sugars 4 g
PROTEIN 35 g
DIETARY EXCHANGES
   3½ starch,
   3 very lean meat

chicken scallops al limone

SERVES 6

This dish is very good over any kind of pasta. It also goes well with Asparagus with Garlic and Parmesan Bread Crumbs (page 416) and Salad Greens with Oranges and Strawberries (page 87).

¼ cup plus 1 tablespoon all-purpose flour
½ teaspoon pepper
¼ teaspoon salt
6 boneless, skinless chicken breast halves (about 4 ounces each), all visible fat discarded, flattened to ¼-inch thickness
2 teaspoons olive oil

1¾ cups fat-free, low-sodium chicken broth, such as on page 43
¼ cup fresh lemon juice
¼ cup dry white wine (regular or nonalcoholic)
1 tablespoon finely snipped fresh parsley
6 thin lemon slices (optional)

In a shallow dish, stir together the flour, pepper, and salt. Dip one piece of chicken in the flour mixture, turning to coat and gently shaking off any excess. Transfer to a plate. Repeat with the remaining chicken.

In a large nonstick skillet, heat the oil over medium-high heat, swirling to coat the bottom. Cook half the chicken for 2 to 3 minutes, turning to brown both sides (the chicken won't be done at this point). Transfer to a plate. Repeat with the remaining chicken.

Pour the broth, lemon juice, and wine into the skillet. Cook for 7 to 8 minutes, or until the sauce is reduced to about 1½ cups, scraping to dislodge any browned bits.

Return the chicken to the skillet. Bring to a simmer. Reduce the heat and simmer for 5 to 7 minutes, or until the chicken is no longer pink in the center and the sauce is slightly thickened, stirring occasionally. Using a slotted spoon or pancake turner, transfer the chicken to plates.

Stir the parsley into the sauce. Pour over the chicken. Garnish with the lemon slices.

COOK'S TIP on flattening chicken breasts

Put a breast with the smooth side up between two pieces of plastic wrap. With the smooth side of a meat mallet or a heavy pan, flatten the chicken to the desired thickness. Be careful not to tear the meat.

PER SERVING

CALORIES 175
TOTAL FAT 3.0 g
  Saturated Fat 0.5 g
  Trans Fat 0.0 g
  Polyunsaturated Fat 0.5 g
  Monounsaturated Fat 1.5 g
CHOLESTEROL 66 mg
SODIUM 179 mg
CARBOHYDRATES 6 g
  Fiber 0 g
  Sugars 0 g
PROTEIN 28 g
DIETARY EXCHANGES
  ½ starch,
  3 very lean meat

italian chicken roll-ups

SERVES 4

Serve these attractive chicken rolls with a simple salad and Strawberry-Raspberry Ice (page 631).

1 cup water
1 6-ounce can no-salt-added tomato paste
1 medium garlic clove, minced
¾ teaspoon dried oregano, crumbled
¾ teaspoon dried basil, crumbled
½ teaspoon dried marjoram, crumbled
¼ teaspoon pepper, or to taste
⅛ teaspoon salt

4 ounces low-fat cottage cheese, drained
4 boneless, skinless chicken breast halves (about 4 ounces each), all visible fat discarded, flattened to ¼-inch thickness
½ cup shredded low-fat mozzarella cheese

Preheat the oven to 350°F.

In a small saucepan, whisk together the water, tomato paste, and garlic.

In a small bowl, stir together the oregano, basil, marjoram, pepper, and salt. Stir three-fourths of the mixture into the tomato paste mixture. Bring to a boil over medium-high heat. Reduce the heat and simmer for 10 minutes, stirring occasionally.

Meanwhile, stir the cottage cheese into the remaining oregano mixture. Leaving a ½-inch edge all around, spread over the chicken. From the narrow end, roll up each breast jelly-roll style.

Spoon half the tomato paste mixture into an 8-inch glass baking dish. Arrange the chicken rolls with the seam side down on the sauce. Spoon the remaining sauce over the chicken rolls. Sprinkle with the mozzarella.

Bake for 45 minutes, or until the chicken is no longer pink in the center. If the chicken is getting too brown, cover for the last 10 minutes of baking.

PER SERVING

CALORIES 211
TOTAL FAT 3.0 g
  Saturated Fat 1.0 g
  Trans Fat 0.0 g
  Polyunsaturated Fat 0.5 g
  Monounsaturated Fat 1.0 g
CHOLESTEROL 72 mg
SODIUM 405 mg
CARBOHYDRATES 10 g
  Fiber 2 g
  Sugars 6 g
PROTEIN 35 g
DIETARY EXCHANGES
  2 vegetable,
  3½ very lean meat

sun-dried tomato and kalamata olive chicken

SERVES 4

Rich-tasting sun-dried tomatoes, Greek olives, and feta come together to make this simple, yet sensational, fare.

10 dry-packed sun-dried tomato halves, chopped
¼ cup boiling water
½ teaspoon dried oregano, crumbled, and ½ teaspoon dried oregano, crumbled, divided use
4 boneless, skinless chicken breast halves (about 4 ounces each), all visible fat discarded, flattened to ¼-inch thickness

⅛ teaspoon salt
12 kalamata olives, finely chopped
¼ cup finely snipped fresh parsley
⅛ teaspoon crushed red pepper flakes
1 ounce fat-free feta cheese, crumbled
2 teaspoons olive oil (extra virgin preferred)

In a small bowl, stir together the tomatoes and water. Let stand for 10 minutes. Drain.

Meanwhile, sprinkle ½ teaspoon oregano over the chicken, using ¼ teaspoon on each side.

In a large nonstick skillet, cook the chicken over medium-high heat for 3 minutes on each side, or until no longer pink in the center. Remove from the heat. Sprinkle the salt over the chicken.

Stir the olives, parsley, red pepper flakes, and remaining ½ teaspoon oregano into the drained tomatoes. Gently stir in the feta. Serve over the chicken. Drizzle with the oil.

chicken columbo

SERVES 4

Seasoned wheat germ coats the chicken and gives it an interesting crunch and a lot of flavor. Whole-grain shell pasta is a good accompaniment—it helps soak up the savory sauce.

½ cup fat-free milk
⅓ cup toasted wheat germ or plain dry bread crumbs (lowest sodium available)
1 teaspoon dried oregano, crumbled
½ teaspoon salt
¼ teaspoon garlic powder
¼ teaspoon onion powder
Pepper to taste

4 boneless, skinless chicken breast halves (about 4 ounces each), all visible fat discarded
1 tablespoon olive oil
8 ounces button mushrooms, sliced
¼ cup dry marsala or dry sherry
¼ cup water
3 tablespoons no-salt-added tomato paste
2 tablespoons snipped fresh parsley

Pour the milk into a shallow dish. In a separate shallow dish, stir together the wheat germ, oregano, salt, garlic powder, onion powder, and pepper. Set the dishes and a plate in a row, assembly-line fashion. Dip one piece of chicken in the milk, turning to coat and letting the excess drip off. Dip in the wheat-germ mixture, gently shaking off any excess. Transfer to the plate. Repeat with the remaining chicken.

In a large nonstick skillet, heat the oil over medium-high heat, swirling to coat the bottom. Cook the chicken for 3 to 4 minutes on each side, or until lightly browned.

In a medium bowl, stir together the remaining ingredients except the parsley. Pour over the chicken. Reduce the heat and simmer for 10 minutes, or until the chicken is no longer pink in the center. Serve sprinkled with the parsley.

COOK'S TIP on wheat germ

Wheat germ contains more nutrients per ounce than any other grain or vegetable and is very high in protein. Eat wheat germ as a cereal or sprinkle it over other cereals and other foods, such as casseroles, to add a nutty flavor, crunch, and nutrients. Store it in an airtight jar in the refrigerator.

PER SERVING

CALORIES 224
TOTAL FAT 5.5 g
  Saturated Fat 1.0 g
  Trans Fat 0.0 g
  Polyunsaturated Fat 1.0 g
  Monounsaturated Fat 3.0 g
CHOLESTEROL 66 mg
SODIUM 395 mg
CARBOHYDRATES 11 g
  Fiber 2 g
  Sugars 4 g
PROTEIN 31 g
DIETARY EXCHANGES
  ½ starch, 1 vegetable, 3 lean meat

chicken with one-minute tomato sauce

SERVES 4

Cooking the tomato sauce for only one minute lets the fresh taste prevail.

¼ cup dry white wine (regular or
   nonalcoholic)
½ teaspoon grated lemon zest
2 tablespoons fresh lemon juice
2 teaspoons dried oregano, crumbled
4 boneless, skinless chicken breast
   halves (about 4 ounces each), all
   visible fat discarded

TOMATO SAUCE
1 medium tomato, seeded, finely
   chopped
3 tablespoons capers, drained
2 tablespoons finely chopped red
   onion
1 tablespoon olive oil (extra virgin
   preferred)
2 medium garlic cloves, minced
¼ teaspoon salt

In a large shallow glass bowl, stir together the wine, lemon zest, lemon juice, and oregano. Add the chicken, turning to coat. Cover and refrigerate for 8 hours, turning occasionally. Remove the chicken from the marinade, letting the excess drip off. Discard the marinade.

In a large nonstick skillet, cook the chicken over medium-high heat for 3 minutes. Turn over. Cook for 2 to 3 minutes, or until no longer pink in the center. Transfer to plates.

In the same skillet, stir together the tomato sauce ingredients. Cook over medium-high heat for 1 minute, or until the tomato is tender, stirring constantly and scraping to dislodge any browned bits. Spoon over the chicken.

PER SERVING

CALORIES 181
TOTAL FAT 5.0 g
   Saturated Fat 1.0 g
   Trans Fat 0.0 g
   Polyunsaturated Fat 0.5 g
   Monounsaturated Fat 3.0 g
CHOLESTEROL 66 mg
SODIUM 413 mg
CARBOHYDRATES 4 g
   Fiber 1 g
   Sugars 1 g
PROTEIN 27 g
DIETARY EXCHANGES
   3 lean meat

chicken with bell peppers and mushrooms

SERVES 6

Add a whole-grain roll and tossed salad with one of our dressings (pages 136–139) for a dinner to please the whole family.

⅓ cup all-purpose flour
¼ teaspoon pepper
¼ teaspoon salt
6 boneless, skinless chicken breast halves (about 4 ounces each), all visible fat discarded, flattened to ¼-inch thickness
1 teaspoon olive oil and 1 teaspoon olive oil, divided use
8 ounces medium button mushrooms, quartered

1½ medium red bell peppers, cut into strips
3 medium garlic cloves, minced
1½ cups fat-free, low-sodium chicken broth, such as on page 43
⅓ cup white wine (regular or nonalcoholic)
2 tablespoons fresh lemon juice
½ cup sliced green onions
Snipped fresh parsley

In a medium shallow dish, stir together the flour, pepper, and salt. Dip one piece of chicken in the flour mixture, turning to coat and gently shaking off any excess. Transfer the chicken to a plate. Repeat with the remaining chicken.

In a large nonstick skillet, heat 1 teaspoon oil over medium-high heat, swirling to coat the bottom. Cook half the chicken for 3 to 4 minutes on each side, or until lightly brown on both sides. Transfer to a plate. Repeat with the remaining 1 teaspoon oil and chicken.

Put the mushrooms, bell pepper, and garlic in the skillet, stirring to combine. Reduce the heat to medium low. Cook, covered, for 7 to 9 minutes, stirring occasionally.

Pour in the broth, wine, and lemon juice. Add the chicken. Increase the heat to medium. Cook for 10 minutes, or until the sauce thickens slightly, stirring occasionally.

Stir in the green onions. Cook for 1 minute, or until the chicken is no longer pink in the center. Serve sprinkled with the parsley.

PER SERVING

CALORIES 200
TOTAL FAT 3.0 g
  Saturated Fat 0.5 g
  Trans Fat 0.0 g
  Polyunsaturated Fat 0.5 g
  Monounsaturated Fat 1.5 g
CHOLESTEROL 66 mg
SODIUM 185 mg
CARBOHYDRATES 10 g
  Fiber 2 g
  Sugars 2 g
PROTEIN 29 g
DIETARY EXCHANGES
  ½ starch,
  3 very lean meat

rosé chicken with artichoke hearts and mushrooms

SERVES 4

Delicious as is, this one-skillet dish is also great over whole-grain penne.

¼ cup all-purpose flour

4 boneless, skinless chicken breast halves (about 4 ounces each), all visible fat discarded

½ teaspoon olive oil and ½ teaspoon olive oil, divided use

8 ounces medium button mushrooms, quartered

2 medium garlic cloves, minced

1 9-ounce package frozen artichoke hearts, thawed and halved

1 14.5-ounce can no-salt-added diced tomatoes, undrained

¼ cup fat-free, low-sodium chicken broth, such as on page 43

¼ cup rosé wine or dry white wine (regular or nonalcoholic)

1 tablespoon fresh lemon juice

1 teaspoon dried oregano, crumbled

¼ teaspoon salt

½ cup thinly sliced green onions (green part only)

Put the flour in a shallow dish. Dip one piece of chicken in the flour, turning to coat and gently shaking off any excess. Transfer to a plate. Repeat with the remaining chicken.

In a large nonstick skillet, heat ½ teaspoon oil over medium heat, swirling to coat the bottom. Cook the chicken for 4 minutes on each side. Transfer to a plate.

Put the mushrooms, garlic, and remaining ½ teaspoon oil in the skillet, stirring to combine. Cook, covered, for 7 minutes.

Stir in the artichoke hearts. Cook, uncovered, for 1 to 2 minutes, or until the liquid has evaporated.

Stir in the chicken and remaining ingredients except the green onions. Cook for 10 minutes, or until the chicken is no longer pink in the center.

Stir in the green onions. Cook for 1 minute.

PER SERVING

CALORIES 247
TOTAL FAT 3.0 g
  Saturated Fat 0.5 g
  Trans Fat 0.0 g
  Polyunsaturated Fat 0.5 g
  Monounsaturated Fat 1.0 g
CHOLESTEROL 66 mg
SODIUM 305 mg
CARBOHYDRATES 21 g
  Fiber 8 g
  Sugars 5 g
PROTEIN 31 g
DIETARY EXCHANGES
  ½ starch, 3 vegetable,
  3 very lean meat

southwestern chicken

SERVES 6

Serve this spicy dish with warm corn tortillas and wedges of ice-cold watermelon. You can adjust the heat level by cutting back on the jalapeño (see Cook's Tip on Handling Hot Chile Peppers, page 21) and chili powder.

1½ cups orange, red, or yellow bell pepper strips, or a combination
2 teaspoons seeded and minced fresh jalapeño
½ cup diagonally sliced green onions
⅓ cup all-purpose flour
1½ teaspoons chili powder and 1 teaspoon chili powder, divided use
¼ teaspoon pepper and ¼ teaspoon pepper, divided use
¼ teaspoon salt

6 boneless, skinless chicken breast halves (about 4 ounces each), all visible fat discarded, flattened to ¼-inch thickness
1 teaspoon canola or corn oil and 1 teaspoon canola or corn oil, divided use
1 28-ounce can no-salt-added whole tomatoes, undrained
1 teaspoon grated lime zest

In a large nonstick skillet, cook the bell pepper and jalapeño over medium-high heat for 4 to 5 minutes, stirring occasionally.

Stir in the green onions. Cook for 1 minute. Transfer to a plate. Set aside.

In a medium shallow dish, stir together the flour, 1½ teaspoons chili powder, ¼ teaspoon pepper, and salt. Dip one piece of chicken in the mixture, turning to coat and gently shaking off any excess. Transfer to a plate. Repeat with the remaining chicken.

In a large nonstick skillet, heat 1 teaspoon oil over medium-high heat, swirling to coat the bottom. Cook half the chicken for 3 to 4 minutes on each side, or until lightly brown on both sides. Transfer to the plate with the bell pepper mixture. Repeat with the remaining 1 teaspoon oil and chicken.

Pour the tomatoes with liquid into the skillet, breaking up the tomatoes with a spoon. Stir in the remaining 1 teaspoon chili powder and remaining ¼ teaspoon pepper. Reduce the heat and simmer for 3 to 4 minutes.

Stir in the lime zest, bell pepper mixture, and chicken. Increase the heat to medium. Cook for 5 to 6 minutes, or until the chicken is no longer pink in the center and the mixture is heated through.

PER SERVING

CALORIES 203
TOTAL FAT 3.5 g
  Saturated Fat 0.5 g
  Trans Fat 0.0 g
  Polyunsaturated Fat 1.0 g
  Monounsaturated Fat 1.5 g
CHOLESTEROL 66 mg
SODIUM 199 mg
CARBOHYDRATES 14 g
  Fiber 3 g
  Sugars 5 g
PROTEIN 28 g
DIETARY EXCHANGES
  ½ starch, 2 vegetable, 3 very lean meat

burgundy chicken with mushrooms

SERVES 4

A sprinkling of fresh parsley and a drizzle of olive oil top chicken smothered in mushrooms with just a hint of burgundy.

4 boneless, skinless chicken breast halves (about 4 ounces each), all visible fat discarded
8 ounces button mushrooms, sliced
¼ cup finely chopped onion (yellow preferred)
2 medium garlic cloves, minced

2 tablespoons burgundy or other dry red wine (regular or nonalcoholic)
¼ teaspoon salt
2 tablespoons finely snipped fresh parsley
2 teaspoons olive oil (extra virgin preferred)

In a large nonstick skillet, cook the chicken over medium-high heat for 5 minutes. Turn over. Cook for 4 to 5 minutes, or until the chicken begins to brown on the outside and is no longer pink in the center. Transfer to a plate.

Scrape the skillet to dislodge any browned bits. Put the mushrooms, onion, garlic, and burgundy in the skillet, stirring to combine. Cook for 2 minutes.

Add the chicken and its juices. Cook for 5 minutes, or until the mushrooms just begin to brown slightly. Spoon the mushroom mixture over the chicken. Sprinkle with the salt and parsley. Drizzle with the oil.

PER SERVING

CALORIES 170
TOTAL FAT 4.0 g
  Saturated Fat 0.5 g
  Trans Fat 0.0 g
  Polyunsaturated Fat 0.5 g
  Monounsaturated Fat 2.0 g
CHOLESTEROL 66 mg
SODIUM 224 mg
CARBOHYDRATES 4 g
  Fiber 1 g
  Sugars 2 g
PROTEIN 28 g
DIETARY EXCHANGES
  3 lean meat

stuffed chicken with blue cheese

SERVES 4

Light the candles and impress everyone with this high-flavor, low-effort dish!

Cooking spray
1 10-ounce package frozen chopped spinach, thawed and squeezed dry
½ cup finely chopped onion
2 teaspoons dried basil, crumbled
⅛ teaspoon crushed red pepper flakes
2 ounces blue cheese, crumbled

4 boneless, skinless chicken breast halves (about 4 ounces each), all visible fat discarded, flattened to ¼-inch thickness
⅛ teaspoon salt
Pepper to taste
Paprika to taste

Preheat the oven to 400°F. Line a baking sheet with aluminum foil. Lightly spray the foil with cooking spray.

In a small bowl, stir together the spinach, onion, basil, and red pepper flakes.

Gently stir the blue cheese into the spinach mixture.

Place the chicken with the smooth side down on the baking sheet. Spoon the spinach mixture down the center of each breast. Press down on the mixture to pack. Roll the breasts jelly-roll style, placing them on a baking sheet with the seam side down. Lightly spray the chicken rolls with cooking spray. Sprinkle with the salt, pepper, and paprika.

Bake for 25 minutes, or until the chicken is no longer pink in the center.

PER SERVING

CALORIES 205
TOTAL FAT 6.0 g
  Saturated Fat 3.0 g
  Trans Fat 0.0 g
  Polyunsaturated Fat 0.5 g
  Monounsaturated Fat 1.5 g
CHOLESTEROL 76 mg
SODIUM 398 mg
CARBOHYDRATES 6 g
  Fiber 3 g
  Sugars 2 g
PROTEIN 32 g
DIETARY EXCHANGES
  1 vegetable,
  3½ lean meat

grilled lemon-sage chicken

SERVES 6

Fresh sage and rosemary impart a wonderfully different flavor to grilled chicken. Tomato halves and corn on the cob can grill along with the chicken.

MARINADE
- 1 teaspoon grated lemon zest
- ¼ cup fresh lemon juice
- ¼ cup chopped fresh sage leaves
- 1 tablespoon chopped fresh rosemary or 1 teaspoon dried rosemary, crushed
- 1 teaspoon olive oil
- 2 or 3 medium garlic cloves, minced

- 1 teaspoon black peppercorns, cracked
- ½ teaspoon salt

- 6 boneless, skinless chicken breast halves (about 4 ounces each), all visible fat discarded, flattened to ¼-inch thickness
- 6 lemon slices, cut in half (optional)
- Fresh sage leaves (optional)

In a large shallow glass dish, stir together the marinade ingredients. Add the chicken, turning to coat. Cover and refrigerate for 30 minutes to 8 hours, turning occasionally. Discard the marinade.

Preheat the grill on medium high.

Grill the chicken for 6 to 7 minutes on each side, or until no longer pink in the center. Serve garnished with the lemon slices and sage leaves.

PER SERVING

CALORIES 125
TOTAL FAT 1.5 g
  Saturated Fat 0.5 g
  Trans Fat 0.0 g
  Polyunsaturated Fat 0.5 g
  Monounsaturated Fat 0.5 g
CHOLESTEROL 66 mg
SODIUM 268 mg
CARBOHYDRATES 0 g
  Fiber 0 g
  Sugars 0 g
PROTEIN 26 g
DIETARY EXCHANGES
  3 very lean meat

sweet-spice glazed chicken

SERVES 4 (PLUS 4 CHICKEN BREAST HALVES RESERVED)

Allspice, cloves, sweet-and-sour sauce, and a hint of bourbon sumptuously jazz up the glaze in this recipe. The extra chicken you cook is the main ingredient in Island Chicken Salad with Fresh Mint (page 126), an easy dinner for later in the week.

Cooking spray

GLAZE

1 cup sweet-and-sour sauce

¼ cup bourbon

1 tablespoon plus 1 teaspoon Worcestershire sauce (lowest sodium available)

1 tablespoon plus 1 teaspoon canola or corn oil

1 tablespoon cider vinegar

½ teaspoon crushed red pepper flakes

½ teaspoon ground allspice

½ teaspoon ground cloves

8 boneless, skinless chicken breast halves (about 4 ounces each), all visible fat discarded

Preheat the broiler. Lightly spray the broiler pan and rack with cooking spray.

In a small bowl, whisk together the glaze ingredients. Pour half the glaze into a cup.

Put the chicken with the smooth side down on the broiler rack. Using a pastry brush, brush lightly with the glaze in the small bowl.

Broil the chicken 2 to 3 inches from the heat for 4 minutes. Turn over. Broil for 3 minutes. Using a clean pastry brush (to avoid cross-contamination), brush the chicken with the remaining glaze in the small bowl. Broil for 2 to 3 minutes, or until the chicken begins to brown and is no longer pink in the center.

Remove the chicken from the broiler. Using a clean pastry brush, brush with the glaze in the cup. Serve 4 pieces of chicken. Refrigerate the remaining pieces in an airtight container for use in Island Chicken Salad with Fresh Mint.

PER SERVING

CALORIES 209
TOTAL FAT 4.0 g
  Saturated Fat 0.5 g
  Trans Fat 0.0 g
  Polyunsaturated Fat 1.0 g
  Monounsaturated Fat 2.0 g
CHOLESTEROL 66 mg
SODIUM 88 mg
CARBOHYDRATES 10 g
  Fiber 0 g
  Sugars 9 g
PROTEIN 26 g
DIETARY EXCHANGES
  ½ carbohydrate,
  3 lean meat

maple-glazed chicken

SERVES 4 (PLUS 12 OUNCES CHICKEN RESERVED)

Making your own tangy, low-salt glaze is an easy, heart-healthy alternative to using bottled brands, which tend to be high in sodium. The reserved marinated and glazed chicken can be used as the base for Sesame Chicken and Vegetable Stir-Fry (page 247).

MARINADE
- ⅔ cup maple syrup
- ⅓ cup plain rice vinegar
- 2 tablespoons finely grated onion
- 2 tablespoons chili sauce
- 2 teaspoons Worcestershire sauce (lowest sodium available)
- 2 large garlic cloves, minced
- 1 teaspoon crushed red pepper flakes

- 1 teaspoon grated peeled gingerroot

- 2 pounds chicken tenders, all visible fat discarded
- 1 teaspoon olive oil and 1 teaspoon olive oil, divided use
- ½ teaspoon cornstarch
- ½ teaspoon pepper

In a large shallow glass dish, stir together the marinade ingredients. Set aside ⅓ cup for glaze. Add the chicken to the remaining marinade, turning to coat. Cover both the reserved glaze and the chicken in the marinade and refrigerate separately for 1 to 12 hours, turning the chicken occasionally. Discard the marinade.

In a large nonstick skillet, heat the oil over medium-high heat, swirling to coat the bottom. Place half the chicken in a single layer in the skillet, being careful not to crowd the pieces. Cook for 8 to 9 minutes, or until the chicken is no longer pink in the center, turning over once halfway through. Let cool slightly. Transfer to an airtight container. Cover and refrigerate for use within three to four days in Sesame Chicken and Vegetable Stir-Fry. Repeat the cooking process with the remaining oil and remaining chicken.

Meanwhile, stir the cornstarch into the reserved ⅓ cup glaze. Once the second batch of chicken is no longer pink in the center, stir in the glaze mixture to coat the chicken. Cook for 2 to 3 minutes, or until the glaze mixture is thickened, stirring constantly. Sprinkle with the pepper.

PER SERVING

CALORIES 186
TOTAL FAT 3.5 g
  Saturated Fat 0.5 g
  Trans Fat 0.0 g
  Polyunsaturated Fat 0.5 g
  Monounsaturated Fat 2.0 g
CHOLESTEROL 66 mg
SODIUM 136 mg
CARBOHYDRATES 11 g
  Fiber 0 g
  Sugars 9 g
PROTEIN 26 g
DIETARY EXCHANGES
  ½ carbohydrate,
  3 very lean meat

COOK'S TIP

If you don't plan to make the stir-fry, you can still enjoy this recipe. Use half the amount of chicken tenders and prepare half the marinade. Reserve ⅓ cup marinade as directed for the glaze and follow the instructions on page 240.

COOK'S TIP on chili sauce

Look in the condiment section of the supermarket for this tomato-based product, which is similar to ketchup with just a bit of spice. It is not the same as Asian condiments such as chili paste.

triple-pepper chicken

SERVES 4 (PLUS 4 CHICKEN BREAST HALVES RESERVED)

Turn up the heat with a spicy paste of cayenne, lemon pepper, and black pepper! This recipe makes enough for two meals—you can use the extra chicken for Cajun Chicken Salad (page 124).

8 boneless, skinless chicken breast halves (about 4 ounces each), all visible fat discarded

SPICE RUB

1 tablespoon chili powder

2 teaspoons fresh lime juice

1½ teaspoons dried oregano, crumbled

2 medium garlic cloves, minced

½ teaspoon salt-free lemon pepper

½ teaspoon pepper

½ teaspoon onion powder

½ teaspoon ground cumin

½ teaspoon Worcestershire sauce (lowest sodium available)

½ teaspoon no-salt-added liquid smoke

¼ teaspoon cayenne

_____

2 teaspoons canola or corn oil and 2 teaspoons canola or corn oil, divided use

Put the chicken in a large shallow glass dish.

In a small bowl, stir together the spice rub ingredients. Spread in a thin paste over the chicken. Cover the baking dish with plastic wrap and refrigerate for 30 minutes to 4 hours.

In a large nonstick skillet, heat 2 teaspoons oil over high heat, swirling to coat the bottom. Add half the chicken. Immediately reduce the heat to medium. Cook for 4 minutes. Turn over. Cook for 3 to 4 minutes, or until no longer pink in the center. Transfer to a plate. Cover to keep warm.

Increase the heat to high. Heat the remaining 2 teaspoons oil, swirling to coat the bottom. Repeat the cooking process with the remaining chicken. Serve 4 pieces of chicken. Refrigerate the remaining chicken in an airtight container for use in Cajun Chicken Salad.

TIME-SAVER

Although you can refrigerate the chicken with the rub for as little as 30 minutes, the flavor intensifies with longer marinating.

PER SERVING

CALORIES 152
TOTAL FAT 4.0 g
  Saturated Fat 0.5 g
  Trans Fat 0.0 g
  Polyunsaturated Fat 1.0 g
  Monounsaturated Fat 2.0 g
CHOLESTEROL 66 mg
SODIUM 85 mg
CARBOHYDRATES 1 g
  Fiber 1 g
  Sugars 0 g
PROTEIN 27 g
DIETARY EXCHANGES
  3 lean meat

lemon-cayenne chicken

SERVES 4

Cayenne and a tart lemon sauce provide the zip for these lightly breaded chicken breasts.

½ cup all-purpose flour
¾ teaspoon paprika
½ teaspoon salt
¼ teaspoon cayenne
⅛ teaspoon pepper
4 boneless, skinless chicken breast halves (about 4 ounces each), all visible fat discarded, flattened to ¼-inch thickness

1 tablespoon olive oil
3 tablespoons water
1 tablespoon light tub margarine
1 teaspoon fresh lemon juice
2 tablespoons finely snipped fresh parsley

In a shallow dish, stir together the flour, paprika, salt, cayenne, and pepper. Dip one piece of chicken in the mixture, turning to coat and gently shaking off any excess. Transfer to a plate. Repeat with the remaining chicken.

In a large nonstick skillet, heat the oil over medium-high heat for 1 minute, or until hot, swirling to coat the bottom. Cook the chicken for 3 to 4 minutes on each side, or until lightly browned on the outside and no longer pink in the center. Transfer to plates.

In the same skillet, stir together the water, margarine, and lemon juice, scraping to dislodge any browned bits. Bring the mixture to a boil. Boil for about 30 seconds, or until the sauce is slightly thickened. Drizzle over the chicken. Sprinkle with the parsley.

PER SERVING

CALORIES 224
TOTAL FAT 6.0 g
    Saturated Fat 1.0 g
    Trans Fat 0.0 g
    Polyunsaturated Fat 1.0 g
    Monounsaturated Fat 3.5 g
CHOLESTEROL 66 mg
SODIUM 389 mg
CARBOHYDRATES 13 g
    Fiber 1 g
    Sugars 0 g
PROTEIN 28 g
DIETARY EXCHANGES
    1 starch, 3 lean meat

spicy chicken and grits

SERVES 4

Cooks who watch both their time and their saturated fat intake love boneless, skinless chicken breasts—they're fast and easy to prepare and are low in saturated fat. This recipe uses a spice rub for lots of flavor, adds soothing grits, and keeps everything savory and moist with a chicken broth sauce.

1 cup uncooked quick-cooking grits
4 cups fat-free, low-sodium chicken broth and 2 cups fat-free low-sodium chicken broth, such as on page 43, divided use
1 teaspoon paprika
1 teaspoon sugar
½ teaspoon pepper

½ teaspoon cayenne
1 pound boneless, skinless chicken breasts, all visible fat discarded
1 tablespoon olive oil
1 small onion, minced
½ medium green bell pepper, minced
1 medium garlic clove, minced

Prepare the grits using the package directions, substituting 4 cups broth for the water and omitting the salt and margarine. Cover to keep warm and set aside.

Meanwhile, in a small bowl, stir together the paprika, sugar, pepper, and cayenne. Sprinkle over both sides of the chicken. Using your fingertips, gently press the mixture so it adheres to the chicken to coat. Transfer to a cutting board.

In a large nonstick skillet, heat the oil over medium heat, swirling to coat the bottom. Cook the onion, bell pepper, and garlic for 10 minutes, stirring occasionally.

Meanwhile, cut the chicken into thin slivers across the grain. Stir into the onion mixture. Increase the heat to high and cook for about 3 minutes, stirring frequently and scraping to dislodge any browned bits. Transfer to a large plate.

Pour the remaining 2 cups broth into the skillet. Boil rapidly for 5 minutes, or until the broth is reduced to ¾ cup.

Stir the chicken mixture into the broth. Cook for 2 minutes, or until heated through. Serve the chicken and broth over the grits.

PER SERVING

CALORIES 337
TOTAL FAT 5.5 g
  Saturated Fat 1.0 g
  Trans Fat 0.0 g
  Polyunsaturated Fat 1.0 g
  Monounsaturated Fat 3.0 g
CHOLESTEROL 66 mg
SODIUM 114 mg
CARBOHYDRATES 37 g
  Fiber 2 g
  Sugars 3 g
PROTEIN 33 g
DIETARY EXCHANGES
  2½ starch,
  3 very lean meat

sweet-and-sour baked chicken

SERVES 4

Serve this dish on a bed of fluffy brown rice so you don't miss a single drop of the fantastic sauce.

1 8.5-ounce can pineapple chunks in their own juice, drained with juice reserved
½ cup jellied cranberry sauce
2 tablespoons light brown sugar
2 tablespoons frozen orange juice concentrate
2 tablespoons plain rice vinegar or cider vinegar
1 tablespoon dry sherry

1 teaspoon soy sauce (lowest sodium available)
¼ teaspoon ground ginger
2 tablespoons cornstarch
2 tablespoons water
1 pound boneless, skinless chicken breasts, all visible fat discarded, cut into ½-inch strips
1 medium green bell pepper, cut into thin strips

Preheat the oven to 350°F.

Set the pineapple chunks aside. Pour the juice into a small saucepan. Put the saucepan over medium heat.

Whisk the cranberry sauce, brown sugar, orange juice concentrate, vinegar, sherry, soy sauce, and ginger into the juice.

Put the cornstarch in a cup. Add the water, stirring to dissolve. Whisk into the cranberry sauce mixture. Increase the heat to medium high. Cook for 3 to 4 minutes, or until thickened, whisking occasionally.

Stir in the pineapple chunks.

Put the chicken in an 8-inch square nonstick baking pan. Pour the cranberry sauce mixture over the chicken.

Bake, covered, for 35 minutes, or until the chicken is no longer pink in the center. Stir in the bell pepper. Baste with the sauce.

Bake, uncovered, for 5 minutes.

PER SERVING

CALORIES 275
TOTAL FAT 1.5 g
  Saturated Fat 0.5 g
  Trans Fat 0.0 g
  Polyunsaturated Fat 0.5 g
  Monounsaturated Fat 0.5 g
CHOLESTEROL 66 mg
SODIUM 123 mg
CARBOHYDRATES 37 g
  Fiber 2 g
  Sugars 27 g
PROTEIN 27 g
DIETARY EXCHANGES
  ½ fruit, 2 carbohydrate,
  3 very lean meat

chicken and mushroom stir-fry

SERVES 6

This colorful blend of vegetables and chicken is delicious over brown rice or whole-grain pasta.

1 tablespoon grated peeled gingerroot
1 tablespoon hot-pepper oil
3 medium garlic cloves, minced
1 teaspoon toasted sesame oil
1 pound boneless, skinless chicken breasts, all visible fat discarded, cut into 1-inch cubes
2 tablespoons light brown sugar
2 tablespoons fat-free, low-sodium chicken broth, such as on page 43

2 tablespoons dry sherry
1 tablespoon soy sauce (lowest sodium available)
1 tablespoon plain rice vinegar
1 teaspoon cornstarch
8 ounces button mushrooms, sliced
1 medium red bell pepper, diced
1 medium zucchini, diced
½ medium onion, sliced
9 cherry tomatoes, halved

In a large bowl, stir together the gingerroot, hot-pepper oil, garlic, and sesame oil. Add the chicken, stirring to coat. Cover and refrigerate for 15 minutes.

Meanwhile, in a small bowl, whisk together the brown sugar, broth, sherry, soy sauce, vinegar, and cornstarch until the sugar and cornstarch are dissolved. Set aside.

In a large nonstick skillet, cook the chicken with the marinade over medium-high heat for about 4 minutes, or until the chicken is lightly browned, stirring constantly.

Stir in the mushrooms, bell pepper, zucchini, and onion. Cook, covered, for 5 minutes, stirring occasionally.

Stir in the brown sugar mixture and tomatoes. Cook for 3 to 4 minutes, or until the sauce is thickened, stirring occasionally.

BEEF-VEGETABLE STIR-FRY
Substitute 1 pound thinly sliced sirloin or eye-of-round steak, all visible fat discarded, for the chicken.

COOK'S TIP on *mise en place*

Mise en place (meez ahn plahs) is the French term for having all your ingredients ready (measured, sliced, melted, and so on) before you start cooking. This advance preparation is very important when stir-frying because you must do the cooking steps very quickly.

sesame chicken and vegetable stir-fry

SERVES 4

Goodbye, take-out! This Asian-influenced dish, which uses the reserved chicken from Maple-Glazed Chicken (page 240), is loaded with vegetables and flavor. And, in the time it takes for fast food to be prepared and delivered to your home, you could be whipping up this healthier version in your own kitchen!

SAUCE
⅓ cup fat-free, low-sodium chicken broth, such as on page 43
2 teaspoons cornstarch
2 teaspoons soy sauce (lowest sodium available)
1 teaspoon grated peeled gingerroot
½ teaspoon crushed red pepper flakes
½ teaspoon toasted sesame oil
1 small garlic clove, minced

STIR-FRY
1 teaspoon canola or corn oil
4 to 5 ounces broccoli florets, broken into bite-size pieces

2 medium carrots, cut diagonally into ⅛-inch slices
1 8-ounce can sliced water chestnuts, drained
1 cup sliced green cabbage, slices ¼ to ½ inch wide
3 ounces snow peas, trimmed
2 medium green onions, sliced
12 ounces cooked chicken from Maple-Glazed Chicken, cut into bite-size pieces
½ cup canned mandarin oranges in juice, drained
½ teaspoon toasted sesame oil
1 teaspoon sesame seeds

In a small bowl, whisk together the sauce ingredients.

In a large nonstick skillet, heat the oil over medium-high heat, swirling to coat the bottom. Cook the broccoli and carrots for 3 minutes, stirring frequently.

Stir in the water chestnuts, cabbage, snow peas, and green onions. Cook for 3 minutes, stirring occasionally.

Stir in the chicken and sauce. Cook for 4 minutes, or until the chicken is heated through and the sauce is thickened, stirring frequently. Remove from the heat.

Stir in the mandarin oranges and sesame oil. Sprinkle with the sesame seeds.

COOK'S TIP

When you cook this dish at home, you avoid the heavy use of oil and MSG usually found in food at Asian restaurants—and you can personalize your stir-fries to your family's tastes by substituting vegetables they prefer.

PER SERVING

CALORIES 232
TOTAL FAT 5.0 g
  Saturated Fat 1.0 g
  Trans Fat 0.0 g
  Polyunsaturated Fat 1.5 g
  Monounsaturated Fat 2.0 g
CHOLESTEROL 66 mg
SODIUM 185 mg
CARBOHYDRATES 17 g
  Fiber 5 g
  Sugars 6 g
PROTEIN 30 g
DIETARY EXCHANGES
  3 vegetable, 3 lean meat

broiled chicken with hoisin-barbecue sauce

SERVES 4

Barbecue sauce acquires an Asian flair in this broiled chicken dish. Surprise your family by serving tonight's dinner on skewers and jazzing up the color and texture of the rice with green peas and turmeric.

Cooking spray
1 cup uncooked instant brown rice
½ teaspoon ground turmeric
HOISIN-BARBECUE SAUCE
¼ cup hoisin sauce
2 tablespoons barbecue sauce (lowest sodium available)
1 teaspoon sugar
1 teaspoon cider vinegar
¾ teaspoon Worcestershire sauce (lowest sodium available)

½ teaspoon grated peeled gingerroot
⅛ teaspoon cayenne
—
1 pound boneless, skinless chicken breasts, all visible fat discarded, cut into 1-inch cubes
1 cup frozen green peas, thawed and patted dry
¼ cup finely snipped fresh cilantro or parsley

If using long metal skewers, lightly spray 8 skewers with cooking spray. If using wooden skewers, soak 8 skewers for at least 10 minutes in cold water to prevent charring.

Preheat the broiler. Line the broiler pan with aluminum foil. Lightly spray the broiler rack with cooking spray.

Prepare the rice using the package directions, omitting the salt and margarine and adding the turmeric.

Meanwhile, in a small bowl, whisk together the sauce ingredients.

Thread the chicken on the skewers. Put on the broiler rack.

Broil 2 to 3 inches from the heat for 3 minutes. Turn the skewers over. Spoon the sauce over all. Broil for 3 minutes, or until the chicken is no longer pink in the center.

Stir the peas into the rice. Spoon onto a platter. Arrange the skewers on the rice. Sprinkle the cilantro over all.

PER SERVING

CALORIES 277
TOTAL FAT 2.5 g
  Saturated Fat 0.5 g
  Trans Fat 0.0 g
  Polyunsaturated Fat 0.5 g
  Monounsaturated Fat 0.5 g
CHOLESTEROL 66 mg
SODIUM 249 mg
CARBOHYDRATES 31 g
  Fiber 3 g
  Sugars 10 g
PROTEIN 30 g
DIETARY EXCHANGES
  1½ starch,
  ½ carbohydrate,
  3 very lean meat

CURRIED SWEET-AND-SOUR CHICKEN

Substitute ⅜ cup sweet-and-sour sauce for the hoisin and barbecue sauces, and substitute 1 teaspoon curry powder for the gingerroot.

COOK'S TIP on skewered food

For a dramatic presentation, poke skewered items into a large, heavy vegetable. Try a butternut squash, an eggplant, or a red cabbage. Slice a thin piece off the bottom so it will sit flat. Surround the vegetable with parsley sprigs or other fresh herbs. If you're serving fruit kebabs, stick them into a pineapple.

italian double toss

SERVES 4

You'll want to dig down deep with every forkful so you don't miss out on any of the layers.

4 ounces dried whole-grain penne
¾ cup cherry tomatoes, quartered
6 kalamata olives, coarsely chopped
2 tablespoons chopped fresh basil
1 tablespoon plus 1 teaspoon capers, drained
8 ounces boneless, skinless chicken breasts, all visible fat discarded, cut into thin strips
½ medium red bell pepper, cut into thin strips
1 small zucchini, cut lengthwise into eighths, then cut crosswise into 2-inch pieces
¼ medium onion, cut into 4 wedges
1 medium garlic clove, minced
Cooking spray
¼ teaspoon salt
1 tablespoon olive oil (extra virgin preferred)
2 ounces fat-free feta cheese, crumbled

Prepare the pasta using the package directions, omitting the salt. Drain well in a colander, reserving ¼ cup pasta water.

Meanwhile, in a small bowl, stir together the tomatoes, olives, basil, and capers. Set aside.

In a large nonstick skillet, cook the chicken over medium-high heat for 3 to 4 minutes, or until no longer pink in the center, stirring frequently. Transfer to a plate.

Put the bell pepper, zucchini, onion, and garlic in the skillet. Lightly spray the vegetables and garlic with cooking spray. Cook for 4 minutes, or until the bell pepper is just tender-crisp, stirring frequently.

Stir in the chicken, reserved pasta water, and salt.

Spoon the pasta onto a serving plate. Top with the chicken mixture, drizzle with the oil, then top with the tomato mixture. Sprinkle with the feta.

PER SERVING

CALORIES 247
TOTAL FAT 6.5 g
  Saturated Fat 1.0 g
  Trans Fat 0.0 g
  Polyunsaturated Fat 1.0 g
  Monounsaturated Fat 4.0 g
CHOLESTEROL 33 mg
SODIUM 587 mg
CARBOHYDRATES 27 g
  Fiber 5 g
  Sugars 5 g
PROTEIN 21 g
DIETARY EXCHANGES
  1½ starch, 1 vegetable,
  2½ lean meat

chicken stufino

SERVES 6

The taste of chicken slowly oven-braised in a tomato-rich sauce with vegetables will end your day on a comforting note.

1 tablespoon all-purpose flour
½ teaspoon salt
¼ teaspoon pepper, or to taste
1½ pounds boneless, skinless chicken breasts, all visible fat discarded, cut into large cubes
Olive oil spray
1 teaspoon olive oil
1 cup dry white wine (regular or nonalcoholic)
2 medium carrots, finely chopped
2 medium ribs of celery, finely chopped

1 medium onion, finely chopped
1 to 2 medium garlic cloves, minced
1 14.5-ounce can no-salt-added stewed tomatoes, crushed, undrained
12 ounces dried tricolor medium pasta shells
1 teaspoon dried Italian seasoning, crumbled
¼ cup snipped fresh parsley (optional)

In a small bowl, stir together the flour, salt, and pepper.

Put the chicken on a plate. Sprinkle with the flour mixture. Gently shake off any excess.

Lightly spray a Dutch oven or heavy ovenproof skillet with olive oil spray. Heat the oil over medium-high heat, swirling to coat the bottom. Cook the chicken for 2 to 3 minutes, stirring occasionally so it cooks evenly on all sides. (The chicken won't be done yet.)

Meanwhile, preheat the oven to 300°F.

Pour the wine into the Dutch oven, scraping to dislodge any browned bits. Stir in the carrots, celery, onion, and garlic. Cook for 2 to 3 minutes, stirring occasionally.

Stir in the tomatoes with liquid. Bring to a boil.

Bake, covered, for 1 hour, or until the chicken is tender and no longer pink in the center.

Meanwhile, prepare the pasta using the package directions, omitting the salt and adding the Italian seasoning. Drain well in a colander. Top with the chicken. Sprinkle with the parsley.

PER SERVING

CALORIES 414
TOTAL FAT 3.0 g
  Saturated Fat 0.5 g
  Trans Fat 0.0 g
  Polyunsaturated Fat 1.0 g
  Monounsaturated Fat 1.0 g
CHOLESTEROL 66 mg
SODIUM 310 mg
CARBOHYDRATES 53 g
  Fiber 4 g
  Sugars 8 g
PROTEIN 35 g
DIETARY EXCHANGES
  3 starch, 2 vegetable,
  3 very lean meat

baked chicken parmesan

SERVES 6

Chicken pieces take a double dip—in buttermilk and in seasoned bread crumbs—then bake on a rack so they stay crisp all over.

Cooking spray
4 slices whole-grain bread (lowest sodium available), processed into fine crumbs
¼ cup plus 2 tablespoons shredded or grated Parmesan cheese
1½ tablespoons finely snipped fresh parsley

1½ teaspoons paprika
¾ teaspoon garlic powder
½ teaspoon dried thyme, crumbled
½ cup low-fat buttermilk
6 boneless, skinless chicken breast halves (about 4 ounces each), all visible fat discarded

Preheat the oven to 450°F. Lightly spray a baking sheet and slightly smaller cooling rack with cooking spray. Put the rack on the baking sheet.

Put the bread crumbs in a shallow dish. Stir in the Parmesan, parsley, paprika, garlic powder, and thyme. Pour the buttermilk into a separate shallow dish. Set the dishes and baking sheet in a row, assembly-line fashion. Dip one piece of chicken in the buttermilk, turning to coat and gently shaking off the excess. Dip in the bread crumb mixture, turning to coat and gently shaking off any excess. Put the chicken on the rack. Repeat with the remaining chicken.

Bake for 15 minutes. Turn over. Bake for 10 minutes, or until no longer pink in the center.

PER SERVING

CALORIES 197
TOTAL FAT 3.5 g
  Saturated Fat 1.5 g
  Trans Fat 0.0 g
  Polyunsaturated Fat 0.5 g
  Monounsaturated Fat 1.0 g
CHOLESTEROL 70 mg
SODIUM 253 mg
CARBOHYDRATES 9 g
  Fiber 2 g
  Sugars 1 g
PROTEIN 31 g
DIETARY EXCHANGES
  ½ starch, 3 lean meat

orange microwave chicken with vegetables

SERVES 6

Use the speediness of microwave cooking to prepare this chicken dish—complete with vegetables—in a snap.

1½ pounds boneless, skinless chicken breasts, all visible fat discarded, cut into 1-inch cubes
2 cups fat-free, low-sodium chicken broth, such as on page 43
1 teaspoon light tub margarine
6 ounces small broccoli florets
1 large onion, finely chopped
1 large carrot, sliced

1 teaspoon grated orange zest
1 cup fresh orange juice
2 tablespoons cornstarch
2 tablespoons dry sherry
1 tablespoon soy sauce (lowest sodium available)
½ teaspoon garlic powder
¼ teaspoon salt
⅓ cup slivered almonds, dry-roasted

Put the chicken and broth in a microwaveable casserole dish. Cook, covered, on 50 percent power (medium) for 5 minutes. Stir. Cook for 5 minutes. Drain the chicken, reserving 1 cup broth for the sauce. Transfer the chicken to a plate.

In the same casserole dish, melt the margarine on 100 percent power (high) for 20 seconds. Stir in the broccoli, onion, and carrot. Cook, covered, on 100 percent power (high) for 7 minutes. Remove from the microwave. Return the chicken to the dish.

In a medium microwaveable bowl, stir together the reserved broth and remaining ingredients except the almonds. Cook on 100 percent power (high) for 5 minutes. Stir into the chicken mixture. Cook, covered, on 50 percent power (medium) for 3 minutes, or until the chicken is no longer pink in the center and the mixture is heated through. Serve sprinkled with the almonds.

PER SERVING

CALORIES 229
TOTAL FAT 5.0 g
    Saturated Fat 0.5 g
    Trans Fat 0.0 g
    Polyunsaturated Fat 1.0 g
    Monounsaturated Fat 2.5 g
CHOLESTEROL 66 mg
SODIUM 270 mg
CARBOHYDRATES 15 g
    Fiber 3 g
    Sugars 7 g
PROTEIN 30 g
DIETARY EXCHANGES
    1 carbohydrate,
    3 lean meat

couscous paella

SERVES 4

Chicken or turkey andouille sausage packs plenty of heat and spice in this easy and delicious skillet dinner. Even the cold leftovers are tempting when tossed with lettuce for a light lunch.

1 cup fat-free, low-sodium chicken broth, such as on page 43
¼ teaspoon saffron threads or ⅛ teaspoon crushed red pepper flakes
1½ teaspoons olive oil and 1½ teaspoons olive oil, divided use
1 small red bell pepper, chopped
1 small onion or 1 large shallot, chopped
1 medium garlic clove, minced
8 ounces boneless, skinless chicken breasts, all visible fat discarded, cut crosswise into ½-inch strips

8 large raw shrimp (about 4 ounces total), peeled, rinsed, and patted dry
3 ounces cooked chicken or turkey andouille sausage link, cut crosswise into ¼-inch pieces
8 cherry tomatoes, halved
1 cup frozen green peas
¾ cup uncooked whole-wheat couscous
¼ teaspoon salt
¼ teaspoon pepper
1 teaspoon grated lemon zest
1 medium lemon, quartered

In a small saucepan, combine the broth and saffron threads. Bring to a simmer over medium-high heat. Reduce the heat to low to keep the mixture heated until needed.

Meanwhile, in a large skillet or a Dutch oven, heat 1½ teaspoons oil over medium-high heat, swirling to coat the bottom. Cook the bell pepper, onion, and garlic for 3 minutes, or until the bell pepper is almost tender, stirring frequently. Push to the side.

Add the remaining 1½ teaspoons oil, swirling to coat the part of the skillet that is uncovered. Add the chicken, shrimp, and sausage. Cook for 3 to 5 minutes, or until the chicken is no longer pink in the center and the shrimp are pink on the outside, stirring and turning frequently.

Stir in the tomatoes and peas. Pour in the hot broth mixture. Bring to a boil, still on medium high.

Stir in the couscous. Remove from the heat and let sit, covered, for 5 minutes, or until the couscous absorbs the broth. Stir gently.

Sprinkle with the salt, pepper, and lemon zest. Stir. Serve garnished with lemon wedges to be squeezed to taste over the dish.

tandoori ginger chicken strips

SERVES 4

This dish features the flavors of tandoori chicken, India's version of barbecued chicken, from the yogurt marinade and traditional spices such as curry and cumin. The recipe gets its name from the clay oven called a tandoor in which the chicken is cooked.

¾ cup coarsely chopped onion
1 tablespoon coarsely chopped peeled gingerroot
2 medium garlic cloves
1 cup fat-free plain yogurt
2 tablespoons fresh lemon juice
1 tablespoon paprika
1½ teaspoons curry powder

½ teaspoon ground cumin
¼ teaspoon salt and ⅛ teaspoon salt, divided use
⅛ teaspoon cayenne
1 pound chicken tenders, all visible fat discarded
Cooking spray

In a food processor or blender, process the onion, ginger-root, and garlic until smooth.

Add the yogurt, lemon juice, paprika, curry powder, cumin, ¼ teaspoon salt, and cayenne. Process until well blended.

Put the chicken in a large shallow glass dish. Pour the yogurt mixture over the chicken. Turn several times to coat. Cover and refrigerate for 4 to 8 hours, turning occasionally.

Preheat the broiler. Lightly spray a broiler pan and rack with cooking spray.

Remove the chicken from the marinade, leaving what clings to the chicken. Discard the marinade in the dish.

Broil the chicken about 4 inches from the heat for 6 minutes on each side, or until no longer pink in the center. Sprinkle with the remaining ⅛ teaspoon salt.

COOK'S TIP

For peak flavor and texture, do not marinate longer than the suggested time.

PER SERVING

CALORIES 140
TOTAL FAT 1.5 g
   Saturated Fat 0.5 g
   Trans Fat 0.0 g
   Polyunsaturated Fat 0.5 g
   Monounsaturated Fat 0.5 g
CHOLESTEROL 66 mg
SODIUM 307 mg
CARBOHYDRATES 3 g
   Fiber 0 g
   Sugars 2 g
PROTEIN 27 g
DIETARY EXCHANGES
   3 very lean meat

chicken gyros with tzatziki sauce

SERVES 4

Chicken tenders are anything but ordinary when you season them with freshly squeezed lemon juice, olive oil, and spices and serve them with Greece's well-loved yogurt-based sauce.

1 pound chicken tenders, all visible fat discarded
1 teaspoon dried oregano, crumbled
1 teaspoon ground cumin
1 teaspoon onion powder
½ teaspoon paprika
⅛ teaspoon cayenne
⅛ teaspoon salt
3 tablespoons fresh lemon juice
2 teaspoons olive oil
2 medium garlic cloves, minced
Cooking spray

TZATZIKI SAUCE
⅓ cup finely chopped peeled cucumber
⅓ cup fat-free plain yogurt
3 tablespoons fat-free sour cream
2 teaspoons snipped fresh dillweed
2 teaspoons fresh lemon juice
1 medium garlic clove, finely chopped
⅛ teaspoon salt
⅛ teaspoon pepper

Put the chicken in a medium glass bowl.

In a small shallow glass dish, stir together the oregano, cumin, onion powder, paprika, cayenne, and ⅛ teaspoon salt. Sprinkle over the chicken. Using your fingertips, press the mixture so it adheres to the chicken.

In the same small dish, stir together 3 tablespoons lemon juice, oil, and 2 minced garlic cloves. Pour over the chicken. Using your fingertips, rub into the chicken. Cover the bowl and refrigerate for 10 minutes.

Meanwhile, preheat the broiler. Line a baking sheet with aluminum foil. Lightly spray with cooking spray.

Remove the chicken from the marinade, discarding the marinade. Transfer the chicken to the baking sheet.

Broil the chicken 4 to 5 inches from the heat for 8 minutes. Turn over. Broil for 3 minutes, or until no longer pink in the center.

Meanwhile, in a small bowl, stir together the sauce ingredients. Serve over the chicken.

PER SERVING

CALORIES 157
TOTAL FAT 1.5 g
  Saturated Fat 0.5 g
  Trans Fat 0.0 g
  Polyunsaturated Fat 0.5 g
  Monounsaturated Fat 0.5 g
CHOLESTEROL 68 mg
SODIUM 246 mg
CARBOHYDRATES 5 g
  Fiber 1 g
  Sugars 3 g
PROTEIN 29 g
DIETARY EXCHANGES
  ½ carbohydrate,
  3 very lean meat

SERVES 6

  1 recipe Chicken Gyros with Tzatziki Sauce (page 256)
  6 6-inch whole-grain pita breads (lowest sodium available)
  2 cups bite-size pieces romaine (about 4 medium leaves)
  2 medium tomatoes, sliced
  ½ cup thinly sliced red onion

Prepare the recipe on page 256 but don't top the chicken with the sauce. Wrap 2 pitas in damp paper towels. Microwave on 100 percent power (high) for 30 seconds, or just until soft and warm. Repeat with the remaining pitas. Spoon the romaine, then the chicken, tomatoes, and onions on top of one-half of each pita. Top that half with the sauce. Fold the bread in half.

COOK'S TIP on tzatziki sauce

This classic Greek sauce is also a great dip. Serve it with baked whole-grain pita triangles or raw veggie dippers.

PER SERVING

CHICKEN GYRO PITAS
CALORIES 278
TOTAL FAT 3.0 g
  Saturated Fat 0.5 g
  Trans Fat 0.0 g
  Polyunsaturated Fat 1.0 g
  Monounsaturated Fat 0.5 g
CHOLESTEROL 45 mg
SODIUM 487 mg
CARBOHYDRATES 40 g
  Fiber 6 g
  Sugars 5 g
PROTEIN 26 g
DIETARY EXCHANGES
  2½ starch,
  2½ very lean meat

boneless buffalo wings

SERVES 4

If it's a challenge to choose between the sauce coatings for these "wings," make a half batch of each sauce and try both!

Olive oil spray
¼ cup all-purpose flour
1 teaspoon salt-free all-purpose seasoning blend
8 chicken breast tenders (about 1 pound), all visible fat discarded, cut in half crosswise

HOT-PEPPER SAUCE COATING
1 tablespoon light tub margarine
1 teaspoon red hot-pepper sauce

OR

BARBECUE SAUCE COATING
¼ cup barbecue sauce (lowest sodium available)
1 teaspoon soy sauce (lowest sodium available)
½ teaspoon toasted sesame oil

Preheat the oven to 350°F. Lightly spray a baking sheet with olive oil spray.

In a large shallow dish, stir together the flour and seasoning blend. Add several chicken tenders, turning to coat and gently shaking off any excess. Repeat in batches with the remaining chicken. Arrange in a single layer on the baking sheet. Lightly spray the chicken with olive oil spray.

Bake for 20 to 25 minutes, or lightly browned on the outside and no longer pink in the center.

Meanwhile, in a medium bowl, stir together the ingredients for the coating of your choice. Add the cooked chicken. Toss to coat.

PER SERVING

WITH HOT-PEPPER SAUCE
CALORIES 164
TOTAL FAT 2.5 g
  Saturated Fat 0.5 g
  Trans Fat 0.0 g
  Polyunsaturated Fat 0.5 g
  Monounsaturated Fat 1.0 g
CHOLESTEROL 66 mg
SODIUM 104 mg
CARBOHYDRATES 6 g
  Fiber 0 g
  Sugars 0 g
PROTEIN 27 g
DIETARY EXCHANGES
  ½ starch, 3 very lean meat

PER SERVING

WITH BARBECUE SAUCE
CALORIES 189
TOTAL FAT 2.0 g
  Saturated Fat 0.5 g
  Trans Fat 0.0 g
  Polyunsaturated Fat 0.5 g
  Monounsaturated Fat 0.5 g
CHOLESTEROL 66 mg
SODIUM 211 mg
CARBOHYDRATES 13 g
  Fiber 0 g
  Sugars 6 g
PROTEIN 27 g
DIETARY EXCHANGES
  ½ starch, ½ carbohydrate, 3 very lean meat

chicken and barley chili

SERVES 4

Dig into a bowl of this chili on a winter night and you'll feel like you've pulled on a cozy sweater. Complete your menu with a salad and Jalapeño Cheese Bread (page 524).

Olive oil spray
2 teaspoons olive oil
1 pound boneless, skinless chicken breasts, all visible fat discarded, cut into ½-inch cubes
1 small onion, chopped
1 small green bell pepper, chopped
1 medium fresh jalapeño, seeds and ribs discarded, minced
3 medium garlic cloves, minced
2 tablespoons chili powder

2 teaspoons ground cumin
3 cups water
1 14.5-ounce can no-salt-added diced tomatoes, undrained
1¾ cups fat-free, low-sodium chicken broth, such as on page 43
½ cup uncooked pearl barley
2 tablespoons yellow cornmeal
¼ cup snipped fresh cilantro
1 tablespoon fresh lime juice

Lightly spray a stockpot with olive oil spray. Add the oil, swirling to coat the bottom. Cook the chicken over medium-high heat for 8 minutes, or until lightly browned on all sides, stirring frequently.

Stir in the onion, bell pepper, jalapeño, and garlic. Cook for 3 minutes, or until the onion and bell pepper are soft, stirring occasionally.

Stir in the chili powder and cumin. Stir in the water, tomatoes with liquid, broth, and barley. Increase the heat to high and bring to a boil. Reduce the heat and simmer, covered, for 30 minutes, or until the barley is tender yet firm to the bite.

Stir in the cornmeal. Increase the heat to medium high and cook, uncovered, for 3 to 5 minutes, or until the chili is thickened, stirring occasionally. Remove from the heat and stir in the cilantro and lime juice.

BEAN AND BARLEY CHILI

To make a vegetarian version of the chili, omit the chicken and use low-sodium vegetable broth, such as on page 44, in place of chicken broth. Stir in one 15.5-ounce can no-salt-added black beans, pinto beans, or kidney beans, rinsed and drained, when you add the barley. Proceed as directed with the recipe.

PER SERVING

CALORIES 309
TOTAL FAT 5.0 g
  Saturated Fat 1.0 g
  Trans Fat 0.0 g
  Polyunsaturated Fat 1.0 g
  Monounsaturated Fat 2.0 g
CHOLESTEROL 66 mg
SODIUM 177 mg
CARBOHYDRATES 36 g
  Fiber 8 g
  Sugars 7 g
PROTEIN 32 g
DIETARY EXCHANGES
  1½ starch, 2 vegetable,
  3 lean meat

PER SERVING

BEAN AND BARLEY CHILI
CALORIES 275
TOTAL FAT 3.5 g
  Saturated Fat 0.5 g
  Trans Fat 0.0 g
  Polyunsaturated Fat 0.5 g
  Monounsaturated Fat 2.0 g
CHOLESTEROL 0 mg
SODIUM 96 mg
CARBOHYDRATES 52 g
  Fiber 13 g
  Sugars 10 g
PROTEIN 11 g
DIETARY EXCHANGES
  2½ starch, 2 vegetable
  1 very lean meat

slow-cooker white chili

SERVES 6

You can easily stretch this cook-while-you-work dish to serve more people by ladling it over brown rice.

CHILI

1 pound dried navy or Great Northern beans, sorted for stones and shriveled beans and rinsed

1 pound skinless chicken thighs with bone, all visible fat discarded

6 cups fat-free, low-sodium chicken broth, such as on page 43

2 4-ounce cans chopped green chiles, drained

1 medium onion, chopped

4 medium garlic cloves, minced

1 medium fresh jalapeño, seeds and ribs discarded, minced

2 teaspoons ground cumin

2 teaspoons dried oregano, crumbled

¼ teaspoon cayenne

⅛ to ¼ teaspoon ground cloves

¼ cup plus 2 tablespoons salsa (lowest sodium available), such as Salsa Cruda (page 508)

¼ cup plus 2 tablespoons fat-free sour cream

In the order listed, put the chili ingredients in a 4- or 4½-quart slow cooker. Don't stir. Cook, covered, on low for 8 to 10 hours, or until the beans and chicken are tender.

Transfer the chicken to a cutting board. Discard the bones. Separate the chicken into bite-size pieces. Stir the chicken into the chili. Serve topped with the salsa and sour cream.

PER SERVING

CALORIES 388
TOTAL FAT 5.5 g
  Saturated Fat 1.5 g
  Trans Fat 0.0 g
  Polyunsaturated Fat 1.5 g
  Monounsaturated Fat 1.5 g
CHOLESTEROL 41 mg
SODIUM 279 mg
CARBOHYDRATES 55 g
  Fiber 20 g
  Sugars 7 g
PROTEIN 31 g
DIETARY EXCHANGES
  3½ starch,
  3 very lean meat

chipotle chicken wraps

SERVES 6

Smoky chicken saved from Mexican Chicken and Vegetables with Chipotle Peppers (page 216) is rolled in flour tortillas with sour cream, red onion, cilantro, black olives, and freshly squeezed lime juice.

4 cooked chicken breast halves from Mexican Chicken and Vegetables with Chipotle Peppers
1 cup tomato mixture from Mexican Chicken and Vegetables with Chipotle Peppers
6 8-inch fat-free flour tortillas (lowest sodium available)

½ cup fat-free sour cream
½ cup finely chopped red onion
¼ cup snipped fresh cilantro (optional)
12 medium black olives, quartered
Pepper to taste
Fresh lime juice to taste

In a small saucepan, warm the reserved chicken and tomato sauce mixture over medium heat for 10 minutes, or until heated through, stirring occasionally.

Using the package directions, warm the tortillas.

To assemble, layer as follows down the center of each tortilla: chicken mixture (use a slotted spoon), sour cream, onion, cilantro, olives, pepper, and lime juice. Fold both sides of each tortilla to the center. Starting from the bottom, roll each wrap to the top to enclose the filling.

PER SERVING

CALORIES 271
TOTAL FAT 3.0 g
  Saturated Fat 0.5 g
  Trans Fat 0.0 g
  Polyunsaturated Fat 0.5 g
  Monounsaturated Fat 1.0 g
CHOLESTEROL 47 mg
SODIUM 587 mg
CARBOHYDRATES 36 g
  Fiber 4 g
  Sugars 6 g
PROTEIN 24 g
DIETARY EXCHANGES
  2 starch, 1 vegetable,
  2½ very lean meat

chicken-spinach manicotti

SERVES 6

This recipe is a great way to use leftover cooked chicken.

Cooking spray
12 dried manicotti shells

FILLING

2 cups diced cooked skinless chicken breasts, cooked without salt
1½ cups fat-free cottage cheese
1 10-ounce package frozen chopped spinach, thawed and squeezed dry
¾ cup egg substitute
⅓ cup shredded or grated Parmesan cheese
2 teaspoons dried basil, crumbled
Pepper to taste

SAUCE

1 teaspoon olive oil
1 large onion, chopped
3 medium garlic cloves, minced
1 14.5-ounce can no-salt-added diced tomatoes, undrained
1 cup water
1 6-ounce can no-salt-added tomato paste
1 teaspoon dried Italian seasoning, crumbled
1 teaspoon dried basil, crumbled

3 tablespoons shredded or grated Parmesan cheese

Lightly spray a 13 x 9 x 2-inch baking pan with cooking spray. Set aside.

Prepare the pasta using the package directions, omitting the salt. Drain well in a colander. Set aside.

Meanwhile, in a large bowl, stir together the filling ingredients. Set aside.

In a medium saucepan, heat the oil over medium-high heat, swirling to coat the bottom. Cook the onion for about 3 minutes, or until soft, stirring occasionally.

Stir in the garlic. Cook for 1 minute, stirring occasionally.

Stir in the remaining sauce ingredients. Crush the tomatoes slightly. Bring to a simmer. Reduce the heat and simmer for 8 to 10 minutes. Spread 1 cup sauce in the pan.

Meanwhile, preheat the oven to 375°F.

Gently stuff the shells with the filling. Place them on the sauce. Spoon the remaining sauce over the shells. Sprinkle with the remaining 3 tablespoons Parmesan.

Bake for 30 minutes, or until heated through.

PER SERVING

CALORIES 359
TOTAL FAT 6.0 g
  Saturated Fat 2.0 g
  Trans Fat 0.0 g
  Polyunsaturated Fat 1.0 g
  Monounsaturated Fat 2.0 g
CHOLESTEROL 47 mg
SODIUM 527 mg
CARBOHYDRATES 43 g
  Fiber 6 g
  Sugars 12 g
PROTEIN 35 g
DIETARY EXCHANGES
  2 starch, 3 vegetable,
  3 lean meat

MICROWAVE METHOD

Prepare the shells as directed. In a 1-quart microwaveable bowl, stir together the oil, onion, and garlic. Microwave on 100 percent power (high) for 3 minutes. Stir in the remaining sauce ingredients. Cook on 50 percent power (medium) for 10 minutes. Put half the sauce in a microwaveable baking dish. Fill the shells as directed. Place them on the sauce. Cover with the remaining sauce. Top with 3 tablespoons Parmesan. Microwave, covered and vented, on 50 percent power (medium) for 25 minutes. Let stand, covered, for 5 minutes.

spaghetti with grilled chicken, mixed bell peppers, and zucchini

SERVES 4

A bit of apple juice gives a subtle sweetness to this colorful all-in-one dish.

8 ounces dried whole-grain spaghetti

1 cup unsweetened apple juice

3 or 4 medium garlic cloves, finely minced

¼ teaspoon crushed red pepper flakes, or to taste

8 to 10 fresh basil leaves

2 boneless, skinless chicken breast halves (about 4 ounces each), all visible fat discarded

1 medium zucchini, quartered lengthwise

1 medium red bell pepper, quartered lengthwise

1 medium green bell pepper, quartered lengthwise

1 medium yellow bell pepper, quartered lengthwise

1 small red onion, cut into ¼-inch wedges

Cooking spray

1 teaspoon dried Italian seasoning, crumbled

2 ounces fat-free feta cheese, crumbled

¼ teaspoon salt

Preheat the grill on medium high.

Prepare the pasta using the package directions, omitting the salt. Drain well in a colander.

As soon as you put the water on to boil, put the apple juice, garlic, and red pepper flakes in a small saucepan and stir together. Cook over high heat for about 5 minutes, or until reduced by half. Remove from the heat. Set aside.

Meanwhile, stack the basil leaves in 2 stacks, then roll up tightly from the tip end to the base. Cut crosswise into very thin strips. Transfer to a large serving bowl. Set aside.

Put the chicken on a small plate. Put the zucchini and bell peppers on a large rimmed baking sheet. Tear off an 18-inch-long piece of aluminum foil. Fold in half crosswise, with the shiny side in, then roll up the edges to make a slightly raised rim. Put the onion on the foil. Spray the chicken, zucchini, bell peppers, and onion with cooking spray, turning to coat both sides. Sprinkle with the Italian seasoning.

PER SERVING

CALORIES 355
TOTAL FAT 2.5 g
 Saturated Fat 0.5 g
 Trans Fat 0.0 g
 Polyunsaturated Fat 1.0 g
 Monounsaturated Fat 0.5 g
CHOLESTEROL 33 mg
SODIUM 414 mg
CARBOHYDRATES 60 g
 Fiber 9 g
 Sugars 14 g
PROTEIN 25 g
DIETARY EXCHANGES
 3 starch, 2 vegetable,
 ½ fruit, 2 very lean meat

Place the chicken, zucchini, bell peppers, and foil with the onions on the grill grate. Handle carefully; the spray will make them quite slippery. Cook, covered, for 10 minutes, or until the chicken is no longer pink in the center and the zucchini and bell peppers are just tender, turning or stirring halfway through. If the food is cooking too fast, adjust the temperature as needed.

Slice the zucchini and peppers crosswise into ¼-inch pieces. Add to the basil. Add the onions, covering to keep the mixture warm. Cut each piece of chicken in half lengthwise, then cut crosswise into ¼-inch strips. Add to the bowl. Add the feta, salt, and the apple juice mixture. Toss gently with tongs. Serve over the pasta.

linguine with chicken and artichokes

SERVES 4

Artichokes add flair to this simple pasta dish. You don't need to thaw them in advance—just cook the frozen artichokes along with the onion and sauce.

4 ounces dried whole-grain linguine
12 ounces boneless, skinless chicken breasts, all visible fat discarded, cut into 1-inch cubes
¼ teaspoon salt
2 teaspoons olive oil
2 medium garlic cloves, finely chopped
12 ounces frozen artichoke quarters

1 cup sliced onion
½ teaspoon crushed red pepper flakes
2 teaspoons cornstarch
¾ cup fat-free, low-sodium chicken broth, such as on page 43
½ teaspoon dried rosemary, crushed
⅓ cup fat-free half-and-half
¼ cup shredded or grated Parmesan cheese

Prepare the pasta using the package directions, omitting the salt and cooking for about 2 minutes less than instructed, until almost tender. Drain well in a colander. Cover and set aside.

Put the chicken in a medium bowl. Sprinkle with the salt.

In a small bowl, stir together the oil and garlic. Using your fingertips, rub into the chicken.

Heat a large nonstick skillet over medium-high heat for 2 minutes. Cook the chicken for about 3 minutes, or until lightly browned on the outside and no longer pink in the center, stirring constantly. Reduce the heat to medium.

Stir in the artichokes and onion. Sprinkle with the red pepper flakes. Cook for 7 minutes, or until the onion begins to turn golden and the artichokes soften and turn light brown in spots, stirring frequently.

Meanwhile, put the cornstarch in a small bowl. Pour in the broth, stirring to dissolve. Stir in the rosemary. When the artichokes and onion have cooked, pour the broth mixture into the skillet. Bring to a simmer, still over medium heat, stirring frequently. Reduce the heat and simmer for 3 minutes, or until the sauce begins to thicken, stirring frequently.

Stir in the half-and-half. Return to a simmer.

Stir in the pasta. Return to a simmer and simmer for 1 to 2 minutes, or until heated through. Serve topped with the Parmesan.

PER SERVING

CALORIES 311
TOTAL FAT 5.5 g
  Saturated Fat 1.5 g
  Trans Fat 0.0 g
  Polyunsaturated Fat 1.0 g
  Monounsaturated Fat 2.5 g
CHOLESTEROL 53 mg
SODIUM 358 mg
CARBOHYDRATES 36 g
  Fiber 10 g
  Sugars 4 g
PROTEIN 29 g
DIETARY EXCHANGES
  1½ starch, 2 vegetable,
  3 lean meat

chicken curry in a hurry

SERVES 4

Serve this quick and easy hit over brown rice or rice pilaf. Add a splash of color by offering small bowls of toppings such as sliced green onions or Cranberry Chutney (page 487).

Cooking spray	1 cup water
1 teaspoon canola or corn oil	1 medium Granny Smith apple, finely
2 cups diced cooked skinless chicken	chopped
or turkey breast, cooked without salt	1 cup fat-free, low-sodium chicken
8 ounces button mushrooms, thinly	broth, such as on page 43
sliced	¾ cup fat-free milk
1 small onion, chopped	¼ cup snipped fresh parsley
3 tablespoons all-purpose flour	1½ teaspoons curry powder

Lightly spray a Dutch oven with cooking spray. Heat the oil over medium-high heat, swirling to coat the bottom. Cook the chicken, mushrooms, and onion for 4 to 5 minutes, or until the chicken is warm and the mushrooms and onion are soft, stirring occasionally.

Put the flour in a small bowl. Add the water, whisking to dissolve. Pour into the pot.

Stir in the remaining ingredients. Bring to a boil over medium-high heat, stirring constantly. Reduce the heat and simmer for 3 minutes, or until the apple pieces are tender-crisp, stirring constantly.

COOK'S TIP on curry powder

If you feel like experimenting and making your own signature curry powder, combine ½ teaspoon each of the ground forms of cardamom, cinnamon, cloves, and turmeric (the last gives curry powder its characteristic yellow color). Then add small smounts to taste of any other spices commonly used in curry powder, such as chiles, coriander, cumin, fennel seed, fenugreek, mace, nutmeg, red and black pepper, poppy and sesame seeds, saffron, and tamarind.

PER SERVING

CALORIES 222
TOTAL FAT 5.0 g
  Saturated Fat 1.0 g
  Trans Fat 0.0 g
  Polyunsaturated Fat 1.0 g
  Monounsaturated Fat 2.0 g
CHOLESTEROL 60 mg
SODIUM 88 mg
CARBOHYDRATES 18 g
  Fiber 3 g
  Sugars 10 g
PROTEIN 27 g
DIETARY EXCHANGES
  ½ starch, ½ fruit,
  3 lean meat

cider-glazed turkey tenderloin with harvest vegetables

SERVES 4

Here's a turkey dinner with heart-healthy fixings that's easy to prepare and roasts while you're busy elsewhere. It's like Thanksgiving without the fuss—or all the extra calories!

Cooking spray
1 1-pound turkey tenderloin, all visible fat discarded
1 teaspoon olive oil and 2 teaspoons olive oil, divided use
1 medium carrot, cut into 1-inch pieces
1 medium parsnip, cut into 1-inch pieces
½ medium onion, cut into 1-inch wedges
¼ small acorn squash, peeled, seeds and strings discarded, cut in 1½-inch cubes
½ teaspoon dried thyme, crumbled
¼ teaspoon salt
¼ teaspoon pepper
¼ teaspoon ground nutmeg
1 cup unsweetened apple cider

Preheat the oven to 425°F.

Line a 13 x 9 x 2-inch baking pan with aluminum foil. Lightly spray the foil with cooking spray. Place the turkey in the pan. Brush the top of the turkey with 1 teaspoon oil.

In a large bowl, combine the carrot, parsnip, onion, and squash. Drizzle with the remaining 2 teaspoons oil. Stir to coat. Place around the turkey.

In a small bowl, stir together the remaining ingredients except the cider. Sprinkle over the turkey and vegetables.

Roast for 30 minutes.

Meanwhile, in a small saucepan, bring the cider to a boil over medium-high heat. Boil for 10 minutes, or until reduced to about ½ cup. Remove from the heat.

Remove the baking pan from the oven after 30 minutes. Stir the vegetables. Pour the cider over the turkey and vegetables. Roast for 10 minutes, or until the turkey is no longer pink in the center and registers 165°F on an instant-read thermometer and the vegetables are tender.

PER SERVING

CALORIES 228
TOTAL FAT 4.0 g
  Saturated Fat 0.5 g
  Trans Fat 0.0 g
  Polyunsaturated Fat 0.5 g
  Monounsaturated Fat 2.5 g
CHOLESTEROL 75 mg
SODIUM 227 mg
CARBOHYDRATES 19 g
  Fiber 3 g
  Sugars 11 g
PROTEIN 28 g
DIETARY EXCHANGES
  2 vegetable, ½ fruit,
  3 lean meat

Remove from the oven. Cover the turkey loosely with aluminum foil. Let stand for 10 minutes. Cut the turkey crosswise into slices about ¾ inch thick. Serve with the vegetables.

COOK'S TIP

Peel and cut the remaining acorn squash into cubes. Cook them in a small amount of water in a covered saucepan over medium-high heat for 15 to 20 minutes, or until tender. Or preheat the oven to 350°F, spread the squash cubes on a baking sheet, lightly spray them with cooking spray, and bake for 25 to 35 minutes, or until tender when tested with the tip of a sharp knife or a fork. Sprinkle the cooked squash with ground ginger or ground nutmeg or brush with unsweetened apple cider or orange juice. If desired, mash the cooked squash, spoon it into freezer containers, and freeze for up to 12 months. The squash is a wonderful accompaniment for main dishes such as roast chicken and grilled pork chops, or a nice addition to many soups and stews.

five-spice turkey medallions

SERVES 4

With its cinnamon, cloves, fennel, anise, and pepper blend, five-spice powder packs a pungent flavor punch.

2 teaspoons toasted sesame oil
1 teaspoon soy sauce and 1 teaspoon soy sauce (lowest sodium available), divided use
1½ teaspoons five-spice powder
1 pound turkey tenderloins, cut crosswise into ¼-inch slices

8 ounces snow peas, trimmed and halved
½ cup chopped red bell pepper
¼ cup slivered red onion
3 tablespoons plain rice vinegar
1 tablespoon grated peeled gingerroot
1 medium garlic clove, minced

In a medium bowl, stir together the oil, 1 teaspoon soy sauce, and five-spice powder.

Add the turkey, stirring to coat.

In a large nonstick skillet, cook the turkey mixture over medium heat for about 5 minutes, or until the turkey is no longer pink in the center, stirring occasionally. Transfer to a plate. Cover to keep warm.

In the same skillet, stir together the snow peas, bell pepper, onion, vinegar, gingerroot, and garlic. Cook over medium heat for 4 to 5 minutes, or until the snow peas are tender-crisp, stirring occasionally.

Stir in the remaining 1 teaspoon soy sauce. Serve the turkey over the snow pea mixture.

PER SERVING

CALORIES 185
TOTAL FAT 3.5 g
  Saturated Fat 0.5 g
  Trans Fat 0.0 g
  Polyunsaturated Fat 1.0 g
  Monounsaturated Fat 1.0 g
CHOLESTEROL 70 mg
SODIUM 125 mg
CARBOHYDRATES 8 g
  Fiber 2 g
  Sugars 3 g
PROTEIN 30 g
DIETARY EXCHANGES
  2 vegetable, 3 lean meat

turkey rolls with garden pesto

SERVES 4

Boldly colored pesto and a honey and soy sauce glaze are great complements to these turkey rolls.

Cooking spray	2 tablespoons shredded or grated
GARDEN PESTO	Parmesan cheese
½ cup packed fresh basil	
1 small tomato, peeled, seeded, and coarsely chopped	2 8-ounce turkey tenderloins, halved lengthwise
1 tablespoon pine nuts, dry-roasted	1 tablespoon honey
1 large garlic clove, minced	1 tablespoon soy sauce (lowest sodium available)

Preheat the oven to 350°F. Lightly spray an 8-inch square baking pan with cooking spray.

In a food processor or blender, process the pesto ingredients except the Parmesan until nearly smooth. Stir in the Parmesan.

Spread 1 rounded tablespoon pesto mixture on a piece of turkey. Roll up from one short end. Repeat with the remaining turkey. Place the turkey rolls with the seam side down in the pan. Set aside any remaining pesto.

In a small bowl, whisk together the honey and soy sauce. Brush on the turkey rolls.

Bake for 40 to 45 minutes, or until the turkey is no longer pink in the center. Top the turkey rolls with the remaining pesto.

COOK'S TIP on peeling tomatoes

Cut a small, shallow X in the bottom end of each tomato. Plunge the tomatoes into boiling water for 10 to 15 seconds, then into ice water for about 1 minute. Use a paring knife to peel off the skin easily.

PER SERVING

CALORIES 166
TOTAL FAT 2.5 g
  Saturated Fat 1.0 g
  Trans Fat 0.0 g
  Polyunsaturated Fat 0.5 g
  Monounsaturated Fat 0.5 g
CHOLESTEROL 76 mg
SODIUM 188 mg
CARBOHYDRATES 6 g
  Fiber 1 g
  Sugars 5 g
PROTEIN 29 g
DIETARY EXCHANGES
  ½ carbohydrate,
  3 very lean meat

turkey fillets with fresh herbs

SERVES 6

No more dry turkey! The buttermilk tenderizes the fillets and keeps them moist as they cook. Refrigerate any leftovers and serve slices of chilled turkey over your favorite salad greens.

MARINADE
- 2 cups low-fat buttermilk
- 1 large onion, finely chopped
- 1 tablespoon finely chopped fresh dillweed
- 1 tablespoon finely chopped fresh tarragon
- 1 tablespoon finely chopped fresh cilantro

- 1 tablespoon finely chopped fresh rosemary
- 1 tablespoon canola or corn oil
- 1 teaspoon pepper
- ¼ teaspoon salt

- 6 skinless turkey fillets (about 4 ounces each), about ¾ inch thick, all visible fat discarded

In a large shallow glass dish, stir together the marinade ingredients. Add the turkey, turning to coat. Cover and refrigerate for 1 to 12 hours, turning several times.

Preheat the grill on medium high or preheat the broiler.

Remove the turkey from the marinade, discarding the marinade.

Grill for 4 to 5 minutes on each side or broil about 6 inches from the heat for 5 to 7 minutes on each side, or until no longer pink in the center.

COOK'S TIP on herbs

In most recipes, such as this one, you can substitute dried herbs for fresh, though the flavor won't be quite as good. Use about one-third as much as you would of fresh herbs.

PER SERVING

CALORIES 121
TOTAL FAT 0.5 g
  Saturated Fat 0.0 g
  Trans Fat 0.0 g
  Polyunsaturated Fat 0.0 g
  Monounsaturated Fat 0.0 g
CHOLESTEROL 74 mg
SODIUM 221 mg
CARBOHYDRATES 0 g
  Fiber 0 g
  Sugars 0 g
PROTEIN 27 g
DIETARY EXCHANGES
  3 very lean meat

turkey sausage patties

SERVES 8

For brunch, serve this tasty, low-fat meat with Southern Raised Biscuits (page 539) and Cranberry Chutney (page 487). After you find out how good these patties are, you'll also want to try them in sandwiches and even as a dinner entrée.

1 pound lean ground skinless turkey breast	½ to ¾ teaspoon cayenne
¼ cup plain fine dry bread crumbs (lowest sodium available)	½ teaspoon ground cumin
	½ teaspoon garlic powder
1 tablespoon dried Italian seasoning, crumbled	¼ teaspoon pepper
	¼ teaspoon salt
1¼ teaspoons ground coriander	½ cup fat-free, low-sodium chicken broth, such as on page 43
1 teaspoon paprika	

In a large bowl, stir together all the ingredients except the broth.

Stir in the broth. Let stand for 15 minutes. Form into 8 patties, about ¾ inch thick.

In a large nonstick skillet, cook the patties over medium heat for 7 to 8 minutes on each side, or until cooked through.

COOK'S TIP on ground turkey breast

Select a piece of skinless turkey breast and ask the butcher to grind it. The ground turkey already in the meat case often contains skin.

PER SERVING

CALORIES 80
TOTAL FAT 0.5 g
  Saturated Fat 0.0 g
  Trans Fat 0.0 g
  Polyunsaturated Fat 0.0 g
  Monounsaturated Fat 0.0 g
CHOLESTEROL 35 mg
SODIUM 127 mg
CARBOHYDRATES 3 g
  Fiber 0 g
  Sugars 0 g
PROTEIN 15 g
DIETARY EXCHANGES
  2 very lean meat

turkey lasagna

SERVES 9

Here's the solution for what to take to potluck dinners.

Cooking spray
8 ounces dried whole-grain lasagna noodles
1 pound lean ground skinless turkey breast
8 ounces button mushrooms, sliced
½ cup chopped onion
3 medium garlic cloves, minced
3 cups no-salt-added tomato sauce

2 teaspoons dried basil, crumbled
½ teaspoon dried oregano, crumbled
Pepper to taste
16 ounces fat-free cottage cheese
1 10-ounce package frozen chopped spinach, thawed and squeezed dry
Dash of nutmeg
2 cups shredded or grated low-fat mozzarella cheese

Preheat the oven to 375°F. Lightly spray a 13 x 9 x 2-inch glass baking dish with cooking spray.

Prepare the noodles using the package directions, omitting the salt.

Meanwhile, in a large nonstick skillet over medium-high heat, stir together the turkey, mushrooms, onion, and garlic. Cook for 8 to 10 minutes, or until the turkey is no longer pink, stirring occasionally to turn and break up the turkey. Reduce the heat to low. Cook, covered, for 3 to 4 minutes, or until the mushrooms have released their liquid. Increase the heat to high. Cook, uncovered, for 2 to 3 minutes, or until the liquid evaporates.

Stir in the tomato sauce, basil, oregano, and pepper. Reduce the heat to low. Cook for 5 to 6 minutes, or until heated through.

In a large bowl, stir together the cottage cheese, spinach, and nutmeg.

In the baking dish, layer one-third of the cooked noodles, one-half of the cottage cheese mixture, one-third of the turkey mixture, and one-third of the mozzarella. Repeat the layers. Finish in order with the remaining noodles, turkey, and mozzarella.

Bake, covered, for 35 to 40 minutes, or until the casserole is heated through and the mozzarella is melted.

PER SERVING

CALORIES 283
TOTAL FAT 3.5 g
  Saturated Fat 1.0 g
  Trans Fat 0.0 g
  Polyunsaturated Fat 0.5 g
  Monounsaturated Fat 1.0 g
CHOLESTEROL 42 mg
SODIUM 413 mg
CARBOHYDRATES 33 g
  Fiber 6 g
  Sugars 9 g
PROTEIN 30 g
DIETARY EXCHANGES
  1½ starch, 2 vegetable,
  3½ very lean meat

turkey enchiladas

SERVES 4; 2 ENCHILADAS PER SERVING

Everything you'd expect from the whole enchilada—and more—is in this Tex-Mex classic. Green chile enchilada sauce and sour cream are the toppers.

Cooking spray
8 ounces lean ground skinless turkey breast
8 6-inch corn tortillas
½ 15.5-ounce can no-salt-added black beans, rinsed and drained
½ cup frozen whole-kernel corn, thawed
½ cup shredded low-fat Cheddar cheese

½ 4-ounce can chopped green chiles, drained
1 teaspoon chili powder
½ teaspoon ground cumin
¼ teaspoon dried oregano, crumbled
⅛ teaspoon salt
4 ounces canned green chile enchilada sauce
½ cup fat-free sour cream

Preheat the oven to 350°F. Lightly spray an 8-inch square baking pan with cooking spray.

In a large nonstick skillet, cook the turkey over medium-high heat for 7 to 8 minutes, or until lightly browned on the outside and no longer pink in the center, stirring occasionally to turn and break up the turkey.

Meanwhile, wrap the tortillas in aluminum foil. Bake for 5 minutes, or until warmed through. Remove the tortillas from the oven, leaving them in the foil.

Stir the beans, corn, Cheddar, chiles, chili powder, cumin, oregano, and salt into the turkey.

Remove the tortillas from the foil. Spoon the turkey mixture down the center of each tortilla. Roll up jelly-roll style and place with the seam side down in the baking pan. Pour the enchilada sauce over all.

Bake, covered, for 25 minutes, or until the filling is warmed through. Spread the sour cream on top. Bake for 5 minutes, or until the sour cream is warmed through and flows over the enchiladas.

PER SERVING

CALORIES 260
TOTAL FAT 3.0 g
  Saturated Fat 1.0 g
  Trans Fat 0.0 g
  Polyunsaturated Fat 0.5 g
  Monounsaturated Fat 0.5 g
CHOLESTEROL 43 mg
SODIUM 475 mg
CARBOHYDRATES 34 g
  Fiber 5 g
  Sugars 5 g
PROTEIN 25 g
DIETARY EXCHANGES
  2 starch,
  2½ very lean meat

turkey loaf

SERVES 8

This meat loaf substitute is so moist that you'll gobble it up! Try it with Spinach-Chayote Salad with Orange Vinaigrette (page 90).

Cooking spray

4 slices whole-grain bread (lowest sodium available), processed into fine crumbs

¼ cup fat-free milk

2 pounds lean ground skinless turkey breast

1 cup grated or finely chopped onion

1 cup canned no-salt-added stewed tomatoes, crushed, undrained

1 medium rib of celery, diced

½ medium red bell pepper, chopped

½ cup egg substitute

¼ cup minced fresh parsley

1 teaspoon seeded and finely minced fresh jalapeño, or to taste

¼ teaspoon salt

¼ teaspoon pepper

2 tablespoons no-salt-added ketchup

Preheat the oven to 350°F. Lightly spray a 10½ x 5½ x 2½-inch loaf pan with cooking spray.

In a shallow dish, stir together the bread crumbs and milk. Let the crumbs soak for 5 minutes.

Meanwhile, put the remaining ingredients except the ketchup in a large bowl. Using your hands or a spoon, combine gently but thoroughly.

Drain the bread crumbs and squeeze out the excess milk to form a paste. Stir into the turkey mixture. Spoon into the loaf pan. Spread the ketchup over the loaf.

Bake for 1 hour 30 minutes, or until the loaf registers 165°F on an instant-read thermometer. Let stand for 5 to 10 minutes before serving.

PER SERVING

CALORIES 195
TOTAL FAT 1.5 g
 Saturated Fat 0.5 g
 Trans Fat 0.0 g
 Polyunsaturated Fat 0.5 g
 Monounsaturated Fat 0.5 g
CHOLESTEROL 71 mg
SODIUM 240 mg
CARBOHYDRATES 12 g
 Fiber 2 g
 Sugars 5 g
PROTEIN 32 g
DIETARY EXCHANGES
 ½ starch, 1 vegetable,
 3 very lean meat

mediterranean turkey burgers

SERVES 4

A dollop of mango chutney is the crowning touch for these just-spicy-enough burgers.

1 teaspoon canola or corn oil	2 tablespoons fresh lemon juice
1 medium Granny Smith apple, peeled and diced	¼ teaspoon pepper
¼ cup chopped red onion	¼ teaspoon ground chipotle pepper
2 tablespoons chopped celery	⅛ teaspoon salt
1 pound lean ground skinless turkey breast	Cooking spray
2 tablespoons panko (Japanese bread crumbs)	¼ cup mango chutney (lowest sodium available)
2 tablespoons coarsely snipped fresh cilantro	4 whole-grain hamburger buns (lowest sodium available)

If using an outside grill (rather than a grill pan), preheat on medium high.

In a small nonstick skillet, heat the oil over medium-high heat, swirling to coat the bottom. Cook the apple, onion, and celery for 6 to 8 minutes, or until the apple and onion are tender, stirring frequently.

In a medium bowl, stir together the apple mixture, turkey, panko, cilantro, lemon juice, pepper, ground chipotle, and salt just until blended. Form into 4 patties ¼ to ½ inch thick. Lightly spray the tops with cooking spray.

Grill the patties with the cooking spray side down on a nonstick grill pan over medium-high heat or on the outdoor grill for 5 to 7 minutes on each side, or until no longer pink in the center. Serve on the buns, topping the patties with the chutney.

COOK'S TIP on sodium in chutney

It is really important to compare nutrition facts labels on chutneys because the sodium varies drastically from one brand to another. The one we used has 55 mg of sodium in each tablespoon.

PER SERVING
CALORIES 309
TOTAL FAT 4.0 g
Saturated Fat 0.5 g
Trans Fat 0.0 g
Polyunsaturated Fat 1.5 g
Monounsaturated Fat 1.5 g
CHOLESTEROL 70 mg
SODIUM 377 mg
CARBOHYDRATES 37 g
Fiber 4 g
Sugars 14 g
PROTEIN 32 g
DIETARY EXCHANGES
2 starch, ½ fruit,
3 very lean meat

southwestern turkey wraps

SERVES 4

These wraps get their kick from salsa and Dijon mustard and give you an easy way to use leftover turkey.

3 ounces light tub cream cheese
2 tablespoons salsa (lowest sodium available), such as Salsa Cruda (page 508)
2 tablespoons sliced green onions
1 teaspoon Dijon mustard
4 6-inch fat-free flour tortillas (lowest sodium available)

1 cup shredded lettuce
6 ounces very thinly sliced or finely chopped roasted turkey breast, cooked without salt, skin and all visible fat discarded
4 strips red bell pepper, about ¼ inch wide

In a small bowl, stir together the cream cheese, salsa, green onions, and mustard.

To assemble, spread the cream cheese mixture over each tortilla. Top with the lettuce, turkey, and bell pepper. Roll to enclose the filling. Wrap tightly in plastic wrap. Refrigerate for several hours or until serving time.

COOK'S TIP

Cut each tortilla roll into fourths to serve as appetizers for eight.

PER SERVING

CALORIES 199
TOTAL FAT 4.0 g
 Saturated Fat 2.0 g
 Trans Fat 0.0 g
 Polyunsaturated Fat 0.0 g
 Monounsaturated Fat 1.0 g
CHOLESTEROL 49 mg
SODIUM 437 mg
CARBOHYDRATES 22 g
 Fiber 1 g
 Sugars 2 g
PROTEIN 17 g
DIETARY EXCHANGES
 1½ starch,
 2 very lean meat

turkey with vegetables and brown rice

SERVES 4

Leftover turkey teams up with broccoli, carrots, brown rice, and a rich-tasting sauce in this stovetop meal-in-one.

1¼ cups fat-free, low-sodium chicken broth, such as on page 43
1 cup uncooked instant brown rice
3 to 4 ounces broccoli florets
1 large carrot, thinly sliced
½ teaspoon dried basil, crumbled
1 10.75-ounce can low-fat condensed cream of chicken soup (lowest sodium available)

1 cup diced cooked skinless turkey breast, cooked without salt (about 4 ounces)
½ cup fat-free half-and-half
2 tablespoons snipped fresh parsley or 2 teaspoons dried parsley, crumbled
½ teaspoon dried oregano, crumbled

In a medium saucepan, bring the broth to a boil over high heat.

Stir in the brown rice, broccoli, carrot, and basil. Reduce the heat and simmer, covered, for 10 minutes, or until the rice, broccoli, and carrot are tender.

Meanwhile, in a separate medium saucepan, stir together the remaining ingredients. Heat over medium heat for 8 to 10 minutes, or until warmed through, stirring occasionally and lowering the heat if necessary so the mixture doesn't come to a simmer rapidly. Serve over the rice mixture.

PER SERVING

CALORIES 213
TOTAL FAT 2.5 g
  Saturated Fat 0.5 g
  Trans Fat 0.0 g
  Polyunsaturated Fat 1.0 g
  Monounsaturated Fat 0.5 g
CHOLESTEROL 27 mg
SODIUM 364 mg
CARBOHYDRATES 32 g
  Fiber 3 g
  Sugars 5 g
PROTEIN 15 g
DIETARY EXCHANGES
  2 starch,
  1½ very lean meat

stuffed cornish hens with orange-brandy sauce

SERVES 12

Petite Cornish hens get four-star treatment with rice stuffing and brandied orange sections. You'll need some extra time for prepping and roasting, but it will be worth the effort because this main course will make any occasion extra special.

Cooking spray
1⅓ cups uncooked long-grain and wild rice, seasoning packet discarded
2 teaspoons light tub margarine
1 medium onion, chopped
1 teaspoon dried sage, thyme, savory, or tarragon, crumbled
6 Cornish hens (about 14 ounces each), all visible fat, tails, and giblets discarded

½ cup fat-free, low-sodium chicken broth, such as on page 43
½ cup water
1 cup orange sections (1 to 2 medium)
¼ cup brandy

Preheat the oven to 350°F. Lightly spray a roasting pan and cooking rack(s) with cooking spray.

Prepare the rice using the package directions, omitting the salt and margarine and cooking until still slightly firm.

In a large skillet over medium-high heat, melt the margarine, swirling to coat the bottom. Cook the onion for 3 to 4 minutes, or until lightly browned, stirring occasionally.

Stir in the rice and sage. Remove from the heat.

Stuff the hens lightly with the rice mixture. Skewer or sew the cavities closed. Lightly spray the hens with cooking spray. Put with the breast side up on the rack in the roasting pan.

Roast for 1 hour, or until the meat near the bone at the thickest part of the hens is no longer pink and the stuffing registers 165°F on an instant-read thermometer, basting occasionally with the broth.

Transfer the hens to cutting boards. Pour the liquid from the pan into a small saucepan. Cut the hens in half along the backbone (kitchen scissors work well). Discard the skin. Place the hens on a platter.

PER SERVING

CALORIES 199
TOTAL FAT 3.5 g
  Saturated Fat 1.0 g
  Trans Fat 0.0 g
  Polyunsaturated Fat 1.0 g
  Monounsaturated Fat 1.0 g
CHOLESTEROL 85 mg
SODIUM 58 mg
CARBOHYDRATES 18 g
  Fiber 1 g
  Sugars 2 g
PROTEIN 21 g
DIETARY EXCHANGES
  1 starch, 3 very lean meat

Heat the liquid over medium-high heat. Pour in the water, scraping to dislodge any browned bits.

Stir in the orange sections and brandy. Cook for 2 minutes, stirring constantly. Serve the sauce over the hens or on the side.

COOK'S TIP on sewing poultry

Keep the stuffing moist in any kind of poultry by skewering or sewing the cavity. Pull it closed and weave a sharp, thin metal or wooden skewer into the skin at the sides of the cavity. (If using wooden skewers, be sure to soak them for at least 10 minutes in cold water to keep them from charring.) If you prefer, buy a large-eyed sewing needle at a craft or carpet store and thread it with thin kitchen twine. Sew the cavity closed.

meats

Fillet of Beef with Herbes de Provence

Pot Roast Ratatouille and Pasta

Beef Roast with Rosemary and Hoisin Sauce

Brisket Stew, Slow and Easy

Zesty Hot-Oven Sirloin

Ginger-Lime Sirloin

Sirloin with Creamy Horseradish Sauce

Steak Marinated in Beer and Green Onions

Smothered Steak with Sangría Sauce

Shredded Beef Soft Tacos

Grilled Stuffed Flank Steak

Grilled Lemongrass Flank Steak

Greek-Style Eye-of-Round Steaks

Beef Bourguignon

Mediterranean Beef and Vegetable Stir-Fry

Portobello Mushrooms and Sirloin Strips over Spinach Pasta

Classic Chinese Beef Stir-Fry

Southwestern Beef Stir-Fry

Braised Sirloin Tips

Steak and Vegetable Kebabs

Asian Beef Skillet

Savory Beef Stew

Yogurt-Marinated Grilled Round Steak

Swiss Steak

Slow-Cooker Round Steak with Mushrooms and Tomatoes

Cube Steak with Mushroom Sauce

Philadelphia-Style Cheese Steak Wrap

Salisbury Steaks with Mushroom Sauce

Grilled Hamburgers with Vegetables and Feta

Ground Beef Stroganoff

Sweet Barbecue Meat Loaf

Mediterranean Meat Loaf

Tex-Mex Lasagna

Slow-Cooker Chili

Beef and Pasta Skillet

Spaghetti with Meat Sauce

Beef and Noodle Casserole Dijon

Greek-Style Beef Skillet Supper

fillet of beef with herbes de provence

SERVES 6

Black pepper, herbes de Provence, and a good measure of garlic flavor this tender cut of beef. Very easy and elegant, it's an excellent dish for company.

Olive oil spray
1 1½-pound beef tenderloin, all visible fat and silver skin discarded
3 medium garlic cloves, minced
2 teaspoons dried herbes de Provence or mixed dried herbs, crumbled

1 teaspoon pepper, or to taste
2 medium carrots, finely diced
1 medium onion, sliced
¼ teaspoon salt

Preheat the oven to 400°F. Lightly spray a roasting pan with olive oil spray.

Tie the roast in three or four places with kitchen twine. Rub the garlic into the roast. Sprinkle with the herbes de Provence and pepper. Transfer to the roasting pan. Lightly spray the roast with olive oil spray. Scatter the carrots and onion on and around the roast.

Bake for 25 to 30 minutes per pound for medium-rare, or until the roast registers 5 to 10 degrees below the desired doneness when tested with an instant-read thermometer. Transfer to a cutting board. Sprinkle with the salt. Cover with aluminum foil. Let stand for 10 to 15 minutes before slicing.

COOK'S TIP on herbes de provence

Herbes de Provence is a combination of herbs used quite frequently in southern France: basil, thyme, rosemary, marjoram, sage, and lavender. If you don't have herbes de Provence, use a combination of at least two of these, blended in equal amounts.

PER SERVING

CALORIES 171
TOTAL FAT 5.0 g
　Saturated Fat 2.5 g
　Trans Fat 0.0 g
　Polyunsaturated Fat 0.5 g
　Monounsaturated Fat 2.5 g
CHOLESTEROL 53 mg
SODIUM 165 mg
CARBOHYDRATES 5 g
　Fiber 1 g
　Sugars 3 g
PROTEIN 24 g
DIETARY EXCHANGES
　1 vegetable,
　3 lean meat

pot roast ratatouille and pasta

SERVES 8

This dish can feature any pasta variety—from angel hair to shells to penne.

Olive oil spray
1 1½-pound eye-of-round roast, all visible fat discarded
½ teaspoon salt-free all-purpose seasoning blend
¼ teaspoon pepper
1 10.75-ounce can tomato puree
10 ounces eggplant, chopped
2 medium zucchini, sliced
5 medium Italian plum (Roma) tomatoes, chopped

1 large onion, chopped
2 medium ribs of celery, sliced
1 teaspoon dried oregano or Italian seasoning, crumbled
1 medium garlic clove, minced
1 medium dried bay leaf
¼ teaspoon dried basil, crumbled
8 ounces dried whole-grain pasta

Preheat the oven to 350°F. Lightly spray a Dutch oven with olive oil spray.

Sprinkle the roast with the seasoning blend and pepper.

Heat the Dutch oven over medium-high heat. Brown the roast for 2 to 3 minutes on each side.

Stir in the remaining ingredients except the pasta.

Bake, covered, for about 2 hours, or until the roast is very tender when tested with a fork.

Shortly before the roast is done, prepare the pasta using the package directions, omitting the salt. Drain well in a colander.

Transfer the roast to a cutting board. Cover with aluminum foil and let stand for 10 to 15 minutes before slicing very thinly across the grain, then slicing into thin strips. Discard the bay leaf from the sauce.

Spoon the pasta onto plates. Arrange the roast slices on the pasta. Top with the sauce.

COOK'S TIP on eye-of-round roast

For maximum tenderness, don't overcook eye-of-round roast, and be sure to cut it into thin strips.

PER SERVING

CALORIES 245
TOTAL FAT 2.5 g
 Saturated Fat 1.0 g
 Trans Fat 0.0 g
 Polyunsaturated Fat 0.5 g
 Monounsaturated Fat 1.0 g
CHOLESTEROL 36 mg
SODIUM 55 mg
CARBOHYDRATES 31 g
 Fiber 6 g
 Sugars 7 g
PROTEIN 24 g
DIETARY EXCHANGES
 1½ starch, 2 vegetable,
 2½ very lean meat

beef roast with rosemary and hoisin sauce

SERVES 8

Ingredients from several countries join forces to deliciously flavor a braised eye-of-round roast. For even more of a treat, prepare mashed potatoes spiked with wasabi or horseradish and top them with thin slices of the roast and gravy.

Olive oil spray
1 2-pound eye-of-round roast, all visible fat discarded
1 cup fat-free, no-salt-added beef broth, such as on page 42
2 tablespoons dry vermouth or dry white wine (regular or nonalcoholic)
2 tablespoons hoisin sauce
1 tablespoon balsamic vinegar
2 teaspoons soy sauce (lowest sodium available)
1 teaspoon dried rosemary, crushed
2 medium garlic cloves, minced
1½ tablespoons cornstarch
¼ cup water

Preheat the oven to 350°F. Lightly spray a Dutch oven with olive oil spray.

Heat the Dutch oven over medium-high heat. Brown the roast for 2 to 3 minutes on each side.

Stir in the broth, vermouth, hoisin sauce, vinegar, soy sauce, rosemary, and garlic. Bring to a simmer.

Bake, covered, for about 2 hours, or until the roast is very tender when tested with a fork. Transfer to a cutting board, leaving the liquid in the pot. Cover the roast with aluminum foil. Let stand for 10 to 15 minutes before slicing across the grain into very thin pieces.

While the roast is standing, put the cornstarch in a small bowl. Add the water, whisking to dissolve. Whisk into the cooking liquid. Bring to a simmer over medium-high heat. Reduce the heat and simmer for 1 to 2 minutes, or until the mixture has thickened, whisking occasionally. Spoon over the roast slices.

COOK'S TIP on wasabi or horseradish mashed potatoes

For mashed potatoes with some firepower, just stir 1 to 2 teaspoons of wasabi paste or wasabi powder or 1 tablespoon bottled white horseradish into 4 cups mashed potatoes (mashed with fat-free milk and 1 tablespoon olive oil instead of butter).

PER SERVING

CALORIES 148
TOTAL FAT 2.0 g
 Saturated Fat 1.0 g
 Trans Fat 0.0 g
 Polyunsaturated Fat 0.0 g
 Monounsaturated Fat 1.0 g
CHOLESTEROL 53 mg
SODIUM 88 mg
CARBOHYDRATES 4 g
 Fiber 0 g
 Sugars 1 g
PROTEIN 26 g
DIETARY EXCHANGES
 3 very lean meat

brisket stew, slow and easy

SERVES 4

Slow cooking and a touch of sherry are the keys to the success of this comfort food. Serve as is or over no-yolk noodles.

2 medium carrots, cut into 1-inch pieces

1 medium onion, cut into ½-inch wedges

1 medium green bell pepper, cut into 1-inch squares

1 medium rib of celery, cut into 1-inch pieces

1 1-pound flat-cut beef brisket, all visible fat discarded

¼ cup dry sherry or dry red wine (regular or nonalcoholic)

1 teaspoon very low sodium beef bouillon granules

1 teaspoon dried oregano, crumbled

2 tablespoons no-salt-added tomato paste

1 tablespoon sugar

1 tablespoon cider vinegar

2 teaspoons Worcestershire sauce (lowest sodium available)

½ teaspoon salt

¼ teaspoon dried basil, crumbled

Put the carrots, onion, bell pepper, and celery in a 3½- or 4-quart slow cooker. Place the roast on top. Pour the sherry over all. Sprinkle with the bouillon granules and oregano.

Cook, covered, on high for 6 hours, or until the roast is tender when tested with a fork. Transfer the roast to a cutting board, leaving the carrot mixture in the slow cooker. Let the roast stand for 10 minutes before slicing.

In a small bowl, whisk together the remaining ingredients. Stir into the carrot mixture. Return the sliced roast to the slow cooker to heat for 5 minutes.

COOK'S TIP

Purchase a brisket that weighs about 2½ pounds. After you trim all the fat, the roast should weigh about 2 pounds. Cut it in half and freeze one piece to use later.

PER SERVING

CALORIES 212
TOTAL FAT 4.5 g
  Saturated Fat 1.5 g
  Trans Fat 0.0 g
  Polyunsaturated Fat 0.5 g
  Monounsaturated Fat 2.0 g
CHOLESTEROL 47 mg
SODIUM 425 mg
CARBOHYDRATES 14 g
  Fiber 3 g
  Sugars 9 g
PROTEIN 26 g
DIETARY EXCHANGES
  3 lean meat, 2 vegetable

zesty hot-oven sirloin

SERVES 4

The marinade in this dish is transformed into an intense sauce that packs a palatable punch. A little sauce goes a long way!

MARINADE
- 2 tablespoons soy sauce (lowest sodium available)
- 2 tablespoons balsamic vinegar
- 2 tablespoons fresh lemon juice
- 1 tablespoon Worcestershire sauce (lowest sodium available)
- 2 teaspoons dried oregano, crumbled
- 2 medium garlic cloves, minced

- 1 1-pound boneless sirloin steak, about 1 inch thick, all visible fat discarded

Cooking spray
- ¼ cup water
- 1½ teaspoons light tub margarine
- ¼ teaspoon salt
- ¼ teaspoon pepper
- 2 tablespoons finely snipped fresh parsley

In a medium glass dish, combine the marinade ingredients. Add the steak, turning to coat. Cover and refrigerate for 8 hours, turning occasionally.

Preheat the oven to 500°F. Lightly spray a rimmed baking sheet with cooking spray.

Transfer the steak to the baking sheet, reserving the marinade.

Roast the steak on the top oven rack for 12 to 14 minutes, or to the desired doneness. Cut into 4 pieces.

Meanwhile, in a small saucepan, bring the marinade and water to a boil over high heat. Reduce the heat and simmer for 3 minutes, or until reduced to ¼ cup. Remove from the heat.

Add the margarine, salt, and pepper to the marinade mixture, stirring until the margarine has melted. Spoon over the steak. Sprinkle with the parsley.

PER SERVING

CALORIES 166
TOTAL FAT 5.0 g
  Saturated Fat 2.0 g
  Trans Fat 0.0 g
  Polyunsaturated Fat 0.5 g
  Monounsaturated Fat 2.5 g
CHOLESTEROL 56 mg
SODIUM 408 mg
CARBOHYDRATES 4 g
  Fiber 0 g
  Sugars 2 g
PROTEIN 25 g
DIETARY EXCHANGES
  3 lean meat

ginger-lime sirloin

SERVES 4

The same tasty combination serves as both marinade and sauce for the broiled steak in this recipe.

MARINADE

3 tablespoons sugar

3 tablespoons soy sauce (lowest sodium available)

2 tablespoons cider vinegar

1 tablespoon fresh lime juice

1 teaspoon grated peeled gingerroot

1 medium garlic clove, minced

½ teaspoon crushed red pepper flakes
_____

1 1-pound boneless sirloin steak, about 1 inch thick, all visible fat discarded

Cooking spray

In a small glass bowl, stir together the marinade ingredients until the sugar is dissolved.

Pour half the marinade into a medium glass dish. Add the steak, turning to coat. Cover and refrigerate for 8 hours, turning occasionally. Cover and refrigerate the remaining marinade.

Preheat the broiler. Lightly spray a broiler pan and rack with cooking spray.

Drain the steak, discarding the marinade in the glass dish.

Broil the steak about 4 inches from the heat for 5 minutes. Turn over. Broil for 8 minutes, or to the desired doneness. Transfer to a cutting board. Let stand for 5 minutes before cutting into thin slices.

Meanwhile, in a small saucepan, bring the reserved marinade to a boil over high heat. Boil for 1 to 2 minutes, or until reduced to about 2 tablespoons, stirring frequently. Spoon over the steak.

COOK'S TIP

The steak is cooked longer on one side to allow it to blacken slightly.

PER SERVING

CALORIES 189
TOTAL FAT 4.5 g
  Saturated Fat 2.0 g
  Trans Fat 0.0 g
  Polyunsaturated Fat 0.0 g
  Monounsaturated Fat 2.0 g
CHOLESTEROL 56 mg
SODIUM 341 mg
CARBOHYDRATES 11 g
  Fiber 0 g
  Sugars 10 g
PROTEIN 25 g
DIETARY EXCHANGES
  ½ carbohydrate,
  3 lean meat

sirloin with creamy horseradish sauce

SERVES 4

Season, sear, and serve—that's all it takes to put this family favorite on the table. Even the special sauce is extra-quick. The pungent sauce also goes well with grilled vegetables and makes a great topping for baked potatoes or dip for fresh vegetables.

1 medium garlic clove, halved crosswise

1 1-pound boneless sirloin steak, all visible fat discarded

½ teaspoon chili powder

½ teaspoon onion powder

1 teaspoon olive oil

⅛ teaspoon salt

CREAMY HORSERADISH SAUCE

½ cup fat-free sour cream

2 teaspoons bottled white horseradish, drained

2 teaspoons olive oil

1 teaspoon Dijon mustard (coarse-grain preferred)

½ medium garlic clove, minced

½ teaspoon Worcestershire sauce (lowest sodium available)

⅛ teaspoon salt

¼ cup water

Pepper, to taste (coarsely ground preferred)

Rub the halved garlic over both sides of the steak.

Sprinkle the chili powder and onion powder on both sides of the steak. Using your fingertips, firmly press so they adhere to the steak.

In a large nonstick skillet, heat 1 teaspoon oil over medium-high heat, swirling to coat the bottom. Cook the steak for 5 minutes. Turn over. Reduce the heat to medium and cook for 5 minutes, or to the desired doneness. Transfer the steak to a cutting board, leaving any browned bits in the skillet.

Sprinkle the steak with ⅛ teaspoon salt. Let stand for 3 minutes before slicing.

Meanwhile, in a small bowl, whisk together the sauce ingredients. Set aside.

Add the water to the skillet, scraping to dislodge any browned bits. Bring to a boil over medium-high heat. Boil for 1 to 1½ minutes, or until the liquid is reduced to 2 tablespoons.

Serve the steak topped with the pan juices and pepper. Serve the sauce on the side.

PER SERVING

CALORIES 202
TOTAL FAT 8.0 g
  Saturated Fat 2.0 g
  Trans Fat 0.0 g
  Polyunsaturated Fat 0.5 g
  Monounsaturated Fat 4.0 g
CHOLESTEROL 47 mg
SODIUM 255 mg
CARBOHYDRATES 6 g
  Fiber 0 g
  Sugars 3 g
PROTEIN 25 g
DIETARY EXCHANGES
  ½ carbohydrate,
  3 lean meat

steak marinated in beer and green onions

SERVES 8

Many Asian hosts serve beer rather than wine for special meals. It's no wonder then that beer is often used in Asian recipes, such as this one.

MARINADE
12 ounces light beer (regular or nonalcoholic)
4 medium green onions, minced
2 tablespoons light brown sugar
2 tablespoons dry sherry
1 tablespoon grated peeled gingerroot
1 tablespoon soy sauce (lowest sodium available)

2 medium garlic cloves, minced
1 teaspoon crushed red pepper flakes
1 teaspoon canola or corn oil
Dash of red hot-pepper sauce

2 pounds boneless top sirloin steak, all visible fat discarded

In a large glass dish, stir together the marinade ingredients until the brown sugar is dissolved. Add the steak, turning to coat. Cover and refrigerate for 1 to 24 hours, turning occasionally.

Preheat the grill on medium high.

Remove the steak from the marinade, discarding the marinade.

Grill the steak for 8 to 12 minutes on each side, or to the desired doneness.

PER SERVING
CALORIES 142
TOTAL FAT 4.5 g
  Saturated Fat 2.0 g
  Trans Fat 0.0 g
  Polyunsaturated Fat 0.0 g
  Monounsaturated Fat 2.0 g
CHOLESTEROL 56 mg
SODIUM 96 mg
CARBOHYDRATES 0 g
  Fiber 0 g
  Sugars 0 g
PROTEIN 24 g
DIETARY EXCHANGES
  3 lean meat

smothered steak with sangria sauce

SERVES 4

Different and easy, this dish is great for company. Serve it over brown rice or whole-grain pasta so you can enjoy all the sauce.

SANGRIA SAUCE
- 1 cup sangria (white preferred)
- 1 medium tomato, chopped
- 1 small green bell pepper, chopped
- ¼ cup golden raisins
- ¼ cup dried apricots, coarsely chopped
- 1 large dried bay leaf
- 1 teaspoon dried basil, crumbled
- ½ teaspoon dried thyme, crumbled
- ¼ teaspoon pepper, or to taste

- Cooking spray
- 4 thin boneless sirloin steaks (about 4 ounces each), all visible fat discarded

In a medium bowl, stir together the sauce ingredients.

Lightly spray a large skillet with cooking spray. Cook the steaks over medium-high heat for 2 to 3 minutes on each side.

Pour the sauce into the skillet. Reduce the heat and simmer, covered, for 30 to 40 minutes, or until the steaks are tender. Discard the bay leaf.

TIME-SAVER
Use cube steaks instead of sirloin steaks and reduce the simmering time to 20 to 25 minutes.

PER SERVING
CALORIES 241
TOTAL FAT 4.5 g
  Saturated Fat 2.0 g
  Trans Fat 0.0 g
  Polyunsaturated Fat 0.5 g
  Monounsaturated Fat 2.0 g
CHOLESTEROL 56 mg
SODIUM 56 mg
CARBOHYDRATES 21 g
  Fiber 2 g
  Sugars 16 g
PROTEIN 25 g
DIETARY EXCHANGES
  1 fruit, ½ carbohydrate,
  3 lean meat

shredded beef soft tacos

SERVES 8

Let your slow cooker fix dinner while you're at work. Then give your family a Mexican feast of sirloin, onions, and bell peppers with cumin, all wrapped in warm tortillas. Serve with plenty of napkins!

1½ pounds boneless top sirloin steak or sirloin tip roast, all visible fat discarded
3 large onions, chopped
1 medium green bell pepper, chopped
½ cup no-salt-added ketchup
¼ cup dry red wine (regular or nonalcoholic)
2 tablespoons cider vinegar
6 medium garlic cloves, minced
2 teaspoons very low sodium beef bouillon granules

2 medium dried bay leaves
¾ teaspoon liquid smoke
½ teaspoon ground cumin and ½ teaspoon ground cumin, divided use
½ teaspoon red hot-pepper sauce
¼ teaspoon pepper
1 teaspoon sugar (dark brown preferred)
8 8-inch fat-free flour tortillas (lowest sodium available)

Put the steak in a 3½- or 4-quart slow cooker. Add the onions and bell pepper.

In a medium bowl, whisk together the ketchup, wine, vinegar, garlic, bouillon granules, bay leaves, liquid smoke, ½ teaspoon cumin, hot-pepper sauce, and pepper. Pour into the slow cooker.

Cook, covered, on low for 9 hours, or until the steak is tender. Transfer the steak to a cutting board. Discard the bay leaves.

Using two forks, shred the steak. Return to the slow cooker to stand (the heat should be off).

Stir in the sugar and remaining ½ teaspoon cumin. Let stand, covered, for 1 hour so the flavors blend.

Warm the tortillas using the package directions.

Spoon the steak mixture down the center of each tortilla. Fold one end and each side of the tortillas toward the center.

COOK'S TIP

Before folding the tortillas over the filling, add chopped tomatoes and shredded lettuce, or try salsa, such as Salsa Cruda (page 508), and fat-free sour cream.

PER SERVING

CALORIES 296
TOTAL FAT 4.0 g
  Saturated Fat 1.5 g
  Trans Fat 0.0 g
  Polyunsaturated Fat 0.5 g
  Monounsaturated Fat 1.5 g
CHOLESTEROL 45 mg
SODIUM 402 mg
CARBOHYDRATES 38 g
  Fiber 4 g
  Sugars 10 g
PROTEIN 25 g
DIETARY EXCHANGES
  1½ starch, 2 vegetable, 2½ lean meat

grilled stuffed flank steak

SERVES 4

If you are a grilling enthusiast, you will enjoy adding this entrée to your repertoire. The moist stuffing is an unusual combination of vegetables, dried apricots, and chutney.

1 slice whole-grain bread (lowest sodium available), torn into small pieces
1 large carrot, shredded
4 medium green onions, thinly sliced
½ cup coarsely chopped button mushrooms
¼ cup coarsely chopped dried apricots

¼ cup egg substitute
2 tablespoons mango chutney
1 teaspoon salt-free all-purpose seasoning blend
Olive oil spray
1 1-pound flank steak, all visible fat and silver skin discarded

In a small bowl, soak six 10-inch pieces of kitchen twine in enough water to cover for 5 minutes (this will help keep the twine from burning on the grill).

Meanwhile, in a medium bowl, stir together the bread, carrot, green onions, mushrooms, apricots, egg substitute, chutney, and seasoning blend until the bread pieces are moistened.

Lightly spray the grill rack with olive oil spray. Preheat the grill on medium high.

Using a long, sharp knife, butterfly the steak. Starting at the widest edge, cut the steak almost in half parallel to your work surface (through the middle of the meat), stopping about ½ inch from the opposite edge so the two halves are still joined. Open the split steak (it will resemble a butterfly) and discard any visible fat or gristle. Place a piece of plastic wrap over the steak. Using the smooth side of a meat mallet or heavy pan, pound the steak to a thickness of ¼ inch. Don't pound thinner than ¼ inch.

Spoon the bread mixture onto the center of the opened steak. Fold the long edges over the stuffing, enclosing it (leave the ends open). Tie the steak at 2-inch intervals with the kitchen twine. Lightly spray the outside with olive oil spray.

PER SERVING

CALORIES 239
TOTAL FAT 7.0 g
  Saturated Fat 3.0 g
  Trans Fat 0.5 g
  Polyunsaturated Fat 0.5 g
  Monounsaturated Fat 3.5 g
CHOLESTEROL 48 mg
SODIUM 131 mg
CARBOHYDRATES 16 g
  Fiber 3 g
  Sugars 9 g
PROTEIN 27 g
DIETARY EXCHANGES
  1 carbohydrate,
  3 lean meat

Grill the steak, turning every 10 minutes, for 40 to 45 minutes, or until the steak is browned on all sides and the stuffing reaches an internal temperature of 160°F. Transfer to a cutting board. Cover with aluminum foil. Let stand for 10 minutes before slicing crosswise into 8 pieces.

TIME-SAVER
Ask the butcher to butterfly a flank steak for you. Usually there is no extra charge for this service.

grilled lemongrass flank steak

SERVES 4 (PLUS 6 OUNCES RESERVED)

Flank steak is marinated in a fragrant lemongrass mixture that also spotlights delicate rice vinegar and zesty chili garlic sauce. Serve four people tonight and refrigerate the extra two servings to use in Grilled Flank Steak Salad with Sweet-and-Sour Sesame Dressing (page 127) later in the week.

MARINADE
- 3 stalks of lemongrass, outer leaves discarded, bottom 6 to 8 inches cut crosswise into ¼-inch pieces, or 3 teaspoons lemongrass powder
- ⅓ cup plain rice vinegar
- 3 medium garlic cloves, minced
- 1 teaspoon chili garlic sauce or chili garlic paste

- 1 teaspoon soy sauce (lowest sodium available)
- 1 teaspoon canola or corn oil

- 1½ pounds flank steak, all visible fat and silver skin discarded

In a large glass dish, stir together the marinade ingredients. Add the steak, turning to coat. Cover and refrigerate for 2 to 12 hours, turning occasionally.

Preheat the grill on medium high.

Remove the steak from the marinade, discarding the marinade.

Grill the steak for 8 to 9 minutes on each side, or to the desired doneness. Transfer to a cutting board. Let stand for 5 minutes before slicing thinly against the grain. Serve 12 ounces (about two-thirds) of the cooked steak slices. Cover and refrigerate the remaining cooked steak (about 6 ounces) for use in Grilled Flank Steak Salad.

PER SERVING
CALORIES 162
TOTAL FAT 6.5 g
  Saturated Fat 3.0 g
  Trans Fat 0.0 g
  Polyunsaturated Fat 0.5 g
  Monounsaturated Fat 3.0 g
CHOLESTEROL 48 mg
SODIUM 98 mg
CARBOHYDRATES 0 g
  Fiber 0 g
  Sugars 0 g
PROTEIN 24 g
DIETARY EXCHANGES
  3 lean meat

greek-style eye-of-round steaks

SERVES 4

When braised until fork-tender with ingredients popular in Greek cooking, lean eye-of-round steaks make an elegant entrée. This dish is even more delicious the day after you make it.

Olive oil spray
4 eye-of-round steaks (about 4 ounces each), all visible fat discarded
1 large green bell pepper, cut into 1-inch squares
1 cup frozen pearl onions, thawed
1 14.5-ounce can no-salt-added diced tomatoes, undrained

½ cup dry red wine (regular or nonalcoholic)
2 tablespoons chopped kalamata olives
1 teaspoon grated lemon zest
1 tablespoon fresh lemon juice
1 teaspoon dried oregano, crumbled
⅛ teaspoon ground cinnamon

Lightly spray a medium skillet with olive oil spray. Cook the steaks over medium-high heat for 3 minutes on each side, or until browned.

Stir in the bell pepper and onions. Cook for 1 to 2 minutes, or until the pepper is tender-crisp.

Stir in the remaining ingredients. Bring to a simmer. Reduce the heat and simmer, covered, for 1 hour 30 minutes, or until the steaks are tender, stirring occasionally.

PER SERVING

CALORIES 229
TOTAL FAT 3.0 g
  Saturated Fat 1.0 g
  Trans Fat 0.0 g
  Polyunsaturated Fat 0.5 g
  Monounsaturated Fat 1.5 g
CHOLESTEROL 53 mg
SODIUM 137 mg
CARBOHYDRATES 16 g
  Fiber 3 g
  Sugars 7 g
PROTEIN 28 g
DIETARY EXCHANGES
  3 vegetable,
  3 very lean meat

beef bourguignon

SERVES 8

Like other stews, Beef Bourguignon tastes best when made ahead so the flavors have time to blend. Serve it on brown rice or whole-grain noodles.

Cooking spray
1 tablespoon olive oil
5 medium onions, sliced
2 pounds boneless top sirloin roast, all visible fat discarded, cut into 1-inch cubes
1½ tablespoons all-purpose flour
½ teaspoon pepper, or to taste
¼ teaspoon dried marjoram, crumbled

¼ teaspoon dried thyme, crumbled
1 cup dry red wine (regular or nonalcoholic) (plus more as needed)
½ cup fat-free, no-salt-added beef broth, such as on page 42 (plus more as needed)
8 ounces button mushrooms, sliced
½ teaspoon salt

Lightly spray a Dutch oven with cooking spray. Add the oil, swirling to coat the bottom. Heat over medium-high heat. Cook the onions for 5 minutes, or until soft, stirring occasionally. Transfer to a plate.

In the same pot, cook the beef for 10 to 12 minutes, or until browned on all sides.

Sprinkle the beef with the flour, pepper, marjoram, and thyme. Stir well. Stir in the wine and broth. Reduce the heat and simmer, covered, for 1 hour 30 minutes to 2 hours, or until the beef is almost tender. Add more wine and broth (2 parts wine to 1 part broth) as necessary to keep the beef barely covered.

Return the onions to the pot. Stir in the mushrooms and salt. Cook, covered, for 30 minutes, stirring occasionally and adding more wine and broth if necessary. The sauce should be thick and dark brown.

COOK'S TIP on marjoram

Available fresh as well as dried, marjoram tastes much like oregano, but is a bit milder. It is especially good with meats and vegetables.

TIME-SAVER

Reduce the simmering time of the beef in the wine and broth mixture to 30 minutes if you are in a hurry. The flavor won't be as full, but it will still be good.

PER SERVING

CALORIES 230
TOTAL FAT 6.5 g
    Saturated Fat 2.0 g
    Trans Fat 0.0 g
    Polyunsaturated Fat 0.5 g
    Monounsaturated Fat 3.5 g
CHOLESTEROL 60 mg
SODIUM 221 mg
CARBOHYDRATES 11 g
    Fiber 2 g
    Sugars 6 g
PROTEIN 27 g
DIETARY EXCHANGES
    2 vegetable, 3 lean meat

mediterranean beef and vegetable stir-fry

SERVES 4

When you spot a vibrant purple eggplant in the grocery, add it to your shopping cart. When you get home, turn to this recipe. A variety of vegetables and lean sirloin round out the dish.

2 teaspoons canola or corn oil
1 pound boneless sirloin steak, all visible fat discarded, cut into thin strips
2 medium shallots, coarsely chopped
1 small eggplant (about 1 pound), cut into ½-inch cubes
2 tablespoons fat-free, low-sodium chicken broth, such as on page 43
1 14.5-ounce can artichoke hearts, drained and coarsely chopped

1 small yellow summer squash, cut into thin slices
1 14.5-ounce can no-salt-added diced tomatoes, undrained
¼ cup coarsely chopped fresh basil
2 tablespoons chopped kalamata olives
¼ teaspoon salt
¼ teaspoon pepper

In a large nonstick skillet, heat the oil over medium-high heat, swirling to coat the bottom. Cook the beef for 4 to 5 minutes, or to the desired doneness, stirring constantly. Transfer to a bowl. Set aside.

In the same pan, cook the shallots for 1 minute, or until tender-crisp, stirring constantly.

Stir in the eggplant and broth. Cook for 4 to 5 minutes, or until the eggplant is tender, stirring constantly.

Stir in the artichoke hearts and squash. Cook for 2 to 3 minutes, or until the squash is tender-crisp, stirring constantly.

Stir in the tomatoes with liquid, basil, olives, salt, and pepper. Cook for 2 to 3 minutes, or until the mixture is almost heated through, stirring constantly.

Stir in the beef. Cook for 1 to 2 minutes, or until heated through, stirring constantly.

COOK'S TIP

For easier slicing, first put the raw beef in the freezer for about 30 minutes.

PER SERVING

CALORIES 261
TOTAL FAT 8.0 g
  Saturated Fat 2.0 g
  Trans Fat 0.0 g
  Polyunsaturated Fat 1.0 g
  Monounsaturated Fat 4.5 g
CHOLESTEROL 60 mg
SODIUM 492 mg
CARBOHYDRATES 19 g
  Fiber 7 g
  Sugars 8 g
PROTEIN 30 g
DIETARY EXCHANGES
  4 vegetable, 3 lean meat

portobello mushrooms and sirloin strips over spinach pasta

SERVES 4

Beef and robust portobello mushrooms, both marinated in red wine and seasonings, make a terrific combination.

MARINADE
- ⅓ cup burgundy or other dry red wine (regular or nonalcoholic)
- 3 tablespoons soy sauce (lowest sodium available)
- 3 tablespoons Worcestershire sauce (lowest sodium available)
- 6 medium garlic cloves, minced
- 2 teaspoons olive oil

- 1½ teaspoons dried oregano, crumbled
- ––––––
- 12 ounces boneless top sirloin steak, all visible fat discarded, cut into thin strips
- 12 ounces portobello mushrooms, sliced
- 8 ounces dried spinach fettuccine

In a medium glass dish, stir together the marinade ingredients. Add the beef and mushrooms, turning to coat. Cover and refrigerate for 30 minutes, turning frequently.

Prepare the pasta using the package directions, omitting the salt. Drain well in a colander.

Drain the beef mixture, discarding the marinade. In a large nonstick skillet, cook half the beef over medium-high heat for 4 minutes, or until no longer pink, stirring frequently. Transfer to a plate. Repeat with the remaining beef mixture, leaving it in the skillet. Return the other half of the beef mixture with any juices to the skillet. Increase the heat to high. Cook for 5 minutes, stirring frequently. Remove from the heat. Spoon over the pasta.

PER SERVING

CALORIES 340
TOTAL FAT 5.0 g
  Saturated Fat 1.5 g
  Trans Fat 0.0 g
  Polyunsaturated Fat 1.0 g
  Monounsaturated Fat 2.0 g
CHOLESTEROL 45 mg
SODIUM 380 mg
CARBOHYDRATES 45 g
  Fiber 3 g
  Sugars 4 g
PROTEIN 30 g
DIETARY EXCHANGES
  3 starch,
  2½ very lean meat

classic chinese beef stir-fry

SERVES 4

For Chinese comfort food at its best, serve lean beef and colorful vegetables in a soy-hoisin sauce over brown rice.

1 cup uncooked instant brown rice
½ cup fat-free, no-salt-added beef broth, such as on page 42
1 tablespoon soy sauce (lowest sodium available)
2 teaspoons cornstarch
1 teaspoon toasted sesame oil
1 pound boneless sirloin steak, all visible fat discarded, cut into thin strips
½ medium red bell pepper, thinly sliced lengthwise

1 cup sugar snap peas, trimmed
4 ounces asparagus, trimmed, cut crosswise into 1-inch pieces
¼ cup canned sliced water chestnuts, drained, or ¼ small jícama, peeled and diced
2 medium green onions, cut into 1-inch pieces
2 tablespoons chopped unsalted peanuts, dry-roasted

Prepare the rice using the package directions, omitting the salt and margarine.

Meanwhile, in a small bowl, whisk together the broth, soy sauce, cornstarch, and oil until the cornstarch is dissolved. Set aside.

Heat a large nonstick skillet over medium-high heat. Cook the beef for 5 minutes, or until no longer pink in the center, stirring constantly. Transfer to a bowl.

In the same skillet, cook the bell pepper for 1 to 2 minutes, or until tender-crisp, stirring constantly.

Stir in the peas, asparagus, water chestnuts, and green onions. Cook for 1 to 2 minutes, or until the peas and asparagus are tender-crisp, stirring constantly.

Stir in the broth mixture and beef. Cook for 2 to 3 minutes, or until the sauce is thickened and the mixture is heated through, stirring constantly. Spoon over the rice. Garnish with the peanuts.

PER SERVING

CALORIES 400
TOTAL FAT 9.5 g
  Saturated Fat 2.5 g
  Trans Fat 0.0 g
  Polyunsaturated Fat 2.0 g
  Monounsaturated Fat 4.5 g
CHOLESTEROL 60 mg
SODIUM 182 mg
CARBOHYDRATES 45 g
  Fiber 6 g
  Sugars 4 g
PROTEIN 33 g
DIETARY EXCHANGES
  2½ starch, 2 vegetable, 3 lean meat

southwestern beef stir-fry

SERVES 4

Try this quick and easy dish if you already know how good chayote squash and tomatillos are—or if you want to find out.

1 cup uncooked instant brown rice

1 pound boneless sirloin steak, all visible fat discarded, cut into thin strips

1 medium chayote, peeled, sliced, and seed discarded

1 medium zucchini, thinly sliced

5 medium tomatillos (about 4 ounces total), paperlike skin discarded, rinsed and quartered

1 14.5-ounce can no-salt-added diced tomatoes, undrained

2 tablespoons canned green chiles, drained

½ teaspoon ground cumin

¼ teaspoon salt

Prepare the rice using the package directions, omitting the salt and margarine.

Meanwhile, heat a large nonstick skillet over medium-high heat. Cook the beef for 4 to 5 minutes, or until no longer pink in the center, stirring constantly. Transfer to a bowl.

In the same skillet, cook the chayote, zucchini, and tomatillos for 3 to 4 minutes, or until the chayote and zucchini are tender-crisp, stirring constantly.

Stir in the tomatoes with liquid, chiles, cumin, and salt. Cook for 3 to 4 minutes, or until the chayote and zucchini are tender, stirring constantly.

Stir in the beef. Cook for 2 minutes, or until heated through, stirring constantly. Serve over the rice.

PER SERVING

CALORIES 286
TOTAL FAT 6.0 g
  Saturated Fat 2.0 g
  Trans Fat 0.0 g
  Polyunsaturated Fat 1.0 g
  Monounsaturated Fat 2.5 g
CHOLESTEROL 60 mg
SODIUM 293 mg
CARBOHYDRATES 28 g
  Fiber 5 g
  Sugars 6 g
PROTEIN 30 g
DIETARY EXCHANGES
  1 starch, 2 vegetable, 3 lean meat

braised sirloin tips

SERVES 8

For a real treat, try this dish with Sweet Lemon Snow Peas (page 458) and no-yolk noodles.

2 pounds sirloin tip, all visible fat discarded, cut into 1-inch cubes	⅓ cup dry red wine (regular or nonalcoholic)
¼ teaspoon pepper	1 tablespoon soy sauce (lowest sodium available)
1 small to medium onion, finely chopped	2 tablespoons cornstarch
2 medium garlic cloves, minced	¼ cup cold water
1¼ cups fat-free, no-salt-added beef broth, such as on page 42	¼ cup snipped fresh parsley

Sprinkle the beef with the pepper.

Heat a large nonstick skillet over medium-high heat. Cook the beef for 8 to 10 minutes, or until well browned on all sides, stirring frequently.

Stir in the onion and garlic. Cook for 3 minutes, or until the onion is soft, stirring frequently.

Stir in the broth, wine, and soy sauce. Bring to a boil. Reduce the heat and simmer, covered, for 1 hour 30 minutes, or until the beef is tender.

Put the cornstarch in a small bowl. Add the water, whisking to dissolve. Slowly pour into the skillet, stirring constantly. Increase the heat to medium high. Cook for 2 to 3 minutes, or until thickened, stirring constantly. Sprinkle with the parsley.

PER SERVING

CALORIES 162
TOTAL FAT 3.0 g
  Saturated Fat 1.0 g
  Trans Fat 0.0 g
  Polyunsaturated Fat 0.5 g
  Monounsaturated Fat 1.5 g
CHOLESTEROL 58 mg
SODIUM 124 mg
CARBOHYDRATES 4 g
  Fiber 1 g
  Sugars 1 g
PROTEIN 26 g
DIETARY EXCHANGES
  3 very lean meat

steak and vegetable kebabs

SERVES 4

The steak for these kebabs marinates for eight hours so it has plenty of time to absorb the hearty flavors.

MARINADE
- 1 small onion, chopped
- ½ cup dry red wine (regular or nonalcoholic)
- 2 tablespoons red wine vinegar
- 1 tablespoon brown sugar
- 4 medium garlic cloves, minced
- 1 teaspoon paprika
- ½ teaspoon pepper

Cooking spray
- 1 large red onion, cut into 16 wedges
- 1 small red bell pepper, cut into 16 squares
- 16 cherry tomatoes
- 1 small yellow bell pepper, cut into 16 squares
- ½ teaspoon salt

- 1 pound sirloin tip steak, all visible fat discarded, cut into 16 cubes

In a large glass dish, stir together the marinade ingredients until the sugar is dissolved. Add the beef, turning to coat. Cover and refrigerate for 8 hours, turning occasionally. Drain the beef, discarding the marinade.

Soak 8 long wooden skewers for at least 10 minutes in cold water to keep them from charring, or use metal skewers.

Lightly spray the grill rack with cooking spray. Preheat the grill on medium high.

On each skewer, thread in order a beef cube, onion wedge, red bell pepper square, cherry tomato, and yellow bell pepper square. Repeat on each skewer. Sprinkle with the salt.

Grill the kebabs for 12 to 15 minutes, or until the desired doneness, turning frequently.

COOK'S TIP

If you don't want to use wine for marinating the steak, you can use fat-free, no-salt-added beef broth, such as on page 42, instead.

PER SERVING
CALORIES 174
TOTAL FAT 3.0 g
  Saturated Fat 1.5 g
  Trans Fat 0.0 g
  Polyunsaturated Fat 0.5 g
  Monounsaturated Fat 1.5 g
CHOLESTEROL 58 mg
SODIUM 366 mg
CARBOHYDRATES 8 g
  Fiber 2 g
  Sugars 5 g
PROTEIN 26 g
DIETARY EXCHANGES
  2 vegetable,
  3 very lean meat

asian beef skillet

SERVES 4

The ingredients in this dish provide a pleasant color and flavor palette. Try this stir-fry over a bed of brown rice.

2 tablespoons dry sherry
2 tablespoons water
1 tablespoon cornstarch
1 tablespoon soy sauce (lowest sodium available)
1½ teaspoons grated peeled gingerroot
⅛ teaspoon red hot-pepper sauce
8 ounces flank steak, all visible fat and silver skin discarded, cut against the grain into strips 2 to 3 inches long and ½ to 1 inch wide

2 teaspoons canola or corn oil
¼ cup chopped onion
1 to 2 medium garlic cloves, minced
2 cups small cauliflower florets (about ½ medium head)
1 cup fat-free, no-salt-added beef broth, such as on page 42
1 small or medium red bell pepper, diced
3 ounces snow peas, trimmed

In a small bowl, whisk together the sherry, water, cornstarch, soy sauce, gingerroot, and hot-pepper sauce. Set aside.

Heat a large nonstick skillet over medium-high heat. Cook half the beef for 3 to 4 minutes, or just until browned, stirring constantly. Transfer to a bowl. Repeat with the remaining beef.

In the same skillet, heat the oil, swirling to coat the bottom. Cook the onion and garlic for 3 minutes, or until the onion is soft, stirring frequently.

Stir in the cauliflower and broth. Cook for 2 minutes.

Stir in the bell pepper and snow peas. Cook for 1 minute.

Stir the sherry mixture and beef into the cauliflower mixture. Cook for 2 to 3 minutes, or until the sauce is thickened.

PER SERVING

CALORIES 156
TOTAL FAT 6.0 g
  Saturated Fat 1.5 g
  Trans Fat 0.0 g
  Polyunsaturated Fat 1.0 g
  Monounsaturated Fat 3.0 g
CHOLESTEROL 24 mg
SODIUM 145 mg
CARBOHYDRATES 10 g
  Fiber 3 g
  Sugars 4 g
PROTEIN 15 g
DIETARY EXCHANGES
  2 lean meat, 2 vegetable

savory beef stew

SERVES 12

The exciting array of seasonings makes this stew interesting. Try serving Whole-Wheat French Bread (page 518) with it.

Cooking spray
2½ pounds eye-of-round roast, all visible fat discarded, cut into bite-size pieces
1 teaspoon olive oil
1 large onion, finely chopped
5½ cups fat-free, no-salt-added beef broth and 2 cups fat-free, no-salt-added beef broth, such as on page 42, divided use
1 teaspoon dried thyme and 1 teaspoon dried thyme, crumbled, divided use
1 teaspoon dried marjoram, crumbled

1 medium dried bay leaf
1 pound red potatoes, cut into chunks
2 large carrots, sliced
8 ounces button mushrooms, quartered
1 medium red bell pepper, diced
4 medium green onions, thinly sliced
¼ cup plus 2 tablespoons cornstarch
¼ cup no-salt-added tomato paste
1 teaspoon dried Italian seasoning, crumbled
¾ teaspoon pepper
½ teaspoon salt

Lightly spray a stockpot with cooking spray. Heat over medium-high heat. Cook the beef for 2 to 3 minutes on each side, or until browned (the beef won't be done at this point). Transfer to a large plate.

In the same pot, heat the oil, swirling to coat the bottom. Cook the onion for 3 to 4 minutes, or until soft, stirring frequently.

Stir in the beef, any pan juices, 5½ cups broth, 1 teaspoon thyme, marjoram, and bay leaf. Increase the heat to high and bring to a boil. Reduce the heat and simmer, covered, for 1 hour 30 minutes, or until the beef is tender.

Stir in the potatoes, carrots, and mushrooms. Simmer, covered, for 30 minutes.

Stir in the bell pepper and green onions.

In a medium bowl, whisk together the cornstarch, tomato paste, remaining 1 teaspoon thyme, Italian seasoning, pepper, salt, and remaining 2 cups broth. Pour into the stew. Increase the heat to high and bring to a boil, stirring constantly. Reduce the heat to low. Cook for 5 minutes, or until the sauce is thickened, stirring constantly. Discard the bay leaf.

PER SERVING

CALORIES 189
TOTAL FAT 2.5 g
  Saturated Fat 1.0 g
  Trans Fat 0.0 g
  Polyunsaturated Fat 0.5 g
  Monounsaturated Fat 1.0 g
CHOLESTEROL 40 mg
SODIUM 168 mg
CARBOHYDRATES 17 g
  Fiber 3 g
  Sugars 4 g
PROTEIN 24 g
DIETARY EXCHANGES
  ½ starch, 1 vegetable, 3 very lean meat

COOK'S TIP on no-salt-added tomato paste

Sometimes you can save money by reading nutrition labels. For instance, a can of tomato paste labeled "No salt added" may cost more than "regular" tomato paste with the same sodium content—about 20 milligrams per serving.

COOK'S TIP on red bell peppers

Buy red bell peppers when they're on sale and roast or broil them for later use. Freeze them in resealable freezer bags for up to four months.

yogurt-marinated grilled round steak

SERVES 4

Round steak usually needs long, slow cooking to become tender. In this recipe the acidity of the yogurt and lemon does the job instead. Let the steak marinate while you're at work or out for the day and then come home and fire up the grill. Serve with grilled red bell pepper and onion strips and whole-grain pita bread.

MARINADE
- 6 ounces fat-free plain yogurt
- ¼ cup thinly sliced green onions
- 2 tablespoons snipped fresh parsley (Italian, or flat-leaf, preferred)
- 2 teaspoons grated lemon zest
- 1 tablespoon fresh lemon juice
- 1 medium garlic clove, minced

- 1 1-pound boneless round steak, all visible fat discarded
- ¼ cup fat-free sour cream
- ¼ teaspoon salt

In a large glass dish, stir together the marinade ingredients. Pour ¼ cup marinade into a small bowl. Set aside. Add the steak to the remaining marinade, turning to coat. Cover the dish and refrigerate the steak for 8 hours, turning occasionally.

Stir the sour cream into the marinade in the small bowl. Cover and refrigerate until ready to serve.

Preheat the grill on medium high.

Scrape the marinade off the steak, discarding the marinade. Sprinkle the steak with the salt.

Grill the steak for 6 to 8 minutes on each side, or to the desired doneness. Thinly slice the steak against the grain. Serve with the sauce.

PER SERVING

CALORIES 158
TOTAL FAT 3.0 g
  Saturated Fat 1.0 g
  Trans Fat 0.0 g
  Polyunsaturated Fat 0.0 g
  Monounsaturated Fat 1.5 g
CHOLESTEROL 61 mg
SODIUM 263 mg
CARBOHYDRATES 4 g
  Fiber 0 g
  Sugars 2 g
PROTEIN 28 g
DIETARY EXCHANGES
  3 very lean meat

swiss steak

SERVES 4

Baking lean round steak makes it fork-tender. Try this classic dish with fluffy mashed potatoes, such as Mashed Potatoes with Parmesan and Green Onions (page 462).

Cooking spray
1 1-pound boneless top round steak, about ¾ inch thick, all visible fat discarded, quartered
¼ teaspoon pepper
⅛ teaspoon salt
1 cup chopped onion
1 medium carrot, chopped
1 medium rib of celery, chopped
¼ small green bell pepper, chopped

3 medium button mushrooms, chopped
1 14.5-ounce can no-salt-added whole tomatoes, drained and chopped
½ cup fat-free, no-salt-added beef broth, such as on page 42
½ teaspoon dried thyme, crumbled
½ teaspoon Worcestershire sauce (lowest sodium available)

Preheat the oven to 350°F. Lightly spray a Dutch oven with cooking spray.

Cook the steaks in the Dutch oven over medium-high heat for about 3 minutes on each side, or until well browned. Drain any liquid.

Sprinkle both sides of the steaks with the pepper and salt. Place the onion, carrot, celery, bell pepper, and mushrooms around the steaks. Cook for 2 to 3 minutes, stirring frequently.

Stir in the remaining ingredients.

Bake, covered, for 45 to 50 minutes, or until the steaks are tender.

PER SERVING

CALORIES 184
TOTAL FAT 3.0 g
  Saturated Fat 1.5 g
  Trans Fat 0.0 g
  Polyunsaturated Fat 0.5 g
  Monounsaturated Fat 1.5 g
CHOLESTEROL 57 mg
SODIUM 209 mg
CARBOHYDRATES 10 g
  Fiber 3 g
  Sugars 6 g
PROTEIN 28 g
DIETARY EXCHANGES
  2 vegetable,
  3 very lean meat

slow-cooker round steak with mushrooms and tomatoes

SERVES 4

Browning the steak strips in olive oil before placing them in the slow cooker adds a more robust flavor to the final dish.

Cooking spray
1 teaspoon garlic powder
¼ teaspoon cayenne
⅛ teaspoon pepper
1 pound boneless top round steak, all visible fat discarded, cut into 2 x 1-inch strips
1 tablespoon olive oil
1 14.5-ounce can no-salt-added stewed tomatoes, undrained
8 ounces button mushrooms, sliced
½ medium onion (sweet, such as Vidalia or Maui, preferred), chopped
1 medium green or red bell pepper, chopped

¼ cup water and 2 tablespoons water, divided use
¼ cup picante sauce (lowest sodium available)
2 tablespoons vinegar
1 tablespoon Worcestershire sauce (lowest sodium available)
1 tablespoon snipped fresh parsley
3 medium garlic cloves, minced
2 teaspoons dried oregano, crumbled
1½ teaspoons firmly packed light brown sugar
1 tablespoon cornstarch
3 ounces dried whole-grain noodles
¼ cup chopped green onions (optional)

Lightly spray a 4- or 4½-quart slow cooker with cooking spray.

In a small bowl, stir together the garlic powder, cayenne, and pepper. Sprinkle over the top side of the beef.

In a large nonstick skillet, heat the oil over medium-high heat, swirling to coat the bottom. Cook the beef for 5 to 7 minutes, or until browned, stirring frequently. Transfer to the slow cooker.

In a large bowl, stir together the stewed tomatoes with liquid, mushrooms, onion, bell pepper, ¼ cup water, picante sauce, vinegar, Worcestershire sauce, parsley, garlic, oregano, and brown sugar. Stir into the beef mixture. Cook, covered, on low for 6 to 7 hours, or until the meat is tender. (If you are in a hurry, you can cook the mixture on high for 3 hours to 3 hours 30 minutes, but the meat will not be quite as tender.)

PER SERVING

CALORIES 324
TOTAL FAT 7.0 g
  Saturated Fat 1.5 g
  Trans Fat 0.0 g
  Polyunsaturated Fat 1.0 g
  Monounsaturated Fat 4.0 g
CHOLESTEROL 58 mg
SODIUM 159 mg
CARBOHYDRATES 33 g
  Fiber 6 g
  Sugars 10 g
PROTEIN 32 g
DIETARY EXCHANGES
  1½ starch, 2 vegetable,
  3 lean meat

Put the cornstarch in a small bowl. Add the remaining 2 tablespoons water, whisking to dissolve. Stir into the meat mixture. Cook, covered, on high for 10 to 15 minutes, or until slightly thickened.

Meanwhile, prepare the noodles using the package directions, omitting the salt. Drain well in a colander. Serve topped with the beef mixture and green onions.

COOK'S TIP on slow cookers

Lifting the lid of a slow cooker to take a quick peek increases the time needed to finish cooking the dish. Because most slow-cooker recipes don't require stirring, taking that peek usually isn't necessary.

cube steak with mushroom sauce

SERVES 4

Shallots impart a wonderful flavor and aroma to this quick-to-prepare steak and mushroom dish, and the grape spread adds a winelike flavor.

½ teaspoon salt-free onion and herb seasoning blend
½ teaspoon garlic powder
½ teaspoon pepper
4 cube steaks (about 4 ounces each), all visible fat discarded
2 teaspoons olive oil

8 ounces button mushrooms, sliced
2 medium shallots, finely chopped
1½ tablespoons all-purpose flour
1 cup fat-free, no-salt-added beef broth, such as on page 42
3 tablespoons all-fruit grape spread

In a small bowl, stir together the seasoning blend, garlic powder, and pepper. Sprinkle over both sides of the steaks.

In a large nonstick skillet, heat the oil over medium-high heat, swirling to coat the bottom. Cook the steaks for 4 to 5 minutes on each side, or until browned. Transfer to a large plate. Cover to keep warm.

In the same skillet, cook the mushrooms and shallots over medium-high heat for 4 to 5 minutes, or until soft, stirring frequently.

Stir in the flour. Stir in the broth and grape spread. Bring to a boil. Reduce the heat and simmer for 1 to 2 minutes, or until thickened, stirring constantly.

Add the steaks, spooning the sauce over them. Simmer for 1 to 2 minutes, or until heated through.

COOK'S TIP on shallots

Shallots resemble garlic bulbs but are actually part of the onion family. A staple of French cooking, they offer a more delicate flavor than other onions.

philadelphia-style cheese steak wrap

SERVES 6

When you wrap marinated beef, onions, and bell peppers in a tortilla with a bit of cheese, you have a twist on a classic.

MARINADE
- 1 tablespoon balsamic vinegar or red wine vinegar
- 2 teaspoons Worcestershire sauce (lowest sodium available)
- 1 teaspoon sugar
- 1 teaspoon dried oregano, crumbled
- 1 teaspoon olive oil
- 2 medium garlic cloves, minced
- ¼ teaspoon pepper

- 12 ounces eye-of-round roast, all visible fat discarded, cut against the grain into ⅛-inch slices

- 1 small onion, thinly sliced
- 1 medium green bell pepper, thinly sliced
- 2 1-ounce slices fat-free sharp Cheddar cheese, each cut into thirds
- 6 6-inch fat-free flour tortillas (lowest sodium available)

In a medium glass dish, stir together the marinade ingredients until the sugar is dissolved. Add the beef, turning to coat. Cover and refrigerate for 10 minutes to 8 hours, turning occasionally.

Preheat the oven to 350°F.

Heat a nonstick griddle or large nonstick skillet over medium-high heat. Drain the steak, discarding the marinade. Cook for 3 to 5 minutes, or until no longer pink, stirring occasionally. Transfer to a bowl. Cover.

Wipe the griddle with paper towels. Cook the onion and bell pepper for about 5 minutes, or until soft, stirring occasionally.

Place the tortillas in a large, shallow baking pan. Spoon the beef down the center of each tortilla. Top with the onion mixture and cheese. Cover with aluminum foil. Heat in the oven for 4 to 5 minutes. Roll up the tortillas jelly-roll style. Secure with toothpicks if desired.

MICROWAVE METHOD

Place tortillas on a microwaveable plate. Add the filling as directed. Microwave on 100 percent power (high) for 30 seconds. Roll up the tortillas as directed.

PER SERVING

CALORIES 159
TOTAL FAT 1.5 g
  Saturated Fat 0.5 g
  Trans Fat 0.0 g
  Polyunsaturated Fat 0.0 g
  Monounsaturated Fat 0.5 g
CHOLESTEROL 26 mg
SODIUM 311 mg
CARBOHYDRATES 17 g
  Fiber 2 g
  Sugars 2 g
PROTEIN 18 g
DIETARY EXCHANGES
  1 starch, 2 very lean meat

salisbury steaks with mushroom sauce

SERVES 4

The sauce for this dressed-up hamburger patty uses the soaking liquid from your favorite dried mushrooms. Complete the meal with Baked Fries with Creole Seasoning (page 463) and sliced tomatoes.

½ to ¾ ounce dried mushrooms, any
  variety or combination
1 cup warm water

BEEF PATTIES

12 ounces extra-lean ground beef
½ medium onion, grated or minced
1½ tablespoons all-purpose flour
1½ teaspoons Worcestershire sauce
  (lowest sodium available)
½ teaspoon salt-free all-purpose
  seasoning blend
¼ teaspoon dried thyme, crumbled

¼ teaspoon salt
⅛ teaspoon pepper
2 tablespoons fat-free milk

────

½ cup (about) fat-free, no-salt-added
  beef broth, such as on page 42
½ cup dry red wine (regular or
  nonalcoholic)
½ medium carrot, grated
2 to 3 tablespoons snipped fresh
  parsley

In a small bowl, soak the mushrooms in the water for 20 to 30 minutes.

Meanwhile, in a large bowl, using your hands or a spoon, combine all the patty ingredients except the milk. Pour in the milk and combine. Shape into 4 patties.

Using a small sieve, scoop out the mushrooms, reserving the liquid. Rinse the mushrooms, then chop. Strain the liquid through a damp coffee filter, paper towel, or cheesecloth into a 2-cup liquid measuring cup to remove any dirt. Add enough broth to the strained liquid to make 1 cup.

Stir the wine into the broth mixture.

In a heavy nonstick skillet, cook the patties over medium-high heat for 5 to 6 minutes on each side, or until they are brown and register 160°F on an instant-read thermometer. Reduce the heat to medium if the patties are browning too quickly. Drain on paper towels. Discard any liquid left in the skillet.

In the same skillet, bring the mushrooms, wine mixture, and carrot to a boil over high heat. Boil for 4 to 5 minutes, or until the liquid is reduced by one-third to one-half.

Add the patties. Reduce the heat and simmer for 10 minutes. Sprinkle with the parsley.

PER SERVING

CALORIES 178
TOTAL FAT 4.5 g
  Saturated Fat 1.5 g
  Trans Fat 0.5 g
  Polyunsaturated Fat 0.5 g
  Monounsaturated Fat 2.0 g
CHOLESTEROL 47 mg
SODIUM 232 mg
CARBOHYDRATES 8 g
  Fiber 2 g
  Sugars 2 g
PROTEIN 21 g
DIETARY EXCHANGES
  1 vegetable,
  2½ lean meat

grilled hamburgers with vegetables and feta

SERVES 6

The vegetables are built right into this hamburger, with a flavor boost from feta cheese.

Cooking spray

HAMBURGERS

1 pound extra-lean ground beef

2 cups shredded broccoli (packaged broccoli slaw)

1 medium portobello mushroom, stem discarded, finely chopped

¼ cup low-fat feta cheese

½ teaspoon salt-free lemon pepper

6 whole-grain hamburger buns (lowest sodium available)

Lightly spray the grill rack with cooking spray. Preheat the grill on medium high.

In a medium bowl, using your hands or a spoon, combine the hamburger ingredients. Shape into 6 patties.

Grill the patties for 4 to 5 minutes on each side, or until they register 160°F on an instant-read thermometer. Serve on the buns.

COOK'S TIP

Rather than the same old ketchup and mustard, try these topping ideas: Dijon mustard flavored with horse-radish, fruit chutney, baby spinach, red onions, or sliced cooked beets (a popular topping in Australia—it's really good, mate!).

PER SERVING

CALORIES 234
TOTAL FAT 6.5 g
    Saturated Fat 2.5 g
    Trans Fat 0.0 g
    Polyunsaturated Fat 1.5 g
    Monounsaturated Fat 2.0 g
CHOLESTEROL 44 mg
SODIUM 353 mg
CARBOHYDRATES 24 g
    Fiber 4 g
    Sugars 4 g
PROTEIN 22 g
DIETARY EXCHANGES
    1½ starch, 2½ lean meat

ground beef stroganoff

SERVES 4

Replacing traditional ingredients with extra-lean beef and light cream cheese makes this stroganoff lighter in saturated fat, so you can enjoy the creamy mushroom sauce without guilt!

5 ounces dried no-yolk noodles	1 cup fat-free evaporated milk
Cooking spray	2 teaspoons all-purpose flour
1 pound extra-lean ground beef	2 tablespoons light chive and onion
½ cup chopped onion	tub cream cheese
2 medium garlic cloves, minced	2 teaspoons Worcestershire sauce
4 to 6 ounces button mushrooms,	(lowest sodium available)
sliced	¼ teaspoon salt
½ cup fat-free, no-salt-added beef	2 tablespoons snipped fresh Italian
broth, such as on page 42	(flat-leaf) parsley

Prepare the noodles using the package directions, omitting the salt. Drain well in a colander. Set aside.

Meanwhile, lightly spray a Dutch oven or large skillet with cooking spray. Cook the beef over medium-high heat for 4 to 5 minutes, or until no longer pink, stirring frequently to turn and break up the beef. Drain if necessary.

Stir in the onion and garlic. Cook for 4 to 5 minutes, or until the onion is soft, stirring occasionally.

Stir in the mushrooms and broth. Reduce the heat and simmer for 5 minutes, stirring occasionally.

In a small bowl, whisk together the evaporated milk and flour until smooth. Stir into the beef mixture. Increase the heat to medium. Bring to a simmer. Reduce the heat and simmer for 2 minutes, or until slightly thickened, stirring constantly.

Stir in the cream cheese, Worcestershire sauce, and salt until well blended. Serve over the noodles. Sprinkle with the parsley.

COOK'S TIP on cleaning mushrooms

Because mushrooms absorb water, clean them by wiping them gently with a damp paper towel or mushroom brush or rinsing them briefly and gently under cold water.

PER SERVING

CALORIES 370
TOTAL FAT 7.5 g
 Saturated Fat 3.0 g
 Trans Fat 0.5 g
 Polyunsaturated Fat 0.5 g
 Monounsaturated Fat 2.5 g
CHOLESTEROL 69 mg
SODIUM 376 mg
CARBOHYDRATES 39 g
 Fiber 2 g
 Sugars 11 g
PROTEIN 36 g
DIETARY EXCHANGES
 2 starch, ½ fat-free milk,
 3 lean meat

sweet barbecue meat loaf

SERVES 4

Bottled barbecue sauce that is spiced up with raspberry spread and a bit of crushed red pepper takes ordinary meat loaf to a new—and delicious—level.

Cooking spray
½ cup barbecue sauce (lowest sodium available)
¼ cup all-fruit raspberry spread, slightly melted
⅛ teaspoon crushed red pepper flakes
1 pound extra-lean ground beef

½ medium green bell pepper, finely chopped
½ medium onion, finely chopped
⅓ cup uncooked quick-cooking oatmeal
2 large egg whites

Preheat the oven to 375°F. Line a baking sheet with aluminum foil. Lightly spray with cooking spray.

In a small bowl, stir together the barbecue sauce, raspberry spread, and pepper flakes.

In a medium bowl, using your hands or a spoon, combine ¼ cup barbecue sauce mixture and the remaining ingredients. Shape the mixture into an oval about 8 x 5 x 5 inches. Place on the baking sheet.

Spoon the remaining barbecue sauce mixture on the top and sides of the meat loaf.

Bake for 50 minutes, or until the meat loaf registers 160°F on an instant-read thermometer. Transfer the baking sheet to a cooling rack and let the meat loaf stand for 5 to 10 minutes before slicing.

COOK'S TIP

One way to slightly melt the all-fruit spread is to put it in a small microwaveable bowl, cover it, and microwave on 100 percent power (high) for about 20 seconds.

PER SERVING

CALORIES 292
TOTAL FAT 6.0 g
  Saturated Fat 2.5 g
  Trans Fat 0.5 g
  Polyunsaturated Fat 0.5 g
  Monounsaturated Fat 2.5 g
CHOLESTEROL 62 mg
SODIUM 325 mg
CARBOHYDRATES 30 g
  Fiber 1 g
  Sugars 22 g
PROTEIN 27 g
DIETARY EXCHANGES
  2 carbohydrate,
  3 lean meat

mediterranean meat loaf

SERVES 4

Here's how to get the taste of meatballs without the work. This meat loaf freezes well (see Timesaver below) so you can make it once and enjoy it twice!

8 ounces extra-lean ground beef
4 ounces low-fat bulk breakfast sausage
1 medium green bell pepper, finely chopped
½ cup finely chopped onion
⅓ cup plain dry bread crumbs (lowest sodium available)

⅓ cup spaghetti sauce and ⅓ cup spaghetti sauce (lowest sodium available), divided use
2 large egg whites
2 teaspoons dried basil, crumbled
1 teaspoon dried oregano, crumbled

Preheat the oven to 350°F.

In a medium bowl, using your hands or a spoon, gently but thoroughly combine all the ingredients except the second ⅓ cup spaghetti sauce.

On a nonstick baking sheet, shape the mixture into a 9 x 5-inch oval loaf. Top with the remaining ⅓ cup spaghetti sauce.

Bake for 50 minutes, or until the loaf registers 160°F on an instant-read thermometer. Let stand for 5 to 10 minutes before slicing.

TIME-SAVER

Save time by doubling this recipe. Bake one loaf and freeze the other (uncooked) to use another day. When it's needed, simply thaw the loaf and bake.

PER SERVING

CALORIES 186
TOTAL FAT 4.5 g
    Saturated Fat 1.5 g
    Trans Fat 0.0 g
    Polyunsaturated Fat 0.5 g
    Monounsaturated Fat 1.0 g
CHOLESTEROL 45 mg
SODIUM 434 mg
CARBOHYDRATES 14 g
    Fiber 2 g
    Sugars 5 g
PROTEIN 21 g
DIETARY EXCHANGES
    1 starch, 2½ lean meat

tex-mex lasagna

SERVES 8

When you're planning a party for a hungry crowd or it's your turn to feed the soccer team, you will appreciate this easy-to-assemble, satisfying meal.

Cooking spray

1 pound extra-lean ground beef

1 14.5-ounce can no-salt-added tomatoes, undrained

½ cup salsa (lowest sodium available), such as Salsa Cruda (page 508)

¼ teaspoon salt

1 cup fat-free ricotta cheese

1 teaspoon chili powder

1 teaspoon ground cumin

16 6-inch corn tortillas, halved

1 cup shredded low-fat Monterey Jack cheese

1 15.5-ounce can no-salt-added pinto beans, rinsed and well drained

1 cup frozen whole-kernel corn, thawed and patted dry

¼ cup sliced black olives

Preheat the oven to 375°F. Lightly spray a 13 x 9 x 2-inch baking pan with cooking spray.

In a large nonstick skillet, cook the beef over medium-high heat for 8 to 10 minutes, or until browned on the outside and no longer pink in the center, stirring occasionally to turn and break up the beef.

Stir in the tomatoes with liquid, salsa, and salt. Reduce the heat to medium low and cook for 5 minutes, or until heated through, stirring occasionally. Turn off the heat, leaving the skillet on the stove.

In a small bowl, stir together the ricotta cheese, chili powder, and cumin.

Arrange 8 tortilla halves in the baking dish. (The tortillas may overlap slightly, and they will not completely cover the bottom.) Spread half the beef mixture over the tortillas. Sprinkle with half the Monterey Jack. Arrange 8 tortilla halves over the cheese. Spoon 1-tablespoon mounds of the ricotta mixture over the tortillas. Using a spatula, flatten each mound slightly. Top the ricotta mixture with the beans and corn. Add another layer of 8 tortilla halves. Spread the remaining beef mixture over the tortillas. Sprinkle with the remaining Monterey Jack. Top with the remaining 8 tortilla halves. Sprinkle with the olives.

Bake, covered, for 30 minutes, or until heated through. Transfer the pan to a cooling rack. Let cool for 5 minutes before cutting.

PER SERVING

CALORIES 288
TOTAL FAT 7.0 g
  Saturated Fat 3.0 g
  Trans Fat 0.0 g
  Polyunsaturated Fat 1.0 g
  Monounsaturated Fat 2.0 g
CHOLESTEROL 42 mg
SODIUM 431 mg
CARBOHYDRATES 31 g
  Fiber 5 g
  Sugars 6 g
PROTEIN 26 g
DIETARY EXCHANGES
  2 starch, 3 lean meat

slow-cooker chili

SERVES 6

This hearty dish blends ground beef with beans, tomatoes, and spices. It's the perfect recipe for a slow cooker.

Cooking spray

CHILI

1 pound extra-lean ground beef
1 cup chopped onion
1 medium green bell pepper, chopped
3 large garlic cloves, minced
1 15.5-ounce can no-salt-added kidney beans, rinsed and drained
1 14.5-ounce can no-salt-added diced tomatoes, undrained
1 8-ounce can no-salt-added tomato sauce

2 to 3 tablespoons chili powder
2 tablespoons water
1 teaspoon sugar (optional)
½ teaspoon dried basil, crumbled
½ teaspoon pepper
¼ teaspoon salt

6 ounces dried whole-grain spaghetti
2 tablespoons shredded or grated Parmesan cheese

Lightly spray a large, heavy skillet and 4- or 4½-quart slow cooker with cooking spray.

In the skillet, cook the beef over medium-high heat for 4 to 5 minutes, or until no longer pink, stirring occasionally to turn and break up the beef. Drain if necessary. Pour the beef into the slow cooker.

Wipe the skillet with paper towels. Lightly spray with cooking spray. Cook the onion and bell pepper over medium-high heat for 3 to 4 minutes, or until soft, stirring frequently.

Stir in the garlic. Cook for 10 seconds, stirring frequently.

Stir the remaining chili ingredients and onion mixture into the beef. Cook, covered, on low for 8 to 10 hours or on high for 4 to 5 hours.

Shortly before serving time, prepare the spaghetti using the package directions, omitting the salt. Drain well in a colander. Serve topped with the chili and Parmesan.

PER SERVING

CALORIES 327
TOTAL FAT 5.5 g
  Saturated Fat 2.0 g
  Trans Fat 0.0 g
  Polyunsaturated Fat 1.0 g
  Monounsaturated Fat 2.0 g
CHOLESTEROL 43 mg
SODIUM 232 mg
CARBOHYDRATES 45 g
  Fiber 9 g
  Sugars 8 g
PROTEIN 27 g
DIETARY EXCHANGES
  2 starch, 3 vegetable,
  2½ very lean meat

COOK'S TIP

To prep the chili up to a day in advance, combine all the chili ingredients in the slow cooker as directed, but don't cook. Remove the insert from the slow cooker, cover, and refrigerate. When you are ready to cook the chili, place the insert in the slow cooker (the slow cooker should be off). Proceed to cook as directed.

beef and pasta skillet

SERVES 6

Serve this family-pleasing dish with steamed zucchini and a dessert of Fruit with Vanilla Cream (page 618).

8 ounces dried tricolor rotini
8 ounces button mushrooms, sliced
8 ounces extra-lean ground beef
1 large onion, chopped
3 medium garlic cloves, minced
1½ teaspoons dried Italian seasoning, crumbled
1½ teaspoons dried basil, crumbled
1 cup water

1 6-ounce can no-salt-added tomato paste
2 tablespoons shredded or grated Parmesan cheese
2 tablespoons finely snipped fresh parsley
1 teaspoon Worcestershire sauce (lowest sodium available)
¼ teaspoon salt

Prepare the pasta using the package directions, omitting the salt. Drain well in a colander.

In a large skillet, stir together the mushrooms, beef, onion, garlic, Italian seasoning, and basil. Cook, covered, over medium-high heat for 8 to 10 minutes, or until the beef is no longer pink and the mushrooms have released their liquid and are fully cooked, stirring occasionally to turn and break up the beef.

In a small bowl, whisk together the remaining ingredients. Stir the mixture and the pasta into the skillet. Cook for 5 minutes.

PER SERVING

CALORIES 246
TOTAL FAT 3.0 g
  Saturated Fat 1.0 g
  Trans Fat 0.0 g
  Polyunsaturated Fat 0.5 g
  Monounsaturated Fat 1.0 g
CHOLESTEROL 22 mg
SODIUM 191 mg
CARBOHYDRATES 39 g
  Fiber 3 g
  Sugars 8 g
PROTEIN 17 g
DIETARY EXCHANGES
  2 starch, 2 vegetable,
  1 very lean meat

spaghetti with meat sauce

SERVES 8

Savory and traditional, this meat sauce is heavy on the vegetables. Team it with fruit for dessert for more heart-healthy benefits.

Cooking spray

MEAT SAUCE

2 large onions, chopped

1½ pounds extra-lean ground beef

4 medium ribs of celery, chopped

1 medium green bell pepper, chopped

1 28-ounce can no-salt-added Italian plum (Roma) tomatoes

1 6-ounce can no-salt-added tomato paste

1 tablespoon Worcestershire sauce (lowest sodium available)

1 teaspoon pepper

1 teaspoon dried oregano, crumbled

1 teaspoon dried basil, crumbled

1 teaspoon garlic powder

2 medium dried bay leaves

———

16 ounces dried whole-grain spaghetti

½ cup shredded or grated Parmesan cheese

Lightly spray a stockpot with cooking spray. Cook the onions over medium-high heat for about 5 minutes, stirring frequently.

Stir in the beef. Cook for 8 to 10 minutes, or until the beef is no longer pink, stirring frequently to turn and break up the beef.

Stir in the celery and bell pepper. Cook for 2 minutes.

Stir in the remaining sauce ingredients. Reduce the heat and simmer, covered, for 30 minutes to 2 hours (the longer, the better), stirring occasionally. Discard the bay leaves.

Near serving time, prepare the pasta using the package directions, omitting the salt. Drain well in a colander. Serve the sauce over the pasta. Sprinkle with the Parmesan.

PER SERVING

CALORIES 399
TOTAL FAT 7.5 g
    Saturated Fat 2.5 g
    Trans Fat 0.5 g
    Polyunsaturated Fat 1.0 g
    Monounsaturated Fat 2.5 g
CHOLESTEROL 50 mg
SODIUM 266 mg
CARBOHYDRATES 56 g
    Fiber 10 g
    Sugars 11 g
PROTEIN 31 g
DIETARY EXCHANGES
    3 starch, 2 vegetable,
    3 lean meat

beef and noodle casserole dijon

SERVES 4

This satisfying casserole requires only one pan from start to finish. With fewer dishes to wash, you'll have the time to take a brisk walk around the block while the casserole bakes.

Cooking spray
8 ounces extra-lean ground beef
8 ounces frozen Italian-style mixed vegetables
1 cup water
1 cup fat-free, no-salt-added beef broth, such as on page 42
½ 10.75-ounce can low-fat condensed cream of mushroom soup (lowest sodium available)
1½ teaspoons Dijon horseradish-flavored mustard, or 1 teaspoon Dijon mustard and ½ teaspoon bottled white horseradish

½ teaspoon dried Italian seasoning, crumbled
½ teaspoon onion powder
¼ teaspoon garlic powder
¼ teaspoon salt
¼ teaspoon pepper
4 ounces dried no-yolk noodles
2 tablespoons plain dry bread crumbs (lowest sodium available)
1 tablespoon shredded or grated Parmesan cheese

Preheat the oven to 350°F.

Lightly spray a Dutch oven with cooking spray. Cook the beef over medium-high heat for 8 to 10 minutes, or until no longer pink, stirring occasionally to turn and break up the beef.

Stir in the vegetables, water, broth, soup, mustard, Italian seasoning, onion powder, garlic powder, salt, and pepper. Bring to a simmer.

Stir in the noodles.

Bake, covered, for 30 to 35 minutes, or until the noodles are tender. Sprinkle with the bread crumbs and Parmesan.

PER SERVING

CALORIES 261
TOTAL FAT 4.5 g
  Saturated Fat 1.5 g
  Trans Fat 0.0 g
  Polyunsaturated Fat 0.5 g
  Monounsaturated Fat 1.5 g
CHOLESTEROL 34 mg
SODIUM 454 mg
CARBOHYDRATES 35 g
  Fiber 4 g
  Sugars 4 g
PROTEIN 19 g
DIETARY EXCHANGES
  2 starch, 1 vegetable,
  2 lean meat

greek-style beef skillet supper

SERVES 4

Classic Greek ingredients transform everyday ground beef into something special.

1 pound extra-lean ground beef	1 teaspoon grated lemon zest
2 cups fat-free, no-salt-added beef broth, such as on page 42	1 teaspoon fresh lemon juice
	½ teaspoon garlic powder
1 14.5-ounce can no-salt-added diced tomatoes, undrained	⅛ teaspoon salt
	¼ teaspoon pepper
2 tablespoons chopped kalamata olives	4 ounces dried whole-grain rotini
	1 10-ounce package frozen chopped spinach, thawed and squeezed dry
1 teaspoon dried oregano, crumbled	
1 teaspoon onion powder	¼ cup crumbled fat-free feta cheese

In a large nonstick skillet, cook the beef over medium-high heat for 8 to 10 minutes, or until no longer pink, stirring occasionally to turn and break up the beef.

Stir in the broth, tomatoes with liquid, olives, oregano, onion powder, lemon zest, lemon juice, garlic powder, salt, and pepper. Bring to a simmer.

Stir in the pasta. Reduce the heat and simmer, covered, for 10 minutes, or until the pasta is tender.

Stir in the spinach. Simmer, covered, for 1 to 2 minutes, or until heated through.

Sprinkle with the feta.

shepherd's pie

SERVES 6

This one-dish meal is for the meat-and-potato lovers in your family.

1 pound extra-lean ground beef
1 cup fat-free, no-salt-added beef broth and ½ cup fat-free, no-salt-added beef broth, such as on page 42, divided use
1 teaspoon pepper
2 medium dried bay leaves
2 whole cloves
Dash of dried thyme, crumbled
2 medium carrots, thinly sliced
1 large onion, thinly sliced
4 ounces button mushrooms, sliced
2 medium ribs of celery, diced

1 cup canned no-salt-added whole-kernel corn, drained
Cooking spray
1 tablespoon plus ¾ teaspoon all-purpose flour
1 pound potatoes, peeled, cooked, and diced
½ cup fat-free milk
1 tablespoon light tub margarine
1 tablespoon very thinly sliced green onions (green part only)
1 cup shredded low-fat mozzarella cheese

In a large skillet, cook the beef over medium-high heat for 8 to 10 minutes, or until no longer pink, stirring frequently to turn and break up the beef.

Stir in 1 cup broth, pepper, bay leaves, cloves, and thyme. Reduce the heat and simmer, covered, for 30 minutes.

Stir in the carrots, onion, mushrooms, celery, and corn. Simmer, covered, for 4 to 5 minutes, or until the vegetables are tender. Discard the bay leaves and cloves.

Meanwhile, preheat the oven to 375°F. Lightly spray a medium casserole dish with cooking spray.

Put the flour in a small bowl. Gradually pour in the remaining ½ cup broth, whisking constantly to form a smooth paste. Stir into the beef mixture. Simmer for 5 minutes, or until slightly thickened. Pour into the casserole dish.

In a large bowl, mash the potatoes with the milk and margarine.

Stir the green onions into the potatoes. Spread over the beef mixture. Sprinkle with the mozzarella.

Bake for 10 minutes.

PER SERVING

CALORIES 277
TOTAL FAT 6.5 g
  Saturated Fat 2.0 g
  Trans Fat 0.0 g
  Polyunsaturated Fat 1.0 g
  Monounsaturated Fat 2.5 g
CHOLESTEROL 49 mg
SODIUM 256 mg
CARBOHYDRATES 30 g
  Fiber 4 g
  Sugars 7 g
PROTEIN 26 g
DIETARY EXCHANGES
  1½ starch, 1 vegetable, 3 lean meat

border beef

SERVES 4

Adding coffee granules to this satisfying dish gives it extra-rich color as well as deep flavor.

Cooking spray
12 ounces extra-lean ground beef
2 medium green bell peppers, chopped
1 large onion, chopped
1 10-ounce can diced tomatoes with lime juice and cilantro, undrained
1½ cups water

2 tablespoons chili powder
1 tablespoon instant coffee granules
1 tablespoon sugar
1½ teaspoons ground cumin and 1 teaspoon ground cumin, divided use
¼ teaspoon salt

Lightly spray a Dutch oven with cooking spray. Cook the beef over medium-high heat for 8 to 10 minutes, or until no longer pink, stirring frequently to turn and break up the beef. Transfer to a plate.

Lightly spray the Dutch oven with cooking spray. Cook the bell peppers and onion for about 5 minutes, or until the onion is soft, stirring frequently.

Return the beef and any accumulated juices to the Dutch oven. Stir in the tomatoes with liquid, water, chili powder, coffee granules, sugar, and 1½ teaspoons cumin. Increase the heat to high and bring to a boil. Reduce the heat and simmer, covered, for 20 minutes. Remove from the heat.

Stir in the salt and remaining 1 teaspoon cumin. Let stand, covered, for 10 minutes so the flavors blend.

PER SERVING

CALORIES 189
TOTAL FAT 5.5 g
  Saturated Fat 2.0 g
  Trans Fat 0.5 g
  Polyunsaturated Fat 1.0 g
  Monounsaturated Fat 2.0 g
CHOLESTEROL 47 mg
SODIUM 370 mg
CARBOHYDRATES 17 g
  Fiber 5 g
  Sugars 10 g
PROTEIN 21 g
DIETARY EXCHANGES
  3 vegetable,
  2½ lean meat

beef tostadas

SERVES 6

Try this Mexican favorite; it's almost as fast as fast food and much better for you.

6 6-inch corn tortillas
Cooking spray

FILLING
1 pound extra-lean ground beef
1 medium onion, finely chopped
1½ to 2 teaspoons chili powder
½ teaspoon ground cumin
½ teaspoon dried oregano, crumbled
½ teaspoon garlic powder
¼ teaspoon salt

Dash of red hot-pepper sauce
————
2 cups shredded lettuce
2 medium Italian plum (Roma) tomatoes or 1 large regular tomato, chopped
¾ cup salsa (lowest sodium available), such as Salsa Cruda (page 508)
¾ cup shredded low-fat Cheddar cheese

Preheat the oven to 450°F.

Put the tortillas on a baking sheet. Lightly spray the tortillas with cooking spray.

Bake for 8 to 10 minutes, or until crisp.

Meanwhile, in a large nonstick skillet, cook the beef and onion over medium-high heat for 8 to 10 minutes, or until the beef is no longer pink, stirring frequently to turn and break up the beef.

Stir in the remaining filling ingredients. Spread over the crisped tortillas.

Top with the remaining ingredients.

PER SERVING

CALORIES 183
TOTAL FAT 5.5 g
  Saturated Fat 2.0 g
  Trans Fat 0.0 g
  Polyunsaturated Fat 0.5 g
  Monounsaturated Fat 2.0 g
CHOLESTEROL 45 mg
SODIUM 393 mg
CARBOHYDRATES 13 g
  Fiber 2 g
  Sugars 4 g
PROTEIN 21 g
DIETARY EXCHANGES
  ½ starch, 1 vegetable,
  2½ lean meat

meat with bell pepper and tomato sauce

SERVES 4

A simple bell pepper and tomato sauce works wonders with leftover lean steak or roast—or try it over cooked pork, chicken, or pasta.

BELL PEPPER AND TOMATO SAUCE
- 1 teaspoon olive oil and 2 teaspoons olive oil (extra virgin preferred), divided use
- 1 medium green bell pepper, thinly sliced lengthwise
- 1 medium onion, thinly sliced crosswise
- 1 teaspoon dried oregano, crumbled
- 1 medium garlic clove, minced

- ½ cup no-salt-added tomato sauce
- ½ cup water
- ½ teaspoon sugar
- 1 teaspoon vinegar
- ½ teaspoon salt

- 12 ounces cooked lean beef, cooked without salt, all visible fat discarded, cut diagonally into thin slices

In a large nonstick skillet, heat 1 teaspoon oil over medium-high heat. Cook the bell pepper, onion, oregano, and garlic for about 4 minutes, or until the onion is soft, stirring frequently.

Stir in the tomato sauce, water, and sugar. Reduce the heat and simmer, covered, for 10 minutes, or until reduced to 1 cup. Remove from the heat.

Stir in the vinegar, salt, and remaining 2 teaspoons oil.

Add the beef to the skillet, spooning the sauce over the slices. Increase the heat to medium and cook, covered, for 5 minutes, or until heated through.

COOK'S TIP

Make the sauce ahead and store it in the freezer so you'll be ready for a lightning-fast meal.

PER SERVING

CALORIES 167
TOTAL FAT 6.5 g
  Saturated Fat 2.0 g
  Trans Fat 0.0 g
  Polyunsaturated Fat 0.5 g
  Monounsaturated Fat 4.0 g
CHOLESTEROL 42 mg
SODIUM 333 mg
CARBOHYDRATES 7 g
  Fiber 2 g
  Sugars 5 g
PROTEIN 19 g
DIETARY EXCHANGES
  1 vegetable,
  2½ lean meat

crustless ham and spinach tart

SERVES 6

This is a great brunch dish. Serve it with Southern Raised Biscuits (page 539) and Claret-Spiced Oranges (page 622).

Cooking spray
2 tablespoons shredded or grated Parmesan cheese and ¼ cup shredded or grated Parmesan cheese, divided use
1 teaspoon olive oil
1 large onion, finely chopped
2 medium garlic cloves, minced
1 10-ounce package frozen chopped spinach, thawed and squeezed dry

3 ½-ounce slices lower-sodium, low-fat ham, all visible fat discarded, cut into strips
1¼ cups fat-free milk
¾ cup egg substitute
1½ tablespoons all-purpose flour
1 tablespoon finely chopped fresh basil or 2 teaspoons dried, crumbled
½ teaspoon pepper
Dash of nutmeg

Preheat the oven to 350°F. Lightly spray a 9-inch glass pie pan with cooking spray. Dust with 2 tablespoons Parmesan.

In a medium nonstick skillet, heat the oil over medium-high heat, swirling to coat the bottom. Cook the onion for 3 to 4 minutes, or until soft, stirring frequently.

Stir in the garlic. Cook for 1 minute, stirring frequently.

Stir in the spinach and ham. Spread the mixture in the pie pan.

In a medium bowl, whisk together the milk, egg substitute, flour, basil, pepper, nutmeg, and remaining ¼ cup Parmesan. Pour over the spinach mixture.

Bake for 50 to 55 minutes, or until a knife inserted in the center comes out clean.

PER SERVING

CALORIES 102
TOTAL FAT 2.5 g
  Saturated Fat 1.0 g
  Trans Fat 0.0 g
  Polyunsaturated Fat 0.0 g
  Monounsaturated Fat 1.0 g
CHOLESTEROL 7 mg
SODIUM 257 mg
CARBOHYDRATES 11 g
  Fiber 2 g
  Sugars 6 g
PROTEIN 10 g
DIETARY EXCHANGES
  ½ starch, 1 vegetable,
  1 lean meat

bayou red beans and rice

SERVES 8

This recipe will show you how easy it is to prepare one of Louisiana's most popular comfort foods.

---

3 15.5-ounce cans no-salt-added red kidney beans, rinsed and drained

3 cups fat-free, low-sodium chicken broth, such as on page 43

1 14.5-ounce can no-salt-added stewed tomatoes, undrained

1 cup chopped lower-sodium, low-fat ham, all visible fat discarded

1 large onion, chopped

2 medium ribs of celery with leaves, chopped

2 teaspoons red hot-pepper sauce

1 medium garlic clove, minced

¼ teaspoon pepper

1 cup uncooked brown rice

In a Dutch oven, stir together all the ingredients except the rice. Bring to a boil over high heat. Reduce the heat and simmer, covered, for 1 hour, stirring occasionally.

Meanwhile, prepare the rice using the package directions, omitting the salt and margarine.

Using a potato masher, mash about one-fourth of the bean mixture while it is in the pot. Stir the mixture. Cook over low heat for 10 minutes, stirring occasionally. Serve over the rice.

PER SERVING

CALORIES 266
TOTAL FAT 0.5 g
    Saturated Fat 0.0 g
    Trans Fat 0.0 g
    Polyunsaturated Fat 0.0 g
    Monounsaturated Fat 0.5 g
CHOLESTEROL 8 mg
SODIUM 186 mg
CARBOHYDRATES 51 g
    Fiber 8 g
    Sugars 7 g
PROTEIN 16 g
DIETARY EXCHANGES
    3 starch, 1 vegetable,
    1 very lean meat

savory black-eyed peas and pasta

SERVES 4

Here's what you can do with a little bit of the ham left over from your holiday dinner.

½ cup minced baked lower-sodium, low-fat ham, all visible fat discarded
1 medium carrot, finely chopped
1 small onion, finely chopped
¼ cup minced fresh parsley
1 medium garlic clove, minced
2 cups fat-free, low-sodium chicken broth, such as on page 43

1 15.5-ounce can no-salt-added black-eyed peas, rinsed and drained
½ teaspoon dried thyme, crumbled
½ teaspoon dried basil, crumbled
½ teaspoon dried oregano, crumbled
½ teaspoon pepper
Dash of cayenne, or to taste
8 ounces dried whole-grain medium pasta shells

In a large nonstick skillet, cook the ham, carrot, onion, parsley, and garlic over medium-high heat for 15 minutes, stirring occasionally.

Stir in the remaining ingredients except the pasta. Bring to a boil. Reduce the heat and simmer for 15 minutes.

Meanwhile, prepare the pasta using the package directions, omitting the salt. Drain well in a colander. Return the pasta to the pot.

Stir the ham mixture into the pasta.

PER SERVING

CALORIES 351
TOTAL FAT 1.5 g
  Saturated Fat 0.5 g
  Trans Fat 0.0 g
  Polyunsaturated Fat 0.5 g
  Monounsaturated Fat 0.5 g
CHOLESTEROL 8 mg
SODIUM 179 mg
CARBOHYDRATES 65 g
  Fiber 7 g
  Sugars 8 g
PROTEIN 18 g
DIETARY EXCHANGES
  4 starch, 1 vegetable, 1 very lean meat

marinated pork tenderloin

SERVES 4

Hot and Spicy Watercress and Romaine Salad (page 85) and brown rice go well with this Asian-flavored pork.

MARINADE
- 1 small onion, grated or minced
- ¼ cup soy sauce (lowest sodium available)
- 1 tablespoon toasted sesame oil
- 2 teaspoons grated peeled gingerroot or ¾ teaspoon ground ginger
- 2 medium garlic cloves, crushed

- 1 teaspoon grated lemon zest

- 1 1-pound pork tenderloin, all visible fat and silver skin discarded
- ¼ cup dry white wine (regular or nonalcoholic)
- ¼ cup honey
- 1 tablespoon dark brown sugar

In a large glass dish, stir together the marinade ingredients. Add the pork, turning to coat. Cover and refrigerate for about 8 hours, turning occasionally.

Preheat the oven to 375°F.

Transfer the pork to a nonstick baking pan, discarding the marinade.

In a small bowl, whisk together the wine, honey, and brown sugar. Pour over the pork, turning to coat.

Bake for 25 to 30 minutes, or until the pork registers 150°F on an instant-read thermometer or is slightly pink in the very center. Transfer to a cutting board. Let stand for about 10 minutes before slicing. The pork will continue to cook during the standing time, reaching about 160°F.

COOK'S TIP on pork tenderloin

Pork tenderloin is long, cylindrical, and usually 2 to 3 inches in diameter. Do not confuse it with the larger pork loin. Be sure to select tenderloin that has not been previously seasoned or marinated.

PER SERVING
CALORIES 247
TOTAL FAT 5.0 g
  Saturated Fat 2.0 g
  Trans Fat 0.0 g
  Polyunsaturated Fat 0.5 g
  Monounsaturated Fat 2.0 g
CHOLESTEROL 75 mg
SODIUM 445 mg
CARBOHYDRATES 22 g
  Fiber 0 g
  Sugars 21 g
PROTEIN 25 g
DIETARY EXCHANGES
  1½ carbohydrate,
  3 lean meat

herb-rubbed pork tenderloin with dijon-apricot mop sauce

SERVES 8

A dry herb rub flavors the pork and makes a nice crust. You may want to stop right there, or you can go one step further and add the tangy mop sauce. Serve the pork with sweet potatoes and green beans.

HERB RUB
- 1 tablespoon dried rosemary, crushed
- 1 tablespoon dried thyme, crumbled
- 1 tablespoon ground cumin
- 2 teaspoons pepper (coarsely ground preferred)
- 2 teaspoons paprika
- 2 teaspoons celery seeds

- 2 1-pound pork tenderloins, all visible fat and silver skin discarded
- Cooking spray

DIJON-APRICOT MOP SAUCE (OPTIONAL)
- 1 teaspoon canola or corn oil
- 1 small onion, finely chopped
- ½ cup cider vinegar
- ¼ cup honey
- ¼ cup all-fruit apricot spread
- 2 tablespoons Dijon mustard
- 1 teaspoon grated lemon zest
- 1 tablespoon fresh lemon juice

In a small bowl, stir together the rub ingredients. Using your fingertips, firmly press the mixture so it adheres to the pork. Set aside.

Preheat the oven to 350°F or lightly spray the grill rack with cooking spray and preheat the grill on medium high.

For the mop sauce, in a small saucepan, heat the oil over medium-high heat, swirling to coat the bottom. Cook the onion for 3 minutes, or until soft, stirring occasionally.

Stir in the remaining sauce ingredients. Bring to a boil. Reduce the heat and simmer for 5 minutes, stirring occasionally. (You may wish to reserve ½ cup sauce to use as a dipping sauce for the cooked pork.)

If baking, lightly spray a broiling pan and rack with cooking spray. Put the tenderloins on the rack in the pan. Bake for 30 minutes. Using a pastry brush or basting mop, baste on all sides. Bake for 10 minutes, then baste again with a clean pastry brush or basting mop. Bake for 10 to 15 minutes, or until the pork registers 150°F on an instant-read thermometer or is slightly pink in the very center.

PER SERVING

CALORIES 231
TOTAL FAT 6.5 g
  Saturated Fat 2.0 g
  Trans Fat 0.0 g
  Polyunsaturated Fat 0.5 g
  Monounsaturated Fat 2.5 g
CHOLESTEROL 75 mg
SODIUM 133 mg
CARBOHYDRATES 18 g
  Fiber 1 g
  Sugars 14 g
PROTEIN 25 g
DIETARY EXCHANGES
  1 carbohydrate,
  3 lean meat

If grilling, grill the tenderloins for 10 minutes on each side (40 minutes total). Baste with the mop sauce. Grill for 2 to 3 minutes on each side, or until the pork registers 150°F on an instant-read thermometer or is slightly pink in the very center.

Transfer the pork to a cutting board. Let stand for about 10 minutes before slicing. The pork will continue to cook during the standing time, reaching about 160°F.

COOK'S TIP

Chicken, flank steak, and eye-of-round roast are delicious with both the rub and the mop sauce. Try the mop sauce on its own over vegetable kebabs, beef, poultry, firm fish fillets, or shrimp.

PER SERVING

WITHOUT SAUCE
CALORIES 160
TOTAL FAT 5.5 g
  Saturated Fat 2.0 g
  Trans Fat 0.0 g
  Polyunsaturated Fat 0.5 g
  Monounsaturated Fat 2.0 g
CHOLESTEROL 75 mg
SODIUM 55 mg
CARBOHYDRATES 2 g
  Fiber 1 g
  Sugars 0 g
PROTEIN 25 g
DIETARY EXCHANGES
  3 lean meat

orange pork medallions

SERVES 4

An unusual combination of flavors enhances this dish. It's very good served with Couscous with Vegetables (page 447).

SAUCE
⅔ to 1 cup fresh orange juice
2½ tablespoons fresh lemon juice
2 tablespoons finely snipped fresh parsley
2 tablespoons all-fruit orange marmalade
1 tablespoon cornstarch
2 teaspoons toasted sesame oil
¾ teaspoon bottled white horseradish
½ teaspoon ground cinnamon

½ teaspoon dried rosemary, crushed
¼ teaspoon pepper
———
1 pound pork tenderloin, all visible fat and silver skin discarded, cut into slices ½ inch thick, flattened to ¼-inch thickness
4 medium green onions, thinly sliced
1 11-ounce can mandarin orange slices in juice, drained
4 large sprigs of fresh parsley (optional)

In a small bowl, whisk together the sauce ingredients.

Heat a large nonstick skillet over medium-high heat. Cook the pork for about 2 minutes on each side, or until browned.

Add the green onions. Cook for 1 minute, or until tender.

Stir in the sauce. Cook for 2 to 3 minutes, or until the pork is slightly pink in the center and the sauce is thickened, stirring constantly.

Serve the sauce over the pork. Spoon the mandarin oranges over or beside the pork. Garnish with the parsley.

PER SERVING
CALORIES 253
TOTAL FAT 7.5 g
    Saturated Fat 2.0 g
    Trans Fat 0.0 g
    Polyunsaturated Fat 1.5 g
    Monounsaturated Fat 3.0 g
CHOLESTEROL 75 mg
SODIUM 65 mg
CARBOHYDRATES 20 g
    Fiber 2 g
    Sugars 14 g
PROTEIN 25 g
DIETARY EXCHANGES
    1 fruit, ½ carbohydrate,
    3 lean meat

slow-cooker pork roast with orange-cranberry sauce

SERVES 4

This fork-tender pork roast features a built-in savory, slightly tart sauce.

1 1-pound boneless pork loin roast, all visible fat discarded	2 tablespoons cider vinegar
1 16-ounce can whole-berry cranberry sauce	2 medium shallots, coarsely chopped
2 teaspoons grated orange zest	1 tablespoon fresh rosemary, coarsely chopped, or 1 teaspoon dried, crushed
1 cup fresh orange juice	¼ teaspoon salt
½ cup water	¼ teaspoon pepper

In the order listed, put all the ingredients in a 3½- or 4-quart slow cooker. Cook, covered, on high for 4 to 5 hours or on low for 8 to 10 hours, or until the pork registers 150°F on an instant-read thermometer or is slightly pink in the very center. Transfer the pork to a cutting board, reserving the sauce. Let stand for about 10 minutes before slicing. The pork will continue to cook during the standing time, reaching about 160°F. Serve topped with the sauce or serve the sauce on the side.

COOK'S TIP

If you have any pork roast left over, try chopping it and combining it with whole-grain pasta and broccoli with the sauce spooned on top.

PER SERVING

CALORIES 364
TOTAL FAT 8.0 g
  Saturated Fat 3.0 g
  Trans Fat 0.0 g
  Polyunsaturated Fat 0.5 g
  Monounsaturated Fat 3.5 g
CHOLESTEROL 64 mg
SODIUM 219 mg
CARBOHYDRATES 50 g
  Fiber 2 g
  Sugars 33 g
PROTEIN 23 g
DIETARY EXCHANGES
  3½ carbohydrate,
  3 lean meat

harvest pork stew

SERVES 4

This stew combines subtle spices with the sweetness of apples and sweet potatoes.

1 pound pork tenderloin, all visible fat and silver skin discarded, cut into 1-inch cubes
2 teaspoons ground ginger
¼ teaspoon salt
¼ teaspoon cayenne
Cooking spray
3 medium garlic cloves, finely chopped
1 tablespoon cider vinegar
¾ pound sweet potatoes, peeled and cut into 1-inch cubes

2 medium unpeeled Granny Smith apples, cut into 1-inch cubes
1 8-ounce red onion, halved lengthwise and cut crosswise into ½-inch slices
1 tablespoon cornstarch
½ teaspoon paprika
¼ teaspoon ground nutmeg
½ cup apple cider
½ cup fat-free, low-sodium chicken broth, such as on page 43

Put the pork in a medium bowl.

In a small bowl, stir together the ginger, salt, and cayenne. Sprinkle over the pork, stirring to coat.

Lightly spray a medium skillet with cooking spray. Cook the pork over medium-high heat for 3 to 5 minutes, or until browned on all sides, stirring frequently.

Lightly spray a 3½- or 4-quart slow cooker with cooking spray. Transfer the pork to the slow cooker. Sprinkle the garlic over the pork. Using a spoon, press the garlic into the pork. Drizzle the vinegar over the pork, turning to coat.

Add the sweet potatoes, apples, and onion to the pork. Using a large spoon or tongs, gently combine.

In a measuring cup (this works well for easy pouring), stir together the cornstarch, paprika, and nutmeg. Pour in the apple cider and broth, stirring to dissolve. Pour into the slow cooker. Stir. Cook, covered, on low for 7 hours, or until the pork is tender. (The high setting is not recommended for this recipe.)

COOK'S TIP

The cider vinegar used here helps tenderize the lean pork tenderloin.

PER SERVING

CALORIES 300
TOTAL FAT 3.0 g
  Saturated Fat 1.0 g
  Trans Fat 0.0 g
  Polyunsaturated Fat 0.5 g
  Monounsaturated Fat 1.0 g
CHOLESTEROL 74 mg
SODIUM 263 mg
CARBOHYDRATES 42 g
  Fiber 6 g
  Sugars 20 g
PROTEIN 27 g
DIETARY EXCHANGES
  1½ starch, 1 fruit,
  1 vegetable,
  3 very lean meat

pork and vegetable lo mein

SERVES 4

No need to get take-out Chinese when you can prepare this dish simply at home and skip the MSG!

4 ounces dried whole-grain linguine	4 medium green onions, chopped, and
Cooking spray	2 medium green onions, chopped
12 ounces boneless center-cut pork	(optional), divided use
loin chops, all visible fat discarded,	2 medium garlic cloves, minced
cut into thin, bite-size strips	1 tablespoon cornstarch
1 8-ounce can sliced water chestnuts,	1 cup fat-free, no-salt-added beef
drained	broth, such as on page 42
¾ cup shredded carrot	1 tablespoon soy sauce (lowest
1 small green bell pepper, diced	sodium available)
1 medium rib of celery, sliced	1 teaspoon grated peeled gingerroot

Prepare the pasta using the package directions, omitting the salt. Drain well in a colander. Set aside.

Meanwhile, lightly spray a large skillet with cooking spray. Cook the pork over medium-high heat for 3 minutes, or until slightly pink in the center, stirring frequently. Transfer to a medium plate. Set aside.

Reduce the heat to medium and cook the water chestnuts, carrot, bell pepper, celery, 4 green onions, and garlic for 4 to 5 minutes, or until the bell pepper and celery are tender, stirring frequently.

Put the cornstarch in a small bowl. Pour in the broth and soy sauce, whisking to dissolve. Add the broth mixture and gingerroot to the water chestnut mixture. Bring to a simmer, still over medium heat, stirring constantly.

Gently stir in the pork and pasta to heat through. Sprinkle with the remaining 2 green onions.

sweet-and-sour pork

SERVES 4

You don't even need a wok to create this classic at home.

1 15-ounce can pineapple chunks in their own juice, drained with juice reserved

1 tablespoon plus 1 teaspoon plain rice vinegar

2 teaspoons dry sherry

2 teaspoons soy sauce (lowest sodium available)

⅛ teaspoon ground ginger

⅛ teaspoon ground allspice

⅛ teaspoon hot-pepper oil

2 teaspoons cornstarch

¼ cup water

12 ounces pork tenderloin, all visible fat and silver skin discarded, cut into 2 x ¼-inch strips

½ cup sliced green bell pepper

1 small onion, sliced

2 tablespoons minced leeks or green onions

2 teaspoons snipped fresh parsley

⅛ teaspoon pepper

Add enough water to the reserved pineapple juice to make 1 cup. Set the pineapple aside.

In a small saucepan, whisk together the pineapple juice mixture, vinegar, sherry, soy sauce, ginger, allspice, and hot-pepper oil. Cook over medium-high heat for 3 to 4 minutes, or until the sauce comes just to a boil, whisking occasionally.

Meanwhile, put the cornstarch in a small bowl. Add ¼ cup water, whisking to dissolve.

Whisk the cornstarch mixture into the pineapple juice mixture. Reduce the heat to medium and cook for 1 to 2 minutes, or until the sauce begins to thicken, whisking constantly. Remove from the heat.

In a large nonstick skillet, cook the pork over medium-high heat for 4 to 5 minutes, or until no longer pink on the outside, stirring frequently. Push to the side.

Reduce the heat to medium. Put the bell pepper, onion, and leeks in the skillet. Top with the pork. Sprinkle with the parsley and pepper. Cook for 4 to 5 minutes, or until the bell pepper and onion are tender-crisp and the pork is slightly pink in the center, stirring occasionally.

Stir in the sauce and pineapple. Cook for 3 minutes.

PER SERVING

CALORIES 199
TOTAL FAT 4.0 g
  Saturated Fat 1.5 g
  Trans Fat 0.0 g
  Polyunsaturated Fat 0.5 g
  Monounsaturated Fat 1.5 g
CHOLESTEROL 56 mg
SODIUM 116 mg
CARBOHYDRATES 20 g
  Fiber 2 g
  Sugars 15 g
PROTEIN 19 g
DIETARY EXCHANGES
  1 fruit, 1 vegetable,
  2½ lean meat

slow-cooker chile verde pork chops

SERVES 4

In this tangy take on a Mexican classic, tomatillos, lime, and fresh cilantro put the *verde* in this dish.

4 boneless center-cut pork loin chops (about 4 ounces each), all visible fat discarded	1 pound fresh tomatillos, husks discarded, chopped
1 teaspoon ground cumin	1 medium onion, chopped
¼ teaspoon salt	1 teaspoon grated lime zest
¼ teaspoon pepper	1 tablespoon fresh lime juice
2 teaspoons olive oil	4 medium garlic cloves, minced
	2 tablespoons snipped fresh cilantro

Sprinkle the pork chops with the cumin, salt, and pepper.

In a large nonstick skillet, heat the oil over medium heat, swirling to coat the bottom. Brown the pork chops for 2 minutes on each side.

In a 3½- or 4-quart slow cooker, stir together the remaining ingredients except the cilantro. Add the pork chops, spooning some sauce over them. Cook, covered, on high for 2 to 3 hours or on low for 4 to 5 hours, or until the tomatillos are tender and the pork is slightly pink in the center. Transfer the pork chops to plates. Using a slotted spoon, spoon the tomatillo mixture on top. Sprinkle with the cilantro.

COOK'S TIP on tomatillos

Tomatillos look like a cross between a green tomato and a gooseberry and have a tart, applelike flavor. When buying, look for firm, bright green tomatillos. Peel off and discard the papery husks, then rinse the tomatillos under cold water before chopping.

PER SERVING

CALORIES 218
TOTAL FAT 9.5 g
   Saturated Fat 2.0 g
   Trans Fat 0.0 g
   Polyunsaturated Fat 1.5 g
   Monounsaturated Fat 4.0 g
CHOLESTEROL 66 mg
SODIUM 194 mg
CARBOHYDRATES 11 g
   Fiber 3 g
   Sugars 7 g
PROTEIN 23 g
DIETARY EXCHANGES
   2 vegetable, 3 lean meat

asian-style barbecue pork

SERVES 4

Kiwifruit helps tenderize the pork and adds a layer of sweetness to this interesting dish.

1 firm kiwifruit, peeled and coarsely grated

¼ cup coarsely grated onion

2 teaspoons ground ginger

2 teaspoons honey

1 pound pork tenderloin, all visible fat and silver skin discarded, cut on the diagonal into ⅛-inch slices

SAUCE

3 tablespoons finely sliced green onions

2 tablespoons soy sauce (lowest sodium available)

2 tablespoons plain rice vinegar

1 tablespoon sugar

4 medium garlic cloves, minced

2 teaspoons honey

1 teaspoon olive oil

1 teaspoon toasted sesame oil

1 teaspoon crushed red pepper flakes

———

Cooking spray

2 teaspoons soy sauce (lowest sodium available)

1 teaspoon plain rice vinegar

2 medium green onions, thinly sliced

1 teaspoon sesame seeds, dry-roasted

In a medium bowl, stir together the kiwifruit, grated onion, ginger, and 2 teaspoons honey. Add the pork. Using your fingertips, gently press the marinade so it adheres to the pork. Cover and refrigerate for 20 minutes.

Meanwhile, in a small glass bowl, stir together the sauce ingredients. Set aside.

Shortly before the pork finishes marinating, preheat the broiler. Lightly spray the rack of the broiler pan with cooking spray.

Pour the sauce over the marinated pork, turning to coat. Place the pork slices in a single layer on the rack. Discard any remaining sauce.

Broil the pork about 4 inches from the heat for 5 to 7 minutes, or until slightly pink in the center (no turning needed).

Meanwhile, in a small bowl, stir together the remaining 2 teaspoons soy sauce and remaining 1 teaspoon vinegar.

Transfer the pork to a platter. Drizzle the soy sauce mixture over the top. Sprinkle with the green onions and sesame seeds.

PER SERVING

CALORIES 217
TOTAL FAT 5.5 g
  Saturated Fat 1.0 g
  Trans Fat 0.0 g
  Polyunsaturated Fat 1.5 g
  Monounsaturated Fat 2.5 g
CHOLESTEROL 74 mg
SODIUM 327 mg
CARBOHYDRATES 16 g
  Fiber 1 g
  Sugars 12 g
PROTEIN 25 g
DIETARY EXCHANGES
  1 carbohydrate,
  3 lean meat

easy barbecue-sauced pork chops

SERVES 4

This is a great recipe for those harried days when you need something easy for your dinner entrée. It takes almost no time to put together and cooks very quickly.

4 boneless center-cut pork loin chops (about 4 ounces each), all visible fat discarded

⅓ cup barbecue sauce (lowest sodium available)

2 tablespoons all-fruit blackberry spread

2 teaspoons Worcestershire sauce (lowest sodium available)

1 teaspoon grated orange zest

½ teaspoon grated peeled gingerroot

Heat a large nonstick skillet over medium-high heat. Cook the pork for 4 minutes on each side, or until slightly pink in the center. Transfer to plates. Remove the skillet from the heat.

In the same skillet, stir together the remaining ingredients. Bring to a boil, scraping the bottom of the pan to dislodge any browned bits. Reduce the heat to medium. Cook for 2 minutes, or until reduced to ¼ cup. Spoon over the pork.

PER SERVING

CALORIES 205
TOTAL FAT 6.0 g
  Saturated Fat 1.5 g
  Trans Fat 0.0 g
  Polyunsaturated Fat 0.5 g
  Monounsaturated Fat 2.0 g
CHOLESTEROL 66 mg
SODIUM 191 mg
CARBOHYDRATES 14 g
  Fiber 0 g
  Sugars 12 g
PROTEIN 21 g
DIETARY EXCHANGES
  1 carbohydrate,
  3 lean meat

pork chops stuffed with apricots and walnuts

SERVES 4

Slightly sweet, slightly tart filling permeates pork chops as they cook, and walnuts add a delicate crunch. Serve with whole-grain pasta and steamed green beans garnished with lemon zest.

4 boneless pork loin chops (about 4 ounces each), all visible fat discarded
½ cup chopped dried apricots
2 tablespoons chopped walnuts
1 tablespoon light brown sugar
1 tablespoon cider vinegar

1 teaspoon dried marjoram, crumbled
½ cup unsweetened apple juice
½ cup fat-free, low-sodium chicken broth, such as on page 43
1 tablespoon maple syrup
¼ teaspoon pepper

With a sharp knife, make a lengthwise cut into the side of each pork chop to form a pocket for stuffing. Be careful not to cut through to the other side.

In a small bowl, stir together the apricots, walnuts, brown sugar, vinegar, and marjoram. Spoon about 2 tablespoons of the mixture into the pocket of each pork chop. Secure with wooden toothpicks.

In a large nonstick skillet, cook the pork over medium heat for 1 minute on each side, or until golden brown. (Watch carefully. The brown sugar in the filling may seep out, which can make the pork burn more easily.)

Stir in the remaining ingredients. Increase the heat to medium high and bring to a simmer. Reduce the heat and simmer, covered, for 30 minutes, or until the pork is slightly pink in the center and the stuffing is heated through. Transfer to a serving plate. Discard the toothpicks. Cover the plate to keep warm.

Increase the heat to medium high and bring the cooking liquid to a simmer. Reduce the heat and simmer for 5 minutes, or until reduced to about ½ cup. Spoon over the pork.

PER SERVING

CALORIES 264
TOTAL FAT 9.0 g
  Saturated Fat 2.5 g
  Trans Fat 0.0 g
  Polyunsaturated Fat 2.5 g
  Monounsaturated Fat 3.0 g
CHOLESTEROL 67 mg
SODIUM 56 mg
CARBOHYDRATES 21 g
  Fiber 2 g
  Sugars 18 g
PROTEIN 25 g
DIETARY EXCHANGES
  1 fruit, ½ carbohydrate,
  3 lean meat

jollof rice

SERVES 8

Jollof rice is a way of cooking rice with meat, vegetables, and different spices. Popular in western Africa, this dish will be a hit in your home as well.

Cooking spray
1 pound boneless center-cut pork loin chops (about 4 ounces each), all visible fat discarded, cut into ¾-inch cubes
1 medium bell pepper, diced (any color) (optional)
1 large carrot, thinly sliced
1 medium onion, chopped
2 medium garlic cloves, minced
2 cups fat-free, low-sodium chicken broth, such as on page 43
1 14.5-ounce can no-salt-added diced tomatoes, undrained
1 cup water
¼ cup no-salt-added tomato paste
¼ cup diced lower-sodium, low-fat ham (about 2 ounces), all visible fat discarded

1 fresh medium jalapeño, seeds and ribs discarded, diced
1 teaspoon curry powder
½ teaspoon salt
¼ teaspoon pepper
1 medium dried bay leaf
2 cups uncooked instant brown rice
2 cups frozen green beans
1 cup frozen green peas
GARNISHES (OPTIONAL)
¼ cup snipped fresh parsley
1 cup chopped cooked cabbage
Whites of 4 large hard-cooked eggs, chopped

Lightly spray a Dutch oven with cooking spray. Cook the pork over medium-high heat for 5 to 6 minutes, or until browned, stirring occasionally.

Stir in the bell pepper, carrot, onion, and garlic. Cook for about 3 minutes, or until the onion is soft, stirring occasionally.

Stir in the broth, tomatoes with liquid, water, tomato paste, ham, jalapeño, curry powder, salt, pepper, and bay leaf. Simmer, covered, for 30 minutes to 1 hour, or until the pork is tender and slightly pink in the center.

Stir in the rice, beans, and peas. Increase the heat to medium high and return to a simmer. Simmer, covered, for 10 minutes, or until the rice is tender. Discard the bay leaf. Serve with the garnishes.

PER SERVING

CALORIES 288
TOTAL FAT 5.5 g
  Saturated Fat 1.5 g
  Trans Fat 0.0 g
  Polyunsaturated Fat 1.0 g
  Monounsaturated Fat 2.0 g
CHOLESTEROL 47 mg
SODIUM 349 mg
CARBOHYDRATES 38 g
  Fiber 6 g
  Sugars 7 g
PROTEIN 22 g
DIETARY EXCHANGES
  2 starch, 2 vegetable,
  2 lean meat

boneless pork ribs with black cherry barbecue sauce

SERVES 4

If you crave tender pork ribs, you'll enjoy this boneless version. Lean pork loin with a zesty rub is braised to perfection and served with kicked-up barbecue sauce.

½ teaspoon ground cumin
½ teaspoon chili powder
½ teaspoon onion powder
½ teaspoon garlic powder
¼ teaspoon pepper
1 pound boneless pork loin chops, all visible fat discarded, cut into 16 strips, each about 1 inch wide

Cooking spray
8 ounces beer (light or nonalcoholic)
¼ cup barbecue sauce (lowest sodium available)
¼ cup all-fruit black cherry spread

In a medium bowl, stir together the cumin, chili powder, onion powder, garlic powder, and pepper. Add the pork, turning to coat.

Lightly spray a large skillet with cooking spray. Cook the pork over medium-high heat for 3 minutes on each side, or until browned.

Pour the beer into the skillet. Bring to a simmer. Reduce the heat and simmer, covered, for 1 hour to 1 hour 30 minutes, or until the pork is tender and slightly pink in the center (no stirring needed). Transfer the pork strips to a serving plate, leaving the liquid. Cover the plate to keep warm.

Stir the barbecue sauce and black cherry spread into the cooking liquid. Increase the heat to medium low and cook for 2 to 3 minutes, or until heated through, stirring occasionally. Spoon over the pork.

PER SERVING

CALORIES 251
TOTAL FAT 6.5 g
  Saturated Fat 2.5 g
  Trans Fat 0.0 g
  Polyunsaturated Fat 0.5 g
  Monounsaturated Fat 3.0 g
CHOLESTEROL 67 mg
SODIUM 159 mg
CARBOHYDRATES 19 g
  Fiber 0 g
  Sugars 14 g
PROTEIN 24 g
DIETARY EXCHANGES
  1 carbohydrate,
  3 lean meat

louisiana skillet pork

SERVES 4

Deeply browned veggies with a hint of olive oil complement these Cajun-seasoned pork chops.

4 boneless center-cut pork chops (about 4 ounces each), all visible fat discarded
1 teaspoon salt-free Creole or Cajun seasoning blend, such as on page 463
Cooking spray
1 cup frozen whole-kernel corn

1 medium red bell pepper, chopped
1 small zucchini, chopped
½ cup finely chopped onion
1 medium rib of celery, finely chopped
¼ teaspoon pepper
1 teaspoon olive oil (extra virgin preferred)
½ teaspoon salt

Sprinkle the pork on both sides with the seasoning blend.

In a large nonstick skillet, cook the pork over medium-high heat for 6 minutes on each side, or until slightly pink in the center. Remove from the heat. Transfer the pork to a plate. Cover to keep warm. Lightly spray any browned bits in the skillet with cooking spray.

Put the corn, bell pepper, zucchini, onion, celery, and pepper in the skillet, stirring to combine. Cook over medium-high heat for 4 minutes, or until the celery is tender-crisp and the vegetables begin to brown on the edges, stirring frequently. Remove from the heat.

Stir in the oil and salt. Spoon over the pork or serve on the side.

COOK'S TIP

Be sure to remove the skillet from the heat before adding the small amount of olive oil so the oil isn't absorbed.

PER SERVING
CALORIES 232
TOTAL FAT 8.0 g
  Saturated Fat 2.5 g
  Trans Fat 0.0 g
  Polyunsaturated Fat 1.0 g
  Monounsaturated Fat 4.0 g
CHOLESTEROL 67 mg
SODIUM 354 mg
CARBOHYDRATES 15 g
  Fiber 3 g
  Sugars 4 g
PROTEIN 26 g
DIETARY EXCHANGES
  ½ starch, 1 vegetable,
  3 lean meat

vegetarian entrées

Artichoke-Tomato Pita Pockets

Zucchini Linguine with Walnuts

Pecan-Topped Pasta with Vegetables

Spaghetti Cheese Amandine

Sesame-Peanut Pasta

Spaghetti with Zesty Marinara Sauce

Spaghetti with Perfect Pesto

Mediterranean Linguine

Thai-Style Vegetables with Pasta

Two-Cheese Sour Cream Noodles

Three-Cheese Macaroni

Tortellini and Vegetable Kebabs with Italian Pesto Salsa

Vegetable Biryani

Bulgur-Mushroom Burgers

Portobellos with Polenta and Tomatoes

Stuffed Zucchini

Stuffed Peppers

Barley Risotto with Mushrooms and Asparagus

Barley with Braised Squash and Swiss Chard

Cheese-Topped Anaheim Peppers with Pinto Rice

Rice Sticks with Asian Vegetables (Pad Thai)

Butternut, Broccoli, and Brown Rice Stir-Fry

Hoppin' John

Mediterranean Lentils and Rice

Chickpea Pilaf

Slow-Cooker Chickpea Stew

Green Chile and Rice Pie

Bulgur, Brown Rice, and Beans

Vegetable and Pinto Bean Enchiladas

Enchilada Bake

Black Bean Polenta with Avocado Salsa

Cuban Black Beans

Red Beans and Couscous

Mediterranean Toasted Quinoa and Spinach

Quinoa with Black Beans and Seared Bell Pepper

Cumin and Ginger Lentils on Quinoa

Quinoa Pilaf with Tofu and Vegetables

Curried Cauliflower and Tofu with Basmati Rice

Edamame Fried Rice

Edamame and Vegetable Stir-Fry

Meatless Moussaka

Ratatouille with Cannellini Beans and Brown Rice

Eggplant Parmesan

Eggplant Zucchini Casserole

Spinach Artichoke Gratin

Spinach Ricotta Swirls

Asparagus and Artichoke Quiche

Meatless Lasagna with Zucchini and Red Wine

Three-Cheese Vegetable Strudel

Tomato Quiche in Couscous Crust

Spinach Soufflé

Farmstand Frittata

Portobello Mushroom Wrap with Yogurt Curry Sauce

Open-Face Swiss Cheese, Spinach, and Tomato Sandwiches

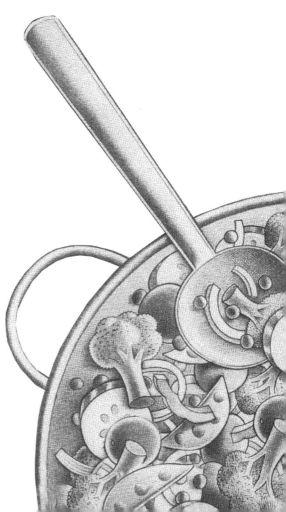

artichoke-tomato pita pockets

SERVES 6

You can use pita pockets to combine veggies and melted cheese inside whole-grain goodness.

Olive oil spray

6 ounces shredded low-fat mozzarella cheese

1 9-ounce package frozen artichoke hearts, thawed, drained, and chopped

3 medium Italian plum (Roma) tomatoes, chopped

½ cup thinly sliced red onion

1 teaspoon balsamic vinegar

1 medium garlic clove, minced

½ teaspoon dried Italian seasoning, crumbled

6 6-inch whole-grain pita pockets, each split into 2 pockets

Preheat the oven to 375°F. Lightly spray a baking sheet with olive oil spray.

In a medium bowl, stir together all the ingredients except the pita pockets. Stuff the pita pockets with the filling.

Place the pitas on the baking sheet. Lightly spray the tops with olive oil spray.

Bake for 8 to 10 minutes, or until the filling is heated through and the mozzarella is melted.

PER SERVING

CALORIES 246
TOTAL FAT 4.0 g
  Saturated Fat 1.5 g
  Trans Fat 0.0 g
  Polyunsaturated Fat 0.5 g
  Monounsaturated Fat 1.0 g
CHOLESTEROL 10 mg
SODIUM 544 mg
CARBOHYDRATES 41 g
  Fiber 9 g
  Sugars 3 g
PROTEIN 14 g
DIETARY EXCHANGES
  2 starch, 2 vegetable,
  1 lean meat

zucchini linguine with walnuts

SERVES 4

The generous amount of toasted walnuts gives this one-dish meal a warm and rustic character—just right for a cold or rainy night.

8 ounces dried whole-grain linguine	4 medium garlic cloves, minced
Olive oil spray	¼ teaspoon crushed red pepper flakes
2 medium zucchini, sliced	½ cup chopped walnuts, dry-roasted
1 medium onion, thinly sliced	2 teaspoons olive oil (extra virgin
8 ounces button mushrooms, sliced	preferred)
1 tablespoon dried oregano, crumbled	½ teaspoon salt

Prepare the pasta using the package directions, omitting the salt. Drain well in a colander, reserving ½ cup pasta water.

Meanwhile, lightly spray a large skillet or Dutch oven with olive oil spray. Cook the zucchini and onion over medium-high heat for 8 minutes, or until beginning to lightly brown on the edges, stirring frequently. Remove the pan from the heat. Transfer the zucchini mixture to a plate.

Lightly spray the pan with olive oil spray. Cook the mushrooms, oregano, garlic, and red pepper flakes for 4 minutes, or until the mushrooms begin to lightly brown, stirring occasionally.

Stir the zucchini mixture into the mushroom mixture. Stir in the pasta and reserved pasta water. Cook for 30 seconds, or until most of the liquid has evaporated. Remove from the heat.

Stir in the walnuts, oil, and salt.

PER SERVING

CALORIES 366
TOTAL FAT 13.5 g
  Saturated Fat 1.5 g
  Trans Fat 0.0 g
  Polyunsaturated Fat 8.0 g
  Monounsaturated Fat 3.5 g
CHOLESTEROL 0 mg
SODIUM 306 mg
CARBOHYDRATES 54 g
  Fiber 10 g
  Sugars 7 g
PROTEIN 13 g
DIETARY EXCHANGES
  3 starch, 2 vegetable,
  2 fat

pecan-topped pasta with vegetables

SERVES 4

This pasta is piled high with sizzling veggies and a sprinkling of toasted pecans.

8 ounces dried whole-grain rotini
1½ cups finely chopped onion
1 medium red bell pepper, thinly sliced
1 cup matchstick-size carrot strips
6 ounces button mushrooms, thinly sliced

Cooking spray
½ teaspoon ground cumin
½ teaspoon salt
⅓ cup finely chopped pecan pieces, dry-roasted

Prepare the pasta using the package directions, omitting the salt. Drain well in a colander.

Put the onion, bell pepper, carrots, and mushrooms in a large nonstick skillet. Lightly spray them with cooking spray. Cook over medium-high heat for 10 to 12 minutes, or until the onion is deeply browned, stirring frequently.

Stir in the cumin and salt. Cook for 30 seconds. Serve over the pasta. Sprinkle with the pecans.

PER SERVING

CALORIES 332
TOTAL FAT 9.5 g
  Saturated Fat 0.5 g
  Trans Fat 0.0 g
  Polyunsaturated Fat 3.0 g
  Monounsaturated Fat 4.5 g
CHOLESTEROL 0 mg
SODIUM 319 mg
CARBOHYDRATES 55 g
  Fiber 10 g
  Sugars 8 g
PROTEIN 11 g
DIETARY EXCHANGES
  3 starch, 2 vegetable, 1½ fat

spaghetti cheese amandine

SERVES 4

The texture of the sauce is one of the features that stands out in this dish. Serve with sliced tomatoes, a tossed salad, or fresh fruit.

8 ounces dried whole-grain spaghetti, broken into small pieces
1 cup fat-free cottage cheese
1 cup frozen green peas, thawed
2 medium green onions (green part only), sliced
2 tablespoons shredded or grated Parmesan cheese

2 tablespoons fat-free milk
½ teaspoon dried Italian seasoning, crumbled
1 tablespoon light tub margarine
Pepper to taste
¼ cup slivered almonds, dry-roasted

Prepare the spaghetti using the package directions, omitting the salt. Drain well in a colander.

Meanwhile, in a medium bowl, stir together the cottage cheese, peas, green onions, Parmesan, milk, and Italian seasoning.

In the pot used for the spaghetti, melt the margarine over medium-low heat, swirling to coat the bottom. Return the spaghetti to the pot. Stir. When the spaghetti is warm, stir in the cottage cheese mixture. Cook for 3 to 4 minutes, or until heated through, stirring occasionally. Stir in the pepper. Sprinkle with the almonds.

PER SERVING

CALORIES 335
TOTAL FAT 7.0 g
    Saturated Fat 0.5 g
    Trans Fat 0.0 g
    Polyunsaturated Fat 1.5 g
    Monounsaturated Fat 3.5 g
CHOLESTEROL 5 mg
SODIUM 322 mg
CARBOHYDRATES 53 g
    Fiber 9 g
    Sugars 7 g
PROTEIN 18 g
DIETARY EXCHANGES
    3½ starch, 1 lean meat

sesame-peanut pasta

SERVES 4

While the pasta is cooking, you can prepare the super simple seven-ingredient sauce and have this dish put together in minutes! It's delicious either hot or cold.

8 ounces dried whole-grain spaghetti
½ cup low-sodium vegetable broth, such as on page 44
2 medium green onions, thinly sliced
3 tablespoons peanut butter

1 tablespoon plus 1 teaspoon cider vinegar or plain rice vinegar
1 teaspoon toasted sesame oil
⅛ to ¼ teaspoon cayenne
⅛ teaspoon salt

Prepare the spaghetti using the package directions, omitting the salt. Drain well in a colander. Transfer to a platter.

Meanwhile, in a medium bowl, whisk together the remaining ingredients. Stir into the spaghetti. Serve for a hot entrée or cover and refrigerate for a cold entrée.

PER SERVING

CALORIES 290
TOTAL FAT 8.5 g
  Saturated Fat 1.5 g
  Trans Fat 0.0 g
  Polyunsaturated Fat 2.5 g
  Monounsaturated Fat 4.0 g
CHOLESTEROL 0 mg
SODIUM 132 mg
CARBOHYDRATES 45 g
  Fiber 7 g
  Sugars 4 g
PROTEIN 10 g
DIETARY EXCHANGES
  3 starch, ½ very lean meat, 1 fat

spaghetti with zesty marinara sauce

SERVES 8

This aromatic sauce turns any meal into an Italian feast. Since it freezes well, you might want to cook half the amount of spaghetti to serve four and then freeze the remaining half of the sauce for a later use; it'll keep for up to six months.

MARINARA SAUCE
- 1 teaspoon olive oil
- 1 large onion, finely chopped
- 2 large garlic cloves, crushed
- 1 6-ounce can no-salt-added tomato paste
- 2 tablespoons minced fresh parsley
- 2 teaspoons sugar
- 1¼ teaspoons dried Italian seasoning, crumbled
- ½ teaspoon dried basil, crumbled
- ¼ teaspoon pepper, or to taste
- ⅛ teaspoon crushed red pepper flakes, or to taste

- ⅛ teaspoon salt
- 1 14.5-ounce can no-salt-added tomatoes, crushed, undrained
- 1 cup water
- 1 8-ounce can no-salt-added tomato sauce
- ¼ cup dry red wine (regular or nonalcoholic)
- 1 medium dried bay leaf

- 16 ounces dried whole-grain spaghetti
- ½ cup shredded or grated Parmesan cheese

In a medium saucepan, heat the oil over medium-high heat, swirling to coat the bottom. Cook the onion and garlic for 3 minutes, or until the onion is soft, stirring occasionally.

Whisk in the tomato paste, parsley, sugar, Italian seasoning, basil, pepper, red pepper flakes, and salt. Reduce the heat to medium low. Cook for 4 minutes, stirring frequently.

Stir in the remaining sauce ingredients. Increase the heat to high and bring to a boil. Reduce the heat and simmer, partially covered, for 1 hour to 1 hour 30 minutes, stirring occasionally. Discard the bay leaf.

Meanwhile, prepare the spaghetti using the package directions, omitting the salt. Drain well in a colander. Transfer to a large serving bowl.

Stir in the Parmesan. Top with the sauce.

PER SERVING

CALORIES 297
TOTAL FAT 3.5 g
  Saturated Fat 1.0 g
  Trans Fat 0.0 g
  Polyunsaturated Fat 0.5 g
  Monounsaturated Fat 1.5 g
CHOLESTEROL 4 mg
SODIUM 156 mg
CARBOHYDRATES 56 g
  Fiber 9 g
  Sugars 10 g
PROTEIN 12 g
DIETARY EXCHANGES
  3 starch, 2 vegetable

spaghetti with perfect pesto

SERVES 6

This sauce includes the traditional pesto ingredients and adds spinach—a nutrition bonus—to boost the vitamins and minerals in this dish!

12 ounces dried whole-grain thin spaghetti

PESTO SAUCE

2 cups firmly packed fresh spinach (3 to 4 ounces)

½ cup firmly packed fresh basil

½ cup firmly packed fresh parsley

¼ cup low-sodium vegetable broth, such as on page 44

¼ cup shredded or grated Parmesan cheese, or 2 tablespoons shredded or grated Parmesan cheese and 2 tablespoons shredded or grated Romano cheese

2 tablespoons pine nuts, dry-roasted

1 tablespoon olive oil

2 medium garlic cloves

Pepper to taste

1 to 2 tablespoons water (if needed)

Prepare the spaghetti using the package directions, omitting the salt. Drain well in a colander. Transfer to a large serving bowl.

Meanwhile, in a food processor or blender, process the sauce ingredients except the water until almost smooth. If the mixture is too thick, add the water. Serve over the spaghetti.

COOK'S TIP on pine nuts

Native to many parts of the world, pine nuts are the seeds found in particular varieties of pine trees. The difficulty in harvesting makes them rather expensive, but you use them in small quantities. Pine nuts—also called *pignoli* or *piñons*—are traditionally used in pesto sauce and are very popular in southwestern cuisine. Store them in the refrigerator or freezer to keep them from turning rancid.

PER SERVING

CALORIES 257
TOTAL FAT 6.0 g
 Saturated Fat 1.0 g
 Trans Fat 0.0 g
 Polyunsaturated Fat 1.5 g
 Monounsaturated Fat 3.0 g
CHOLESTEROL 2 mg
SODIUM 73 mg
CARBOHYDRATES 43 g
 Fiber 7 g
 Sugars 2 g
PROTEIN 10 g
DIETARY EXCHANGES
 3 starch, ½ fat

mediterranean linguine

SERVES 4

If you're a fan of kalamata olives and capers, you'll rave about this all-in-one dinner.

Cooking spray
6 ounces dried whole-grain linguine
1 medium green bell pepper, thinly sliced
1 medium red bell pepper, thinly sliced
1 medium onion, cut into ¼-inch wedges
1 medium zucchini, cut lengthwise into eighths, then crosswise into 2-inch pieces

8 dry-packed sun-dried tomato halves, chopped
¼ cup finely snipped fresh parsley
3 tablespoons capers, drained
12 kalamata olives, chopped
1½ tablespoons dried basil, crumbled
1 medium garlic clove, minced
¾ cup shredded low-fat mozzarella cheese
2 tablespoons shredded or grated Parmesan cheese

Preheat the broiler. Lightly spray a broiler pan with cooking spray.

Prepare the pasta using the package directions, omitting the salt. Drain well in a colander, reserving ½ cup pasta water.

Meanwhile, arrange the bell peppers, onion, and zucchini in a single layer in the broiler pan. Lightly spray the tops with cooking spray.

Broil for 10 minutes. Stir. Broil for 4 minutes, or until the edges begin to deeply brown.

Meanwhile, in a small bowl, stir together the tomatoes, parsley, capers, olives, basil, and garlic.

In a large shallow dish, gently stir together the pasta, reserved pasta water, bell pepper mixture, and tomato mixture. Gently stir in the mozzarella and Parmesan.

PER SERVING

CALORIES 297
TOTAL FAT 7.0 g
  Saturated Fat 1.5 g
  Trans Fat 0.0 g
  Polyunsaturated Fat 1.0 g
  Monounsaturated Fat 3.5 g
CHOLESTEROL 9 mg
SODIUM 580 mg
CARBOHYDRATES 46 g
  Fiber 9 g
  Sugars 8 g
PROTEIN 15 g
DIETARY EXCHANGES
  2 starch, 3 vegetable,
  1 very lean meat, 1 fat

thai-style vegetables with pasta

SERVES 4

Popular ingredients of Thai cuisine—such as lemongrass, bok choy, basil, and tofu—blend well with whole-grain pasta in this one-skillet dish. Serve it with juicy grapefruit segments on the side.

1 teaspoon canola or corn oil

½ medium red bell pepper, cut into 1-inch squares

1 cup sliced mushrooms, such as shiitake (stems discarded if using shiitake)

2 medium shallots, coarsely chopped

1½ cups low-sodium vegetable broth, such as on page 44

2 teaspoons fish sauce or soy sauce (lowest sodium available)

2 teaspoons fresh lime juice

1 teaspoon light brown sugar

1 teaspoon ground dried lemongrass or 1 tablespoon finely chopped fresh lemongrass (cut from bottom end of stalk) (optional)

¼ to ½ teaspoon crushed red pepper flakes

2 tablespoons chopped fresh basil or ½ teaspoon dried, crumbled

3 ounces dried whole-grain angel hair

12 ounces light firm tofu, drained, cut into ½-inch cubes

2 medium stalks of bok choy, stems and leaves coarsely chopped

1 cup fresh or frozen snow peas, trimmed if fresh

In a large skillet, heat the oil over medium-high heat, swirling to coat the bottom. Cook the bell pepper, mushrooms, and shallots for 2 to 3 minutes, or until the bell pepper is tender-crisp, stirring occasionally.

Stir in the broth, fish sauce, lime juice, brown sugar, lemongrass, red pepper flakes, and dried basil, if using. Bring to a simmer. Reduce the heat and simmer, covered, for 3 minutes.

Stir in the pasta. Simmer, covered, for 4 to 5 minutes, or until the pasta is tender.

Gently stir in the tofu, bok choy, snow peas, and fresh basil, if using. Simmer, covered, for 1 to 2 minutes, or until the tofu is heated through and the bok choy and snow peas are tender-crisp.

PER SERVING

CALORIES 165
TOTAL FAT 3.0 g
  Saturated Fat 0.5 g
  Trans Fat 0.0 g
  Polyunsaturated Fat 0.5 g
  Monounsaturated Fat 1.0 g
CHOLESTEROL 0 mg
SODIUM 109 mg
CARBOHYDRATES 24 g
  Fiber 3 g
  Sugars 4 g
PROTEIN 12 g
DIETARY EXCHANGES
  1 starch, 1 vegetable,
  1 lean meat

two-cheese sour cream noodles

SERVES 4

You'll need to save the empty containers to prove you didn't use high-fat ingredients to make this rich-tasting dish. For a nonvegetarian entrée to serve to more people, add cooked ground beef or steamed shrimp.

Cooking spray	1 teaspoon Worcestershire sauce
8 ounces dried yolk-free noodles	(lowest sodium available)
1½ cups fat-free sour cream	⅛ teaspoon pepper (white preferred)
1 cup fat-free cottage cheese, drained	¼ cup shredded or grated Parmesan
¼ cup fat-free milk	cheese
2 medium garlic cloves, minced	1 tablespoon poppy seeds

Preheat the oven to 350°F. Lightly spray a 2-quart casserole dish with cooking spray.

Prepare the noodles using the package directions, omitting the salt. Drain well in a colander.

Meanwhile, in a large bowl, stir together the sour cream, cottage cheese, milk, garlic, Worcestershire sauce, and pepper.

Stir in the noodles. Spoon into the casserole dish.

Bake for 15 minutes. Sprinkle with the Parmesan and poppy seeds. Bake for 5 minutes.

PER SERVING

CALORIES 380
TOTAL FAT 3.0 g
  Saturated Fat 1.0 g
  Trans Fat 0.0 g
  Polyunsaturated Fat 0.5 g
  Monounsaturated Fat 0.5 g
CHOLESTEROL 21 mg
SODIUM 412 mg
CARBOHYDRATES 63 g
  Fiber 3 g
  Sugars 11 g
PROTEIN 22 g
DIETARY EXCHANGES
  4 starch,
  1½ very lean meat

three-cheese macaroni

SERVES 6

This jazzed-up version of an old favorite is easy to put together. You don't even have to cook the pasta before adding it to the casserole.

Cooking spray
16 ounces canned tomato puree
1 cup water
2 teaspoons dried Italian seasoning, crumbled
2 medium garlic cloves, minced, and 1 medium garlic clove, minced, divided use

24 ounces low-fat cottage cheese
1 large shallot, finely chopped
8 ounces dried whole-grain elbow macaroni
1 tablespoon shredded or grated Parmesan cheese
¼ cup shredded low-fat mozzarella cheese

Preheat the oven to 350°F. Lightly spray a 9-inch square casserole dish with cooking spray.

In a medium bowl, stir together the tomato puree, water, Italian seasoning, and 2 garlic cloves.

In another medium bowl, stir together the cottage cheese, shallot, and remaining 1 garlic clove.

Spread one-third of the tomato mixture in the casserole dish. In order, layer half the pasta, all the cottage cheese mixture, one-third of the tomato mixture, all the Parmesan, the remaining pasta, and the remaining tomato mixture.

Bake, covered, for 1 hour. Uncover and top with the mozzarella. Bake, uncovered, for 5 minutes, or until the mozzarella is melted. Let stand for 10 minutes before serving.

PER SERVING

CALORIES 248
TOTAL FAT 2.0 g
  Saturated Fat 1.0 g
  Trans Fat 0.0 g
  Polyunsaturated Fat 0.5 g
  Monounsaturated Fat 0.5 g
CHOLESTEROL 7 mg
SODIUM 375 mg
CARBOHYDRATES 36 g
  Fiber 4 g
  Sugars 5 g
PROTEIN 22 g
DIETARY EXCHANGES
  2 starch, 1 vegetable,
  2 very lean meat

tortellini and vegetable kebabs with italian pesto salsa

SERVES 4

These make-ahead kebabs of pasta and vegetables are perfect food to serve dinner guests. Once assembled, the kebabs are ready to go without any last-minute cooking.

KEBABS
- 24 fresh cheese tortellini (about 4½ ounces)
- 24 small broccoli florets
- 24 cherry tomatoes

PESTO SALSA
- 1 14.5-ounce can no-salt-added diced tomatoes, undrained
- ½ cup loosely packed fresh basil
- ¼ cup pine nuts or chopped walnuts, dry-roasted
- 2 tablespoons shredded or grated Parmesan cheese
- 1 tablespoon balsamic vinegar
- 1 medium garlic clove, minced

Prepare the tortellini using the package directions, omitting the salt. One minute before the end of their cooking time, stir in the broccoli. Cook for 1 minute, or until the broccoli is tender-crisp. Drain well in a colander.

Using twelve 8-inch wooden skewers, thread one tortellini, one broccoli floret, and one cherry tomato on each skewer. Repeat. (Cover and refrigerate the kebabs at this point for up to two days if desired.)

In a food processor or blender, process the salsa ingredients for 30 to 40 seconds, or until slightly chunky. Transfer to a small serving bowl. Place the bowl of salsa in the middle of a platter. Arrange the kebabs around the bowl.

PER SERVING

CALORIES 209
TOTAL FAT 7.0 g
  Saturated Fat 2.0 g
  Trans Fat 0.0 g
  Polyunsaturated Fat 2.0 g
  Monounsaturated Fat 1.5 g
CHOLESTEROL 14 mg
SODIUM 256 mg
CARBOHYDRATES 30 g
  Fiber 5 g
  Sugars 9 g
PROTEIN 11 g
DIETARY EXCHANGES
  1 starch, 3 vegetable,
  ½ very lean meat, 1 fat

vegetable biryani

SERVES 6

Add a leafy green salad with soothing Chunky Cucumber and Garlic Dressing (page 138) to complement the spiciness of this dish, and you have a wonderful meal.

2 cups uncooked basmati rice
2 tablespoons canola or corn oil
1 large potato, peeled and cut into ½-inch cubes
2 medium carrots, cut into ½-inch pieces
12 to 14 cauliflower florets
1½ teaspoons whole cumin seeds, dry-roasted
3 tablespoons finely snipped fresh cilantro

½ medium fresh jalapeño, seeds and ribs discarded, finely chopped
1½ teaspoons ground cumin
1 teaspoon finely grated peeled gingerroot
1 medium garlic clove, mashed
1 teaspoon salt
½ teaspoon ground turmeric
¼ to ½ teaspoon cayenne
2¾ cups water
¼ cup chopped cashews

Put the rice in a sieve and rinse. Drain and put in a medium bowl. Add enough water to cover. Let soak for 20 minutes. Drain again in the sieve. Leave in the sieve for 20 minutes to soften.

In a Dutch oven or large heavy saucepan, heat the oil over medium-high heat, swirling to coat the bottom. Cook the potato, carrots, cauliflower, and cumin seeds for 1 minute. Reduce the heat to medium.

Stir in the rice, cilantro, jalapeño, ground cumin, gingerroot, garlic, salt, turmeric, and cayenne. Cook for 2 minutes.

Stir in the water. Bring to a boil. Reduce the heat and simmer, covered, for 25 minutes, or until the water is absorbed. Turn off the heat. Let stand, covered, for 5 minutes (don't stir). Sprinkle with the cashews and fluff with a fork before serving.

PER SERVING

CALORIES 367
TOTAL FAT 8.0 g
  Saturated Fat 1.0 g
  Trans Fat 0.0 g
  Polyunsaturated Fat 2.0 g
  Monounsaturated Fat 4.5 g
CHOLESTEROL 0 mg
SODIUM 422 mg
CARBOHYDRATES 69 g
  Fiber 4 g
  Sugars 3 g
PROTEIN 7 g
DIETARY EXCHANGES
  4 starch, 1 vegetable,
  1 fat

bulgur-mushroom burgers

SERVES 4

Juicy tomato slices and dollops of tangy yogurt top these earthy grain-and-veggie burgers.

½ cup low-sodium vegetable broth, such as on page 44
⅓ cup uncooked bulgur
2 teaspoons olive oil
1½ cups chopped cremini or baby bella mushrooms
½ cup sliced green onions
1 tablespoon balsamic vinegar

⅓ cup chopped walnuts, dry-roasted
¼ cup panko (Japanese bread crumbs)
3 tablespoons egg substitute
½ teaspoon dried thyme, crumbled
¼ teaspoon red hot-pepper sauce
4 slices tomato
¼ cup fat-free plain yogurt

In a small saucepan, bring the broth to a boil over high heat. Stir in the bulgur. Remove from the heat and set aside, covered, for 20 minutes. Drain well, discarding the broth.

Meanwhile, in a medium nonstick skillet, heat the oil over medium heat. Cook the mushrooms and green onions for 6 to 8 minutes, or until the mushrooms are tender, stirring occasionally.

Stir in the vinegar. Spread on a plate and let cool to room temperature, about 30 minutes. (If you don't cool the mushroom mixture to room temperature, it might start cooking the egg substitute when you blend it in.)

Preheat the broiler. Line a baking sheet with aluminum foil.

Put the mushroom mixture and walnuts in a food processor. Pulse until coarsely chopped. Scrape down the side of the processor bowl.

Add the bulgur, panko, egg substitute, thyme, and hot-pepper sauce. Process until combined, scraping the side of the processor bowl if necessary.

Using a heaping ⅓ cup for each, form the bulgur mixture into four ½-inch-thick patties (the mixture may seem a little wet). Place the patties on the baking sheet.

Broil the patties 4 to 6 inches from the heat for 4 minutes on each side, or until browned. Serve the burgers topped with the tomato slices and yogurt.

PER SERVING

CALORIES 174
TOTAL FAT 9.0 g
  Saturated Fat 1.0 g
  Trans Fat 0.0 g
  Polyunsaturated Fat 5.0 g
  Monounsaturated Fat 2.5 g
CHOLESTEROL 0 mg
SODIUM 55 mg
CARBOHYDRATES 19 g
  Fiber 4 g
  Sugars 4 g
PROTEIN 6 g
DIETARY EXCHANGES
  1 starch, 1 vegetable, 1½ fat

portobellos with polenta and tomatoes

SERVES 4

Layered meaty mushrooms, velvety polenta, and juicy red tomato slices give this vegetarian entrée an intriguing texture. Two mushrooms make a satisfying main dish for one person, or serve one mushroom each as a side dish for eight.

1 teaspoon olive oil, 1 teaspoon olive oil, and 1 teaspoon olive oil, divided use
8 large portobello mushrooms (about 4½ inches in diameter), stems and gills discarded
⅛ teaspoon salt
⅓ cup finely diced onion
1 medium garlic clove, minced
2 cups low-sodium vegetable broth, such as on page 44

¼ teaspoon dried basil, crumbled
½ cup yellow cornmeal
½ cup shredded or grated Parmesan cheese and 2 tablespoons shredded or grated Parmesan cheese, divided use
⅛ teaspoon pepper
1 large tomato, cut into 8 slices

In a large nonstick skillet, heat 1 teaspoon oil over medium-high heat, swirling to coat the bottom. Cook 4 of the mushrooms, covered, for 6 to 8 minutes, or until tender, turning once. Place the mushrooms with the cap side down in a single layer in a broiler-proof baking pan, such as a rimmed metal baking sheet. Repeat with 1 teaspoon oil and the remaining 4 mushrooms. Sprinkle the salt over all the mushrooms.

Meanwhile, preheat the broiler.

In a medium saucepan, heat the final 1 teaspoon oil over medium heat, swirling to coat the bottom. Cook the onion for 3 to 4 minutes, or until soft, stirring occasionally. Stir in the garlic. Cook for 1 minute, stirring occasionally.

Add the broth and basil. Increase the heat to high and bring to a boil. Using a long-handled whisk, carefully stir the broth mixture to create a swirl. Slowly pour the cornmeal in a steady stream into the swirl, whisking constantly. Holding the pan steady, continue whisking for 1 to 2 minutes, or until the polenta is very thick. Remove from the heat. Stir in ½ cup Parmesan and the pepper.

PER SERVING

CALORIES 189
TOTAL FAT 7.5 g
  Saturated Fat 3.0 g
  Trans Fat 0.0 g
  Polyunsaturated Fat 1.0 g
  Monounsaturated Fat 3.5 g
CHOLESTEROL 9 mg
SODIUM 298 mg
CARBOHYDRATES 24 g
  Fiber 3 g
  Sugars 4 g
PROTEIN 10 g
DIETARY EXCHANGES
  1 starch, 2 vegetable,
  ½ lean meat, 1 fat

Spoon ¼ cup polenta into each mushroom cap. Top each with a tomato slice. Sprinkle with the remaining 2 tablespoons Parmesan.

Broil about 5 inches from the heat for 1 to 2 minutes, or until the Parmesan melts. Serve immediately for the best texture.

COOK'S TIP

You can give this dish a smoky flavor by grilling the mushrooms. To save time when you are preparing dinner, you can grill them a day ahead and refrigerate them in an airtight container. Reheat the mushrooms in the microwave before filling them with the polenta.

stuffed zucchini

SERVES 4

Brown rice flecked with color is used to stuff zucchini and transform it from its usual side-dish status to main-dish prominence. The chipotle pepper adds a rich, smoky flavor and a bit of heat to spice up the stuffing.

STUFFING
- ½ cup uncooked instant brown rice
- 2 teaspoons olive oil
- 1 medium red onion, finely chopped
- 1 medium tomato, finely chopped
- 1 chipotle pepper canned in adobo sauce, finely chopped
- 1 large garlic clove, coarsely chopped
- ⅛ teaspoon salt
- 2 cups coarsely chopped fresh spinach (about 2 ounces) or 1 10-ounce package frozen chopped spinach, thawed, drained, and squeezed dry

- 4 large pimiento-stuffed green olives, coarsely chopped
- 2 tablespoons coarsely snipped fresh cilantro
- 2 tablespoons white wine vinegar
- ¾ teaspoon dried oregano, crumbled
- ¼ teaspoon ground cumin

- 4 small to medium zucchini
- 1 cup water
- ½ cup shredded low-fat 4-cheese Mexican blend

Preheat the oven to 400°F.

Prepare the rice using the package directions, omitting the salt and margarine.

Meanwhile, in a large, deep skillet, heat the oil over medium-low heat, swirling to coat the bottom. Cook the onion, tomato, chipotle, garlic, and salt for 5 to 7 minutes, or until the onion has softened, stirring occasionally.

Stir in the remaining stuffing ingredients. Cook for 4 minutes, stirring frequently.

While the stuffing cooks, cut the zucchini in half lengthwise. Using a teaspoon, scrape out the seeds and just enough flesh to make a cavity for stuffing.

Stir the rice into the stuffing mixture. Spoon into the zucchini. Place the zucchini in a single layer in a large baking pan. Carefully pour the water around—not over—the zucchini.

Bake, covered, for 35 to 40 minutes, or until the zucchini is tender when tested with a fork inserted into the center. Sprinkle with the cheese.

PER SERVING

CALORIES 165
TOTAL FAT 6.5 g
 Saturated Fat 2.0 g
 Trans Fat 0.0 g
 Polyunsaturated Fat 1.0 g
 Monounsaturated Fat 3.0 g
CHOLESTEROL 9 mg
SODIUM 345 mg
CARBOHYDRATES 20 g
 Fiber 4 g
 Sugars 5 g
PROTEIN 8 g
DIETARY EXCHANGES
 ½ starch, 2 vegetable,
 ½ lean meat, 1 fat

COOK'S TIP on chipotle peppers

Chipotle peppers are smoked jalapeños, so expect a little heat. Buy them dried or packed in cans with flavorful adobo sauce (made of chiles, herbs, and vinegar). You can refrigerate leftover canned chipotle peppers for several months in a jar with a tight-fitting lid.

stuffed peppers

SERVES 4

Stuff any color or colors of bell pepper halves with a crunchy combination of vegetables, brown rice, and water chestnuts.

½ cup uncooked instant brown rice
1 teaspoon olive oil
2 medium tomatoes, chopped
1 medium yellow summer squash, diced
1 medium zucchini, diced
1 medium onion, diced

2 medium garlic cloves, minced
½ cup grated low-fat Cheddar cheese
¼ cup sliced water chestnuts, drained
4 large bell peppers, any color or combination, halved lengthwise, stems, seeds, and ribs discarded
1 cup no-salt-added tomato juice

Preheat the oven to 375°F.

Prepare the rice using the package directions, omitting the salt and margarine.

In a large skillet, heat the oil over medium heat, swirling to coat the bottom. Cook the tomatoes, yellow squash, zucchini, onion, and garlic for 3 to 4 minutes, or until the zucchini is tender-crisp, stirring occasionally. Don't overcook.

In a medium bowl, stir together the rice, Cheddar, and water chestnuts. Gently stir into the tomato mixture. Stuff the bell pepper halves. Place in a 9-inch casserole dish.

Carefully pour the tomato juice around—not over—the bell peppers.

Bake for 30 minutes.

PER SERVING

CALORIES 165
TOTAL FAT 3.0 g
　Saturated Fat 1.0 g
　Trans Fat 0.0 g
　Polyunsaturated Fat 0.5 g
　Monounsaturated Fat 1.5 g
CHOLESTEROL 3 mg
SODIUM 112 mg
CARBOHYDRATES 30 g
　Fiber 7 g
　Sugars 12 g
PROTEIN 9 g
DIETARY EXCHANGES
　½ starch, 4 vegetable,
　½ fat

barley risotto with mushrooms and asparagus

SERVES 4

The fiber-rich barley in this creamy combination has a satisfying nutlike taste and offers more nutrition bang than the arborio rice usually used for risottos. If asparagus isn't in season, try sliced zucchini, yellow summer squash, or bell peppers instead.

4 cups low-sodium vegetable broth, such as on page 44
1½ cups water
2 teaspoons olive oil
2 cups diced onion
1 pound button mushrooms, sliced

1¼ cups uncooked pearl barley
1 pound asparagus spears, trimmed and cut into 2-inch pieces
¾ cup shredded or grated Parmesan cheese
½ teaspoon pepper

In a large saucepan, heat the broth and water over medium-high heat for about 5 minutes, or until hot. Reduce the heat to low to keep the broth hot.

Meanwhile, in another large saucepan, heat the oil over medium-high heat, swirling to coat the bottom. Cook the onion for 3 minutes, or until soft, stirring occasionally.

Stir the mushrooms into the onion. Cook for 8 minutes, or until they exude their liquid, stirring occasionally. Stir in the barley.

Ladle ½ cup broth into the pan. Cook for 1 to 2 minutes, or until the broth is absorbed, stirring occasionally. Repeat, adding ½ cup broth at a time and cooking until the broth is absorbed after each addition, stirring in the asparagus after 15 minutes of cooking time. (The total cooking time will be about 30 minutes.) Remove from the heat.

Stir in the Parmesan and pepper. Serve immediately for the best texture.

COOK'S TIP on asparagus

To remove the tough ends from asparagus spears, bend one spear at a time until you find the point where it naturally snaps in two, usually about 1 inch from the bottom.

PER SERVING

CALORIES 389
TOTAL FAT 7.5 g
  Saturated Fat 3.0 g
  Trans Fat 0.0 g
  Polyunsaturated Fat 1.0 g
  Monounsaturated Fat 3.0 g
CHOLESTEROL 11 mg
SODIUM 282 mg
CARBOHYDRATES 66 g
  Fiber 15 g
  Sugars 9 g
PROTEIN 19 g
DIETARY EXCHANGES
  3½ starch, 3 vegetable, 1 lean meat

barley with braised squash and swiss chard

SERVES 4

Although it is very nutritious—high in fiber, vitamins, and minerals—chard may not have made it into your cooking repertory yet. This dish would be the perfect introduction.

4 cups water
¾ cup uncooked pearl barley
1 tablespoon olive oil
¼ cup sliced shallots
3 medium garlic cloves, minced
⅛ teaspoon crushed red pepper flakes
1 pound butternut squash, peeled and cut into ½-inch cubes

1 cup low-sodium vegetable broth, such as on page 44
1 small bunch Swiss chard (about 12 ounces), stems discarded and leaves coarsely chopped
¼ cup shredded or grated Parmesan cheese

In a medium saucepan, bring the water to a boil over high heat. Stir in the barley. Reduce the heat and simmer, covered, for 45 to 50 minutes, or until the barley is tender. Drain well. Transfer to plates.

Meanwhile, about 30 minutes after the barley starts cooking, heat the oil over medium heat in a large skillet, swirling to coat the bottom. Cook the shallots for 2 minutes, stirring occasionally.

Stir in the garlic and red pepper flakes. Cook for 30 seconds.

Stir in the squash and broth. Increase the heat to medium high and bring to a boil. Reduce the heat and simmer, covered, for 8 to 10 minutes, or until the squash is just tender.

Stir in the Swiss chard. Cook, covered, for 4 to 6 minutes, or until the Swiss chard is wilted. Using a slotted spoon, spoon over the barley. Sprinkle with the Parmesan.

COOK'S TIP

You can get a lot of flavor bang for your buck by using a high-quality, highly flavored cheese, such as Parmigiano-Reggiano. Although it is expensive, you don't need to use much.

PER SERVING

CALORIES 262
TOTAL FAT 5.5 g
  Saturated Fat 1.5 g
  Trans Fat 0.0 g
  Polyunsaturated Fat 0.5 g
  Monounsaturated Fat 3.0 g
CHOLESTEROL 4 mg
SODIUM 284 mg
CARBOHYDRATES 48 g
  Fiber 10 g
  Sugars 4 g
PROTEIN 9 g
DIETARY EXCHANGES
  3 starch, ½ fat

cheese-topped anaheim peppers with pinto rice

SERVES 4

Instead of stuffing mild Anaheim peppers for this dish, you simplify and place the slit peppers on the filling. A splash of fresh lime juice adds just the right touch.

1 cup uncooked instant brown rice
Cooking spray
1 15.5-ounce can no-salt-added pinto beans, rinsed and drained
¾ cup finely chopped green onions
1 tablespoon chili powder
2 teaspoons ground cumin
⅛ teaspoon salt and ⅛ teaspoon salt, divided use

4 medium fresh Anaheim or poblano peppers, halved lengthwise, stems, seeds, and ribs discarded
1 cup shredded low-fat mozzarella cheese
1 medium lime, quartered

Prepare the rice using the package directions, omitting the salt and margarine.

Meanwhile, preheat the oven to 350°F. Lightly spray an 11 x 7 x 2-inch baking pan with cooking spray.

In the pan, stir together the rice, beans, green onions, chili powder, cumin, and ⅛ teaspoon salt. Alternating the wide and narrow ends, arrange the peppers with the cut side down on top of the rice mixture. Sprinkle with the mozzarella.

Bake, covered with aluminum foil, for 45 minutes, or until the peppers are tender when pierced with a fork.

Sprinkle with the remaining ⅛ teaspoon salt. Squeeze the lime juice over all.

COOK'S TIP

If the peppers are too long for the pan, cut off any excess and use for another dish or freeze.

PER SERVING

CALORIES 267
TOTAL FAT 4.0 g
    Saturated Fat 1.0 g
    Trans Fat 0.0 g
    Polyunsaturated Fat 0.5 g
    Monounsaturated Fat 1.5 g
CHOLESTEROL 10 mg
SODIUM 383 mg
CARBOHYDRATES 42 g
    Fiber 9 g
    Sugars 7 g
PROTEIN 16 g
DIETARY EXCHANGES
    2½ starch, 1 vegetable,
    1½ very lean meat

rice sticks with asian vegetables (pad thai)

SERVES 4

You don't need to go out to enjoy this popular dish from Thailand. An exciting blend of taste, color, texture, and aroma awakens your senses. And to complete the dining experience, serve with chopsticks!

8 ounces dried flat rice sticks (rice-flour noodles)
1 tablespoon sugar
2 tablespoons fresh lime juice
2 teaspoons fish sauce or soy sauce (lowest sodium available)
12 ounces light firm tofu, drained and diced
1 teaspoon canola or corn oil
2 medium garlic cloves, minced
½ teaspoon crushed red pepper flakes
4 medium stalks of bok choy, stems and leaves thinly sliced

1 large carrot, cut into matchstick-size strips
1 cup fresh sugar snap peas, trimmed
½ cup canned whole baby corn, drained
1 tablespoon dry sherry (optional)
¼ cup chopped peanuts
2 medium green onions, thinly sliced (optional)
1 large lime, cut into 6 wedges (optional)
6 sprigs of fresh cilantro (optional)

Put the noodles in a large bowl with enough hot tap water to cover by 1 inch. Cover the bowl with plastic wrap and let the noodles soak for 15 to 20 minutes. Drain well in a colander.

Meanwhile, in a small bowl, stir together the sugar, lime juice, and fish sauce. Set aside.

In a large nonstick skillet, cook the tofu over medium-high heat for 2 to 3 minutes, or until heated through, stirring occasionally. Transfer to a separate small bowl.

Pour the oil into the skillet, swirling to coat the bottom. Cook the garlic and red pepper flakes for 10 seconds.

Add the bok choy, carrot, peas, and corn. Cook for 1 to 2 minutes, or until tender-crisp, stirring occasionally.

Stir the noodles, tofu, lime juice mixture, and sherry into the bok choy mixture. Cook for 2 to 3 minutes, or until the noodles are heated through, stirring occasionally (the noodles will get mushy if overcooked).

Transfer to a platter. Sprinkle with the peanuts. Garnish with the green onions, lime, and cilantro.

PER SERVING

CALORIES 364
TOTAL FAT 7.0 g
  Saturated Fat 1.0 g
  Trans Fat 0.0 g
  Polyunsaturated Fat 1.5 g
  Monounsaturated Fat 3.0 g
CHOLESTEROL 0 mg
SODIUM 174 mg
CARBOHYDRATES 60 g
  Fiber 5 g
  Sugars 6 g
PROTEIN 15 g
DIETARY EXCHANGES
  3½ starch, 1 vegetable, 1 lean meat

COOK'S TIP on rice sticks

Asian markets and some grocery and health food stores carry rice sticks, noodles made of rice flour and water. You can buy round or flat rice sticks in a variety of widths and even in some flavors. If you can't find the width you want, substitute a comparable pasta.

COOK'S TIP on fish sauce

Look in the Asian section of the grocery for fish sauce. A common ingredient in classic Thai and Vietnamese dishes, fish sauce has a very pungent aroma and adds a salty, fermented flavor. Only a little is needed to enhance the flavor of a dish.

butternut, broccoli, and brown rice stir-fry

SERVES 4

This unusual combo packs in flavor and nutrients from colorful veggies, a whole grain, and omega-rich sunflower seeds. The warm lemon-honey mixture that tops the dish is infused with just a hint of vanilla and nutmeg.

½ cup uncooked instant brown rice
1 cup low-sodium vegetable broth, such as on page 44
2 cups water
1 cup frozen shelled edamame (green soybeans)
2 teaspoons olive oil
6 ounces broccoli florets
1 10-ounce package frozen cubed butternut squash, thawed

1 teaspoon grated lemon zest
2 tablespoons fresh lemon juice
2 tablespoons honey
½ teaspoon vanilla extract
¼ teaspoon pepper
⅛ teaspoon ground nutmeg
2 tablespoons hulled unsalted sunflower seeds

Prepare the rice using the package directions, omitting the salt and margarine and substituting the broth for the water.

In a medium saucepan, bring the water to a boil over high heat. Add the edamame. Reduce the heat to medium high and cook for 5 minutes, or until tender. Drain well in a colander.

Meanwhile, in a large nonstick skillet, heat the oil over medium-high heat, swirling to coat the bottom. Cook the broccoli for 3 to 4 minutes, or until tender-crisp, stirring constantly.

Gently stir in the butternut squash and edamame, being careful not to mash the squash. Cook for 3 to 5 minutes, or until heated through, stirring occasionally. Reduce the heat to low to keep warm, stirring occasionally.

In a small microwaveable bowl, stir together the remaining ingredients except the sunflower seeds. Microwave on 100 percent power (high) for 20 to 30 seconds, or until heated through.

PER SERVING

CALORIES 238
TOTAL FAT 7.5 g
  Saturated Fat 1.0 g
  Trans Fat 0.0 g
  Polyunsaturated Fat 3.0 g
  Monounsaturated Fat 2.5 g
CHOLESTEROL 0 mg
SODIUM 26 mg
CARBOHYDRATES 36 g
  Fiber 6 g
  Sugars 12 g
PROTEIN 9 g
DIETARY EXCHANGES
  2 starch, 1 vegetable,
  ½ very lean meat, 1 fat

Spoon the rice into shallow dishes or onto plates. Top with the butternut mixture. Drizzle the lemon mixture over all. Sprinkle with the sunflower seeds.

COOK'S TIP on butternut squash

If your supermarket doesn't carry frozen cubed butternut squash, feel free to substitute a 10-ounce package of frozen cooked winter squash. Cook as directed on page 374. Although the texture will be different and not as attractive, the flavor of the dish will be just as delicious.

hoppin' john

SERVES 4

The certainty is that Hoppin' John always combines black-eyed peas with rice, onion, and herbs. The uncertainties are the history of the name and whether eating Hoppin' John on New Year's Day really brings good luck throughout the year. Regardless, your family will definitely feel lucky when you serve this southern dish.

1 cup uncooked rice	1 teaspoon chopped fresh basil
1 teaspoon canola or corn oil	or ¼ teaspoon dried, crumbled
1 medium rib of celery, diced	½ teaspoon dried rosemary, crushed
1 small onion, sliced	Pepper to taste
2½ cups canned no-salt-added	1 15.5-ounce can no-salt-added
tomatoes, undrained	black-eyed peas, rinsed and drained

Prepare the rice using the package directions, omitting the salt and margarine.

Meanwhile, in a large skillet, heat the oil over medium heat, swirling to coat the bottom. Cook the celery and onion for about 3 minutes, or until the onion is soft, stirring frequently.

Stir in the remaining ingredients except the peas. Reduce the heat and simmer for 20 minutes, stirring occasionally.

Add the peas and cook, covered, over low heat for 5 minutes, or until heated through. Serve the peas over the rice.

COOK'S TIP on mortar and pestle

The mortar is a heavy bowl, and the pestle is a grinding tool—a handle with a large knob on one end. Put spices such as caraway seeds or herbs such as rosemary in the mortar and mash them against the bottom and side with the pestle until they are as fine as you want.

PER SERVING

CALORIES 336
TOTAL FAT 1.5 g
  Saturated Fat 0.0 g
  Trans Fat 0.0 g
  Polyunsaturated Fat 0.5 g
  Monounsaturated Fat 1.0 g
CHOLESTEROL 0 mg
SODIUM 73 mg
CARBOHYDRATES 68 g
  Fiber 8 g
  Sugars 10 g
PROTEIN 12 g
DIETARY EXCHANGES
  4 starch, 2 vegetable

mediterranean lentils and rice

SERVES 4

Middle Eastern cuisine often combines sweet ingredients, such as cinnamon and currants, with more-savory ingredients, such as cumin and onion. That sweet and savory pairing "makes" this dish. Although the currants are so small that they aren't readily apparent, they add an important depth and richness.

1 medium onion, minced	¾ cup dried lentils, sorted for stones
2 teaspoons ground cumin	and shriveled lentils and rinsed
2 teaspoons ground cinnamon	1 14.5-ounce can no-salt-added
½ teaspoon cayenne	crushed tomatoes, undrained
2 cups low-sodium vegetable broth	1 cup uncooked rice
and 2 cups low-sodium vegetable	½ cup water
broth, such as on page 44, or 2 cups	⅓ cup dried currants
water and 2 cups water, divided use	¼ cup crumbled fat-free feta cheese

In a large nonstick skillet, cook the onion, cumin, cinnamon, and cayenne over medium heat for 10 minutes, stirring occasionally.

Stir in 2 cups broth and the lentils. Increase the heat to medium high and bring to a boil. Reduce the heat and simmer, covered, for 20 minutes.

Stir in the tomatoes with liquid, rice, ½ cup water, currants, and remaining 2 cups broth. Increase the heat to medium high and bring to a boil. Reduce the heat and simmer, covered, for 20 minutes, or until the rice and lentils are tender. Sprinkle with the feta.

PER SERVING

CALORIES 386
TOTAL FAT 0.5 g
  Saturated Fat 0.0 g
  Trans Fat 0.0 g
  Polyunsaturated Fat 0.0 g
  Monounsaturated Fat 0.0 g
CHOLESTEROL 0 mg
SODIUM 182 mg
CARBOHYDRATES 81 g
  Fiber 9 g
  Sugars 17 g
PROTEIN 19 g
DIETARY EXCHANGES
  4 starch, 2 vegetable,
  ½ fruit, 1 very lean meat

chickpea pilaf

SERVES 6

Quinoa replaces the usual rice in this pilaf. If you want to serve more people, double the amount of the quinoa, but not of the other ingredients.

½ to ¾ cup dry-packed sun-dried
   tomatoes
1 cup boiling water
1 cup uncooked quinoa, rinsed and
   drained
1½ teaspoons olive oil
1 10-ounce package frozen green
   peas, thawed

1 large garlic clove, minced
1 to 1½ teaspoons dried oregano,
   crumbled
½ teaspoon crushed red pepper flakes
1 15.5-ounce can no-salt-added
   chickpeas, rinsed and drained
3 ounces fat-free feta cheese

Put the tomatoes in a small bowl and add the boiling water. Set aside for about 10 minutes to soften. Drain the tomatoes, saving the liquid in a 2-cup measuring cup. Chop the tomatoes and set aside. Add enough water to the tomato liquid to equal 2 cups. Pour into a medium saucepan.

Stir the quinoa into the tomato liquid. Bring to a boil over high heat. Reduce the heat and simmer, covered, for 15 minutes, or until all the liquid is absorbed.

Meanwhile, in a large nonstick skillet, heat the oil over medium heat, swirling to coat the bottom. Cook the peas, garlic, oregano, and red pepper flakes for 2 minutes, stirring occasionally.

Stir in the chickpeas. Cook for 5 minutes, or until heated through.

In a large bowl, stir together the tomatoes, quinoa, and chickpea mixture. Crumble the feta on top.

PER SERVING

CALORIES 259
TOTAL FAT 4.0 g
   Saturated Fat 0.5 g
   Trans Fat 0.0 g
   Polyunsaturated Fat 1.0 g
   Monounsaturated Fat 1.5 g
CHOLESTEROL 0 mg
SODIUM 293 mg
CARBOHYDRATES 42 g
   Fiber 8 g
   Sugars 4 g
PROTEIN 14 g
DIETARY EXCHANGES
   3 starch,
   1 very lean meat

slow-cooker chickpea stew

SERVES 6

Toasted cumin seeds impart a unique flavor to this hearty vegetarian stew.

2 15.5-ounce cans no-salt-added chickpeas, rinsed and drained
1 14.5-ounce can no-salt-added diced tomatoes, undrained
8 ounces unpeeled baby red potatoes, coarsely chopped
1 medium zucchini, quartered lengthwise and sliced
1 medium onion, chopped
1 medium garlic clove, minced
1 teaspoon cumin seeds and 1 teaspoon cumin seeds, all dry-roasted, divided use
½ teaspoon paprika
⅛ teaspoon cayenne or ¼ teaspoon pepper
3 cups low-sodium vegetable broth, such as on page 44, or water

In a 3½- or 4-quart slow cooker, stir together the chickpeas, tomatoes with liquid, potatoes, zucchini, onion, garlic, 1 teaspoon cumin seeds, paprika, and cayenne. Pour in the broth, stirring to combine. Cook, covered, on high for 4½ to 5 hours or on low for 8 to 9 hours, or until the potatoes are tender. Sprinkle with the remaining 1 teaspoon cumin seeds.

COOK'S TIP on dry-roasting cumin seeds

Add an extra dimension of flavor to cumin seeds by spreading them in a skillet and cooking them over medium heat for 2 to 3 minutes, or until they are toasted and aromatic, shaking the skillet occasionally. Transfer the seeds to a plate immediately so they do not burn.

PER SERVING

CALORIES 207
TOTAL FAT 1.5 g
    Saturated Fat 0.0 g
    Trans Fat 0.0 g
    Polyunsaturated Fat 0.5 g
    Monounsaturated Fat 0.5 g
CHOLESTEROL 0 mg
SODIUM 54 mg
CARBOHYDRATES 39 g
    Fiber 8 g
    Sugars 6 g
PROTEIN 10 g
DIETARY EXCHANGES
    2 starch, 2 vegetable,
    1 very lean meat

green chile and rice pie

SERVES 4

Perfect for any time of the day, this quichelike pie has south-of-the-border flair.

Cooking spray

PIE

1 teaspoon olive oil
2 cups sliced button mushrooms
½ cup chopped onion
2 medium garlic cloves, minced
1½ cups fat-free milk
1 14.5-ounce can no-salt-added diced tomatoes, well drained, patted dry with paper towels
1 cup uncooked instant brown rice
½ cup shredded low-fat 4-cheese Mexican blend
½ cup egg substitute

1 4-ounce can diced green chiles, drained
¼ cup shredded or grated Parmesan cheese
¾ teaspoon ground cumin

TOPPING

¼ cup fat-free sour cream
1 tablespoon plus 1 teaspoon salsa (lowest sodium available), such as Salsa Cruda (page 508)
1 tablespoon plus 1 teaspoon snipped fresh cilantro

Preheat the oven to 350°F. Lightly spray a 9-inch deep-dish pie pan with cooking spray.

In a large nonstick skillet, heat the oil over medium-high heat, swirling to coat the bottom. Cook the mushrooms and onion for 3 minutes, or until soft, stirring frequently.

Stir in the garlic. Cook for 30 seconds, stirring frequently.

Pour in the milk. Cook for 1½ to 2 minutes, or until hot but not boiling, stirring occasionally. Remove from the heat.

Stir in the remaining pie ingredients. Carefully pour into the pie pan.

Bake for 30 to 35 minutes, or until a knife inserted in the center comes out clean, the top is golden, and the edges are browned. Spoon the sour cream and salsa on top. Sprinkle with the cilantro.

PER SERVING

CALORIES 266
TOTAL FAT 6.5 g
  Saturated Fat 2.5 g
  Trans Fat 0.0 g
  Polyunsaturated Fat 0.5 g
  Monounsaturated Fat 2.5 g
CHOLESTEROL 17 mg
SODIUM 452 mg
CARBOHYDRATES 35 g
  Fiber 3 g
  Sugars 11 g
PROTEIN 17 g
DIETARY EXCHANGES
  1 starch, ½ fat-free milk,
  2 vegetable, 1 lean meat

bulgur, brown rice, and beans

SERVES 4

Although this dish won't win any beauty contests, it provides a nice variety of tastes and textures.

2 cups water
½ cup uncooked instant brown rice
½ cup uncooked bulgur
1 15.5-ounce can no-salt-added navy beans, rinsed and drained
⅓ cup pine nuts, dry-roasted
1 tablespoon finely snipped fresh oregano or 1 teaspoon dried, crumbled

1 tablespoon olive oil (extra virgin preferred)
2 medium garlic cloves, minced
¾ teaspoon salt
¾ teaspoon finely snipped fresh rosemary or ¼ teaspoon dried, crushed
4 rosemary sprigs (optional)

In a medium saucepan, bring the water to a boil over high heat. Stir in the rice and bulgur. Reduce the heat and simmer, covered, for 10 minutes, or until most of the water has evaporated. Remove from the heat.

Stir in the remaining ingredients except the rosemary sprigs. Use the sprigs for a garnish.

PER SERVING

CALORIES 281
TOTAL FAT 9.0 g
    Saturated Fat 1.5 g
    Trans Fat 0.0 g
    Polyunsaturated Fat 3.0 g
    Monounsaturated Fat 4.5 g
CHOLESTEROL 0 mg
SODIUM 450 mg
CARBOHYDRATES 41 g
    Fiber 8 g
    Sugars 4 g
PROTEIN 12 g
DIETARY EXCHANGES
    2½ starch, ½ lean meat, 1 fat

vegetable and pinto bean enchiladas

SERVES 8

These filling enchiladas offer not only vitamin-rich spinach and plump pinto beans but julienned vegetables as well. Chilled slices of fresh jícama with a squeeze of lime would make a nice accompaniment.

16 6-inch corn tortillas
1 teaspoon olive oil
1 medium carrot, cut into matchstick-size strips
2 medium leeks (white part only), thinly sliced, or ½ cup sliced onion
1 medium zucchini, cut into matchstick-size strips
1 15.5-ounce can no-salt-added pinto beans, rinsed and drained
1 10-ounce package frozen chopped spinach, cooked, well drained, and squeezed dry

4 ounces light tub cream cheese
½ cup salsa (lowest sodium available), such as Salsa Cruda (page 508)
1 teaspoon fresh lime juice
½ teaspoon salt
½ cup fat-free half-and-half
1 teaspoon ground cumin
1 cup shredded or grated low-fat Cheddar cheese

Preheat the oven to 350°F.

Wrap the tortillas in aluminum foil.

Bake for 5 minutes, or until heated through. Set aside, still in the foil, to keep warm.

Meanwhile, in a large nonstick skillet, heat the oil over medium-high heat, swirling to coat the bottom. Cook the carrot and leeks for 2 to 3 minutes, or until the carrot is tender-crisp, stirring occasionally.

Stir in the zucchini. Cook for 2 to 3 minutes, or until the zucchini is tender-crisp.

Stir in the beans, spinach, cream cheese, salsa, lime juice, and salt. Reduce the heat to medium low. Cook for 2 to 3 minutes, or until heated through, stirring occasionally.

Spoon about ¼ cup filling down the center of a tortilla. Roll up jelly-roll style and place with the seam side down in a nonstick 13 x 9 x 2-inch baking pan. Repeat with the remaining filling and tortillas.

In a small bowl, stir together the half-and-half and cumin. Pour over the enchiladas. Sprinkle with the Cheddar.

Bake for 15 to 20 minutes, or until heated through.

enchilada bake

SERVES 6

Layers of vegetables, creamy sauce, beans, and tortillas make a tasty casserole that's even better the day after you prepare it.

SAUCE

1 teaspoon light tub margarine

1 medium onion, chopped

½ medium green bell pepper, chopped

8 ounces medium button mushrooms, quartered

1 to 2 medium garlic cloves, minced

2 cups canned no-salt-added black or pinto beans, rinsed and drained

1 14.5-ounce can no-salt-added stewed tomatoes, undrained

½ cup dry red wine (regular or nonalcoholic)

2 to 3 teaspoons chili powder

1 to 2 teaspoons ground cumin

¼ teaspoon salt

———

Cooking spray

¾ cup fat-free ricotta cheese

½ cup fat-free plain yogurt

6 6-inch corn tortillas, quartered

½ cup grated low-fat mozzarella cheese

6 medium black olives, sliced

In a large saucepan, melt the margarine over medium-high heat, swirling to coat the bottom. Cook the onion, bell pepper, mushrooms, and garlic for about 3 minutes, or until the onion is soft.

Stir in the remaining sauce ingredients. Reduce the heat and simmer for 30 minutes.

Preheat the oven to 350°F. Lightly spray a 1½-quart casserole dish with cooking spray.

In a small bowl, whisk together the ricotta and yogurt.

Place 3 tortillas (12 quarters) in the casserole dish. Top with half the sauce, half the mozzarella, and half the ricotta mixture. Repeat the layers. Top with the olives.

Bake, covered, for 15 to 20 minutes, or until heated through.

PER SERVING

CALORIES 224
TOTAL FAT 2.5 g
   Saturated Fat 0.5 g
   Trans Fat 0.0 g
   Polyunsaturated Fat 0.5 g
   Monounsaturated Fat 1.0 g
CHOLESTEROL 6 mg
SODIUM 324 mg
CARBOHYDRATES 32 g
   Fiber 7 g
   Sugars 11 g
PROTEIN 15 g
DIETARY EXCHANGES
   1½ starch, 2 vegetable,
   1 very lean meat

black bean polenta with avocado salsa

SERVES 6

Try thick pieces of polenta stuffed with black beans and topped with fresh avocado salsa for a stick-to-your-ribs Tex-Italian dinner.

POLENTA

4 cups water
1 teaspoon olive oil
½ teaspoon ground cumin
½ teaspoon ground ancho chile powder
¼ teaspoon salt
1½ cups yellow cornmeal
1 15.5-ounce can no-salt-added black beans, rinsed and drained

AVOCADO SALSA

2 medium avocados, finely chopped
¼ cup finely chopped red onion
2 tablespoons snipped fresh cilantro
2 tablespoons fresh lime juice
¼ teaspoon salt

In a medium saucepan, stir together the water, oil, cumin, chile powder, and salt. Bring to a boil over high heat.

Slowly add the cornmeal, whisking constantly. When all the cornmeal is incorporated, reduce the heat and simmer for 5 minutes, stirring occasionally (a wooden spoon works well). Remove the pan from the heat.

Stir in the beans. Spread in an 8-inch square baking pan. Let cool to room temperature, about 30 minutes, then cover and chill for at least 2 hours.

Preheat the broiler. Line a baking sheet with aluminum foil. Cut the polenta into 6 pieces. Transfer to the baking sheet.

Broil the polenta 4 to 6 inches from the heat for 4 to 5 minutes on each side, or until it is lightly browned and heated through.

Meanwhile, finely chop the avocados. In a medium bowl, stir together the avocado and the remaining salsa ingredients. Serve over the polenta.

cuban black beans

SERVES 8

The green onions and vinegar give this dish its Cuban flavor. Serve with a crisp green salad and Easy Refrigerator Rolls (page 538) for a colorful meatless meal. If you have leftover beans, save a cup of them and give Southwestern Pork Salad (page 129) a try.

2 cups dried black beans (about 1 pound), sorted for stones and shriveled beans and rinsed
Cooking spray
1 teaspoon light tub margarine
2 medium onions, chopped
½ medium rib of celery, diced
½ medium lemon, quartered
1 tablespoon chopped fresh savory or 1 teaspoon dried, crumbled

2 medium garlic cloves, minced
1 medium dried bay leaf
¾ teaspoon salt
Pinch of ground ginger
1½ cups uncooked brown rice
4 medium green onions, chopped (optional)
3 tablespoons red wine vinegar (optional)
2 medium oranges, sliced (optional)

Soak the beans using the package directions. Drain well in a colander.

Lightly spray a stockpot with cooking spray. Heat the margarine over medium-high heat, swirling to coat the bottom. Cook the onions and celery for about 3 minutes, or until the onions are soft.

Add the beans, lemon, savory, garlic, bay leaf, salt and ginger. Add water to cover by 2 inches. Stir well. Increase the heat to high and bring to a boil. Reduce the heat and simmer, covered, for 1 hour to 1 hour 30 minutes, or until the beans are tender. Discard the lemon and bay leaf.

Meanwhile, prepare the rice using the package directions, omitting the salt and margarine.

Spoon the rice into bowls. Spoon the beans over the rice. Sprinkle with the green onions and vinegar, or garnish with the orange slices.

PER SERVING

CALORIES 305
TOTAL FAT 1.0 g
 Saturated Fat 0.0 g
 Trans Fat 0.0 g
 Polyunsaturated Fat 0.5 g
 Monounsaturated Fat 0.5 g
CHOLESTEROL 0 mg
SODIUM 231 mg
CARBOHYDRATES 60 g
 Fiber 7 g
 Sugars 7 g
PROTEIN 13 g
DIETARY EXCHANGES
 4 starch,
 ½ very lean meat

red beans and couscous

SERVES 4

Go for a new spin on the classic red beans and rice with this quick and easy recipe. Serve the dish with slices of tomato and cucumbers.

1 teaspoon olive oil
½ medium green bell pepper, chopped
1 medium rib of celery, chopped
½ medium onion, chopped
2 medium garlic cloves, chopped
2 cups low-sodium vegetable broth, such as on page 44

1 15.5-ounce can no-salt-added red beans, rinsed and drained
2 tablespoons imitation bacon bits
1½ to 2 teaspoons salt-free Creole or Cajun seasoning blend, such as on page 463
1½ cups uncooked whole-wheat couscous

In a medium nonstick saucepan, heat the oil over medium-high heat, swirling to coat the bottom. Cook the bell pepper, celery, onion, and garlic for 3 to 4 minutes, or until tender, stirring occasionally.

Stir in the broth, beans, bacon bits, and seasoning blend. Bring to a simmer. Reduce the heat and simmer for 1 to 2 minutes, or until the bacon bits are tender.

Stir in the couscous. Remove from the heat. Let stand, covered, for 5 minutes, or until the couscous has absorbed the liquid. Fluff with a fork.

PER SERVING

CALORIES 432
TOTAL FAT 3.5 g
  Saturated Fat 0.5 g
  Trans Fat 0.0 g
  Polyunsaturated Fat 0.5 g
  Monounsaturated Fat 1.0 g
CHOLESTEROL 0 mg
SODIUM 108 mg
CARBOHYDRATES 85 g
  Fiber 15 g
  Sugars 3 g
PROTEIN 19 g
DIETARY EXCHANGES
  5½ starch,
  ½ very lean meat

mediterranean toasted quinoa and spinach

SERVES 4

Feta cheese and lemon give a Mediterranean twist to this dish, made colorful with shreds of deep green spinach and slivers of purplish-red onion.

1½ cups uncooked quinoa, rinsed and drained

3 cups low-sodium vegetable broth, such as on page 44

4 cups shredded spinach, stems discarded

1 ounce fat-free feta cheese, crumbled

½ teaspoon grated lemon zest

1 tablespoon fresh lemon juice

1 tablespoon olive oil

¼ teaspoon pepper

¼ cup slivered red onion

In a large skillet, dry-roast the quinoa over medium-high heat for 3 to 4 minutes, or until it is lightly toasted and any excess water has evaporated, stirring frequently (the quinoa won't turn golden brown).

In a medium saucepan, bring the broth to a boil over high heat. Stir in the quinoa. Return to a boil. Reduce the heat and simmer for 15 to 20 minutes, or until the water is absorbed and the quinoa is tender.

Stir in the remaining ingredients except the red onion. Sprinkle with the red onion.

COOK'S TIP on quinoa

Although most packaged quinoa has already been rinsed, it is a good idea to rinse it yourself to be sure the bitter coating is removed. One way is to swirl it around in a bowl of water and drain it in a fine-mesh strainer. Replacing the water each time, repeat several times until the water remains clear. To enhance the flavor, dry-roast the quinoa.

PER SERVING

CALORIES 287
TOTAL FAT 7.5 g
  Saturated Fat 1.0 g
  Trans Fat 0.0 g
  Polyunsaturated Fat 2.5 g
  Monounsaturated Fat 3.5 g
CHOLESTEROL 0 mg
SODIUM 148 mg
CARBOHYDRATES 44 g
  Fiber 5 g
  Sugars 1 g
PROTEIN 12 g
DIETARY EXCHANGES
  3 starch, 1 fat

quinoa with black beans and seared bell pepper

SERVES 4

Pine nuts add a bit of crunch and pizzazz to this filling dish.

1⅓ cups water
⅔ cup uncooked quinoa, rinsed and drained
1 15.5-ounce can no-salt-added black beans, rinsed and drained
¾ cup frozen whole-kernel corn, thawed
Cooking spray
2 medium onions, cut into thin strips
1 large red bell pepper, cut into thin strips
1 medium garlic clove, minced
2 tablespoons pine nuts, dry-roasted
1 tablespoon olive oil (extra virgin preferred)
1 teaspoon ground cumin
¾ teaspoon salt
¼ teaspoon crushed red pepper flakes

In a medium saucepan, bring the water to a boil over high heat. Stir in the quinoa. Return to a boil. Reduce the heat and simmer, covered, for about 12 minutes, or until the water is absorbed and the quinoa is just tender.

Stir in the beans and corn. Remove from the heat. Cover to keep warm.

Meanwhile, lightly spray a large skillet with cooking spray. Cook the onions, bell pepper, and garlic over medium-high heat for 8 minutes, or until deeply browned, stirring frequently.

Stir the bell pepper mixture and remaining ingredients into the quinoa mixture.

COOK'S TIP on dry-roasting pine nuts

To dry-roast pine nuts, heat a small skillet over medium-high heat. Dry-roast the pine nuts for 1 to 2 minutes, or until they begin to brown lightly, stirring constantly. Watch carefully so the nuts don't burn.

PER SERVING

CALORIES 312
TOTAL FAT 7.5 g
  Saturated Fat 1.0 g
  Trans Fat 0.0 g
  Polyunsaturated Fat 2.0 g
  Monounsaturated Fat 3.5 g
CHOLESTEROL 0 mg
SODIUM 447 mg
CARBOHYDRATES 51 g
  Fiber 10 g
  Sugars 11 g
PROTEIN 13 g
DIETARY EXCHANGES
  3 starch, 1 vegetable,
  ½ lean meat, 1 fat

cumin and ginger lentils on quinoa

SERVES 4

Ground cumin is the key ingredient in this dish, tying all the other flavors together. Serve as a meatless entrée for four or as a side with grilled lamb chops or pork for eight.

1 teaspoon olive oil
1½ cups diced onion
1 cup thinly sliced carrots
½ cup thinly sliced celery
2 medium garlic cloves, minced
2 cups water and 1¼ cups water, divided use
½ cup dried lentils, sorted for stones and shriveled lentils and rinsed

½ cup uncooked quinoa, rinsed and drained
¼ cup finely chopped green onions
⅓ cup pine nuts, dry-roasted
2 teaspoons grated peeled gingerroot
¾ to 1 teaspoon ground cumin
½ teaspoon salt
⅛ teaspoon cayenne (optional)

In a large nonstick skillet, heat the oil over medium-high heat, swirling to coat the bottom. Cook the onion, carrots, and celery for 6 minutes, or until beginning to brown on the edges, stirring frequently.

Stir in the garlic. Cook for 15 seconds.

Stir in 2 cups water and the lentils. Bring to a boil, still on medium high. Reduce the heat and simmer, covered, for 25 minutes, or until the lentils are tender. Remove from the heat.

Meanwhile, in a medium saucepan, bring the remaining 1¼ cups water to a boil over high heat. Add the quinoa. Return to a boil. Reduce the heat and simmer, covered, for about 12 minutes, or until the water is absorbed and the quinoa is just tender. Remove from the heat.

Stir the green onions into the quinoa. Set aside, uncovered.

When the lentil mixture is cooked, gently stir in the remaining ingredients.

Spoon the quinoa mixture onto a serving plate. Spoon the lentil mixture over the quinoa. Serve immediately for the most pronounced flavor.

PER SERVING

CALORIES 267
TOTAL FAT 8.0 g
  Saturated Fat 1.0 g
  Trans Fat 0.0 g
  Polyunsaturated Fat 3.0 g
  Monounsaturated Fat 3.0 g
CHOLESTEROL 0 mg
SODIUM 337 mg
CARBOHYDRATES 39 g
  Fiber 10 g
  Sugars 7 g
PROTEIN 13 g
DIETARY EXCHANGES
  2 starch, 2 vegetable,
  1 very lean meat, 1 fat

quinoa pilaf with tofu and vegetables

SERVES 4

The delicate flavor of quinoa is a nice change of pace in this Asian-inspired pilaf.

½ cup uncooked quinoa, rinsed and drained

1 1-pound package frozen mixed stir-fry vegetables

12 ounces light firm tofu, drained and cubed

1 cup low-sodium vegetable broth, such as on page 44

2 teaspoons soy sauce (lowest sodium available)

1 teaspoon chili paste

1 teaspoon toasted sesame oil

2 tablespoons slivered almonds, dry-roasted

In a large nonstick skillet, dry-roast the quinoa over medium-high heat for 3 to 4 minutes, or until lightly toasted and any excess water has evaporated (the quinoa won't turn golden brown), stirring occasionally.

Stir in the remaining ingredients except the almonds. Bring to a simmer. Reduce the heat and simmer, covered, for about 15 minutes, or until the liquid is absorbed and the quinoa is just tender.

Stir in the almonds. Fluff the mixture with a fork.

COOK'S TIP

Quinoa contains protein and all eight essential amino acids.

PER SERVING

CALORIES 198
TOTAL FAT 5.5 g
  Saturated Fat 0.5 g
  Trans Fat 0.0 g
  Polyunsaturated Fat 1.5 g
  Monounsaturated Fat 2.0 g
CHOLESTEROL 0 mg
SODIUM 171 mg
CARBOHYDRATES 23 g
  Fiber 4 g
  Sugars 3 g
PROTEIN 13 g
DIETARY EXCHANGES
  1 starch, 1 vegetable,
  1 very lean meat, 1 fat

curried cauliflower and tofu with basmati rice

SERVES 6

The light and delicate curry flavor along with the unusual combination of ingredients such as mango chutney, apple, cauliflower, green beans, and tofu make this dish a must-try. Although the list of ingredients is long, the preparation isn't complicated, and it all cooks in one pot.

1 cup uncooked basmati rice
1 tablespoon plus 2 teaspoons olive oil
1 small head cauliflower, coarsely chopped
12 medium asparagus spears, trimmed and cut into 1-inch pieces
12 green beans, trimmed and cut into 1-inch pieces
2 large tomatoes, cut into 1-inch wedges
1 large sweet onion, such as Vidalia, Maui, or OsoSweet, coarsely chopped
¼ cup coarsely chopped fresh Italian (flat-leaf) parsley

1 tablespoon curry powder, or to taste
⅛ teaspoon cayenne, or to taste
1 cup fat-free evaporated milk
1 medium apple (Fuji preferred), finely diced
2 tablespoons mango chutney or honey
¼ teaspoon salt
Pepper to taste
1 pound light firm tofu, drained and cut into ½-inch cubes
1 cup frozen green peas
¼ cup coarsely snipped fresh cilantro
2 tablespoons cashews, dry-roasted

Prepare the rice using the package directions, omitting the salt and margarine.

In a stockpot, heat the oil over medium-low heat, swirling to coat the bottom. Add the cauliflower, asparagus, green beans, tomatoes, onion, parsley, curry, and cayenne, stirring to combine. Cook, covered, for 15 minutes, or until the vegetables release their liquids, stirring occasionally.

Stir the evaporated milk, apple, chutney, salt, and pepper into the cauliflower mixture. Cook, covered, for 10 to 12 minutes, or until the green beans are tender-crisp, stirring occasionally.

Gently stir in the tofu, peas, and cilantro. Cook, uncovered, for 5 minutes. Spoon over the rice. Sprinkle with the cashews.

PER SERVING

CALORIES 330
TOTAL FAT 7.0 g
  Saturated Fat 1.0 g
  Trans Fat 0.0 g
  Polyunsaturated Fat 1.0 g
  Monounsaturated Fat 4.0 g
CHOLESTEROL 2 mg
SODIUM 218 mg
CARBOHYDRATES 53 g
  Fiber 7 g
  Sugars 17 g
PROTEIN 16 g
DIETARY EXCHANGES
  2 starch, 2 vegetable,
  1 carbohydrate,
  1 very lean meat, 1 fat

edamame fried rice

SERVES 4

Use this versatile recipe as a base for many combinations. For instance, try peas instead of edamame and add tofu, cooked chicken, or cooked pork strips.

½ cup uncooked instant brown rice
1 teaspoon toasted sesame oil
1 medium garlic clove, minced
⅔ cup egg substitute
1½ cups frozen shelled edamame (green soybeans), thawed
½ cup slivered red bell pepper

½ cup shredded carrot
½ cup water
1 tablespoon soy sauce (lowest sodium available)
¼ cup sliced green onions
1 tablespoon snipped fresh cilantro

Prepare the rice using the package directions, omitting the salt and margarine.

Meanwhile, in a large nonstick skillet, heat the oil over medium heat, swirling to coat the bottom. Cook the garlic for 1 minute, stirring frequently.

Pour in the egg substitute. Cook for 2 to 3 minutes, or until the egg mixture is no longer wet, stirring constantly. Transfer the mixture to a cutting board and coarsely chop. Set aside.

Wipe the skillet with paper towels. Put the edamame, bell pepper, carrot, and water in the skillet. Stir together. Cook over medium-high heat for 5 to 6 minutes, or until the edamame, bell pepper, and carrot are tender and the water has almost evaporated, stirring occasionally.

Stir in the rice and soy sauce. Cook for 2 to 3 minutes, or until heated through, stirring frequently. Stir in the chopped egg substitute mixture, green onions, and cilantro.

edamame and vegetable stir-fry

SERVES 4

Jade-green edamame and vibrant cherry tomatoes really make this a show-stopper in a skillet, and a nutritious one to boot! Serve with Wilted Baby Spinach with Pear and Goat Cheese (page 89).

½ cup low-sodium vegetable broth, such as on page 44
1 tablespoon hoisin sauce
2 teaspoons soy sauce (lowest sodium available)
1½ teaspoons cornstarch
1 teaspoon wasabi powder
1 teaspoon toasted sesame oil

16 ounces frozen shelled edamame (green soybeans)
1 teaspoon canola or corn oil
1 cup diced baby pattypan squash
½ cup matchstick-size carrot strips, halved crosswise
1 cup cherry tomatoes
2 medium green onions, thinly sliced

In a small bowl, whisk together the broth, hoisin sauce, soy sauce, cornstarch, wasabi powder, and sesame oil. Set aside.

Prepare the edamame using the package directions, omitting the salt. Drain well in a colander.

Meanwhile, in a large nonstick skillet, heat the canola oil over medium-high heat, swirling to coat the bottom. Cook the squash and carrots for 2 to 3 minutes, or until tender-crisp, stirring constantly.

Stir in the broth mixture and edamame. Cook for 2 to 3 minutes, or until the mixture is thickened, stirring occasionally.

Stir in the tomatoes and green onions.

PER SERVING

CALORIES 195
TOTAL FAT 7.5 g
    Saturated Fat 0.5 g
    Trans Fat 0.0 g
    Polyunsaturated Fat 1.0 g
    Monounsaturated Fat 1.0 g
CHOLESTEROL 0 mg
SODIUM 109 mg
CARBOHYDRATES 18 g
    Fiber 7 g
    Sugars 9 g
PROTEIN 15 g
DIETARY EXCHANGES
    1 starch, 1 vegetable,
    2 lean meat

meatless moussaka

SERVES 8

Traditional moussaka goes meatless in this tasty version.

Cooking spray
2 pounds eggplant, peeled and thickly sliced crosswise

SAUCE
1 teaspoon olive oil
1 large onion, finely chopped
3 medium garlic cloves, minced
1 14.5-ounce can diced no-salt-added tomatoes, undrained
1 cup water
1 6-ounce can no-salt-added tomato paste
2 teaspoons dried rosemary, crushed

2 tablespoons snipped fresh parsley
2 tablespoons snipped fresh mint

FILLING
16 ounces fat-free cottage cheese
½ cup egg substitute
2 tablespoons shredded or grated Parmesan cheese
1 teaspoon dried rosemary, crushed
½ teaspoon dried oregano, crumbled
½ teaspoon pepper, or to taste
_____
¼ cup shredded or grated Parmesan cheese

Preheat the broiler. Lightly spray a 13 x 9 x 2-inch glass baking dish with cooking spray.

Lightly spray both sides of the eggplant slices with cooking spray. Put on 2 large baking sheets.

Broil about 6 inches from the heat for 5 minutes on each side, or until the eggplant is browned and tender.

Preheat the oven to 375°F.

In a large skillet, heat the oil over medium-high heat, swirling to coat the bottom. Cook the onion and garlic for 3 minutes, or until the onion is soft, stirring frequently.

Stir in the tomatoes with liquid, water, tomato paste, and rosemary. Bring to a simmer. Reduce the heat and simmer for 10 minutes. Stir in the parsley and mint. Remove from the heat.

In a medium bowl, whisk together the filling ingredients.

Layer as follows in the baking dish: half the sauce, half the eggplant, all the filling, the remaining eggplant, and the remaining sauce. Top with the Parmesan.

Bake, covered, for 45 minutes. Bake, uncovered, for 10 minutes.

PER SERVING
CALORIES 129
TOTAL FAT 2.0 g
  Saturated Fat 1.0 g
  Trans Fat 0.0 g
  Polyunsaturated Fat 0.0 g
  Monounsaturated Fat 1.0 g
CHOLESTEROL 5 mg
SODIUM 340 mg
CARBOHYDRATES 19 g
  Fiber 6 g
  Sugars 11 g
PROTEIN 12 g
DIETARY EXCHANGES
  3 vegetable,
  1 very lean meat

ratatouille with cannellini beans and brown rice

SERVES 6

This chunky French stew is a simple combination of vegetables and legumes—comfort food at its best.

RATATOUILLE
- 1 teaspoon olive oil
- 8 ounces button mushrooms, sliced
- ½ medium onion (sweet onion, such as Vidalia or Maui, preferred), sliced into rings and halved
- 2 medium zucchini, cut into ¼-inch slices
- 3 medium garlic cloves, minced
- 2 14.5-ounce cans no-salt-added stewed tomatoes, undrained
- 1 15.5-ounce can no-salt-added cannellini beans, rinsed and drained
- ½ large red bell pepper, diced

- ¼ cup shredded or grated Parmesan cheese
- 2 teaspoons dried oregano, crumbled
- 1 teaspoon dried basil, crumbled
- ½ teaspoon dried thyme, crumbled
- ⅛ teaspoon pepper

- 2 cups uncooked instant brown rice
- 1¾ cups low-sodium vegetable broth, such as on page 44
- 2 tablespoons shredded or grated Parmesan cheese
- Crushed red pepper flakes (optional)

In a large, heavy nonstick skillet, heat the oil over medium-high heat, swirling to coat the bottom. Cook the mushrooms and onion for 5 to 7 minutes, or until the onion starts to brown, stirring occasionally.

Stir in the zucchini and garlic. Cook for 8 to 10 minutes, or until the zucchini is soft, stirring frequently.

Stir in the remaining ratatouille ingredients, breaking up the tomatoes into smaller pieces. Simmer for 15 to 20 minutes, or until the bell pepper is tender, stirring occasionally to prevent sticking.

Meanwhile, prepare the rice using the package directions, omitting the salt and margarine and substituting the broth for the water. Spoon into bowls and top with the ratatouille, remaining 2 tablespoons Parmesan, and red pepper flakes.

PER SERVING

CALORIES 269
TOTAL FAT 4.0 g
  Saturated Fat 1.0 g
  Trans Fat 0.0 g
  Polyunsaturated Fat 0.5 g
  Monounsaturated Fat 1.5 g
CHOLESTEROL 4 mg
SODIUM 144 mg
CARBOHYDRATES 47 g
  Fiber 8 g
  Sugars 9 g
PROTEIN 12 g
DIETARY EXCHANGES
  2 starch, 3 vegetable,
  ½ lean meat

eggplant parmesan

SERVES 4

Cut out lots of saturated fat, cholesterol, and sodium by eating homemade eggplant Parmesan instead of paying more for the far less healthy restaurant version.

Cooking spray

EGGPLANT

2 large egg whites

2 tablespoons fat-free milk

½ cup plain dried bread crumbs (lowest sodium available)

2 tablespoons shredded or grated Parmesan cheese

½ teaspoon dried basil, crumbled

½ teaspoon dried oregano, crumbled

1 1½-pound eggplant, cut crosswise into 12 slices

SAUCE

2 teaspoons olive oil

1 small onion, diced

1 medium garlic clove, minced

2 14-ounce cans no-salt-added Italian plum (Roma) tomatoes, chopped, liquid reserved

¼ teaspoon dried basil, crumbled

¼ teaspoon dried oregano, crumbled

½ cup shredded low-fat mozzarella cheese

1 tablespoon shredded or grated Parmesan cheese

Preheat the oven to 350°F. Lightly spray a large rimmed baking sheet and 15 x 10-inch glass baking dish with cooking spray.

In a shallow dish, whisk together the egg whites and milk. In another shallow dish, stir together the bread crumbs, 2 tablespoons Parmesan, ½ teaspoon basil, and ½ teaspoon oregano. Set the bowls and the baking sheet in a row, assembly-line fashion. Dip one slice of eggplant in the egg white mixture, turning to coat and letting the excess drip off. Dip in the bread crumb mixture, turning to coat. Using your fingertips, gently press so the crumbs adhere. Put the eggplant on the baking sheet. Lightly spray the top side of the eggplant with cooking spray. Repeat with the remaining eggplant, placing the slices in a single layer.

Bake for 25 to 30 minutes, or until the eggplant is browned on the bottom. Turn and bake for 10 to 15 minutes, or until browned. Transfer the baking sheet to a cooling rack. Leave the oven on.

PER SERVING

CALORIES 216
TOTAL FAT 6.0 g
  Saturated Fat 1.5 g
  Trans Fat 0.0 g
  Polyunsaturated Fat 1.0 g
  Monounsaturated Fat 2.5 g
CHOLESTEROL 8 mg
SODIUM 318 mg
CARBOHYDRATES 32 g
  Fiber 9 g
  Sugars 12 g
PROTEIN 13 g
DIETARY EXCHANGES
  ½ starch, 4 vegetable,
  ½ very lean meat, 1 fat

Meanwhile, in a large nonstick skillet, heat the oil over medium-high heat, swirling to coat the bottom. Cook the onion for 3 minutes, or until soft, stirring frequently.

Stir in the garlic. Cook for 1 minute, stirring constantly.

Stir in the tomatoes with liquid, remaining ¼ teaspoon basil, and remaining ¼ teaspoon oregano. Bring to a boil. Reduce the heat and simmer for 15 minutes, or until the sauce is thickened.

Spread 2 cups sauce in the baking dish. Arrange the eggplant slices in slightly overlapping layers on the sauce. Spoon the remaining sauce over the eggplant. Sprinkle with the mozzarella and Parmesan.

Bake for 15 to 20 minutes, or until the sauce is bubbly and the cheese is melted.

COOK'S TIP

If you don't have a 15 x 10-inch glass baking dish, use a 13 x 9 x 2-inch glass baking dish and overlap the eggplant slices as needed.

eggplant zucchini casserole

SERVES 8

Put uncooked spaghetti right in the casserole. Everything bakes together—no spaghetti pot to wash!

Cooking spray

SAUCE

  2 8-ounce cans no-salt-added tomato sauce

  2 medium garlic cloves, crushed

  2 teaspoons Worcestershire sauce (lowest sodium available)

  1 teaspoon dried oregano, crumbled

  ½ teaspoon dried basil, crumbled

  ½ teaspoon dried marjoram, crumbled

    Pepper to taste

1 medium eggplant, peeled and sliced crosswise

2 medium zucchini, sliced crosswise

4 ounces dried whole-grain spaghetti, broken into thirds (about 1 cup)

3 medium ribs of celery, chopped

1 medium onion, chopped

1 medium green bell pepper, chopped

8 ounces low-fat mozzarella cheese, cut into 18 small slices

Preheat the oven to 350°F. Lightly spray a 13 x 9 x 2-inch casserole dish with cooking spray.

In a medium bowl, stir together the sauce ingredients.

In the casserole dish, arrange half the eggplant slices in a single layer. Top with half of each of the following, in order: zucchini, spaghetti, celery, onion, bell pepper, mozzarella, and tomato sauce mixture. Repeat the layers.

Bake, covered, for 1 hour, or until the vegetables are tender.

PER SERVING

CALORIES 165
TOTAL FAT 3.5 g
  Saturated Fat 1.0 g
  Trans Fat 0.0 g
  Polyunsaturated Fat 0.5 g
  Monounsaturated Fat 1.0 g
CHOLESTEROL 10 mg
SODIUM 227 mg
CARBOHYDRATES 24 g
  Fiber 6 g
  Sugars 8 g
PROTEIN 11 g
DIETARY EXCHANGES
  1 starch, 2 vegetable,
  1 lean meat

spinach artichoke gratin

SERVES 6

Spinach, artichokes, and cheese—a perfect combination. As the mixture bakes to bubbly richness, prepare steamed carrots and a tossed salad with one of our salad dressings (pages 136–139) to complete your meal.

Cooking spray
16 ounces fat-free cottage cheese
½ cup egg substitute
3 tablespoons shredded or grated Parmesan cheese and
2 tablespoons shredded or grated Parmesan cheese, divided use
1 tablespoon fresh lemon juice
⅛ teaspoon pepper (white preferred)

⅛ teaspoon ground nutmeg
2 10-ounce packages frozen chopped spinach, thawed and squeezed dry
3 medium green onions, thinly sliced (green part only)
1 9-ounce package frozen artichoke hearts, thawed, drained, halved, and patted dry

Preheat the oven to 375°F. Lightly spray a 1½-quart glass baking dish with cooking spray.

In a food processor or blender, process the cottage cheese, egg substitute, 3 tablespoons Parmesan, lemon juice, pepper, and nutmeg until smooth. Transfer to a large bowl.

Stir the spinach and green onions into the cottage cheese mixture. Spread half in the baking dish.

Place the artichoke hearts in a single layer on the cottage cheese mixture. Sprinkle with the remaining 2 tablespoons Parmesan. Cover with the remaining cottage cheese mixture.

Bake, covered, for 25 minutes, or until heated through.

PER SERVING

CALORIES 130
TOTAL FAT 1.5 g
  Saturated Fat 1.0 g
  Trans Fat 0.0 g
  Polyunsaturated Fat 0.0 g
  Monounsaturated Fat 0.5 g
CHOLESTEROL 6 mg
SODIUM 472 mg
CARBOHYDRATES 14 g
  Fiber 6 g
  Sugars 5 g
PROTEIN 16 g
DIETARY EXCHANGES
  2 vegetable,
  ½ carbohydrate,
  2 very lean meat

spinach ricotta swirls

SERVES 4

Whether for family or guests, this dish will be a showstopper!

8 dried lasagna noodles
Olive oil spray

SAUCE
1 teaspoon olive oil
1 small or medium onion, finely chopped
2 large garlic cloves, minced
2 cups low-sodium vegetable broth, such as on page 44
1 6-ounce can no-salt-added tomato paste
1 teaspoon dried Italian seasoning, crumbled

¼ teaspoon salt

FILLING
2 10-ounce packages frozen chopped spinach, thawed and squeezed dry
1 cup fat-free ricotta cheese
2 tablespoons shredded or grated Parmesan cheese
¼ teaspoon pepper (white preferred)
⅛ teaspoon ground nutmeg

Prepare the noodles using the package directions, omitting the salt. Drain well in a colander. Pat dry. Place in a single layer on wax paper. Set aside.

Preheat the oven to 350°F. Lightly spray an 8-inch square glass baking dish with olive oil spray.

In a small nonstick saucepan, heat the oil over medium-high heat, swirling to coat the bottom. Cook the onion and garlic for about 3 minutes, or until the onion is soft, stirring frequently.

Stir in the remaining sauce ingredients. Reduce the heat and simmer for 5 minutes, or until slightly thickened, stirring occasionally. Remove from the heat. Set aside.

In a large bowl, stir together the filling ingredients.

Spread the filling lengthwise down each noodle, leaving a border on all sides. Roll up each noodle from a short end and place it on its side in the baking dish. (The rolled noodles shouldn't touch each other.) Pour the sauce over the noodles.

Bake, covered, for 25 to 30 minutes, or until heated through.

PER SERVING
CALORIES 361
TOTAL FAT 4.0 g
Saturated Fat 1.0 g
Trans Fat 0.0 g
Polyunsaturated Fat 1.0 g
Monounsaturated Fat 1.5 g
CHOLESTEROL 7 mg
SODIUM 464 mg
CARBOHYDRATES 61 g
Fiber 8 g
Sugars 12 g
PROTEIN 24 g
DIETARY EXCHANGES
3 starch, 3 vegetable, 1½ very lean meat

asparagus and artichoke quiche

SERVES 4

This vegetable quiche sports a brown rice crust, which is very easy to assemble. Serve the wedges of quiche with chilled slices of honeydew melon.

1¼ cups low-sodium vegetable broth, such as on page 44

1 teaspoon salt-free all-purpose seasoning blend

1 cup uncooked instant brown rice
Cooking spray

1 large egg white, lightly beaten with a fork

8 medium asparagus spears, trimmed and cut into ¼-inch slices

1 cup chopped canned artichoke hearts, drained

2 medium Italian plum (Roma) tomatoes, thinly sliced

1 cup fat-free half-and-half

½ cup egg substitute

¼ cup shredded or grated Parmesan cheese

¼ teaspoon pepper

In a medium saucepan, bring the broth and seasoning blend to a simmer over medium-high heat. Stir in the rice. Reduce the heat and simmer, covered, for 10 minutes, or until the rice is tender. Transfer to a medium bowl. Refrigerate for 10 minutes to cool.

Preheat the oven to 400°F. Lightly spray a 9-inch pie pan with cooking spray.

Stir the egg white into the cooled rice. Form a crust by pressing the mixture on the bottom and up the side of the pie pan.

Bake for 6 to 7 minutes, or until the rice is golden brown. Remove the crust from the oven. Reduce the oven temperature to 325°F.

Arrange the asparagus in the warm crust. Top with the artichokes, then the tomatoes.

In a medium bowl, whisk together the remaining ingredients. Pour over the vegetables.

Bake for 40 to 45 minutes, or until the center is set (doesn't jiggle when the quiche is gently shaken). Let cool for 10 minutes before cutting into wedges.

PER SERVING

CALORIES 199
TOTAL FAT 2.0 g
  Saturated Fat 1.0 g
  Trans Fat 0.0 g
  Polyunsaturated Fat 0.5 g
  Monounsaturated Fat 0.5 g
CHOLESTEROL 4 mg
SODIUM 356 mg
CARBOHYDRATES 32 g
  Fiber 2 g
  Sugars 6 g
PROTEIN 14 g
DIETARY EXCHANGES
  1½ starch, 1 vegetable,
  1½ very lean meat

meatless lasagna with zucchini and red wine

SERVES 9

After enjoying a meal of this hearty lasagna, freeze single portions of any that is left over. You'll be ready for dinner on those busy days or for lunch anytime.

Cooking spray
8 ounces dried whole-grain lasagna noodles
1 teaspoon olive oil and 1 tablespoon plus 2 teaspoons olive oil (extra virgin preferred), divided use
2 medium zucchini, thinly sliced
1 medium onion, chopped
4 medium garlic cloves, minced
3 8-ounce cans no-salt-added tomato sauce
⅓ cup dry red wine (regular or nonalcoholic)
1 tablespoon cider vinegar
2 teaspoons dried Italian seasoning, crumbled

¼ teaspoon crushed red pepper flakes (optional)
1 cup fat-free ricotta cheese
1 large egg white
2 tablespoons dried basil, crumbled
8 ounces vegetarian sausage patties or links (soy- or bean-based, about 6), finely chopped
⅛ teaspoon salt and ¼ teaspoon salt, divided use
1 cup shredded low-fat mozzarella cheese
⅓ cup shredded or grated Parmesan cheese

Preheat the oven to 350°F. Lightly spray a 13 x 9 x 2-inch nonstick baking pan with cooking spray.

Prepare the pasta using the package directions, omitting the salt. Drain well in a colander. Pat dry. Place in a single layer on wax paper. Set aside.

Meanwhile, in a large nonstick skillet, heat 1 teaspoon oil over medium heat, swirling to coat the bottom. Cook the zucchini for 4 minutes, or until just beginning to brown, stirring frequently.

Stir in the onion. Cook for 3 minutes, stirring frequently.

Stir in the garlic. Cook for 15 seconds.

Stir in the tomato sauce, wine, vinegar, Italian seasoning, and red pepper flakes. Increase the heat to medium high and bring to a boil. Reduce the heat and simmer for 5 minutes. Remove from the heat.

Stir in the remaining 1 tablespoon plus 2 teaspoons oil.

In a small bowl, whisk together the ricotta, egg white, and basil.

Make a layer of one-third of the noodles. Spoon one-third of the tomato sauce mixture over the noodles. Using a teaspoon (for more even distribution), spoon half the ricotta mixture over the sauce. Sprinkle with half the vegetarian sausage. Repeat the layers. Top with the remaining noodles, remaining sauce, 1/8 teaspoon salt, and mozzarella.

Bake, covered, for 40 minutes, or until the mozzarella melts. Let stand, uncovered, on a cooling rack for 10 minutes. Sprinkle with the remaining 1/4 teaspoon salt, then the Parmesan.

three-cheese vegetable strudel

SERVES 4

Vegetables are cooked quickly in a skillet, seasoned and combined with beans, rolled with wafer-thin layers of phyllo dough, and baked. With dinner all wrapped up, you may even have time to prepare a healthy dessert (pages 564–639).

1 teaspoon olive oil	1 cup fat-free ricotta cheese
1 1-pound package frozen mixed vegetables (any combination)	1 cup shredded low-fat mozzarella cheese
¼ cup coarsely chopped fresh basil	¼ cup shredded or grated Romano cheese
2 tablespoons snipped fresh dillweed	
¼ teaspoon salt-free lemon pepper	6 14 x 18-inch sheets frozen phyllo dough, thawed
1 15.5-ounce can no-salt-added navy beans, rinsed and drained	Cooking spray

In a large nonstick skillet, heat the oil over medium-high heat, swirling to coat the bottom. Cook the vegetables for 8 to 10 minutes, or until tender and heated through, stirring occasionally. (If there is excess liquid in the pan, increase the heat to high. Leaving the vegetables in the pan, cook for 2 to 3 minutes, or until the liquid has almost evaporated, stirring occasionally.) Remove from the heat.

Stir in the basil, dillweed, and lemon pepper. Let cool for 5 minutes.

In a medium bowl, stir together the beans, ricotta, mozzarella, and Romano cheese. Stir in the vegetable mixture. Set aside.

Preheat the oven to 350°F.

Place one sheet of phyllo dough on a cutting board. Lightly spray the top with cooking spray. Place another sheet of phyllo on top. Lightly spray with cooking spray. Repeat with a third sheet of phyllo. Leaving a 2-inch border along one wide end of the phyllo, spoon half the filling along that end. Fold the edge closest to the filling over the filling. Fold the short ends slightly toward the center and roll up from the wide end to enclose the filling. Place the strudel with the seam side down on a large nonstick baking sheet. Repeat with the remaining phyllo and filling, placing the second strudel about 2 inches from the first.

PER SERVING

CALORIES 388
TOTAL FAT 6.0 g
  Saturated Fat 1.5 g
  Trans Fat 0.0 g
  Polyunsaturated Fat 0.5 g
  Monounsaturated Fat 2.0 g
CHOLESTEROL 18 mg
SODIUM 523 mg
CARBOHYDRATES 57 g
  Fiber 9 g
  Sugars 11 g
PROTEIN 27 g
DIETARY EXCHANGES
  3½ starch, 1 vegetable,
  2½ very lean meat

Lightly spray the tops and sides of the strudels with cooking spray. Cut diagonal slits in the tops about 2 inches apart and about ½ inch deep.

Bake for 30 to 35 minutes, or until the crust is golden brown and the filling is heated through. Transfer the baking sheet to a cooling rack. Let the strudel cool for 10 minutes before cutting each in half.

tomato quiche in couscous crust

SERVES 4

Serve a wedge of this dill-flavored quiche with fresh strawberries.

Cooking spray

CRUST

½ cup low-sodium vegetable broth, such as on page 44

½ cup water

½ cup uncooked whole-wheat couscous

⅛ teaspoon ground turmeric

1 medium egg white

FILLING

1 teaspoon olive oil

4 ounces button mushrooms, chopped

6 medium green onions, chopped

2 medium garlic cloves, minced

6 medium Italian plum (Roma) tomatoes, thickly sliced

2 tablespoons shredded or grated Parmesan cheese

¾ cup egg substitute

1 5-ounce can fat-free evaporated milk

1 tablespoon fresh dillweed or 1 teaspoon dried, crumbled

¼ teaspoon pepper

Preheat the oven to 400°F. Lightly spray a 9-inch pie pan with cooking spray.

In a medium saucepan, bring the broth and water to a boil over medium-high heat. Stir in the couscous and turmeric. Remove from the heat. Let stand, covered, for 5 minutes.

Stir the egg white into the couscous. Form a crust by pressing the mixture on the bottom and up the side of the pie pan.

Bake for 10 minutes. Remove the crust from the oven. Let cool completely, about 30 minutes.

After the crust has been removed, reduce the oven temperature to 350°F.

In a medium nonstick skillet, heat the oil over medium-high heat, swirling to coat the bottom. Cook the mushrooms, green onions, and garlic for 2 to 3 minutes, or until tender.

Arrange the tomato slices on the crust, cover with the mushroom mixture, and sprinkle with the Parmesan.

In a medium bowl, whisk together the remaining ingredients. Pour over the vegetables.

Bake for 40 to 45 minutes, or until a knife inserted in the center comes out clean.

PER SERVING

CALORIES 224
TOTAL FAT 2.5 g
  Saturated Fat 0.5 g
  Trans Fat 0.0 g
  Polyunsaturated Fat 0.5 g
  Monounsaturated Fat 1.0 g
CHOLESTEROL 3 mg
SODIUM 212 mg
CARBOHYDRATES 36 g
  Fiber 7 g
  Sugars 10 g
PROTEIN 15 g
DIETARY EXCHANGES
  2 starch, 1 vegetable,
  1 very lean meat

spinach soufflé

SERVES 4

Complement this airy soufflé with brilliantly colored Harvard Beets (page 427) and crunchy corn on the cob.

Cooking spray
2 tablespoons canola or corn oil
2 tablespoons whole-wheat flour
½ cup fat-free milk
1 10-ounce package frozen chopped spinach, cooked, drained, and squeezed dry

2 tablespoons finely chopped onion
¼ heaping teaspoon ground nutmeg
¼ heaping teaspoon pepper, or to taste
6 medium egg whites
3 tablespoons shredded or grated Parmesan cheese

Preheat the oven to 350°F. Lightly spray a 1¾-quart casserole dish with cooking spray. Set aside.

In a small, heavy saucepan, heat the oil over medium-high heat, swirling to coat the bottom. Whisk in the flour. Cook for 1 minute, or until the mixture is smooth and bubbly, whisking constantly. Remove from the heat.

Gradually whisk in the milk. Return to the heat and cook for 1 minute, whisking constantly. Remove from the heat.

In a large bowl, stir together the spinach, onion, nutmeg, and pepper. Stir in the milk mixture.

In a large mixing bowl, beat the egg whites until stiff peaks form. Using a rubber scraper, fold gently into the spinach mixture. Gently transfer to the casserole dish. Sprinkle with the Parmesan.

Bake for 35 minutes, or until the center is set (doesn't jiggle when the casserole is gently shaken). Serve immediately.

PER SERVING

CALORIES 144
TOTAL FAT 8.5 g
    Saturated Fat 1.5 g
    Trans Fat 0.0 g
    Polyunsaturated Fat 2.0 g
    Monounsaturated Fat 5.0 g
CHOLESTEROL 4 mg
SODIUM 198 mg
CARBOHYDRATES 8 g
    Fiber 3 g
    Sugars 3 g
PROTEIN 10 g
DIETARY EXCHANGES
    ½ carbohydrate,
    1 lean meat, 1 fat

farmstand frittata

SERVES 4

Frittatas are an Italian creation—basically an omelet that's not folded. Veggies, low-fat cheese, and seasonings are whisked into the egg substitute base to make a satisfying meal.

1½ cups egg substitute
½ cup shredded low-fat mozzarella cheese
2 tablespoons fat-free half-and-half
2 medium garlic cloves, finely chopped
½ teaspoon dried Italian seasoning, crumbled
¼ teaspoon crushed red pepper flakes
1 medium red bell pepper, chopped

½ cup chopped onion
Cooking spray
1 6-ounce zucchini, halved lengthwise, then cut crosswise into ¼-inch slices
1 teaspoon olive oil
1 tablespoon shredded or grated Parmesan cheese
Pepper or crushed red pepper flakes to taste (optional)

Preheat the oven to 350°F.

In a medium bowl, whisk together the egg substitute, mozzarella, half-and-half, garlic, Italian seasoning, and ¼ teaspoon crushed red pepper flakes. Set aside.

Select a 10-inch nonstick skillet with an oven-safe handle or wrap the handle in aluminum foil. Heat the skillet over medium-high heat for 2 minutes. Remove the skillet from the burner, leaving the heat on. Spread the bell pepper and onion in the skillet. Lightly spray the mixture with cooking spray. Cook for 3 minutes, or until just beginning to soften, stirring frequently.

Reduce the heat to medium. Stir in the zucchini. Cook for 4 minutes, or until the zucchini begins to soften and the onion begins to turn golden, stirring frequently.

Reduce the heat to low. Stir in the oil. Spread the mixture in the skillet.

Whisk the egg substitute mixture to recombine. Pour over the bell pepper mixture. Cook for 1 to 2 minutes, or until partially set, lifting the edge of the frittata with a spatula and tilting the skillet so the uncooked portion flows under the edge.

PER SERVING

CALORIES 119
TOTAL FAT 3.0 g
  Saturated Fat 1.0 g
  Trans Fat 0.0 g
  Polyunsaturated Fat 0.0 g
  Monounsaturated Fat 1.5 g
CHOLESTEROL 6 mg
SODIUM 324 mg
CARBOHYDRATES 9 g
  Fiber 2 g
  Sugars 5 g
PROTEIN 15 g
DIETARY EXCHANGES
  2 vegetable, 2 lean meat

Transfer the skillet to the oven and bake for 5 minutes. Remove from the oven and gently lift the edge of the frittata to allow a little of the uncooked mixture to flow underneath. Bake for 7 to 8 minutes, or until firm, puffy, and golden. Serve sprinkled with the Parmesan and pepper.

portobello mushroom wrap with yogurt curry sauce

SERVES 8

Enhanced by a creamy, curry-flavored sauce, this wrap features tomato, cheese, asparagus, rice, and grilled portobellos as its main attractions.

YOGURT CURRY SAUCE
- 8 ounces fat-free plain yogurt
- 2 teaspoons fresh lemon juice
- 1 teaspoon sugar
- 1 teaspoon curry powder

- 2 tablespoons balsamic vinegar
- 1 tablespoon olive oil
- 2 medium garlic cloves, minced
- 2 medium portobello mushrooms, each cut into 8 slices
- ½ cup uncooked instant brown rice

- 2 medium green onions, thinly sliced
- ¼ cup shredded fat-free mozzarella cheese
- 1 medium Italian plum (Roma) tomato, diced
- 1 teaspoon light brown sugar
- 1 teaspoon plain rice vinegar
- 8 6-inch fat-free flour tortillas (lowest sodium available)
- 16 medium asparagus spears, trimmed and cooked until tender-crisp

In a small bowl, stir together the sauce ingredients. Cover and refrigerate for 30 minutes to two days.

In a shallow glass dish, stir together the balsamic vinegar, oil, and garlic. Add the mushrooms, turning to coat. Cover and refrigerate for 10 to 15 minutes.

Meanwhile, prepare the rice using the package directions, omitting the salt and margarine.

Preheat the grill on medium high.

In a medium bowl, stir together the rice, green onions, mozzarella, tomato, brown sugar, and rice vinegar.

Discard the marinade, leaving what clings to the mushrooms.

Grill the mushrooms for 1 to 2 minutes on each side, or until tender.

Put a tortilla on a microwaveable plate. Put 2 mushroom slices in the center of the tortilla. Top with 2 asparagus spears and ¼ cup rice mixture. Microwave on 100 percent power (high) for 30 seconds. Roll the tortilla jelly-roll style. Repeat with the remaining ingredients. Serve with the sauce.

PER SERVING

CALORIES 168
TOTAL FAT 2.0 g
  Saturated Fat 0.5 g
  Trans Fat 0.0 g
  Polyunsaturated Fat 0.5 g
  Monounsaturated Fat 1.5 g
CHOLESTEROL 1 mg
SODIUM 313 mg
CARBOHYDRATES 31 g
  Fiber 3 g
  Sugars 6 g
PROTEIN 7 g
DIETARY EXCHANGES
  2 starch

open-face swiss cheese, spinach, and tomato sandwiches

SERVES 4

Cheese sandwiches don't need to be boring! Reinvent them with fresh veggies, fat slices of crusty bread, and a different look.

8 ½-inch-thick slices whole-grain Italian bread from a 4½ x 2½-inch loaf (lowest sodium available), lightly toasted
4 1-ounce slices low-fat Swiss cheese, halved
2 teaspoons olive oil (extra virgin preferred)

1 teaspoon red wine vinegar
⅛ teaspoon salt
  Pinch of pepper
2 medium tomatoes, each cut into 8 slices
2 ounces baby spinach or thinly sliced regular spinach

Preheat the oven to 350°F.

Put the bread slices on a baking sheet. Place the cheese slices on the bread.

Bake for 5 minutes, or until the cheese melts.

Meanwhile, in a medium bowl, whisk together the oil, vinegar, salt, and pepper. Dip each tomato slice in the mixture, turning to coat. Let any excess oil drip back into the bowl. Transfer the tomatoes to a plate.

Add the spinach to the remaining oil mixture, tossing to coat. Arrange the spinach over the cheese. Top with the tomato. Serve immediately for the best texture.

COOK'S TIP

Any favorite low-fat cheese will work in this easy combination. Remember, however, that softer cheeses, such as brie and goat cheese, tend to be high in saturated fat.

PER SERVING

CALORIES 235
TOTAL FAT 6.5 g
  Saturated Fat 2.0 g
  Trans Fat 0.0 g
  Polyunsaturated Fat 1.5 g
  Monounsaturated Fat 2.5 g
CHOLESTEROL 10 mg
SODIUM 399 mg
CARBOHYDRATES 29 g
  Fiber 5 g
  Sugars 6 g
PROTEIN 17 g
DIETARY EXCHANGES
  2 starch, 1 very lean meat, 1 fat

vegetables and side dishes

Artichoke Hearts Riviera

Asparagus with Lemon and Capers

Asparagus with Garlic and Parmesan Bread Crumbs

Mixed Squash with Garlic and Lemon Bread Crumbs

Barley, Squash, and Bell Pepper Medley

Braised Barley and Corn with Tomatoes

Edamame with Walnuts

Fresh Green Beans with Water Chestnuts

French-Style Green Beans with Pimiento and Dill Seeds

Green Beans and Rice with Hazelnuts

Louisiana Beans Oregano

Baked Beans

Mediterranean Lima Beans

Roasted Beets

Harvard Beets

Stir-Fried Bok Choy with Green Onion Sauce

Broccoli with Plum Sauce

Pecan Broccoli

Crunchy Broccoli Casserole

Roasted Brussels Sprouts

Brussels Sprouts and Pecans

Apricot Bulgur with Pine Nuts

Cabbage with Mustard-Caraway Sauce

Spiced Red Cabbage

Honeyed Carrots

Tangy Carrots

Baked Grated Carrots with Sherry

Baked Cauliflower and Carrots with Nutmeg

Cauliflower and Roasted Corn with Chili Powder and Lime

Creole Celery and Peas

Roasted Chayote Squash

Grilled Corn on the Cob

Southwestern Creamy Corn

Couscous with Raisins and Almonds

Couscous with Vegetables

Grits Casserole with Cheese and Chiles

Kale Crisps

Mushrooms with Red Wine

Mushrooms with White Wine and Shallots

Baked Okra Bites

Parmesan Parsnip Puree with Leeks and Carrots

Asian Linguine

Oven-Fried Onion Rings

Black-Eyed Peas with Canadian Bacon

French Peas

Sweet Lemon Snow Peas

Stir-Fried Sugar Snap Peas

Basil Roasted Peppers

Scalloped Potatoes

Mashed Potatoes with Parmesan and Green Onions

Baked Fries with Creole Seasoning

Rustic Potato Patties

Baked Sweet Potato Chips

Orange Sweet Potatoes

Lemon-Basil Rice

Risotto Milanese

Risotto with Broccoli and Leeks

Middle Eastern Brown Rice

Mexican Fried Rice

Asian Spinach and Mushrooms

Spinach and Brown Rice Casserole

Acorn Squash Stuffed with Cranberries and Walnuts

Butternut Mash

Maple-Glazed Butternut Squash

Pattypan Squash with Apple-Nut Stuffing

Yellow Summer Squash Casserole

Scalloped Squash

Sautéed Red Swiss Chard

Italian Vegetable Bake

Roasted Veggies with Sesame Seeds

Vegetable Stir-Fry

Southwestern Ratatouille

Apple Dressing

Dressing with Mixed Dried Fruits

Cranberry Chutney

Baked Curried Fruit

Baked Pears with Honey Almonds

Microwave Baked Apple Slices

Grilled Pineapple

artichoke hearts riviera

SERVES 6

This elegant side dish is ready in minutes. You can prepare the sauce while the artichoke hearts cook.

2 9-ounce packages frozen artichoke hearts

SAUCE
½ cup dry white wine (regular or nonalcoholic)
2 tablespoons light tub margarine
1 tablespoon snipped fresh parsley

1 tablespoon fresh lemon juice
1 medium garlic clove, crushed
½ teaspoon dry mustard
½ teaspoon dried tarragon, crumbled
Pepper to taste (white preferred)

——

Snipped fresh parsley (optional)

Prepare the artichoke hearts using the package directions, omitting the salt and margarine. Drain well in a colander. Transfer to a serving bowl.

Meanwhile, in a small saucepan, stir together the sauce ingredients. Bring to a boil over medium-high heat. Reduce the heat and simmer, covered, for 5 minutes.

Pour the sauce over the artichoke hearts. Sprinkle with the remaining parsley.

PER SERVING

CALORIES 71
TOTAL FAT 1.5 g
　Saturated Fat 0.0 g
　Trans Fat 0.0 g
　Polyunsaturated Fat 0.5 g
　Monounsaturated Fat 1.0 g
CHOLESTEROL 0 mg
SODIUM 77 mg
CARBOHYDRATES 9 g
　Fiber 6 g
　Sugars 1 g
PROTEIN 2 g
DIETARY EXCHANGES
　2 vegetable, ½ fat

asparagus with lemon and capers

SERVES 4

Lemon and capers turn fresh asparagus into a Mediterranean culinary delight.

½ cup water
1 pound medium asparagus spears, trimmed
1 tablespoon olive oil (extra virgin preferred)

1 tablespoon capers, drained
½ teaspoon grated lemon zest
2 teaspoons fresh lemon juice
¼ teaspoon pepper

In a large skillet, bring the water to a boil over medium-high heat. Add the asparagus. Reduce the heat and simmer, covered, for 3 to 5 minutes, or just until tender. Drain, discarding the water and leaving the asparagus in the skillet.

Gently stir the remaining ingredients into the asparagus.

COOK'S TIP on asparagus

Try to use crisp asparagus spears that are about as big around as your little finger. If the spears are thicker and tougher than you'd like, use a vegetable peeler to remove the outer layer.

PER SERVING

CALORIES 54
TOTAL FAT 3.5 g
   Saturated Fat 0.5 g
   Trans Fat 0.0 g
   Polyunsaturated Fat 0.5 g
   Monounsaturated Fat 2.5 g
CHOLESTEROL 0 mg
SODIUM 66 mg
CARBOHYDRATES 5 g
   Fiber 3 g
   Sugars 2 g
PROTEIN 3 g
DIETARY EXCHANGES
   1 vegetable, ½ fat

asparagus with garlic and parmesan bread crumbs

SERVES 6

Seasoned bread crumbs blanket steamed asparagus spears in this easy side dish.

BREAD CRUMBS
- 2 slices whole-grain bread (lowest sodium available), torn into 1-inch pieces
- 1 tablespoon light tub margarine
- 2 medium garlic cloves, minced
- 1½ teaspoons dried oregano, crumbled

- 2 tablespoons shredded or grated Parmesan cheese

- 1¼ pounds medium asparagus spears, trimmed
- ⅛ teaspoon salt
- Fat-free spray margarine

Put the bread in a food processor or blender and pulse until the texture of commercial bread crumbs.

In a large nonstick skillet, melt the margarine over medium-high heat, swirling to coat the bottom. Cook the garlic for 10 seconds, stirring constantly.

Stir in the bread crumbs and oregano. Cook for 5 minutes, or until the crumbs are golden brown, stirring frequently. Remove from the heat.

Stir in the Parmesan.

Meanwhile, in a medium saucepan, steam the asparagus for 3 minutes, or until just tender-crisp.

Arrange the asparagus on a platter. Sprinkle with the salt. Lightly spray with the spray margarine. Top with the bread crumb mixture.

MIXED SQUASH WITH GARLIC AND LEMON BREAD CRUMBS

Substitute 2 medium yellow summer squash, thinly sliced, and 2 medium zucchini, thinly sliced, for the asparagus, and 1 tablespoon grated lemon zest for the Parmesan cheese.

PER SERVING

CALORIES 58
TOTAL FAT 1.5 g
  Saturated Fat 0.5 g
  Trans Fat 0.0 g
  Polyunsaturated Fat 0.5 g
  Monounsaturated Fat 0.5 g
CHOLESTEROL 1 mg
SODIUM 130 mg
CARBOHYDRATES 8 g
  Fiber 3 g
  Sugars 2 g
PROTEIN 4 g
DIETARY EXCHANGES
  ½ starch

PER SERVING

MIXED SQUASH WITH GARLIC AND LEMON BREAD CRUMBS
CALORIES 54
TOTAL FAT 1.5 g
  Saturated Fat 0.0 g
  Trans Fat 0.0 g
  Polyunsaturated Fat 0.5 g
  Monounsaturated Fat 0.5 g
CHOLESTEROL 0 mg
SODIUM 108 mg
CARBOHYDRATES 9 g
  Fiber 2 g
  Sugars 3 g
PROTEIN 3 g
DIETARY EXCHANGES
  ½ starch

barley, squash, and bell pepper medley

SERVES 4

When you combine whole grains and colorful veggies, as in this dish, you can dress up even the simplest entrée.

½ cup uncooked quick-cooking barley
1 teaspoon olive oil and 2 teaspoons olive oil (extra virgin preferred), divided use
1 medium yellow summer squash or zucchini, chopped
½ medium green or red bell pepper, thinly sliced lengthwise, then sliced crosswise into 2-inch pieces

½ teaspoon dried thyme, crumbled
⅛ teaspoon crushed red pepper flakes
⅛ teaspoon pepper (coarsely ground preferred)
2 tablespoons snipped fresh parsley or basil
¼ teaspoon salt

Prepare the barley using the package directions, omitting the salt and oil. Drain well in a colander.

Meanwhile, in a large nonstick skillet, heat 1 teaspoon oil over medium heat, swirling to coat the bottom. Add the squash, bell pepper, thyme, red pepper flakes, and pepper, stirring to combine. Cook for 5 minutes, or until the squash begins to brown on the edges, stirring frequently. Remove from the heat.

Stir the barley, parsley, salt, and remaining 2 teaspoons oil into the squash mixture.

PER SERVING

CALORIES 130
TOTAL FAT 4.0 g
  Saturated Fat 0.5 g
  Trans Fat 0.0 g
  Polyunsaturated Fat 0.5 g
  Monounsaturated Fat 2.5 g
CHOLESTEROL 0 mg
SODIUM 150 mg
CARBOHYDRATES 22 g
  Fiber 5 g
  Sugars 2 g
PROTEIN 3 g
DIETARY EXCHANGES
  1½ starch, ½ fat

braised barley and corn with tomatoes

SERVES 4

Chase the winter blues away with this side dish of plump kernels of corn and barley stewed with tomatoes.

1 teaspoon olive oil
¼ medium onion, chopped
1 cup fat-free, low-sodium chicken broth, such as on page 43
½ 14.5-ounce can no-salt-added diced tomatoes, undrained
½ teaspoon salt-free all-purpose seasoning blend
⅛ teaspoon pepper
⅛ teaspoon crushed red pepper flakes (optional)
¼ cup uncooked pearl barley
1 cup frozen whole-kernel corn

In a medium saucepan, heat the oil over medium-high heat, swirling to coat the bottom. Cook the onion for about 3 minutes, or until soft, stirring occasionally.

Stir in the broth, tomatoes with liquid, seasoning blend, pepper, and red pepper flakes. Bring to a simmer, stirring occasionally.

Stir in the barley. Reduce the heat and simmer, covered, for 30 minutes.

Stir in the corn. Simmer, covered, for 15 to 20 minutes, or until the barley is tender and the corn is heated through.

edamame with walnuts

SERVES 6

This delicious and nutritious side dish will become one of your go-to recipes. It's quick, it complements almost any entrée, and the ingredients are easy to keep on hand.

1 tablespoon olive oil	¼ cup panko (Japanese bread crumbs)
16 ounces frozen shelled edamame (green soybeans)	¼ cup chopped walnuts
	¼ teaspoon pepper
3 medium garlic cloves, minced	⅛ teaspoon salt

In a large skillet, heat the oil over medium heat, swirling to coat the bottom. Cook the edamame and garlic for 8 to 10 minutes, or just until tender, stirring occasionally.

Stir in the panko and walnuts. Cook for 3 to 4 minutes, or until the crumbs are golden, stirring occasionally.

Stir in the pepper and salt.

PER SERVING

CALORIES 152
TOTAL FAT 8.5 g
   Saturated Fat 0.5 g
   Trans Fat 0.0 g
   Polyunsaturated Fat 2.5 g
   Monounsaturated Fat 2.0 g
CHOLESTEROL 0 mg
SODIUM 57 mg
CARBOHYDRATES 9 g
   Fiber 4 g
   Sugars 3 g
PROTEIN 10 g
DIETARY EXCHANGES
   ½ starch, 1½ lean meat, 1 fat

fresh green beans
with water chestnuts

SERVES 6

Wondering what to serve with an Asian entrée besides steamed rice? Here's your answer.

1½ pounds fresh green beans, trimmed and cut diagonally into 1½-inch pieces	1 8-ounce can sliced water chestnuts, drained
1½ teaspoons canola or corn oil	1 tablespoon sesame seeds, dry-roasted
1 teaspoon hot-pepper oil	¼ teaspoon salt

In a large saucepan over high heat, bring to a boil enough water to cover the beans. Add the beans and boil for 4 minutes. With a large slotted spoon, remove the beans from the pan. Plunge them into a bowl of ice water to stop the cooking process. Drain well in a colander.

In a large skillet, heat the oils over high heat, swirling to coat the bottom. Cook the water chestnuts for 1 minute, stirring constantly.

Stir in the beans, sesame seeds, and salt. Cook until heated through, stirring constantly.

COOK'S TIP on water chestnuts

Grown in water and frequently used in Chinese cooking, water chestnuts are the underground stems of a marsh plant. Fresh and unpeeled, they do resemble chestnuts. You can find the fresh ones in Chinese markets. Peel them and use either raw or cooked to add crunch to salads and stir-fry dishes. Water chestnuts are also available whole or sliced in cans.

PER SERVING

CALORIES 74
TOTAL FAT 3.0 g
  Saturated Fat 0.5 g
  Trans Fat 0.0 g
  Polyunsaturated Fat 1.0 g
  Monounsaturated Fat 1.5 g
CHOLESTEROL 0 mg
SODIUM 107 mg
CARBOHYDRATES 11 g
  Fiber 5 g
  Sugars 2 g
PROTEIN 3 g
DIETARY EXCHANGES
  ½ starch, ½ fat

french-style green beans with pimiento and dill seeds

SERVES 4

A touch of cider vinegar and dill seeds, plus a trio of chopped vegetables, adds sparkle to this side dish.

1 tablespoon light tub margarine
1 tablespoon water
1 9-ounce package frozen French-style green beans
1 medium rib of celery, finely chopped
¼ cup finely chopped onion

2 tablespoons chopped pimiento, drained
1 tablespoon cider vinegar
¼ teaspoon dill seeds
Pepper to taste

In a medium saucepan, heat the margarine and water over medium heat until the margarine melts, swirling to coat the bottom.

Add the beans. Cook for 1 to 2 minutes, separating them with a fork. Reduce the heat to low. Cook, covered, for 5 to 6 minutes, or until tender-crisp.

Stir in the remaining ingredients. Cook for 2 to 3 minutes, or until heated through. (The celery and onion should remain crisp.)

PER SERVING

CALORIES 41
TOTAL FAT 1.0 g
  Saturated Fat 0.0 g
  Trans Fat 0.0 g
  Polyunsaturated Fat 0.5 g
  Monounsaturated Fat 0.5 g
CHOLESTEROL 0 mg
SODIUM 32 mg
CARBOHYDRATES 6 g
  Fiber 2 g
  Sugars 2 g
PROTEIN 1 g
DIETARY EXCHANGES
  1 vegetable

green beans and rice with hazelnuts

SERVES 8

Green onions and lemon enhance fluffy rice and green beans. Chopped hazelnuts and roasted red bell pepper provide the crowning touch.

½ cup uncooked instant brown rice
1 9-ounce package frozen French-style green beans
1½ tablespoons light tub margarine
3 tablespoons sliced green onions
½ to 1 teaspoon fresh lemon juice
½ teaspoon salt

Pepper to taste
¼ cup chopped or sliced hazelnuts, dry-roasted
¼ cup chopped roasted red bell peppers, rinsed and drained if bottled

Prepare the rice using the package directions, omitting the salt and margarine.

Meanwhile, prepare the green beans using the package directions, omitting the salt and margarine. Drain well in a colander.

In a large saucepan, melt the margarine over medium heat, swirling to coat the bottom. Stir in the beans, rice, green onions, lemon juice, salt, and pepper. Cook until heated through, stirring occasionally. Serve sprinkled with the hazelnuts and chopped bell pepper.

COOK'S TIP on hazelnuts

Traditionally used in many European dishes, hazelnuts, or filberts, have a bitter brown skin that you'll want to remove. Put the nuts in a single layer on a baking pan and dry-roast in a preheated 350°F oven for about 10 minutes. Let them cool for 1 to 2 minutes. While the hazelnuts are still warm, put a handful in a dish towel and rub to remove the skins.

PER SERVING

CALORIES 65
TOTAL FAT 3.0 g
  Saturated Fat 0.0 g
  Trans Fat 0.0 g
  Polyunsaturated Fat 0.5 g
  Monounsaturated Fat 2.0 g
CHOLESTEROL 0 mg
SODIUM 165 mg
CARBOHYDRATES 7 g
  Fiber 2 g
  Sugars 1 g
PROTEIN 2 g
DIETARY EXCHANGES
  ½ starch, ½ fat

louisiana beans oregano

SERVES 4

Try these green beans with blackened redfish or roast chicken.

1½ medium tomatoes, diced
1 medium rib of celery, diced
¼ medium green bell pepper, diced
2 tablespoons chopped onion
⅓ cup water
½ teaspoon garlic powder

½ teaspoon onion powder
½ teaspoon dried oregano, crumbled
⅛ teaspoon pepper (white preferred)
⅛ teaspoon salt
1 9-ounce package frozen green beans (Italian preferred)

In a medium saucepan, stir together all the ingredients except the green beans. Bring to a boil over high heat. Reduce the heat and simmer, covered, for 10 minutes.

Increase the heat to medium. Add the beans, separating them with a fork. Cook, uncovered, for 5 to 8 minutes, or until the beans are tender-crisp, stirring occasionally.

baked beans

SERVES 6

When it's time for a picnic or a potluck supper, try this low-sodium take on a classic side dish.

Cooking spray
2 15.5-ounce cans no-salt-added navy beans, rinsed and drained
¼ cup minced onion
3 tablespoons light molasses

3 tablespoons no-salt-added ketchup
1 tablespoon Dijon mustard
¼ teaspoon pepper
2 slices turkey bacon, each cut into thirds

Preheat the oven to 375°F. Lightly spray a 2-quart glass baking dish with cooking spray.

In a medium bowl, gently stir together the ingredients except the turkey bacon, keeping the beans intact. Pour into the baking dish. Place the turkey bacon on top.

Bake, covered, for 30 minutes. Bake, uncovered, for 30 minutes.

mediterranean lima beans

SERVES 4

Many ingredients typical of Mediterranean cooking—garlic, tomatoes, onion, and mint—flavor this dish.

1 10-ounce package frozen lima beans
1 teaspoon light tub margarine
¼ cup chopped onion
1 medium garlic clove, crushed

1 cup canned no-salt-added
   tomatoes, undrained
½ teaspoon dried mint, crumbled

Prepare the lima beans using the package directions, omitting the salt and margarine. Drain well in a colander.

In a medium skillet, melt the margarine over medium-high heat, swirling to coat the bottom. Cook the onion and garlic for about 3 minutes, or until the onion is soft, stirring frequently.

Stir in the lima beans, tomatoes with liquid, and mint. Heat through.

PER SERVING

CALORIES 98
TOTAL FAT 0.5 g
    Saturated Fat 0.0 g
    Trans Fat 0.0 g
    Polyunsaturated Fat 0.0 g
    Monounsaturated Fat 0.0 g
CHOLESTEROL 0 mg
SODIUM 137 mg
CARBOHYDRATES 18 g
    Fiber 4 g
    Sugars 3 g
PROTEIN 4 g
DIETARY EXCHANGES
    1 starch

roasted beets

SERVES 4

Roasting beets really intensifies their natural sweetness, which is complemented in this dish with a few simple seasonings.

2 pounds fresh beets, stems trimmed to about 1 inch, beets peeled and cut into ½-inch cubes
2 medium shallots, coarsely chopped
1 tablespoon olive oil

½ teaspoon dried thyme or Italian seasoning, crumbled
¼ teaspoon pepper
⅛ teaspoon salt

Preheat the oven to 400°F.

Put the beets and shallots in a single layer on a large rimmed baking sheet. Drizzle with the oil. Stir to coat.

Sprinkle with the thyme, pepper, and salt.

Roast for 35 to 45 minutes, or until the beets are tender and the edges just start to brown and caramelize, stirring once halfway through.

COOK'S TIP on fresh beets

Working with fresh beets while they are raw isn't as messy as working with them after they've been cooked. It will take only a couple of soapings to remove the stains from your fingers after you've cut the raw beets.

PER SERVING

CALORIES 101
TOTAL FAT 3.5 g
  Saturated Fat 0.5 g
  Trans Fat 0.0 g
  Polyunsaturated Fat 0.5 g
  Monounsaturated Fat 2.5 g
CHOLESTEROL 0 mg
SODIUM 192 mg
CARBOHYDRATES 16 g
  Fiber 4 g
  Sugars 11 g
PROTEIN 3 g
DIETARY EXCHANGES
  3 vegetable, ½ fat

harvard beets

SERVES 4

Vibrant reddish-purple beets in a sweet-and-sour sauce is a classic. Try this version with lean pork or chicken and add your favorite green vegetable on the side.

2 pounds fresh beets, stems trimmed to 1 to 2 inches, root ends left uncut, or 2 15-ounce cans no-salt-added beets, drained and diced

SAUCE
⅓ cup fresh orange juice
½ teaspoon grated lemon zest
2 tablespoons fresh lemon juice
2 tablespoons cider vinegar
1½ tablespoons sugar
1 teaspoon cornstarch
⅛ teaspoon garlic powder
⅛ teaspoon salt

If using fresh beets, put them in a large saucepan. Cover with water. Bring to a boil over medium-high heat. Reduce the heat and simmer, covered, for 30 to 40 minutes, or until a knife easily pierces the beets. Drain well in a colander. Let cool slightly. Wearing disposable plastic gloves (to keep from staining your fingers), slip the skins off. Dice the beets.

In a large saucepan, whisk together the sauce ingredients. Bring to a boil over medium-high heat. Cook for 3 to 5 minutes, or until thickened, whisking occasionally.

Stir in the beets. Cook for 2 minutes, or until heated through.

PER SERVING

CALORIES 100
TOTAL FAT 0.5 g
    Saturated Fat 0.0 g
    Trans Fat 0.0 g
    Polyunsaturated Fat 0.0 g
    Monounsaturated Fat 0.0 g
CHOLESTEROL 0 mg
SODIUM 192 mg
CARBOHYDRATES 23 g
    Fiber 4 g
    Sugars 17 g
PROTEIN 3 g
DIETARY EXCHANGES
    3 vegetable,
    ½ carbohydrate

stir-fried bok choy with green onion sauce

SERVES 8

Vitamin-rich bok choy is cooked quickly, then stirred together with an Asian-influenced pestolike sauce. This side dish is great with grilled steak or lean pork loin chops.

GREEN ONION SAUCE
- 4 medium green onions, thinly sliced
- ¼ cup fat-free, low-sodium chicken broth, such as on page 43
- 2 tablespoons snipped fresh cilantro or parsley
- 1 tablespoon slivered almonds
- 1 teaspoon toasted sesame oil
- 1 teaspoon soy sauce (lowest sodium available)

- ½ teaspoon cornstarch
- ½ teaspoon red chili paste (optional)

- 1 teaspoon canola or corn oil
- 8 medium stalks of bok choy (green and white parts), cut into 1-inch pieces

In a food processor or blender, process the sauce ingredients for 10 to 15 seconds, or until almost smooth.

In a large nonstick skillet, heat the oil over medium-high heat, swirling to coat the bottom. Cook the bok choy for 2 to 3 minutes, or until tender-crisp, stirring constantly.

Stir in the sauce. Cook for 1 to 2 minutes, or until the sauce is slightly thickened, stirring constantly.

PER SERVING

CALORIES 23
TOTAL FAT 1.5 g
  Saturated Fat 0.0 g
  Trans Fat 0.0 g
  Polyunsaturated Fat 0.5 g
  Monounsaturated Fat 1.0 g
CHOLESTEROL 0 mg
SODIUM 29 mg
CARBOHYDRATES 2 g
  Fiber 1 g
  Sugars 1 g
PROTEIN 1 g
DIETARY EXCHANGES
  ½ fat

broccoli with plum sauce

SERVES 4

Coriander seeds intensify the delightful lemonlike flavor of this side dish.

1 medium lemon, thinly sliced

1 1-inch piece unpeeled gingerroot, thinly sliced

8 ounces broccoli florets

½ teaspoon coriander seeds, crushed

2 tablespoons Chinese plum sauce

1 teaspoon soy sauce (lowest sodium available)

½ teaspoon toasted sesame oil

2 teaspoons sesame seeds

In a medium saucepan, bring about ½ inch of water to a simmer over high heat. Add the lemon and gingerroot.

Put the broccoli in a steamer basket. Sprinkle with the coriander seeds. Put the steamer basket in the saucepan. Reduce the heat and simmer, covered, for 6 to 8 minutes, or until the broccoli is tender-crisp.

Meanwhile, in a medium bowl, stir together the plum sauce, soy sauce, and sesame oil.

Add the broccoli to the plum sauce mixture, stirring to coat. Sprinkle with the sesame seeds.

PER SERVING

CALORIES 47
TOTAL FAT 1.5 g
  Saturated Fat 0.0 g
  Trans Fat 0.0 g
  Polyunsaturated Fat 0.5 g
  Monounsaturated Fat 0.5 g
CHOLESTEROL 0 mg
SODIUM 96 mg
CARBOHYDRATES 7 g
  Fiber 2 g
  Sugars 3 g
PROTEIN 2 g
DIETARY EXCHANGES
  1 vegetable, ½ fat

pecan broccoli

SERVES 6

It takes only a few dry-roasted nuts to add a crunchy punch to vegetables, such as this citrusy broccoli.

1 pound fresh or frozen broccoli florets	2 tablespoons fresh orange juice
½ teaspoon grated orange zest	⅛ teaspoon salt
	¼ cup chopped pecans, dry-roasted

In a medium saucepan, steam the broccoli for 6 to 8 minutes, or until tender-crisp.

Meanwhile, in a medium bowl, stir together the orange zest, orange juice, and salt. Gently stir in the broccoli. Sprinkle with the pecans.

crunchy broccoli casserole

SERVES 8

Put this attractive casserole together early in the day, refrigerate, then bake just in time for dinner.

Cooking spray
1 bunch broccoli (about 1¾ pounds), any tough stems peeled, stems and florets cut into 4-inch pieces

SAUCE
2 tablespoons fat-free, low-sodium chicken broth and 2 cups fat-free, low-sodium chicken broth, such as on page 43, divided use
1 large onion, finely chopped
½ medium red bell pepper, diced
¼ cup all-purpose flour
1 cup fat-free milk

¼ cup shredded or grated Romano or Parmesan cheese
1 tablespoon finely chopped fresh basil or 1 teaspoon dried, crumbled
⅛ teaspoon salt
⅛ teaspoon ground nutmeg
⅛ teaspoon pepper (white preferred)

————

1 cup unseasoned croutons, coarsely crushed
2 tablespoons finely chopped walnuts, dry-roasted

Preheat the oven to 400°F. Lightly spray a 13 x 9 x 2-inch glass baking dish with cooking spray.

In a large saucepan, steam the broccoli for 4 minutes. Arrange in lengthwise rows in the baking dish. Set aside.

In a medium saucepan, heat 2 tablespoons broth over medium-high heat. Cook the onion and bell pepper for about 3 minutes, or until the onion is soft.

Put the flour in a small bowl. Pour in the milk, whisking to dissolve. Whisk the milk mixture and remaining 2 cups broth into the onion mixture. Reduce the heat to medium and cook until thickened, whisking constantly.

Whisk in the remaining sauce ingredients. Pour over the broccoli.

Sprinkle the croutons and walnuts over the broccoli and sauce.

Bake for 20 to 25 minutes, or until the sauce is bubbly.

PER SERVING

CALORIES 113
TOTAL FAT 2.5 g
  Saturated Fat 0.5 g
  Trans Fat 0.0 g
  Polyunsaturated Fat 1.0 g
  Monounsaturated Fat 0.5 g
CHOLESTEROL 2 mg
SODIUM 169 mg
CARBOHYDRATES 18 g
  Fiber 4 g
  Sugars 5 g
PROTEIN 7 g
DIETARY EXCHANGES
  1 starch, 1 vegetable,
  ½ fat

roasted brussels sprouts

SERVES 4

Roasting brussels sprouts really enhances their flavor—even sprouts-phobes will be convinced to change their minds!

Cooking spray
1 tablespoon olive oil
2 teaspoons balsamic vinegar
3 medium garlic cloves, minced
¼ teaspoon dried thyme, crumbled

⅛ teaspoon salt
⅛ teaspoon pepper
1 pound fresh brussels sprouts (about 16), trimmed, halved lengthwise, and loose outer leaves discarded

Preheat the oven to 400°F. Lightly spray a medium baking sheet with cooking spray.

In a medium bowl, stir together all the ingredients except the brussels sprouts. Add the brussels sprouts, stirring until coated. Place on the baking sheet in a single layer with the cut side up.

Roast for 15 to 20 minutes, or until browned on the outside and tender on the inside, turning over once halfway through the cooking time.

COOK'S TIP

Portions of the brussels sprouts may become very dark, appearing almost burned; actually those spots are caramelized, adding flavor. After making this dish a time or two, you may decide to cook the sprouts longer, until they are even darker and have crisper outside leaves.

PER SERVING

CALORIES 85
TOTAL FAT 3.5 g
  Saturated Fat 0.5 g
  Trans Fat 0.0 g
  Polyunsaturated Fat 0.5 g
  Monounsaturated Fat 2.5 g
CHOLESTEROL 0 mg
SODIUM 102 mg
CARBOHYDRATES 12 g
  Fiber 4 g
  Sugars 3 g
PROTEIN 4 g
DIETARY EXCHANGES
  2 vegetable, 1 fat

brussels sprouts and pecans

SERVES 8

In this change-of-pace dish, a creamy sauce envelops tender brussels sprouts.

Cooking spray

1½ pounds fresh brussels sprouts, trimmed and loose outer leaves discarded, or 2 10-ounce packages frozen brussels sprouts

SAUCE

1 cup fat-free, low-sodium chicken broth, such as on page 43

⅔ cup fat-free evaporated milk

¼ cup all-purpose flour

¼ teaspoon salt

⅛ teaspoon pepper

2 tablespoons chopped pecans, dry-roasted

2 teaspoons chopped fresh sage or ½ teaspoon dried

½ cup plain dry bread crumbs

Preheat the oven to 400°F. Lightly spray a 1½-quart casserole dish with cooking spray.

In a medium saucepan, steam the fresh brussels sprouts for 6 to 8 minutes, or until tender, uncovering briefly after 2 to 3 minutes to release the odor, or prepare the frozen sprouts using the package directions, omitting the salt and margarine. Transfer to the casserole dish.

In the same saucepan, whisk together the sauce ingredients except the pecans. Cook over medium-high heat for 3 to 4 minutes, or until the sauce comes to a boil and thickens, whisking occasionally. Remove from the heat.

Whisk the pecans into the sauce. Pour over the brussels sprouts. Sprinkle with the sage and bread crumbs. Lightly spray with cooking spray.

Bake for 10 minutes, or until the topping is lightly browned.

PER SERVING

CALORIES 107
TOTAL FAT 2.0 g
  Saturated Fat 0.5 g
  Trans Fat 0.0 g
  Polyunsaturated Fat 0.5 g
  Monounsaturated Fat 1.0 g
CHOLESTEROL 1 mg
SODIUM 171 mg
CARBOHYDRATES 18 g
  Fiber 4 g
  Sugars 5 g
PROTEIN 6 g
DIETARY EXCHANGES
  ½ starch, 2 vegetable,
  ½ fat

apricot bulgur with pine nuts

SERVES 4

The combination of a small amount of dry-roasted pine nuts and richly browned onion gives this dish an intensely nutty flavor.

½ cup uncooked quick-cooking bulgur
1 teaspoon canola or corn oil
½ medium onion, diced
5 or 6 dried apricot halves, thinly sliced

¼ cup pine nuts, dry-roasted
¼ teaspoon salt

Prepare the bulgur using the package directions, omitting the salt and oil.

Meanwhile, in a large nonstick skillet, heat the oil over medium heat, swirling to coat the bottom. Cook the onion for 6 minutes, or until very richly browned (this is important), stirring frequently. Remove from the heat.

Stir the bulgur, apricots, pine nuts, and salt into the onion. Cook for 1 to 2 minutes, or until heated through, stirring occasionally.

PER SERVING

CALORIES 126
TOTAL FAT 5.0 g
  Saturated Fat 0.5 g
  Trans Fat 0.0 g
  Polyunsaturated Fat 2.0 g
  Monounsaturated Fat 2.0 g
CHOLESTEROL 0 mg
SODIUM 150 mg
CARBOHYDRATES 19 g
  Fiber 4 g
  Sugars 5 g
PROTEIN 4 g
DIETARY EXCHANGES
  1½ starch, 1 fat

cabbage with mustard-caraway sauce

SERVES 8

The distinctive flavor of caraway combines with spicy mustard and tangy yogurt in a sauce that goes nicely with both cabbage and brussels sprouts. Poached fish or chicken is a nice contrast to this robust dish.

8 cups coarsely shredded cabbage (about 1 2-pound head or 1 1-pound package shredded cabbage) or 1½ pounds fresh brussels sprouts, trimmed and loose outer leaves discarded

MUSTARD-CARAWAY SAUCE

2 cups fat-free, low-sodium chicken broth, such as on page 43

1 tablespoon plus 1 teaspoon spicy brown mustard

1 tablespoon cornstarch (2 tablespoons for brussels sprouts)

½ teaspoon caraway seeds, crushed

⅓ cup fat-free plain yogurt

½ teaspoon grated lemon zest

¼ teaspoon salt

¼ teaspoon pepper

In a medium saucepan, steam the cabbage for 5 minutes (6 to 8 minutes for brussels sprouts), or until tender-crisp. Remove the steamer from the saucepan. Set aside.

Meanwhile, in a large saucepan, whisk together the broth, mustard, cornstarch, and caraway seeds. Bring to a boil over medium-high heat, stirring occasionally. Cook for 1 to 2 minutes, or until thickened.

Stir in the remaining sauce ingredients. Reduce the heat to low. Cook for 2 to 3 minutes.

Stir in the cabbage until well coated. Cook for 2 to 3 minutes, or until heated through. Don't overcook.

COOK'S TIP on caraway seeds

The fruit of an herb in the carrot family, caraway seeds are very popular in German, Austrian, and Hungarian foods. To release their flavor, crush them in a mortar and pestle. In many recipes, you can substitute other seeds, such as fennel, cumin, or dill.

PER SERVING

CALORIES 33
TOTAL FAT 0.0 g
  Saturated Fat 0.0 g
  Trans Fat 0.0 g
  Polyunsaturated Fat 0.0 g
  Monounsaturated Fat 0.0 g
CHOLESTEROL 0 mg
SODIUM 125 mg
CARBOHYDRATES 6 g
  Fiber 2 g
  Sugars 3 g
PROTEIN 2 g
DIETARY EXCHANGES
  1 vegetable

spiced red cabbage

SERVES 4

Celebrate Oktoberfest or any other fall occasion with this festive dish of red cabbage, apples, and spices. Try it with roasted pork tenderloin.

3 cups shredded red cabbage (about 12 ounces)
½ cup water (plus more as needed)
¼ cup cider vinegar
¼ teaspoon ground allspice
¼ teaspoon ground cinnamon
⅛ teaspoon ground nutmeg
2 medium tart apples, peeled and diced
1 tablespoon sugar

In a large saucepan, stir together the cabbage, water, vinegar, allspice, cinnamon, and nutmeg. Cook, covered, over low heat for 15 minutes, stirring occasionally and adding 2 to 3 tablespoons water if needed during cooking.

Stir in the apples. Cook, covered, for 5 minutes. If necessary, uncover and cook until all the moisture has cooked away.

Stir in the sugar.

COOK'S TIP on apples

Tart apples include Granny Smith and Gravenstein. Among the varieties that are tart but have a hint of sweetness are Braeburn, Jonathan, McIntosh, pippin (or Newton pippin), and Winesap.

PER SERVING

CALORIES 71
TOTAL FAT 0.0 g
  Saturated Fat 0.0 g
  Trans Fat 0.0 g
  Polyunsaturated Fat 0.0 g
  Monounsaturated Fat 0.0 g
CHOLESTEROL 0 mg
SODIUM 16 mg
CARBOHYDRATES 18 g
  Fiber 2 g
  Sugars 13 g
PROTEIN 1 g
DIETARY EXCHANGES
  ½ fruit, 1 vegetable

honeyed carrots

SERVES 4

A tantalizing glaze of honey and brown sugar coats tender carrots.

2 cups water
10 to 12 small carrots (about 12 ounces total)
2 tablespoons light tub margarine

1 tablespoon light brown sugar
1 tablespoon honey
2 tablespoons finely snipped fresh parsley or fresh mint

In a large saucepan, bring the water to a boil over high heat. Reduce the heat to medium-high and cook the carrots for 15 minutes, or until tender. Drain well in a colander.

Dry the pan. Melt the margarine over medium heat, swirling to coat the bottom. Stir in the brown sugar, honey, and carrots. Reduce the heat to low. Cook for 2 to 3 minutes, stirring frequently to coat the carrots with the glaze. Serve sprinkled with the parsley.

PER SERVING

CALORIES 85
TOTAL FAT 2.5 g
    Saturated Fat 0.0 g
    Trans Fat 0.0 g
    Polyunsaturated Fat 0.5 g
    Monounsaturated Fat 1.5 g
CHOLESTEROL 0 mg
SODIUM 106 mg
CARBOHYDRATES 16 g
    Fiber 3 g
    Sugars 12 g
PROTEIN 1 g
DIETARY EXCHANGES
    2 vegetable,
    ½ carbohydrate, ½ fat

tangy carrots

SERVES 6

The sharp flavors of mustard and pepper meet the tang of lime juice in this unusual side. Serve it hot or cold.

1 pound medium carrots, halved lengthwise, then halved crosswise
1 large shallot, very thinly sliced
SAUCE
1 tablespoon light tub margarine
1 tablespoon coarse-grain mustard

2 teaspoons fresh lime juice
Generous sprinkle of pepper
2 tablespoons finely snipped fresh parsley

In a medium saucepan, steam the carrots and shallot for 8 to 10 minutes, or until tender. Set aside.

In a small skillet, melt the margarine over medium heat, swirling to coat the bottom. Stir in the mustard, lime juice, and pepper. Cook until heated through, stirring constantly.

In a medium bowl, stir together all the ingredients. Serve hot or cover and refrigerate to serve chilled.

MICROWAVE METHOD

Put the carrots and shallot in a microwave steamer with 2 tablespoons water. Cook on 100 percent power (high) for 6 to 7 minutes, or until tender. Remove from the microwave. Set aside. Put the remaining ingredients except the parsley in a microwaveable dish. Cook on 100 percent power (high) for 10 to 15 seconds, or just until hot. In a medium bowl, stir together the parsley, carrots, shallot, and sauce.

PER SERVING
CALORIES 44
TOTAL FAT 1.5 g
  Saturated Fat 0.0 g
  Trans Fat 0.0 g
  Polyunsaturated Fat 0.0 g
  Monounsaturated Fat 0.5 g
CHOLESTEROL 0 mg
SODIUM 75 mg
CARBOHYDRATES 7 g
  Fiber 2 g
  Sugars 4 g
PROTEIN 1 g
DIETARY EXCHANGES
  1 vegetable, ½ fat

COOK'S TIP on shallots

Shallots combine the flavor of onions and garlic but are milder than either. You can substitute 1 tablespoon minced onion for 1 large shallot.

baked grated carrots with sherry

SERVES 6

Pop this casserole into the oven while you roast a chicken. Fix a salad to round out an easy meal.

3 cups grated carrots	1 tablespoon fresh lemon juice
2 tablespoons light tub margarine, melted	1 tablespoon chopped green onions (green part only)
2 tablespoons dry sherry	

Preheat the oven to 350°F.

In a 1-quart casserole dish, stir together all the ingredients except the green onions. Sprinkle with the green onions.

Bake, covered, for 30 minutes.

PER SERVING

CALORIES 40
TOTAL FAT 1.5 g
  Saturated Fat 0.0 g
  Trans Fat 0.0 g
  Polyunsaturated Fat 0.5 g
  Monounsaturated Fat 1.0 g
CHOLESTEROL 0 mg
SODIUM 68 mg
CARBOHYDRATES 6 g
  Fiber 2 g
  Sugars 3 g
PROTEIN 1 g
DIETARY EXCHANGES
  1 vegetable, ½ fat

baked cauliflower and carrots with nutmeg

SERVES 4

Nutmeg gives a mellow, slightly nutty taste to this dish without overpowering the other flavors. Once you pop this vegetable combo in the oven, you can forget it for 45 minutes.

8 ounces cauliflower florets, broken into bite-size pieces
2 medium carrots, thinly sliced
2 tablespoons water

2 tablespoons light tub margarine
⅛ teaspoon ground nutmeg
Dash of cayenne (optional)
⅛ teaspoon salt

Preheat the oven to 375°F.

In a 9-inch or 2-quart glass baking dish, stir together the cauliflower and carrots. Spoon the water on top. Dot with small pieces of the margarine. Sprinkle with the nutmeg and cayenne.

Bake, covered, for 45 minutes, or until tender. Sprinkle with the salt.

cauliflower and roasted corn with chili powder and lime

SERVES 8

The roasted corn combined with the spiciness of the chili powder and the tanginess of the lime juice provides your palate with an intense flavor sensation. Try this side dish with Turkey Loaf (page 276).

2 medium ears of corn, husks and silks discarded	1 2-ounce jar diced pimientos, drained
4 cups cauliflower florets (about ½ medium head)	1 tablespoon fresh lime juice
¼ cup fat-free, low-sodium chicken broth, such as on page 43	1 tablespoon light tub margarine
	¼ teaspoon chili powder
	¼ teaspoon salt
	⅛ teaspoon pepper

Preheat the oven to 400°F.

Put the corn on a baking sheet. Roast for 15 minutes. Let cool on a cooling rack for 5 to 10 minutes. Slice the corn off the cobs. Discard the cobs. Set the kernels aside.

Meanwhile, in a large saucepan, bring the cauliflower and broth to a boil over medium-high heat. Reduce the heat to medium low. Cook, covered, for 10 to 15 minutes, or until the cauliflower is tender. Discard any remaining liquid.

In a small bowl, stir together the remaining ingredients.

Stir the pimiento mixture and roasted corn into the cauliflower. Cook, uncovered, over medium-low heat for 1 to 2 minutes, or until heated through, stirring occasionally.

PER SERVING

CALORIES 40
TOTAL FAT 1.0 g
  Saturated Fat 0.0 g
  Trans Fat 0.0 g
  Polyunsaturated Fat 0.5 g
  Monounsaturated Fat 0.5 g
CHOLESTEROL 0 mg
SODIUM 105 mg
CARBOHYDRATES 8 g
  Fiber 2 g
  Sugars 2 g
PROTEIN 2 g
DIETARY EXCHANGES
  ½ starch

creole celery and peas

SERVES 10

Different colors, shapes, and textures combine to add interest to this side dish.

1 teaspoon light tub margarine
1 medium onion, chopped
1 14.5-ounce can no-salt-added tomatoes, drained, liquid reserved
½ teaspoon red hot-pepper sauce
¼ teaspoon dried thyme, crumbled
8 medium ribs of celery, cut on the diagonal into bite-size pieces
1 10-ounce package frozen green peas

In a large skillet, melt the margarine over medium-high heat, swirling to coat the bottom. Cook the onion for about 3 minutes, or until soft, stirring frequently.

Stir the liquid from the tomatoes (set the tomatoes aside), hot-pepper sauce, and thyme into the onion. Bring to a boil.

Stir in the celery and peas. Reduce the heat and simmer, covered, for 10 minutes, or until the celery is barely tender.

Stir in the tomatoes, crushing slightly with a spoon. Heat through.

PER SERVING

CALORIES 40
TOTAL FAT 0.5 g
  Saturated Fat 0.0 g
  Trans Fat 0.0 g
  Polyunsaturated Fat 0.0 g
  Monounsaturated Fat 0.0 g
CHOLESTEROL 0 mg
SODIUM 65 mg
CARBOHYDRATES 7 g
  Fiber 2 g
  Sugars 4 g
PROTEIN 2 g
DIETARY EXCHANGES
  ½ starch

roasted chayote squash

SERVES 4

Assertive seasonings, such as the lemon and the red pepper flakes in this dish, are great complements to the very mild, slightly sweet chayote squash.

2 8-ounce chayote squash, halved lengthwise, pits discarded, and skin pierced several places with a fork
Cooking spray
1 tablespoon plus 1 teaspoon olive oil (extra virgin preferred)

½ teaspoon grated lemon zest
2 teaspoons fresh lemon juice
½ teaspoon dried oregano, crumbled
⅛ teaspoon crushed red pepper flakes
⅛ teaspoon salt

Preheat the oven to 400°F. Cover a baking sheet with aluminum foil.

Lightly spray both sides of the squash with cooking spray. Place with the cut side down on the baking sheet.

Bake for 40 to 45 minutes, or until tender when the skin is pierced with a fork. Transfer the squash with the cut side up to plates.

In a small bowl, stir together the remaining ingredients except the salt. Spoon into the cavity of each squash half. Sprinkle with the salt.

PER SERVING

CALORIES 63
TOTAL FAT 4.5 g
  Saturated Fat 0.5 g
  Trans Fat 0.0 g
  Polyunsaturated Fat 0.5 g
  Monounsaturated Fat 3.5 g
CHOLESTEROL 0 mg
SODIUM 75 mg
CARBOHYDRATES 6 g
  Fiber 2 g
  Sugars 2 g
PROTEIN 1 g
DIETARY EXCHANGES
  1 vegetable, 1 fat

grilled corn on the cob

SERVES 4

We bet everyone in the family will love this corn on the cob! Grilling the corn deepens its flavor.

4 small ears of corn, husks and silks discarded
Cooking spray
2 tablespoons light tub margarine, melted
2 tablespoons fat-free, low-sodium chicken broth, such as on page 43

¼ teaspoon paprika
⅛ teaspoon pepper
⅛ teaspoon salt
1 tablespoon snipped fresh cilantro

Put the corn in a large bowl. Fill with cold water to cover the corn. Soak for 30 minutes. Drain well.

Meanwhile, lightly spray the grill rack with cooking spray. Preheat the grill on medium high.

Stir together the remaining ingredients except the cilantro. Brush the corn generously with the mixture, reserving any that remains.

Grill the corn for 10 to 12 minutes, or until tender, turning to grill evenly and brushing frequently with the margarine mixture. Sprinkle with the cilantro before serving.

PER SERVING

CALORIES 84
TOTAL FAT 3.0 g
  Saturated Fat 0.0 g
  Trans Fat 0.0 g
  Polyunsaturated Fat 1.0 g
  Monounsaturated Fat 1.5 g
CHOLESTEROL 0 mg
SODIUM 130 mg
CARBOHYDRATES 14 g
  Fiber 2 g
  Sugars 2 g
PROTEIN 2 g
DIETARY EXCHANGES
  1 starch, ½ fat

southwestern creamy corn

SERVES 6

Try this creamy dish, flecked with color from red bell peppers, green chiles, and cilantro, as a side for Beef Tostadas (page 328).

1 teaspoon light tub margarine	¼ cup fat-free milk
½ large onion, finely chopped	½ teaspoon pepper
½ medium red bell pepper, diced	½ teaspoon chili powder
4 ounces fat-free block cream cheese	2 cups frozen whole-kernel corn
¼ cup diced canned green chiles, drained	2 teaspoons finely snipped fresh cilantro

In a large nonstick skillet, melt the margarine over medium-high heat, swirling to coat the bottom. Cook the onion and bell pepper for about 3 minutes, or until the onion is soft, stirring frequently.

Reduce the heat to low. Stir in the cream cheese, green chiles, milk, pepper, and chili powder. Cook for 2 to 3 minutes, or until the mixture is smooth, stirring constantly.

Stir in the corn. Cook for 2 to 3 minutes, or just until the corn is heated through. Stir in the cilantro.

PER SERVING

CALORIES 92
TOTAL FAT 1.0 g
 Saturated Fat 0.0 g
 Trans Fat 0.0 g
 Polyunsaturated Fat 0.5 g
 Monounsaturated Fat 0.5 g
CHOLESTEROL 4 mg
SODIUM 187 mg
CARBOHYDRATES 17 g
 Fiber 2 g
 Sugars 5 g
PROTEIN 5 g
DIETARY EXCHANGES
 1 starch

couscous with raisins and almonds

SERVES 4

This spice-infused side dish goes nicely with beef or chicken skewers, such as Steak and Vegetable Kebabs on page 304, or with grilled salmon.

1 cup fat-free, low-sodium chicken broth, such as on page 43
¼ cup golden or regular raisins
¼ teaspoon ground cumin
⅛ teaspoon ground cinnamon
¾ cup uncooked whole-wheat couscous

2 tablespoons snipped Italian (flat-leaf) parsley
2 tablespoons sliced almonds, dry-roasted

In a medium saucepan, stir together the broth, raisins, cumin, and cinnamon. Bring to a boil over medium-high heat.

Stir in the couscous. Remove from the heat. Let stand, covered, for 5 minutes.

Add the parsley and almonds. Fluff with a fork.

couscous with vegetables

SERVES 4

The green peas, velvety mushrooms, and fresh parsley in this side dish are a terrific combination.

½ cup uncooked whole-wheat couscous	2 tablespoons dry white wine (regular or nonalcoholic)
1 cup frozen green peas or any other quick-cooking vegetable, thawed and drained	½ teaspoon crushed garlic or ¼ teaspoon garlic powder
½ cup minced onion	2 tablespoons finely snipped fresh parsley
2 medium button mushrooms, thinly sliced	½ teaspoon dried basil, crumbled
	⅛ teaspoon pepper

Prepare the couscous using the package directions, omitting the salt.

Meanwhile, in a medium nonstick saucepan, cook the peas, onion, mushrooms, wine, and garlic over medium-high heat for 3 to 5 minutes, stirring frequently.

Stir in the parsley, basil, and pepper. Transfer to a medium bowl.

Stir in the couscous.

COOK'S TIP on couscous

If your supermarket doesn't have whole-wheat couscous, look in the ethnic food sections or bulk food bins of natural food supermarkets. Almost all couscous takes only about 5 minutes to prepare; avoid any brand that calls for long steaming.

PER SERVING

CALORIES 148
TOTAL FAT 0.5 g
  Saturated Fat 0.0 g
  Trans Fat 0.0 g
  Polyunsaturated Fat 0.5 g
  Monounsaturated Fat 0.0 g
CHOLESTEROL 0 mg
SODIUM 39 mg
CARBOHYDRATES 30 g
  Fiber 6 g
  Sugars 3 g
PROTEIN 6 g
DIETARY EXCHANGES
  2 starch

grits casserole
with cheese and chiles

SERVES 8

Grill pork tenderloins and a medley of fresh vegetables, add this filling side dish of cheesy grits, and you'll have an easy dinner for eight. The casserole is also excellent as a brunch dish.

Cooking spray
2 cups fat-free, low-sodium chicken broth, such as on page 43
2 cups water
1 cup uncooked quick grits
½ cup fat-free milk
¼ cup shredded or grated Parmesan cheese
2 ¾-ounce slices fat-free Swiss cheese, diced

2 ounces canned chopped green chiles, drained
1 tablespoon light tub margarine
2 medium garlic cloves, minced
¼ teaspoon salt
⅛ teaspoon pepper
½ cup egg substitute
½ teaspoon chili powder

Preheat the oven to 375°F. Lightly spray a 13 x 9 x 2-inch baking pan with cooking spray. Set aside.

In a large saucepan, bring the broth and water to a boil over medium-high heat. Gradually whisk in the grits. Reduce the heat to low. Cook, covered, for 5 minutes, whisking occasionally. Remove the saucepan from the heat.

Stir the milk, Parmesan and Swiss cheeses, green chiles, margarine, garlic, salt, and pepper into the grits.

Stir in the egg substitute. Pour into the baking pan, smoothing the top.

Sprinkle with the chili powder.

Bake for 45 minutes. Remove from the oven. Let cool for 5 to 10 minutes before serving.

PER SERVING

CALORIES 113
TOTAL FAT 1.5 g
 Saturated Fat 0.5 g
 Trans Fat 0.0 g
 Polyunsaturated Fat 0.5 g
 Monounsaturated Fat 0.5 g
CHOLESTEROL 3 mg
SODIUM 241 mg
CARBOHYDRATES 18 g
 Fiber 1 g
 Sugars 1 g
PROTEIN 7 g
DIETARY EXCHANGES
 1 starch, ½ very lean meat

kale crisps

SERVES 4

Small pieces of kale baked until crisp make a nice accompaniment to a sandwich or other entrée—and even do double duty as an unusual healthy snack.

Cooking spray
8 ounces kale, heavy stems discarded, chopped (about 5 cups)
1 tablespoon olive oil
1 teaspoon vinegar

¼ cup shredded or grated Parmesan cheese
¼ teaspoon garlic powder
⅛ teaspoon smoked paprika

Place a rack on the lowest shelf of the oven and preheat the oven to 350°F. Lightly spray a large rimmed baking sheet with cooking spray.

Thoroughly dry the kale in a salad spinner or by blotting with paper towels or dish towels. (Moisture will keep the kale from getting crisp.) Transfer the kale to a large bowl.

Add the oil and vinegar to the kale, stirring to coat. Spread the kale in a single layer on the baking sheet. Lightly spray the top side of the kale with cooking spray.

Bake for 10 minutes. Transfer the baking sheet to a cooling rack.

Meanwhile, in a small bowl, stir together the Parmesan, garlic powder, and paprika. Sprinkle over the kale, stirring gently to combine thoroughly.

Bake for 15 to 20 minutes, or until the desired crispness, turning with tongs every 5 minutes. As pieces get crisp, remove them from the baking sheet and continue cooking the remaining kale. Serve immediately for maximum crispness.

PER SERVING

CALORIES 80
TOTAL FAT 5.0 g
    Saturated Fat 1.5 g
    Trans Fat 0.0 g
    Polyunsaturated Fat 0.5 g
    Monounsaturated Fat 3.0 g
CHOLESTEROL 4 mg
SODIUM 109 mg
CARBOHYDRATES 6 g
    Fiber 1 g
    Sugars 0 g
PROTEIN 4 g
DIETARY EXCHANGES
    1 vegetable, 1 fat

mushrooms with red wine

SERVES 4

Dress up mushrooms in a snap by cooking them quickly, then letting them absorb a delicate red wine sauce.

1 pound medium button mushrooms, quartered

2 tablespoons dry red wine (regular or nonalcoholic)

2 teaspoons very low sodium beef bouillon granules

1 medium garlic clove, minced

½ teaspoon sugar

½ teaspoon dried thyme, crumbled

¼ cup snipped fresh parsley

2 teaspoons olive oil (extra virgin preferred)

⅛ teaspoon salt

In a large nonstick skillet, cook the mushrooms over medium-high heat for 4 minutes, or until soft.

Meanwhile, in a small bowl, stir together the wine, bouillon granules, garlic, sugar, and thyme.

Stir the wine mixture into the mushrooms. Increase the heat to high and bring to a boil. Remove from the heat.

Stir in the parsley, oil, and salt. Let stand, covered, for 3 minutes before serving.

PER SERVING

CALORIES 61
TOTAL FAT 2.5 g
  Saturated Fat 0.5 g
  Trans Fat 0.0 g
  Polyunsaturated Fat 0.5 g
  Monounsaturated Fat 1.5 g
CHOLESTEROL 0 mg
SODIUM 84 mg
CARBOHYDRATES 6 g
  Fiber 1 g
  Sugars 3 g
PROTEIN 4 g
DIETARY EXCHANGES
  1 vegetable, ½ fat

mushrooms with white wine and shallots

SERVES 4

Cook succulent mushrooms with shallots and white wine, then reduce the juices to intensify the flavor. Serve as a side dish or spoon the mushrooms over lean broiled steak.

2 tablespoons light tub margarine
½ cup finely chopped shallots (about 8 large)
1 pound medium button mushrooms, quartered
½ cup dry white wine (regular or nonalcoholic)
1 tablespoon finely snipped fresh parsley
Pepper to taste

In a large nonstick skillet, melt the margarine over medium-high heat, swirling to coat the bottom. Cook the shallots for about 3 minutes, stirring constantly.

Stir in the mushrooms and wine. Reduce the heat to medium. Cook, covered, for 7 to 9 minutes. Increase the heat to high. Cook, uncovered, for 5 to 6 minutes, or until the juices have evaporated.

Stir in the parsley and pepper.

PER SERVING

CALORIES 80
TOTAL FAT 2.5 g
  Saturated Fat 0.0 g
  Trans Fat 0.0 g
  Polyunsaturated Fat 0.5 g
  Monounsaturated Fat 1.5 g
CHOLESTEROL 0 mg
SODIUM 55 mg
CARBOHYDRATES 7 g
  Fiber 1 g
  Sugars 3 g
PROTEIN 4 g
DIETARY EXCHANGES
  1 vegetable, ½ fat

baked okra bites

SERVES 4

Once you've enjoyed these crisp okra bites as a side dish with grilled fish or as part of a southern-style menu, try them also as "croutons" for a spinach and romaine salad or sprinkle them on top of baked casseroles.

Cooking spray
¼ cup egg substitute
½ cup yellow cornmeal
¼ cup all-purpose flour
½ teaspoon onion powder
½ teaspoon garlic powder
½ teaspoon salt-free Creole or Cajun seasoning blend, such as on page 463, or ½ teaspoon salt-free spicy seasoning blend

8 ounces fresh okra, stems discarded, cut into ½-inch slices, or 2 cups frozen sliced okra, thawed

Preheat the oven to 400°F. Lightly spray a large baking sheet with cooking spray.

Put the egg substitute in a medium bowl. In a shallow dish, stir together the cornmeal, flour, onion powder, garlic powder, and seasoning blend. Set the bowl, dish, and baking sheet in a row, assembly-line fashion. Add the okra to the egg substitute, stirring to coat. Using a slotted spoon, transfer the okra in batches to the cornmeal mixture. Stir to coat. After all the okra has been coated, discard any remaining egg substitute. Arrange the okra in a single layer on the baking sheet (leave space between the pieces so they brown evenly). Lightly spray with cooking spray.

Bake for 20 to 25 minutes, or until crisp on the outside and tender on the inside. Transfer the baking sheet to a cooling rack. Let the okra cool for 2 to 3 minutes before serving.

PER SERVING

CALORIES 117
TOTAL FAT 0.5 g
  Saturated Fat 0.0 g
  Trans Fat 0.0 g
  Polyunsaturated Fat 0.0 g
  Monounsaturated Fat 0.0 g
CHOLESTEROL 0 mg
SODIUM 37 mg
CARBOHYDRATES 25 g
  Fiber 3 g
  Sugars 1 g
PROTEIN 5 g
DIETARY EXCHANGES
  1½ starch, 1 vegetable

parmesan parsnip puree with leeks and carrots

SERVES 6

Process sweet, slightly peppery parsnips with carrots, leeks, and Parmesan cheese for a pale gold side dish similar in texture to mashed potatoes.

1 pound parsnips, peeled and cut into ½-inch pieces

2 large leeks (white part only), thinly sliced

2 small carrots, cut into ½-inch pieces

½ cup fat-free, low-sodium chicken broth and ½ cup fat-free, low-sodium chicken broth, such as on page 43, divided use

2 tablespoons shredded or grated Parmesan cheese

1 tablespoon light tub margarine

¼ teaspoon salt

2 tablespoons thinly sliced almonds, dry-roasted

In a large saucepan, bring the parsnips, leeks, carrots, and ½ cup broth to a boil over high heat. Reduce the heat to medium low. Cook, covered, for 10 minutes, or until tender.

In a food processor or blender, process the parsnip mixture, Parmesan, margarine, salt, and remaining ½ cup broth until smooth. Serve sprinkled with the almonds.

COOK'S TIP on parsnips

Parsnips look like pale carrots and are in the same family. Whether you bake, sauté, roast, steam, or boil them, parsnips are sweet and aromatic. Be careful not to over-cook them, though, as they tend to turn mushy quickly. Look for firm parsnips without pitting. Don't worry if they're large—bigger size doesn't mean parsnips won't be tender. Wrapped in plastic and refrigerated, parsnips will keep for several weeks to several months.

PER SERVING

CALORIES 108
TOTAL FAT 2.5 g
    Saturated Fat 0.5 g
    Trans Fat 0.0 g
    Polyunsaturated Fat 0.5 g
    Monounsaturated Fat 1.0 g
CHOLESTEROL 1 mg
SODIUM 169 mg
CARBOHYDRATES 20 g
    Fiber 5 g
    Sugars 6 g
PROTEIN 3 g
DIETARY EXCHANGES
    1 starch, 1 vegetable,
    ½ fat

asian linguine

SERVES 4

Serve this sassy side dish to dress up the simplest cuts of meats or poultry.

1¾ cups fat-free, low-sodium chicken broth, such as on page 43

2 ounces dried whole-grain linguine, broken in half

1 large onion, thinly sliced

2 medium carrots, cut into matchstick-size strips

2 tablespoons soy sauce (lowest sodium available)

2 tablespoons cider vinegar

1½ tablespoons sugar

⅛ teaspoon garlic powder

3 tablespoons slivered almonds, dry-roasted

In a medium saucepan, bring the broth to a boil over high heat. Stir in the pasta. Return to a boil. Reduce the heat to medium. Cook for 5 minutes, or until the pasta is tender. Don't drain.

Meanwhile, in a large nonstick skillet, cook the onion and carrots over medium-high heat for 6 minutes, or until the carrots are tender-crisp, stirring frequently.

In a small bowl, stir together the remaining ingredients except the almonds.

Add the pasta and any remaining liquid to the onion mixture. Pour in the soy sauce mixture. Toss gently to blend. Serve sprinkled with the almonds.

PER SERVING

CALORIES 144
TOTAL FAT 3.0 g
  Saturated Fat 0.0 g
  Trans Fat 0.0 g
  Polyunsaturated Fat 1.0 g
  Monounsaturated Fat 1.5 g
CHOLESTEROL 0 mg
SODIUM 233 mg
CARBOHYDRATES 25 g
  Fiber 4 g
  Sugars 10 g
PROTEIN 5 g
DIETARY EXCHANGES
  1 starch, 2 vegetable,
  ½ fat

oven-fried onion rings

SERVES 4

Crumbled melba toasts make these onion rings so crisp your family will think they're fried.

Cooking spray
2 tablespoons all-purpose flour
½ teaspoon paprika
⅛ teaspoon cayenne
2 large sweet onions, cut into ½-inch slices and separated into 24 large rings (reserve small inner rings for another use)

3 large egg whites
¾ teaspoon red hot-pepper sauce
16 unsalted whole-grain melba toasts, processed to fine crumbs

Preheat the oven to 400°F. Line 2 large rimmed baking sheets with aluminum foil. Place a cooling rack in each pan. Lightly spray the racks with cooking spray.

In a large resealable plastic bag, combine the flour, paprika, and cayenne. Put the onion rings, a few at a time, in the bag. Seal the bag. Carefully shake the bag to coat the onion rings.

In a shallow dish, whisk together the egg whites and hot-pepper sauce. Put the melba toast crumbs in another shallow dish. Set the dishes and baking sheets in a row, assembly-line fashion. Dip each onion ring in the egg white mixture, letting any excess drip off. Dip each in the crumbs, pressing gently with your fingertips so the crumbs adhere. Arrange the rings in a single layer on the racks. Lightly spray the tops of the onion rings with cooking spray.

Bake for 12 to 15 minutes, or until browned (don't turn).

PER SERVING

CALORIES 143
TOTAL FAT 0.5 g
   Saturated Fat 0.0 g
   Trans Fat 0.0 g
   Polyunsaturated Fat 0.0 g
   Monounsaturated Fat 0.0 g
CHOLESTEROL 0 mg
SODIUM 54 mg
CARBOHYDRATES 28 g
   Fiber 4 g
   Sugars 6 g
PROTEIN 7 g
DIETARY EXCHANGES
   1 starch, 2 vegetable

black-eyed peas with canadian bacon

SERVES 8

In the South, black-eyed peas are traditionally served on New Year's Day to bring good luck throughout the coming year. This tasty version will bring you compliments no matter when you serve it. Just be sure to prepare this dish on a day you're home for awhile so the beans can simmer long enough to get tender.

8 ounces dried black-eyed peas, sorted for stones and shriveled peas and rinsed
1 medium onion, chopped
1 medium rib of celery, chopped
3 ounces no-salt-added tomato paste

2 ounces Canadian bacon, diced
1 small dried bay leaf
1 small garlic clove, chopped
⅛ teaspoon cayenne
Pepper to taste

Put the peas in a large saucepan and add water to cover. Let soak for 45 minutes. Drain well in a colander. Return the peas to the saucepan. Add enough fresh water to just cover.

Stir in the remaining ingredients. Bring to a boil over medium-high heat. Reduce the heat and simmer, covered, for 3 hours, or until tender. Discard the bay leaf.

french peas

SERVES 6

Tender peas, wilted lettuce, and crunchy water chestnuts provide a variety of textures in this side dish. For a Parisian dinner, serve with Burgundy Chicken with Mushrooms (page 236).

1 10-ounce package frozen green peas
1 tablespoon canola or corn oil
1 cup finely shredded lettuce
2 medium green onions, diced
1 teaspoon all-purpose flour

3 tablespoons fat-free, low-sodium chicken broth, such as on page 43
1 8-ounce can sliced water chestnuts, drained
Pepper to taste

Prepare the peas using the package directions, omitting the salt and margarine. Drain well in a colander. Set aside.

Meanwhile, in a large saucepan, heat the oil over low heat, swirling to coat the bottom. Cook the lettuce and green onions for 1 to 2 minutes, stirring occasionally.

Put the flour in a small bowl. Add the broth, stirring to dissolve. Stir into the lettuce mixture. Increase the heat to medium. Cook for 2 to 3 minutes, or until thickened, stirring occasionally.

Stir in the peas, water chestnuts, and pepper. Heat through.

PER SERVING

CALORIES 76
TOTAL FAT 2.5 g
  Saturated Fat 0.0 g
  Trans Fat 0.0 g
  Polyunsaturated Fat 0.5 g
  Monounsaturated Fat 1.5 g
CHOLESTEROL 0 mg
SODIUM 57 mg
CARBOHYDRATES 11 g
  Fiber 4 g
  Sugars 3 g
PROTEIN 3 g
DIETARY EXCHANGES
  ½ starch, ½ fat

sweet lemon snow peas

SERVES 4

Chinese snow pea pods are quickly steamed (just two minutes), then splashed with a spicy-sweet, lemony soy sauce mixture.

2 tablespoons sugar
2 tablespoons soy sauce (lowest sodium available)
1 teaspoon grated lemon zest

2 tablespoons fresh lemon juice
¼ teaspoon crushed red pepper flakes
9 ounces fresh or frozen snow peas, trimmed if fresh

In a small bowl, stir together all the ingredients except the snow peas until the sugar is dissolved.

In a medium saucepan, steam the snow peas for 2 minutes, or until just tender-crisp. Transfer to a rimmed plate or shallow dish.

Pour the sauce over the snow peas. Don't stir.

COOK'S TIP on lemon zest

You can grate the zest of several lemons at one time—especially when they are on sale—and freeze what you don't use.

PER SERVING

CALORIES 59
TOTAL FAT 0.0 g
  Saturated Fat 0.0 g
  Trans Fat 0.0 g
  Polyunsaturated Fat 0.0 g
  Monounsaturated Fat 0.0 g
CHOLESTEROL 0 mg
SODIUM 198 mg
CARBOHYDRATES 12 g
  Fiber 2 g
  Sugars 9 g
PROTEIN 2 g
DIETARY EXCHANGES
  1 starch

stir-fried sugar snap peas

SERVES 4

Crispy-sweet sugar snap peas with an Asian-style sauce and toasted almonds are a snap to make and a real treat at any meal. Serve with grilled pork or poached fish, as well as with Asian entrées.

3 tablespoons fat-free, low-sodium chicken broth, such as on page 43
1 teaspoon soy sauce (lowest sodium available)
½ teaspoon cornstarch
½ teaspoon light brown sugar
¼ teaspoon toasted sesame oil
⅛ teaspoon crushed red pepper flakes (optional)
8 ounces sugar snap peas
1 medium garlic clove, minced
1 tablespoon sliced almonds, dry-roasted

In a small bowl, whisk together the broth, soy sauce, cornstarch, brown sugar, oil, and red pepper flakes until the cornstarch is dissolved.

In a medium nonstick skillet, cook the peas and garlic over medium-high heat for 1 to 2 minutes, or until tender-crisp, stirring constantly.

Pour the broth mixture into the skillet. Reduce the heat and simmer until thickened, stirring occasionally. Serve sprinkled with the almonds.

PER SERVING

CALORIES 42
TOTAL FAT 1.0 g
  Saturated Fat 0.0 g
  Trans Fat 0.0 g
  Polyunsaturated Fat 0.5 g
  Monounsaturated Fat 0.5 g
CHOLESTEROL 0 mg
SODIUM 34 mg
CARBOHYDRATES 7 g
  Fiber 2 g
  Sugars 3 g
PROTEIN 2 g
DIETARY EXCHANGES
  ½ starch

basil roasted peppers

SERVES 8

You'll find many uses for these roasted peppers in your cooking, or serve them cold as a garnish.

Cooking spray
6 firm medium red bell peppers
¼ cup plus 1 tablespoon olive oil
¼ cup red wine vinegar
2 tablespoons finely chopped fresh basil

3 or 4 medium garlic cloves, minced
½ teaspoon pepper, or to taste
¼ teaspoon salt

Preheat the broiler. Lightly spray a broiler pan and rack with cooking spray.

Broil the bell peppers on the rack about 4 inches from the heat for 1 to 2 minutes on each side, or until lightly charred. Transfer to a large bowl. Cover with plastic wrap. Let cool for 5 to 10 minutes. (It won't hurt the peppers to stand for as long as 20 minutes.) Rinse the peppers with cold water, removing and discarding the skin, ribs, seeds, and stem. Blot the peppers dry with paper towels. Cut into strips ½ inch wide.

In a medium bowl, stir together the remaining ingredients. Stir in the peppers. Cover and refrigerate for 30 minutes to 8 hours. Drain well in a colander, discarding the marinade. Refrigerate the drained peppers in an airtight container for up to five days or freeze for up to four months.

PER SERVING

CALORIES 28
TOTAL FAT 0.5 g
  Saturated Fat 0.0 g
  Trans Fat 0.0 g
  Polyunsaturated Fat 0.0 g
  Monounsaturated Fat 0.0 g
CHOLESTEROL 0 mg
SODIUM 76 mg
CARBOHYDRATES 5 g
  Fiber 2 g
  Sugars 4 g
PROTEIN 1 g
DIETARY EXCHANGES
  1 vegetable

scalloped potatoes

SERVES 6

Just out of the oven, these potatoes are a beautiful golden brown with a slight crunch on top. Serve with lean grilled pork chops and Asparagus with Lemon and Capers (page 415) or take to a potluck for plenty of rave reviews.

Cooking spray
2 tablespoons light tub margarine
1 large onion, finely chopped
¼ cup all-purpose flour
2 cups fat-free milk
¼ cup fat-free half-and-half
3 tablespoons finely snipped fresh parsley
⅛ teaspoon salt and ⅛ teaspoon salt, divided use

⅛ to ¼ teaspoon pepper (white preferred) and ⅛ teaspoon pepper (white preferred), divided use
2 pounds baking potatoes, peeled and thinly sliced
2 tablespoons shredded or grated Romano or Parmesan cheese

Preheat the oven to 325°F. Lightly spray an 8-inch square glass baking dish with cooking spray. Set aside.

In a medium saucepan, melt the margarine over medium-high heat, swirling to coat the bottom. Cook the onion for about 3 minutes, or until soft, stirring frequently.

Whisk in the flour. Cook for 1 minute.

Whisk in the milk. Cook for 3 to 4 minutes, or until the sauce is thickened, whisking constantly.

Whisk in the half-and-half, parsley, ⅛ teaspoon salt, and ⅛ to ¼ teaspoon pepper. Remove from the heat.

Arrange the potatoes in the baking dish. Sprinkle with the remaining ⅛ teaspoon salt and remaining ⅛ teaspoon pepper. Pour the sauce over the potatoes. Sprinkle with the Romano.

Bake for 1 hour 30 minutes.

PER SERVING

CALORIES 198
TOTAL FAT 2.0 g
  Saturated Fat 0.5 g
  Trans Fat 0.0 g
  Polyunsaturated Fat 0.5 g
  Monounsaturated Fat 1.0 g
CHOLESTEROL 3 mg
SODIUM 194 mg
CARBOHYDRATES 39 g
  Fiber 3 g
  Sugars 8 g
PROTEIN 7 g
DIETARY EXCHANGES
  2½ starch

mashed potatoes with parmesan and green onions

SERVES 4

For maximum flavors, try topping your mashed potatoes with add-ons instead of mixing them all in.

---

8 ounces red potatoes, unpeeled, cut into ½-inch cubes

2 medium green onions, finely chopped

¼ cup plus 2 tablespoons fat-free evaporated milk

⅛ teaspoon pepper

1 tablespoon plus 1 teaspoon light tub margarine, melted

⅛ teaspoon salt

2 teaspoons shredded or grated Parmesan cheese

In a medium saucepan, steam the potatoes for 8 to 10 minutes, or until tender. Drain. If you have a hand mixer or immersion (handheld) blender, return the potatoes to the pan (off the heat) and beat or blend until no lumps remain (the skins will keep the mixture from being smooth). Otherwise, transfer them to a large mixing bowl. Using an electric mixer, beat on medium.

Set 2 tablespoons green onion aside. Add the remaining green onion, milk, and pepper to the potatoes. Beat until well blended. Transfer to a serving bowl.

Drizzle the potatoes with the margarine. Sprinkle, in order, with the salt, Parmesan, and reserved 2 table-spoons green onion.

PER SERVING

CALORIES 78
TOTAL FAT 2.0 g
 Saturated Fat 0.0 g
 Trans Fat 0.0 g
 Polyunsaturated Fat 0.5 g
 Monounsaturated Fat 1.0 g
CHOLESTEROL 2 mg
SODIUM 149 mg
CARBOHYDRATES 12 g
 Fiber 1 g
 Sugars 4 g
PROTEIN 3 g
DIETARY EXCHANGES
 1 starch

baked fries with creole seasoning

SERVES 4

These spice-flecked, crisp fries will perk up your taste buds. Serve them with extra-lean hamburgers, such as Grilled Hamburgers with Vegetables and Feta (page 315).

4 medium unpeeled russet potatoes (1¼ to 1½ pounds total)	½ teaspoon garlic powder
	½ teaspoon paprika
CREOLE OR CAJUN SEASONING BLEND	½ teaspoon pepper
½ teaspoon chili powder	⅛ teaspoon cayenne (optional)
½ teaspoon ground cumin	
½ teaspoon onion powder	Cooking spray

Cut the potatoes into long strips about ½ inch wide. Put them in a large bowl. Pour in enough cold water to cover by 1 inch. Soak for 15 minutes.

Meanwhile, in a small bowl, stir together the seasoning blend ingredients.

Preheat the oven to 450°F. Lightly spray a large baking sheet with cooking spray.

Drain the potatoes. Pat dry with paper towels. Spread the potatoes in a single layer on the baking sheet. Lightly spray the tops with cooking spray. Sprinkle with the seasoning blend.

Bake for 30 to 35 minutes, or until crisp.

COOK'S TIP on creole or cajun seasoning

To save time in the future, double or triple the seasonings in this recipe and keep the blend in a container with a shaker top. This seasoning blend is excellent on seafood, poultry, meat, and vegetables.

PER SERVING

CALORIES 129
TOTAL FAT 0.5 g
    Saturated Fat 0.0 g
    Trans Fat 0.0 g
    Polyunsaturated Fat 0.0 g
    Monounsaturated Fat 0.0 g
CHOLESTEROL 0 mg
SODIUM 12 mg
CARBOHYDRATES 29 g
    Fiber 2 g
    Sugars 1 g
PROTEIN 4 g
DIETARY EXCHANGES
    2 starch

rustic potato patties

SERVES 5

Black pepper and cayenne heat up these potato patties, which get their texture from the skins.

4 cups water
1 pound red potatoes, unpeeled, diced
½ cup minced onion
¼ cup plus 2 tablespoons fat-free evaporated milk
1 large egg white

¼ teaspoon salt
⅛ teaspoon pepper
⅛ teaspoon cayenne
¼ cup all-purpose flour
1½ teaspoons canola or corn oil and 1½ teaspoons canola or corn oil, divided use

Preheat the oven to warm or 140°F.

In a medium saucepan, bring the water to a boil over high heat. Add the potatoes and return to a boil. Reduce the heat and simmer for 7 to 8 minutes, or until tender but not mushy. Drain well in a colander. If you have a hand mixer or immersion (handheld) blender, return the potatoes to the pan (off the heat) and beat or blend until no lumps remain (the skins will keep the mixture from being smooth). Otherwise, transfer the potatoes to a large mixing bowl. Using an electric mixer, beat on medium.

Beat in the onion, milk, egg white, salt, pepper, and cayenne until well blended.

Beat in the flour.

In a large nonstick skillet, heat 1½ teaspoons oil over medium-high heat for about 2 minutes, or until hot, swirling to coat the bottom. Spoon five ⅓-cup mounds of the potato mixture (about half) into the skillet. Using the back of a fork, flatten slightly until about ½ inch thick. Cook for about 9 minutes, turning once halfway through. Put the patties on an oven-safe platter. Put in the oven. Heat the remaining 1½ teaspoons oil over medium-high heat for 30 seconds. Repeat the process, making 5 more patties.

Since you'll beat the cooked potatoes, you may wonder why you dice them first. It doesn't take long to dice them in the food processor, and using small pieces saves cooking time.

baked sweet potato chips

SERVES 4

When you want to add a bit of flair to your meal, these sweet potato chips do it in a colorful, nutritious way. They're a great side dish for Baked Catfish (page 143).

Cooking spray
1 teaspoon dried rosemary, crushed
1 teaspoon dried parsley, crumbled
½ teaspoon dry mustard
¼ teaspoon paprika

¼ teaspoon salt
¼ teaspoon pepper
2 medium sweet potatoes, unpeeled, cut crosswise into ⅛-inch slices

Preheat the oven to 450°F. Lightly spray a baking sheet with cooking spray.

In a small bowl, stir together the remaining ingredients except the sweet potatoes.

Put the potatoes in a single layer on the baking sheet. Lightly spray the tops with cooking spray. Sprinkle with the rosemary mixture.

Bake for 25 minutes, or until tender-crisp.

orange sweet potatoes

SERVES 6

No matter the season, a sweet potato casserole is a colorful dish to complement a wide variety of entrées.

4 medium sweet potatoes, unpeeled, or 2 16-ounce cans sweet potatoes, packed without liquid or in water	2 tablespoons light brown sugar
	¼ to ½ teaspoon grated orange zest
	¼ teaspoon ground cinnamon
Cooking spray	2 dashes of bitters (optional)
½ cup fresh orange juice	

If using fresh sweet potatoes, fill a stockpot with enough water to just cover them. Bring to a boil over high heat. Boil for 30 minutes, or until tender. Discard the skins. If using canned potatoes in water, drain well.

Preheat the oven to 350°F. Lightly spray a 1-quart casserole dish with cooking spray.

In a large mixing bowl, mash the sweet potatoes.

Add the remaining ingredients. Using an electric mixer on medium, beat until fluffy. Spread the mixture in the casserole dish.

Bake, covered, for 25 minutes, or until heated through.

PER SERVING

CALORIES 125
TOTAL FAT 0.0 g
  Saturated Fat 0.0 g
  Trans Fat 0.0 g
  Polyunsaturated Fat 0.0 g
  Monounsaturated Fat 0.0 g
CHOLESTEROL 0 mg
SODIUM 64 mg
CARBOHYDRATES 30 g
  Fiber 4 g
  Sugars 11 g
PROTEIN 2 g
DIETARY EXCHANGES
  2 starch

lemon-basil rice

SERVES 4

This fragrant dish is great with grilled salmon or chicken breasts.

¾ cup uncooked instant brown rice
1½ cups fat-free, low-sodium chicken
 broth, such as on page 43
2 teaspoons finely grated lemon zest
1 tablespoon plus 2 teaspoons fresh
 lemon juice

2 teaspoons olive oil (extra virgin
 preferred)
¼ teaspoon pepper
¼ cup chopped fresh basil (about
 ½ ounce)

In a 2-quart saucepan, prepare the rice using the package directions, substituting the broth for water and omitting the salt and margarine. Remove from the heat.

Add the lemon zest and lemon juice. Fluff with a fork.

Add the oil and pepper. Fluff again. Let cool slightly, about 5 minutes (this will help keep the basil greener when added).

Sprinkle with the basil. Fluff again.

COOK'S TIP on basil

Basil can easily turn brown when washed and chopped. To help keep it green, store it carefully so it doesn't bruise. Fill a bowl with cool water to wash. Remove the leaves from the stems. Swish the leaves in the water. Gently pat dry with paper towels (a salad spinner can bruise the delicate leaves). Finally, chop with a very sharp knife.

PER SERVING

CALORIES 90
TOTAL FAT 3.0 g
 Saturated Fat 0.5 g
 Trans Fat 0.0 g
 Polyunsaturated Fat 0.5 g
 Monounsaturated Fat 2.0 g
CHOLESTEROL 0 mg
SODIUM 14 mg
CARBOHYDRATES 14 g
 Fiber 1 g
 Sugars 0 g
PROTEIN 2 g
DIETARY EXCHANGES
 1 starch, ½ fat

risotto milanese

SERVES 8

Unlike most other risotto recipes, this one doesn't require constant stirring—all the creamy goodness without all the work!

2 tablespoons light tub margarine
1½ cups uncooked arborio rice
3 medium green onions, finely chopped
¼ cup dry white wine (regular or nonalcoholic)
4 cups fat-free, low-sodium chicken broth, such as on page 43

2 medium button mushrooms, chopped
⅛ teaspoon saffron or ½ teaspoon ground turmeric
2 tablespoons shredded or grated Parmesan cheese

In a large, heavy saucepan, melt the margarine over medium heat, swirling to coat the bottom. Stir in the rice and green onions. Cook for 2 to 3 minutes, or until the rice is milky, stirring constantly.

Stir in the wine. Continue to cook for 2 to 3 minutes, or until the wine is absorbed, stirring constantly.

Stir in the broth, mushrooms, and saffron. Increase the heat to medium high and bring to a boil, stirring occasionally. Reduce the heat to low. Cook, covered, for 20 minutes, or until the liquid is absorbed. Sprinkle with the Parmesan.

COOK'S TIP on arborio rice

While there are several types of rice particularly suited for use in risotto, arborio is perhaps the most popular due to its high starch content, giving risotto and other dishes a particular creaminess that no other rice provides.

COOK'S TIP on saffron

Saffron comes from the pistil of a certain crocus. Each flower has three threads called stigmas, and it takes more than 14,000 stigmas to make one ounce of saffron, which accounts for its very high cost. You can buy saffron in powder form or in threads; the threads are fresher and more flavorful. Crush them just before you use them.

PER SERVING

CALORIES 158
TOTAL FAT 2.0 g
  Saturated Fat 0.0 g
  Trans Fat 0.0 g
  Polyunsaturated Fat 0.5 g
  Monounsaturated Fat 1.0 g
CHOLESTEROL 1 mg
SODIUM 59 mg
CARBOHYDRATES 30 g
  Fiber 2 g
  Sugars 1 g
PROTEIN 5 g
DIETARY EXCHANGES
  2 starch

risotto with broccoli and leeks

SERVES 8

The key to making risotto delectably creamy is using arborio rice. This version gets its flavor from thyme and garlic.

2 medium leeks
3½ cups fat-free, low-sodium chicken broth, such as on page 43
½ cup dry white wine (regular or nonalcoholic) or fat-free, low-sodium chicken broth
2 teaspoons chopped fresh thyme or ½ teaspoon dried, crumbled
¼ teaspoon salt

⅛ teaspoon pepper
1 teaspoon olive oil
3 medium garlic cloves, minced
1 cup uncooked arborio rice
1 pound fresh or frozen broccoli florets, cut into bite-size pieces, cooked, and drained
¼ cup shredded or grated Parmesan or Romano cheese

Trim and discard the root ends from the leeks. Cut a 2- to 3-inch section of the white part from each leek. Cut the sections in half lengthwise, then cut crosswise into thin slices. Put the leeks in a small colander. Rinse well under cold water. Drain well.

In a large liquid measuring cup or other container with a handle and pouring spout, stir together the broth, wine, thyme, salt, and pepper. Set aside.

In a deep skillet, heat the oil over medium-high heat, swirling to coat the bottom. Cook the leeks and garlic for 2 to 3 minutes, or until the leeks are tender, stirring frequently.

Stir in the rice. Cook for 1 to 2 minutes, or until lightly toasted, stirring constantly.

Pour about ½ cup broth mixture into the skillet. Cook until the liquid is absorbed, stirring occasionally. Repeat the procedure until you've used all the liquid (the process takes 20 to 30 minutes). Reduce the heat to medium if the rice begins to stick excessively to the skillet.

Stir in the broccoli and Parmesan. Cook over medium heat for 2 to 3 minutes, or until the broccoli is heated through, stirring occasionally.

PER SERVING

CALORIES 150
TOTAL FAT 2.0 g
  Saturated Fat 0.5 g
  Trans Fat 0.0 g
  Polyunsaturated Fat 0.0 g
  Monounsaturated Fat 0.5 g
CHOLESTEROL 2 mg
SODIUM 150 mg
CARBOHYDRATES 27 g
  Fiber 3 g
  Sugars 2 g
PROTEIN 6 g
DIETARY EXCHANGES
  1½ starch, 1 vegetable

middle eastern brown rice

SERVES 8

Oranges and golden raisins add a Middle Eastern touch to wholesome brown rice.

1½ teaspoons light tub margarine
½ medium onion, minced
1 medium rib of celery, minced
1 cup uncooked brown rice
1½ cups water
1 cup fat-free, low-sodium chicken broth, such as on page 43

⅓ cup golden raisins
Zest of ½ medium orange, minced
1 medium orange, peeled and cut into small pieces
Dash of ground cloves
Fresh mint sprigs (optional)

In a medium saucepan, melt the margarine over medium-high heat, swirling to coat the bottom. Cook the onion and celery for 3 minutes, stirring occasionally.

Stir in the rice. Cook for 2 minutes.

Stir in the water, broth, raisins, and orange zest. Bring to a boil. Reduce the heat and simmer, covered, for 40 to 45 minutes, or until the liquid is absorbed.

Stir in the orange pieces and cloves. Garnish with the mint.

COOK'S TIP on raisins

Seedless raisins are made from seedless grapes. Golden raisins and dark raisins are made from the same grape but are dried differently. The golden ones are dried by artificial heat, and dark raisins are left in the sun for several weeks to achieve their deep color. This means that golden raisins are moister. Freezing raisins makes them easier to cut. If you're baking with raisins, coat them with some of the flour before adding to the batter. This will keep them from sinking to the bottom.

PER SERVING

CALORIES 123
TOTAL FAT 1.0 g
  Saturated Fat 0.0 g
  Trans Fat 0.0 g
  Polyunsaturated Fat 0.5 g
  Monounsaturated Fat 0.5 g
CHOLESTEROL 0 mg
SODIUM 19 mg
CARBOHYDRATES 26 g
  Fiber 2 g
  Sugars 7 g
PROTEIN 3 g
DIETARY EXCHANGES
  1 starch, ½ fruit

mexican fried rice

SERVES 6

Slightly browning the rice before cooking it imparts a mildly toasted flavor. Serve this traditional dish with fat-free refried beans and Shredded Beef Soft Tacos (page 293) for a Tex-Mex feast.

1 teaspoon canola or corn oil
1 cup uncooked rice
2 cups fat-free, low-sodium chicken broth, such as on page 43
⅔ cup canned chopped green chiles, drained

4 to 5 medium green onions, thinly sliced
½ cup diced tomatoes
1 medium garlic clove, minced

In a large, heavy nonstick skillet, heat the oil over medium-high heat, swirling to coat the bottom. Cook the rice for 2 to 3 minutes, or until golden brown, stirring constantly.

Stir in the remaining ingredients. Reduce the heat and simmer, covered, for 30 minutes, or until the rice is tender and the liquid is absorbed. Fluff with a fork.

PER SERVING

CALORIES 149
TOTAL FAT 1.0 g
  Saturated Fat 0.0 g
  Trans Fat 0.0 g
  Polyunsaturated Fat 0.5 g
  Monounsaturated Fat 0.5 g
CHOLESTEROL 0 mg
SODIUM 112 mg
CARBOHYDRATES 30 g
  Fiber 2 g
  Sugars 1 g
PROTEIN 3 g
DIETARY EXCHANGES
  2 starch

asian spinach and mushrooms

SERVES 4

Just a little sesame oil adds rich flavor to this vegetable combo.

2 teaspoons toasted sesame oil
1 cup sliced button mushrooms
¼ cup chopped shallots
1 tablespoon grated peeled gingerroot
1 tablespoon plain rice vinegar

8 cups loosely packed spinach, stems discarded
¼ teaspoon pepper
⅛ teaspoon salt

In a large skillet, heat the oil over medium heat, swirling to coat the bottom. Cook the mushrooms, shallots, gingerroot, and vinegar for 4 to 5 minutes, or until the mushrooms are tender, stirring occasionally.

Using tongs, combine the spinach with the mushroom mixture. Cook for 2 to 3 minutes, or just until the spinach is wilted, turning frequently with the tongs. Do not overcook.

Add the pepper and salt, turning to combine.

PER SERVING

CALORIES 46
TOTAL FAT 2.5 g
  Saturated Fat 0.5 g
  Trans Fat 0.0 g
  Polyunsaturated Fat 1.0 g
  Monounsaturated Fat 1.0 g
CHOLESTEROL 0 mg
SODIUM 123 mg
CARBOHYDRATES 5 g
  Fiber 2 g
  Sugars 1 g
PROTEIN 3 g
DIETARY EXCHANGES
  1 vegetable, ½ fat

spinach and brown rice casserole

SERVES 8

This casserole is quite filling, so you may want to serve it with a light entrée.

½ cup uncooked instant brown rice
Cooking spray
1 cup fat-free cottage cheese
2 tablespoons egg substitute
1½ teaspoons all-purpose flour
1½ teaspoons shredded or grated Parmesan cheese and 1½ tablespoons shredded or grated Parmesan cheese, divided use
¼ teaspoon dried thyme, crumbled
Pepper to taste

1 teaspoon light tub margarine
1 medium onion, chopped
1 or 2 medium garlic cloves, minced
5 ounces fresh spinach, stems discarded and leaves torn into bite-size pieces, or 5 ounces frozen chopped spinach, thawed and squeezed dry
4 ounces button mushrooms, sliced
1 tablespoon hulled unsalted sunflower seeds

Prepare the rice using the package directions, omitting the salt and margarine. Set aside.

Preheat the oven to 375°F. Lightly spray an 8-inch-square baking pan with cooking spray.

In a medium bowl, stir together the rice, cottage cheese, egg substitute, flour, 1½ teaspoons Parmesan, thyme, and pepper.

In a large saucepan, melt the margarine over medium-high heat, swirling to coat the bottom. Cook the onion and garlic for about 3 minutes, or until the onion is soft, stirring frequently.

Reduce the heat to low. Stir in the spinach and mushrooms. Cook, covered, for 3 minutes.

Stir in the rice mixture. Spoon into the baking pan. Sprinkle with the remaining 1½ tablespoons Parmesan and sunflower seeds.

Bake for 25 to 30 minutes.

PER SERVING

CALORIES 71
TOTAL FAT 1.5 g
  Saturated Fat 0.5 g
  Trans Fat 0.0 g
  Polyunsaturated Fat 0.5 g
  Monounsaturated Fat 0.5 g
CHOLESTEROL 2 mg
SODIUM 157 mg
CARBOHYDRATES 10 g
  Fiber 1 g
  Sugars 3 g
PROTEIN 6 g
DIETARY EXCHANGES
  ½ starch, ½ very lean meat

acorn squash stuffed with cranberries and walnuts

SERVES 6

A bounty of ingredients, including wine-red dried cranberries, fills mellow squash for a delectable dish.

STUFFING
- ¼ cup uncooked instant brown rice
- 1 cup unseasoned croutons
- 1 medium onion, finely chopped
- ½ cup fat-free, low-sodium chicken broth, such as on page 43
- ¼ cup sweetened dried cranberries
- 2 tablespoons chopped walnuts, dry-roasted
- 1 tablespoon light tub margarine

- 1 teaspoon dried sage
- ½ teaspoon dried thyme, crumbled
- ¼ teaspoon dried oregano, crumbled
- ¼ teaspoon salt
- ¼ teaspoon pepper

  ———
- 3 small acorn squash (about 4 inches in diameter), halved lengthwise, seeds and strings discarded
- ¼ cup water

Prepare the rice using the package directions, omitting the salt and margarine.

Preheat the oven to 400°F.

In a large bowl, stir together the rice and remaining stuffing ingredients. Fill the squash halves loosely with the stuffing mixture.

Pour the water into a 13 x 9 x 2-inch casserole dish. Place the squash halves with the filled side up in the dish.

Bake for 1 hour to 1 hour 15 minutes, or until the squash is tender when pierced with the tip of a sharp knife or a fork.

MICROWAVE METHOD

Put the acorn squash halves (unstuffed) with the cut side down in a microwaveable dish. Add ¼ cup water. Microwave, covered, on 100 percent power (high) for 5 minutes. Carefully remove the covering to avoid steam burns. Remove the squash from the dish, leaving the water. Fill the squash halves loosely with the stuffing mixture. Return to the dish. Microwave, covered, on 100 percent power (high) for 10 to 12 minutes, or until the squash is tender when pierced with the tip of a sharp knife.

PER SERVING

CALORIES 171
TOTAL FAT 3.0 g
  Saturated Fat 0.0 g
  Trans Fat 0.0 g
  Polyunsaturated Fat 1.5 g
  Monounsaturated Fat 0.5 g
CHOLESTEROL 0 mg
SODIUM 171 mg
CARBOHYDRATES 37 g
  Fiber 5 g
  Sugars 11 g
PROTEIN 4 g
DIETARY EXCHANGES
  2½ starch

butternut mash

SERVES 8

Savory spices and a spark of lime boost the flavor of yellow-orange butternut squash. Serve this side dish with a pork roast or seared chicken breasts.

1 2½-pound butternut squash, halved lengthwise, seeds and strings discarded
1 cup water
¼ cup fat-free half-and-half
2 medium garlic cloves, minced

2 teaspoons fresh lime juice
1 teaspoon ground cumin
1 teaspoon olive oil
¼ teaspoon salt
¼ teaspoon pepper

Place the squash with the cut side up in a large microwaveable dish. Pour the water around the squash. Microwave, covered, on 100 percent power (high) for 14 to 15 minutes, or until the squash is tender when tested with the tip of a sharp knife or a fork. Let cool for 3 to 4 minutes.

Meanwhile, in a small saucepan, cook the remaining ingredients over low heat for 2 to 3 minutes, stirring occasionally. Cover the pan.

Scoop the flesh from the squash into a medium bowl. Pour in the half-and-half mixture. Mash with a potato masher until smooth.

COOK'S TIP

To roast the squash instead, cut it in half vertically (see Cook's Tip on Cutting Winter Squash, page 56) and scoop out the seeds and strings. Place the squash with the cut sides up on a nonstick baking sheet. Bake in a preheated 350°F oven for 1 hour, or until tender when tested with the tip of a sharp knife or a fork.

PER SERVING

CALORIES 51
TOTAL FAT 0.5 g
    Saturated Fat 0.0 g
    Trans Fat 0.0 g
    Polyunsaturated Fat 0.0 g
    Monounsaturated Fat 0.5 g
CHOLESTEROL 0 mg
SODIUM 85 mg
CARBOHYDRATES 12 g
    Fiber 3 g
    Sugars 3 g
PROTEIN 2 g
DIETARY EXCHANGES
    1 starch

maple-glazed butternut squash

SERVES 4

The light touch of maple syrup and cinnamon makes nutritious squash a real winner.

1 1- to 1½-pound butternut squash, halved lengthwise, seeds and strings discarded
2 teaspoons light tub margarine

1 tablespoon plus 1 teaspoon maple syrup
¼ teaspoon ground cinnamon

Preheat the oven to 425°F.

Put the squash with the cut side up in a shallow baking pan. Put 1 teaspoon margarine in the hollow of each half.

In a small bowl, stir together the maple syrup and cinnamon. Pour into the hollows.

Bake the squash for 40 to 50 minutes, or until tender when tested with the tip of a sharp knife or a fork. Cut each piece in half lengthwise. Brush with the maple syrup mixture from the pan.

PER SERVING

CALORIES 63
TOTAL FAT 1.0 g
  Saturated Fat 0.0 g
  Trans Fat 0.0 g
  Polyunsaturated Fat 0.0 g
  Monounsaturated Fat 0.5 g
CHOLESTEROL 0 mg
SODIUM 20 mg
CARBOHYDRATES 15 g
  Fiber 3 g
  Sugars 6 g
PROTEIN 1 g
DIETARY EXCHANGES
  1 starch

pattypan squash with apple-nut stuffing

SERVES 4

Here's a summertime version of stuffed squash. Like its wintertime counterpart, stuffed acorn squash, it goes especially well with poultry and pork.

4 medium pattypan squash, unpeeled, halved crosswise, seeds discarded
2 medium baking apples, such as Rome Beauty, chopped
¼ cup sweetened dried cranberries

2½ tablespoons light brown sugar
2 tablespoons chopped walnuts or pecans
Fat-free spray margarine

Preheat the oven to 350°F.

Put the squash with the cut side down in a 13 x 9 x 2-inch glass baking dish.

Bake for 30 minutes.

Meanwhile, in a small bowl, stir together the remaining ingredients except the spray margarine. Spoon into the squash halves. Spray with the spray margarine.

Bake with the stuffed side up for 30 minutes, or until tender when tested with the tip of a sharp knife or a fork.

COOK'S TIP on pattypan squash

A white, yellow, or pale green summer squash, pattypan looks something like a scalloped flying saucer with a stem. Its unique shape makes it perfect for stuffing. (You may need to cut a slice from the bottom so the squash won't rock.) Use as you would yellow summer squash or zucchini.

PER SERVING

CALORIES 154
TOTAL FAT 3.0 g
  Saturated Fat 0.5 g
  Trans Fat 0.0 g
  Polyunsaturated Fat 2.0 g
  Monounsaturated Fat 0.5 g
CHOLESTEROL 0 mg
SODIUM 4 mg
CARBOHYDRATES 33 g
  Fiber 5 g
  Sugars 27 g
PROTEIN 3 g
DIETARY EXCHANGES
  1 fruit, 1 vegetable,
  1 carbohydrate, ½ fat

yellow summer squash casserole

SERVES 6

Tender cooked and mashed yellow summer squash enhanced with fresh sage and combined with soft bread crumbs tastes somewhat like bread stuffing.

Olive oil spray
½ teaspoon olive oil and 1 teaspoon olive oil, divided use
½ large onion, thinly sliced
1 pound yellow summer squash, diced
2 tablespoons fat-free, low-sodium chicken broth, such as on page 43
¾ teaspoon chopped fresh sage or ¼ teaspoon dried

1 medium garlic clove, minced
⅛ teaspoon salt
⅛ teaspoon pepper
1¼ cups soft whole-grain bread crumbs (lowest sodium available)
2 tablespoons shredded or grated Parmesan cheese

Lightly spray a medium saucepan with olive oil spray. Heat ½ teaspoon oil over medium-high heat, swirling to coat the bottom. Cook the onion for 8 to 10 minutes, or until golden, stirring occasionally.

Stir in the squash, broth, sage, garlic, salt, and pepper. Bring to a simmer. Reduce the heat and simmer, covered, for 10 to 12 minutes, or until the squash is tender.

Meanwhile, preheat the oven to 375°F.

In a medium bowl, stir together the bread crumbs, Parmesan, and remaining 1 teaspoon oil.

Using a potato masher, mash the squash mixture until slightly chunky. Pour into an 8-inch square baking dish. Spread the bread crumb mixture over the squash. Lightly spray with olive oil spray.

Bake for 25 to 30 minutes, or until the topping is golden brown and the squash mixture is heated through.

PER SERVING

CALORIES 66
TOTAL FAT 2.0 g
   Saturated Fat 0.5 g
   Trans Fat 0.0 g
   Polyunsaturated Fat 0.5 g
   Monounsaturated Fat 1.0 g
CHOLESTEROL 1 mg
SODIUM 135 mg
CARBOHYDRATES 9 g
   Fiber 2 g
   Sugars 3 g
PROTEIN 3 g
DIETARY EXCHANGES
   ½ starch, 1 vegetable, ½ fat

scalloped squash

SERVES 6

Serve this herb-flecked dish with Tilapia Amandine (page 180) and fresh green beans.

1 teaspoon light tub margarine
1 large onion, finely chopped
1½ pounds yellow summer squash, sliced
⅔ cup fat-free, low-sodium chicken broth, such as on page 43

1 teaspoon dried basil, crumbled
1 teaspoon dried thyme, crumbled
1 teaspoon dried marjoram, crumbled
¼ teaspoon salt
1¾ cups unseasoned croutons, crushed
¼ cup snipped fresh chives

In a large saucepan, melt the margarine over medium-high heat, swirling to coat the bottom. Cook the onion for about 3 minutes, or until soft, stirring frequently.

Stir in the squash, broth, basil, thyme, marjoram, and salt. Reduce the heat to medium. Cook, covered, for 10 minutes, or until the squash is tender.

Stir in the croutons. If the mixture is too dry, stir in a small amount of hot water. Stir in the chives.

sautéed red swiss chard

SERVES 4

With its pretty green leaves and ruby-hued stems, red Swiss chard is an especially colorful vegetable. This simple preparation brings out its natural flavor.

1 tablespoon olive oil
1 bunch red Swiss chard (about 12 ounces), stems cut crosswise into ½-inch slices and leaves coarsely chopped

1 medium garlic clove, minced
¼ teaspoon salt-free lemon pepper

In a large skillet, heat the oil over medium heat, swirling to coat the bottom. Cook the chard stems and garlic for 4 to 5 minutes, or until tender-crisp, stirring frequently.

Add the leaves. Using tongs, combine with the stems. Cook for 4 to 5 minutes, or until the leaves are wilted, turning several times with the tongs.

Sprinkle with the lemon pepper, using the tongs to combine.

PER SERVING

CALORIES 47
TOTAL FAT 3.5 g
  Saturated Fat 0.5 g
  Trans Fat 0.0 g
  Polyunsaturated Fat 0.5 g
  Monounsaturated Fat 2.5 g
CHOLESTEROL 0 mg
SODIUM 181 mg
CARBOHYDRATES 4 g
  Fiber 1 g
  Sugars 1 g
PROTEIN 2 g
DIETARY EXCHANGES
  1 vegetable, ½ fat

italian vegetable bake

SERVES 4

Try different kinds of mushroom and vary the herbs and vegetables to "invent" different side dishes from this basic recipe.

Olive oil spray	3 tablespoons light Italian salad
8 to 10 ounces mushrooms, any	dressing
variety or combination, sliced	2 teaspoons chopped fresh basil
1 small zucchini, thinly sliced	or ½ teaspoon dried, crumbled
4 medium Italian plum (Roma)	2 teaspoons chopped fresh oregano
tomatoes, sliced	or ½ teaspoon dried, crumbled
2 small green onions, thinly sliced	½ medium garlic clove, minced

Preheat the oven to 350°F. Lightly spray an 8-inch square glass baking dish with olive oil spray.

Make one layer each of the mushrooms, zucchini, tomatoes, and green onions in the baking dish.

In a small bowl, stir together the remaining ingredients. Drizzle over the vegetables.

Bake, covered, for 25 minutes, or until the vegetables are tender. Using a slotted spoon, remove the vegetables from the liquid.

PER SERVING

CALORIES 45
TOTAL FAT 1.0 g
  Saturated Fat 0.0 g
  Trans Fat 0.0 g
  Polyunsaturated Fat 0.5 g
  Monounsaturated Fat 0.5 g
CHOLESTEROL 1 mg
SODIUM 166 mg
CARBOHYDRATES 7 g
  Fiber 2 g
  Sugars 4 g
PROTEIN 3 g
DIETARY EXCHANGES
  1 vegetable

roasted veggies with sesame seeds

SERVES 4

Roasting carrots, zucchini, and onion brings out their natural richness. A sprinkling of sesame seed adds a nice crunchiness.

2 medium carrots, quartered diagonally	1 tablespoon sesame seeds
1 medium zucchini, quartered and cut into 2-inch pieces, or 1 medium red bell pepper, cut into thin strips	Cooking spray
	1½ tablespoons soy sauce (lowest sodium available)
1 medium onion, cut into ½-inch wedges	1 tablespoon cider vinegar
	1 tablespoon sugar

Preheat the oven to 425°F.

Arrange the carrots, zucchini, and onion in a single layer on a nonstick baking sheet. Sprinkle with the sesame seeds. Lightly spray the vegetables with cooking spray.

Bake for 16 minutes, or until the vegetables begin to brown on the edges, stirring once halfway through.

Meanwhile, in a small bowl, stir together the soy sauce, vinegar, and sugar.

Transfer the vegetables to a small rimmed platter or shallow dish. Spoon the soy sauce mixture over all. Don't stir.

COOK'S TIP on roasting vegetables

It's important to arrange vegetables in a single layer when roasting to allow them to brown properly.

PER SERVING

CALORIES 65
TOTAL FAT 1.5 g
 Saturated Fat 0.0 g
 Trans Fat 0.0 g
 Polyunsaturated Fat 0.5 g
 Monounsaturated Fat 0.5 g
CHOLESTEROL 0 mg
SODIUM 179 mg
CARBOHYDRATES 12 g
 Fiber 3 g
 Sugars 8 g
PROTEIN 2 g
DIETARY EXCHANGES
 2 vegetable, ½ fat

vegetable stir-fry

SERVES 4

This quick side dish features the unusual seasoning combination of nutmeg and thyme.

8 ounces fresh broccoli
1 teaspoon light tub margarine
1 teaspoon canola or corn oil
8 ounces carrots, thinly sliced
6 ounces button mushrooms, thinly sliced
1 to 2 medium green onions, thinly sliced

1 tablespoon dry sherry
1½ teaspoons fresh lemon juice
½ teaspoon ground nutmeg
½ teaspoon dried thyme, crumbled
Pepper to taste

Separate the broccoli florets so they are of a small, uniform size. Peel the tough stems. Cut the stems into 2-inch pieces.

In a large skillet, heat the margarine and oil over medium heat, swirling to coat the bottom. Stir-fry the broccoli, carrots, mushrooms, and green onions for 5 minutes, or until tender-crisp, stirring constantly.

Stir in the remaining ingredients.

PER SERVING

CALORIES 74
TOTAL FAT 2.0 g
  Saturated Fat 0.0 g
  Trans Fat 0.0 g
  Polyunsaturated Fat 0.5 g
  Monounsaturated Fat 1.0 g
CHOLESTEROL 0 mg
SODIUM 69 mg
CARBOHYDRATES 12 g
  Fiber 4 g
  Sugars 5 g
PROTEIN 4 g
DIETARY EXCHANGES
  2 vegetable, ½ fat

southwestern ratatouille

SERVES 8

Southwestern spices combine with traditional Provençal vegetables in this version of ratatouille. It is equally good hot or cold.

1 medium eggplant, peeled and diced
¼ teaspoon salt
1 teaspoon olive oil
1 medium onion, finely chopped
1 medium red or green bell pepper, cut into thin strips
2 tablespoons minced garlic
2 teaspoons dried oregano, crumbled
2 teaspoons chili powder
2 teaspoons ground cumin
3 sprigs of fresh thyme, leaves removed and crushed and stems discarded, or ½ teaspoon dried, crumbled

¼ teaspoon crushed red pepper flakes
4 large tomatoes, seeded and chopped
2 medium zucchini, sliced
2 tablespoons finely snipped fresh parsley
1½ tablespoons shredded or grated Parmesan cheese

Put the eggplant in a colander. Sprinkle with salt. Let stand for 30 minutes. Rinse well. Pat dry with paper towels.

In a large skillet, heat the oil over medium-high heat, swirling to coat the bottom. Cook the onion, bell pepper, and garlic for 2 minutes, or until tender-crisp, stirring frequently.

Stir in the oregano, chili powder, cumin, thyme, and red pepper flakes. Stir in the tomatoes. Reduce the heat and simmer for 4 to 5 minutes.

Stir in the eggplant and zucchini. Simmer, covered, for 20 minutes.

Stir in the parsley and Parmesan. Serve or cover and refrigerate to serve chilled.

COOK'S TIP on eggplant

Salting eggplant and letting it stand awhile before rinsing helps draw out the bitterness and excess moisture.

PER SERVING

CALORIES 65
TOTAL FAT 1.5 g
  Saturated Fat 0.5 g
  Trans Fat 0.0 g
  Polyunsaturated Fat 0.5 g
  Monounsaturated Fat 0.5 g
CHOLESTEROL 1 mg
SODIUM 109 mg
CARBOHYDRATES 12 g
  Fiber 5 g
  Sugars 6 g
PROTEIN 3 g
DIETARY EXCHANGES
  2 vegetable, ½ fat

apple dressing

SERVES 12

For a warming fall or winter meal, serve this apple-sage dressing with Orange Sweet Potatoes (page 467) and roasted turkey breast or pork tenderloin.

Cooking spray
1 teaspoon light tub margarine
¼ cup chopped onion
½ medium rib of celery, chopped
4 cups toasted whole-grain bread cubes or 6 cups fresh whole-grain bread cubes (lowest sodium available)

1 cup diced unpeeled apple
½ teaspoon poultry seasoning
½ teaspoon dried sage
Pepper to taste
½ cup fat-free, low-sodium chicken broth, such as on page 43

Preheat the oven to 350°F. Lightly spray a 13 x 9 x 2-inch glass baking dish with cooking spray.

In a small skillet, melt the margarine over medium-high heat, swirling to coat the bottom. Cook the onion and celery for 5 minutes, or until soft, stirring frequently. Transfer to a large bowl.

Stir the remaining ingredients except the broth into the onion mixture. Gently stir in the broth. Transfer to the baking dish.

Bake, covered, for 45 minutes.

DRESSING WITH MIXED DRIED FRUIT

Omit the apple. In a small saucepan, stir together 1 cup chopped dried fruit, such as apricots, prunes, or peaches, or a combination, and ½ cup sweetened dried cranberries or raisins. Add water to cover. Simmer, covered, for 20 minutes. Drain well in a colander. Let cool slightly. Proceed as directed.

PER SERVING

CALORIES 44
TOTAL FAT 0.5 g
  Saturated Fat 0.0 g
  Trans Fat 0.0 g
  Polyunsaturated Fat 0.0 g
  Monounsaturated Fat 0.5 g
CHOLESTEROL 0 mg
SODIUM 72 mg
CARBOHYDRATES 8 g
  Fiber 1 g
  Sugars 2 g
PROTEIN 2 g
DIETARY EXCHANGES
  ½ starch

PER SERVING

DRESSING WITH MIXED DRIED FRUIT
CALORIES 84
TOTAL FAT 0.5 g
  Saturated Fat 0.0 g
  Trans Fat 0.0 g
  Polyunsaturated Fat 0.0 g
  Monounsaturated Fat 0.5 g
CHOLESTEROL 0 mg
SODIUM 73 mg
CARBOHYDRATES 18 g
  Fiber 2 g
  Sugars 11 g
PROTEIN 2 g
DIETARY EXCHANGES
  ½ starch, 1 fruit

cranberry chutney

SERVES 16

Especially good with curried meat dishes, this chutney also pairs well with turkey and chicken. The serving size is more for a condiment than a true side dish.

1 pound whole fresh cranberries
8 ounces dates, chopped
1¼ cups water
1 cup sugar
1 cup golden raisins
¾ cup cider vinegar
¼ cup fresh orange juice
1 tablespoon grated lemon zest

½ teaspoon salt
½ teaspoon ground cinnamon
½ teaspoon ground ginger
¼ to 1 teaspoon crushed red pepper flakes
¼ teaspoon ground allspice
⅛ teaspoon ground cloves

In a large saucepan, stir together the ingredients. Bring to a boil over medium-high heat. Reduce the heat and simmer, covered, for 15 minutes, stirring occasionally.

Transfer to a glass jar with a tight-fitting lid and refrigerate. Use within two weeks.

COOK'S TIP

For a longer shelf life, spoon the mixture into hot sterilized jars. Follow the jar manufacturer's directions for sealing the jars. Process for 10 minutes in a boiling water bath (the water should cover the jars by 1 to 2 inches). Remove the jars from the water. Let cool for at least 12 hours at room temperature. Then check to be sure the seal is tight (there should be no air pocket when you press the center of the lid).

PER SERVING

CALORIES 140
TOTAL FAT 0.0 g
  Saturated Fat 0.0 g
  Trans Fat 0.0 g
  Polyunsaturated Fat 0.0 g
  Monounsaturated Fat 0.0 g
CHOLESTEROL 0 mg
SODIUM 76 mg
CARBOHYDRATES 36 g
  Fiber 3 g
  Sugars 30 g
PROTEIN 1 g
DIETARY EXCHANGES
  1½ fruit, 1 carbohydrate

baked curried fruit

SERVES 8

When the weather turns cold, serve this spicy fruit for brunch or instead of salad at dinner.

Cooking spray
1 15.25-ounce can pineapple chunks in their own juice, well drained
1 15-ounce can peaches in fruit juice, well drained
1 14.5-ounce can Bing cherries, well drained
1 11-ounce can mandarin oranges in juice, well drained
½ cup firmly packed light brown sugar
1½ teaspoons curry powder
2 tablespoons fresh lemon juice
1 tablespoon plus 1 teaspoon light tub margarine

Preheat the oven to 300°F. Lightly spray a shallow 12 x 8 x 2-inch casserole dish with cooking spray.

Spoon the pineapple, peaches, cherries, and mandarin oranges into the dish, stirring to combine.

In a small bowl, stir together the brown sugar and curry powder. Sprinkle over the fruit.

Sprinkle the fruit with the lemon juice. Dot with the margarine.

Bake, covered, for 45 minutes.

PER SERVING

CALORIES 153
TOTAL FAT 1.0 g
 Saturated Fat 0.0 g
 Trans Fat 0.0 g
 Polyunsaturated Fat 0.0 g
 Monounsaturated Fat 0.5 g
CHOLESTEROL 0 mg
SODIUM 31 mg
CARBOHYDRATES 37 g
 Fiber 2 g
 Sugars 31 g
PROTEIN 1 g
DIETARY EXCHANGES
 1 fruit, 1½ carbohydrate

baked pears with honey almonds

SERVES 4

Curry coupled with drizzles of honey makes these baked pears a great side dish or the perfect ending for any meal.

2 large pears (about 1 pound total), halved and cored
¼ cup finely chopped dried apricots
1 teaspoon light tub margarine
¼ teaspoon curry powder

1 tablespoon fresh lemon juice
2 tablespoons slivered almonds, dry-roasted
1 tablespoon plus 1 teaspoon honey

Preheat the oven to 350°F.

In a pie pan, arrange the pears with the cut side up. Fill each pear half with apricots.

In a small bowl, stir together the margarine and curry powder. Dot on each pear half.

Drizzle the lemon juice over the pears.

Bake, covered, for 40 minutes, or until the pears are tender when pierced with a fork. Sprinkle with the almonds. Drizzle with the honey.

COOK'S TIP

Using almond slivers rather than the thin slices gives a crunchier texture to this dish.

PER SERVING

CALORIES 132
TOTAL FAT 2.0 g
  Saturated Fat 0.0 g
  Trans Fat 0.0 g
  Polyunsaturated Fat 0.5 g
  Monounsaturated Fat 1.5 g
CHOLESTEROL 0 mg
SODIUM 10 mg
CARBOHYDRATES 30 g
  Fiber 5 g
  Sugars 22 g
PROTEIN 2 g
DIETARY EXCHANGES
  2 fruit, ½ fat

microwave baked apple slices

SERVES 4

This dish is so easy, you'll want to make it every time you serve pork chops or pork tenderloin or baked chicken or meat loaf—you get the idea! It's even great as a quick dessert or after-school snack for the kids.

Cooking spray
1 pound unpeeled apples, cored and cut into ½-inch wedges
1½ tablespoons sugar

1 tablespoon light tub margarine
½ teaspoon ground cinnamon
¼ teaspoon vanilla extract

Lightly spray a 9-inch glass baking dish with cooking spray. Spread the apples in the dish. Microwave, covered, on 100 percent (high) for 2½ minutes, or until just tender. Remove from the microwave.

Add the remaining ingredients, stirring until the margarine is melted.

grilled pineapple

SERVES 6

While you're grilling your entrée, put some fruit on to grill for a side dish as well. After you've tried pineapple, branch out to other seasonal fruits (see the Cook's Tip below). You can use the lemon-honey mixture in this recipe for any of these alternatives.

¼ cup honey
½ teaspoon grated lemon zest
1 tablespoon fresh lemon juice

¼ teaspoon ground cinnamon
1 medium pineapple, peeled and cut into 12 spears

Preheat the grill on medium.

In a small bowl, stir together all the ingredients except the pineapple.

Grill the pineapple directly on the grill rack for 6 to 8 minutes, or until tender, turning once halfway through. Transfer to plates. Brush with the honey mixture. Serve immediately.

COOK'S TIP for grilled fruit

For the best results, all fruit for grilling should be ripe but still firm. Peaches should be halved and pitted, then grilled for 8 to 10 minutes. Cut peeled mangoes lengthwise into slabs (about 4 per mango); grill for 4 to 6 minutes. Grill whole bananas or halve them lengthwise, then grill for 4 to 6 minutes. Regardless of the fruit you choose, turn it once about halfway through the grilling time.

PER SERVING
CALORIES 119
TOTAL FAT 0.0 g
  Saturated Fat 0.0 g
  Trans Fat 0.0 g
  Polyunsaturated Fat 0.0 g
  Monounsaturated Fat 0.0 g
CHOLESTEROL 0 mg
SODIUM 2 mg
CARBOHYDRATES 32 g
  Fiber 2 g
  Sugars 26 g
PROTEIN 1 g
DIETARY EXCHANGES
  1 fruit, 1 carbohydrate

sauces and gravies

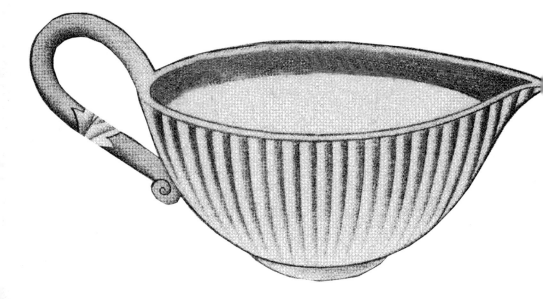

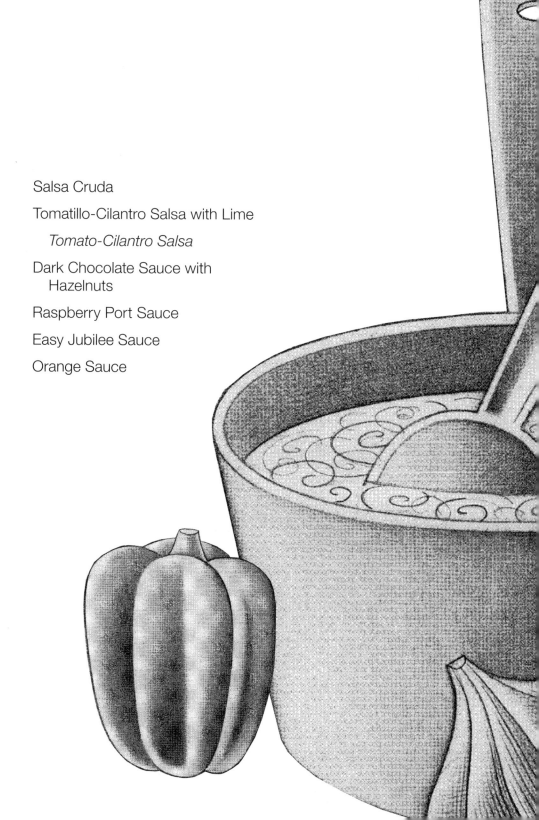

basic gravy

SERVES 4; ¼ CUP PER SERVING

Adjust the amount of flour according to whether you want thin, medium, or thick gravy. This recipe doubles or triples well.

2 to 4 tablespoons all-purpose flour
½ cup fat-free, low-sodium chicken broth or fat-free, no-salt-added beef broth and ½ cup fat-free, low-sodium chicken broth or fat-free, no-salt-added beef broth, such as on pages 43 and 42, divided use

¼ teaspoon salt

In a medium skillet, cook the flour over medium-high heat for 5 to 6 minutes, or until lightly colored, stirring occasionally. Transfer to a small bowl.

Pour ½ cup broth into the flour, whisking until smooth. Pour into the skillet.

Whisk in the salt and remaining ½ cup broth. Bring to a simmer over medium heat. Cook until the desired consistency, whisking constantly.

MUSHROOM GRAVY
In a small skillet over medium heat, cook ¼ cup sliced button mushrooms in 2 tablespoons of the same broth used in the gravy. Stir into the cooked gravy.

PER SERVING

CALORIES 24
TOTAL FAT 0.0 g
  Saturated Fat 0.0 g
  Trans Fat 0.0 g
  Polyunsaturated Fat 0.0 g
  Monounsaturated Fat 0.0 g
CHOLESTEROL 0 mg
SODIUM 152 mg
CARBOHYDRATES 5 g
  Fiber 0 g
  Sugars 0 g
PROTEIN 1 g
DIETARY EXCHANGES
  ½ starch

creamy chicken gravy

SERVES 4; ¼ CUP PER SERVING

Everyone needs a recipe for basic chicken gravy. This one is about as simple as a recipe can be.

1 cup fat-free, low-sodium chicken broth, such as on page 43	2 tablespoons all-purpose flour
¼ cup fat-free milk	½ teaspoon pepper, or to taste
	¼ teaspoon salt

In a medium saucepan, warm the broth over medium heat.

In a small bowl, whisk together the remaining ingredients until smooth. Gradually whisk into the broth. Cook for 3 to 5 minutes, or until thickened, whisking constantly.

PER SERVING

CALORIES 23
TOTAL FAT 0.0 g
  Saturated Fat 0.0 g
  Trans Fat 0.0 g
  Polyunsaturated Fat 0.0 g
  Monounsaturated Fat 0.0 g
CHOLESTEROL 0 mg
SODIUM 158 mg
CARBOHYDRATES 4 g
  Fiber 0 g
  Sugars 1 g
PROTEIN 1 g
DIETARY EXCHANGES
  Free

basic white sauce

SERVES 4; ¼ CUP PER SERVING

Here's an easy, fat-free version of classic white sauce. For the basic sauce, use 2 tablespoons of flour; for a thick sauce, use 3 to 4 tablespoons.

1 cup fat-free milk	¼ teaspoon salt
2 to 4 tablespoons all-purpose flour	Dash of white pepper, or to taste

In a small saucepan, whisk together the ingredients. Bring just to a boil over medium-high heat, whisking occasionally. Reduce the heat to medium and cook for 1 to 2 minutes, or until thickened, whisking occasionally.

COOK'S TIP

For a different flavor, add a hint of curry powder, dried dillweed, or dried nutmeg.

PER SERVING

CALORIES 42
TOTAL FAT 0.0 g
  Saturated Fat 0.0 g
  Trans Fat 0.0 g
  Polyunsaturated Fat 0.0 g
  Monounsaturated Fat 0.0 g
CHOLESTEROL 1 mg
SODIUM 171 mg
CARBOHYDRATES 8 g
  Fiber 0 g
  Sugars 3 g
PROTEIN 3 g
DIETARY EXCHANGES
  ½ starch

walnut cream sauce

SERVES 4; ¼ CUP PER SERVING

A delicious toasted walnut flavor permeates this rich-tasting sauce. It's especially good over poached chicken or grilled fish.

2 tablespoons chopped walnuts	½ teaspoon dried marjoram, crumbled
1 medium shallot, finely chopped	⅛ teaspoon salt
1 cup fat-free milk	2 tablespoons shredded or grated
1½ tablespoons all-purpose flour	Romano or Parmesan cheese
1 teaspoon Creole mustard or coarse-grain mustard	

Put the nuts in a single layer in a medium saucepan. Dry-roast over medium heat for about 4 minutes, or just until fragrant, stirring frequently.

Stir in the shallot. Cook for 2 minutes, or until the shallot is tender-crisp, stirring occasionally.

Whisk in the remaining ingredients except the Romano cheese until the flour is dissolved (there may be a few lumps). Increase the heat to medium high and bring to a simmer, whisking occasionally. Reduce the heat and simmer for 2 to 3 minutes, or until thickened, whisking occasionally. Remove from the heat.

Add the Romano, whisking constantly until the cheese is melted.

PER SERVING

CALORIES 69
TOTAL FAT 3.0 g
   Saturated Fat 0.5 g
   Trans Fat 0.0 g
   Polyunsaturated Fat 2.0 g
   Monounsaturated Fat 0.5 g
CHOLESTEROL 3 mg
SODIUM 163 mg
CARBOHYDRATES 7 g
   Fiber 0 g
   Sugars 3 g
PROTEIN 4 g
DIETARY EXCHANGES
   ½ starch, ½ fat

yogurt-tahini sauce

SERVES 8; 2 TABLESPOONS PER SERVING

Serve this sauce with grilled salmon or tuna, over steamed or grilled vegetables, or even on a burger.

¾ cup low-fat plain Greek yogurt
2 tablespoons snipped fresh cilantro
2 tablespoons tahini
1 tablespoon fresh lemon juice

¼ teaspoon ground cumin
⅛ teaspoon salt
Pinch of cayenne pepper

In a medium bowl, whisk together all the ingredients. Serve or cover and refrigerate for up to two days.

COOK'S TIP on tahini

Tahini, which is made from ground sesame seeds, is a staple of Middle Eastern cooking. It is typically used in preparing hummus and baba ghanouj. Look for it in the ethnic aisles at the supermarket.

COOK'S TIP on greek yogurt

Greek yogurt has had the whey (liquid) drained off, rendering the end product thick and creamy.

PER SERVING

CALORIES 37
TOTAL FAT 2.5 g
　Saturated Fat 0.5 g
　Trans Fat 0.0 g
　Polyunsaturated Fat 1.0 g
　Monounsaturated Fat 1.0 g
CHOLESTEROL 1 mg
SODIUM 45 mg
CARBOHYDRATES 2 g
　Fiber 0 g
　Sugars 1 g
PROTEIN 3 g
DIETARY EXCHANGES
　½ fat

creamy dijon-lime sauce

SERVES 6; 2 TABLESPOONS PER SERVING

Serve this terrifically quick sauce at room temperature over chilled vegetables, such as fresh tomato slices or slightly steamed and chilled asparagus, or heat it to serve over steamed vegetables such as broccoli, cauliflower, lima beans, green beans, or carrots.

⅓ cup fat-free plain yogurt
1 tablespoon plus 1 teaspoon Dijon mustard
1 teaspoon fresh lime juice

⅛ teaspoon salt
1 tablespoon olive oil (extra virgin preferred)

In a small bowl, whisk together all the ingredients except the oil until smooth.

If using over chilled vegetables, stir in the oil. If using over hot vegetables, heat the sauce in a small saucepan over medium-low heat. Don't allow to boil. Remove from the heat. Stir in the oil.

COOK'S TIP

You'll get a more pronounced flavor from the olive oil by adding it after you take the sauce off the heat.

PER SERVING

CALORIES 32
TOTAL FAT 2.5 g
   Saturated Fat 0.5 g
   Trans Fat 0.0 g
   Polyunsaturated Fat 0.0 g
   Monounsaturated Fat 1.5 g
CHOLESTEROL 0 mg
SODIUM 128 mg
CARBOHYDRATES 2 g
   Fiber 0 g
   Sugars 1 g
PROTEIN 1 g
DIETARY EXCHANGES
   ½ fat

sour cream sauce with dill

SERVES 4; ¼ CUP PER SERVING

Enjoy this sauce three ways. Try the dill sauce over grilled or poached salmon, the garlic variation over boiled red potatoes, and the blue cheese version over steamed broccoli.

8 ounces fat-free sour cream
1 tablespoon snipped fresh dillweed
1 tablespoon minced green onions
   (green part only)

½ teaspoon pepper
2 to 3 tablespoons fat-free milk
   (optional)

In a medium bowl, whisk together all the ingredients except the milk. Thin the mixture with the milk, if desired. Cover and refrigerate.

COOK'S TIP on dillweed

Formerly used in charms against witchcraft, dillweed now leads a less exotic existence. It's used primarily to flavor pickles, sauces, and soups. Because its leaves are feathery, fragrant dillweed also makes a pretty garnish.

COOK'S TIP on snipping fresh herbs

Put pieces of a fresh herb in a measuring cup or coffee mug. Using kitchen scissors, snip the herb until the pieces are the desired fineness.

PER SERVING

WITH DILL OR GARLIC
CALORIES 55
TOTAL FAT 0.0 g
   Saturated Fat 0.0 g
   Trans Fat 0.0 g
   Polyunsaturated Fat 0.0 g
   Monounsaturated Fat 0.0 g
CHOLESTEROL 9 mg
SODIUM 45 mg
CARBOHYDRATES 9 g
   Fiber 0 g
   Sugars 4 g
PROTEIN 4 g
DIETARY EXCHANGES
   ½ starch

For each variation, omit the dill and stir the listed ingredients into the sauce on page 500 before refrigerating.

SOUR CREAM SAUCE WITH GARLIC

SERVES 4; ¼ CUP PER SERVING
- 1 tablespoon finely snipped fresh parsley
- ¼ teaspoon garlic powder
- Dash of red hot-pepper sauce

SOUR CREAM SAUCE WITH BLUE CHEESE

SERVES 5; ¼ CUP PER SERVING
- 3 tablespoons crumbled blue cheese
- ¼ teaspoon Worcestershire sauce (lowest sodium available)

PER SERVING

WITH BLUE CHEESE
CALORIES 62
TOTAL FAT 1.5 g
  Saturated Fat 1.0 g
  Trans Fat 0.0 g
  Polyunsaturated Fat 0.0 g
  Monounsaturated Fat 0.5 g
CHOLESTEROL 11 mg
SODIUM 108 mg
CARBOHYDRATES 8 g
  Fiber 0 g
  Sugars 3 g
PROTEIN 4 g
DIETARY EXCHANGES
  ½ starch

mild mustard sauce

SERVES 4; 2 TABLESPOONS PER SERVING

Buttermilk gives this sauce a gentle zing that complements just about any vegetable. Serve it chilled over cold or room-temperature blanched vegetables or warm over hot cooked vegetables.

⅓ cup low-fat buttermilk

2 tablespoons light mayonnaise

1 teaspoon bottled yellow mustard

In a medium bowl, whisk together the ingredients until smooth.

If using over cold or room temperature vegetables, cover and refrigerate the sauce until chilled. If using over hot vegetables, heat the sauce in a small saucepan over low heat for 2 to 3 minutes, or until warm.

PER SERVING

CALORIES 27
TOTAL FAT 2.0 g
  Saturated Fat 0.0 g
  Trans Fat 0.0 g
  Polyunsaturated Fat 1.5 g
  Monounsaturated Fat 0.5 g
CHOLESTEROL 3 mg
SODIUM 101 mg
CARBOHYDRATES 2 g
  Fiber 0 g
  Sugars 1 g
PROTEIN 1 g
DIETARY EXCHANGES
  ½ fat

bourbon barbecue sauce

SERVES 6; ¼ CUP PER SERVING

Chile powder adds deep color and a slight bite to this barbecue sauce.

⅓ cup bourbon
¼ cup finely chopped sweet onion, such as Maui or OsoSweet
2 medium garlic cloves, minced
1 8-ounce can no-salt-added tomato sauce
3 tablespoons cider vinegar
3 tablespoons light or dark molasses
2 tablespoons packed light or dark brown sugar
1 tablespoon no-salt-added tomato paste
1 tablespoon Worcestershire sauce (lowest sodium available)
1 teaspoon chile powder (made with ancho chiles preferred)
1 teaspoon dry mustard
½ teaspoon ground cumin
¼ teaspoon pepper
¼ teaspoon liquid smoke (optional)

In a medium saucepan, stir together the bourbon, onion, and garlic. Bring to a boil over high heat. Reduce the heat and simmer for 4 to 6 minutes, or until the onion is soft and the liquid has nearly evaporated.

Stir in the remaining ingredients. Increase the heat to medium high and return to a boil. Reduce the heat and simmer for 6 to 8 minutes, or until the desired thickness, stirring occasionally. Refrigerate any leftover sauce for up to one week in an airtight container.

PER SERVING

CALORIES 101
TOTAL FAT 0.5 g
　Saturated Fat 0.0 g
　Trans Fat 0.0 g
　Polyunsaturated Fat 0.0 g
　Monounsaturated Fat 0.0 g
CHOLESTEROL 0 mg
SODIUM 22 mg
CARBOHYDRATES 17 g
　Fiber 1 g
　Sugars 14 g
PROTEIN 1 g
DIETARY EXCHANGES
　1 carbohydrate

mock hollandaise sauce

SERVES 4; ¼ CUP PER SERVING

By using chicken broth and a small amount of oil instead of lots of butter, you can prepare a heart-healthy hollandaise sauce that will dress up many dishes in your repertory.

1 tablespoon cornstarch
1 tablespoon canola or corn oil
¾ cup fat-free, low-sodium chicken broth, such as on page 43

2 tablespoons egg substitute
1 to 2 tablespoons fresh lemon juice

In a small saucepan, whisk together the cornstarch and oil. Cook over low heat for 1 minute, or until smooth, whisking constantly.

Whisk in the broth. Increase the heat to medium high. Cook for 3 to 4 minutes, or until thickened, whisking constantly. Remove from the heat.

Slowly whisk the egg substitute into the sauce. Cook over low heat for 1 minute, whisking constantly. Remove from the heat.

Whisk in the lemon juice.

COOK'S TIP on juicing lemons

Before you cut a lemon, let it reach room temperature if it's been refrigerated. Then roll it on the counter while pressing down hard with your hand. This will cause the lemon to release more of its juice.

PER SERVING

CALORIES 46
TOTAL FAT 3.5 g
  Saturated Fat 0.5 g
  Trans Fat 0.0 g
  Polyunsaturated Fat 1.0 g
  Monounsaturated Fat 2.0 g
CHOLESTEROL 0 mg
SODIUM 21 mg
CARBOHYDRATES 3 g
  Fiber 0 g
  Sugars 0 g
PROTEIN 1 g
DIETARY EXCHANGES
  1 fat

mock béarnaise sauce

SERVES 4; ¼ CUP PER SERVING

Turn poached fish or steamed vegetables into something special with this elegant sauce.

¼ cup white wine vinegar
¼ cup dry white wine (regular or nonalcoholic) or dry vermouth
1 tablespoon minced shallot or green onions (green part only)
1 tablespoon minced fresh tarragon or 1 teaspoon dried, crumbled

⅛ teaspoon pepper (white preferred)
1 tablespoon cornstarch
1 tablespoon canola or corn oil
¾ cup fat-free, low-sodium chicken broth, such as on page 43
2 tablespoons egg substitute

In a small saucepan, whisk together the vinegar, wine, shallot, tarragon, and pepper. Bring to a boil over medium-high heat, whisking constantly. Cook for 4 to 5 minutes, or until reduced to about 2 tablespoons. Set aside.

In another small saucepan, whisk together the cornstarch and oil. Cook over low heat for 1 minute, or until smooth, whisking constantly.

Whisk the broth into the cornstarch mixture. Increase the heat to medium high. Cook for 3 to 4 minutes, or until thickened, whisking constantly. Remove from the heat.

Slowly whisk the egg substitute into the cornstarch mixture. Cook over low heat for 1 minute, whisking constantly. Remove from the heat.

Whisk in the vinegar mixture.

PER SERVING

CALORIES 62
TOTAL FAT 3.5 g
   Saturated Fat 0.5 g
   Trans Fat 0.0 g
   Polyunsaturated Fat 1.0 g
   Monounsaturated Fat 2.0 g
CHOLESTEROL 0 mg
SODIUM 22 mg
CARBOHYDRATES 4 g
   Fiber 0 g
   Sugars 0 g
PROTEIN 1 g
DIETARY EXCHANGES
   1 fat

fresh tomato and roasted red bell pepper sauce

SERVES 8; ¼ CUP PER SERVING

If you need a side dish for tonight's meal, serve this great-tasting sauce over whole-grain pasta. For an entrée instead, try it over chicken, fish, or pork.

1 tablespoon olive oil and
   1 tablespoon olive oil (extra virgin preferred), divided use
1 medium onion, finely chopped
4 medium garlic cloves, minced
1 pound Italian plum (Roma) tomatoes, coarsely chopped

3 ounces canned no-salt-added tomato paste
1 cup roasted red bell peppers, rinsed and drained if bottled, chopped
¼ cup chopped fresh basil or 1 tablespoon plus 1 teaspoon dried, crumbled

In a large saucepan, heat 1 tablespoon oil over medium-high heat until hot, swirling to coat the bottom. Cook the onion for 3 minutes, or until soft, stirring frequently.

Stir in the garlic. Cook for 10 seconds, stirring constantly.

Stir in the tomatoes and tomato paste. Bring to a boil. Reduce the heat and simmer, covered, for 25 minutes, or until the tomatoes are soft. Remove the pan from the heat.

Stir in the roasted peppers, basil, and remaining 1 tablespoon oil. Let stand, covered, for 10 minutes so the flavors blend.

COOK'S TIP

The variety of tomato makes a difference, especially when using a large amount, as in this sauce. If you substitute grape tomatoes, the sauce will be sweeter; if you use a regular tomato, the sauce will be thinner.

PER SERVING

CALORIES 118
TOTAL FAT 7.0 g
  Saturated Fat 1.0 g
  Trans Fat 0.0 g
  Polyunsaturated Fat 1.0 g
  Monounsaturated Fat 5.0 g
CHOLESTEROL 0 mg
SODIUM 59 mg
CARBOHYDRATES 14 g
  Fiber 3 g
  Sugars 8 g
PROTEIN 2 g
DIETARY EXCHANGES
  3 vegetable, 1½ fat

tomato sauce

SERVES 16; ¼ CUP PER SERVING

This easy sauce is good over stuffed bell peppers, meat loaf, or stuffed cabbage. Since it makes enough for several meals, freeze what you don't use and try it with a different entrée another time.

1 28-ounce can no-salt-added Italian plum (Roma) tomatoes	2 medium garlic cloves, minced
1 large onion, diced	1 teaspoon salt
3 tablespoons no-salt-added tomato paste	½ teaspoon pepper, or to taste
	½ teaspoon dried oregano, crumbled
	½ teaspoon dried basil, crumbled

In a medium saucepan, stir together the ingredients. Bring to a boil over medium-high heat. Reduce the heat and simmer, covered, for 20 minutes.

CREOLE SAUCE

Add 1 diced medium green bell pepper, 2 ounces sliced button mushrooms, and 1 medium rib of celery, chopped, to the other ingredients. Cook as directed.

PER SERVING

CALORIES 17
TOTAL FAT 0.0 g
   Saturated Fat 0.0 g
   Trans Fat 0.0 g
   Polyunsaturated Fat 0.0 g
   Monounsaturated Fat 0.0 g
CHOLESTEROL 0 mg
SODIUM 154 mg
CARBOHYDRATES 4 g
   Fiber 1 g
   Sugars 2 g
PROTEIN 1 g
DIETARY EXCHANGES
   Free

PER SERVING

CREOLE SAUCE
CALORIES 20
TOTAL FAT 0.0 g
   Saturated Fat 0.0 g
   Trans Fat 0.0 g
   Polyunsaturated Fat 0.0 g
   Monounsaturated Fat 0.0 g
CHOLESTEROL 0 mg
SODIUM 156 mg
CARBOHYDRATES 5 g
   Fiber 1 g
   Sugars 3 g
PROTEIN 1 g
DIETARY EXCHANGES
   Free

salsa cruda

SERVES 6; ¼ CUP PER SERVING

Serve this zippy salsa as a dip or as a terrific topping for many Mexican dishes, such as Beef Tostadas (page 328).

2 large tomatoes, diced
¼ cup finely chopped onion
2 teaspoons chopped fresh jalapeño, seeds and ribs discarded

2 teaspoons finely snipped fresh cilantro, or to taste
2 to 4 teaspoons fresh lime juice
¼ teaspoon salt

In a medium bowl, stir together the ingredients. Cover and refrigerate.

COOK'S TIP

For a different texture, combine the ingredients in a food processor or blender and process until fairly smooth.

PER SERVING

CALORIES 15
TOTAL FAT 0.0 g
  Saturated Fat 0.0 g
  Trans Fat 0.0 g
  Polyunsaturated Fat 0.0 g
  Monounsaturated Fat 0.0 g
CHOLESTEROL 0 mg
SODIUM 100 mg
CARBOHYDRATES 3 g
  Fiber 1 g
  Sugars 2 g
PROTEIN 1 g
DIETARY EXCHANGES
  Free

tomatillo-cilantro salsa with lime

SERVES 4; ¼ CUP PER SERVING

Small green tomato-like fruits known as tomatillos (tohm-ah-TEE-ohs) join fresh cilantro, lime juice, and a bit of jalapeño for this winning salsa. Serve it as a dip for baked tortillas or over food from the grill, such as fish fillets or pork cutlets.

8 ounces tomatillos, papery skin discarded
½ cup snipped fresh cilantro
2 tablespoons chopped green onions
1 tablespoon fresh lime juice

1 medium fresh jalapeño, seeds and ribs discarded, quartered
⅛ teaspoon salt
1 tablespoon olive oil (extra virgin preferred)

In a food processor or blender, process all the ingredients except the oil until smooth. Pour into a small bowl.

Stir in the oil. Serve or, for a stronger flavor, cover and refrigerate for up to two days.

TOMATO-CILANTRO SALSA
Replace the tomatillos with 8 ounces finely chopped tomatoes and replace the lime juice with 2 tablespoons cider vinegar. Don't use a food processor or blender with this variation; the color will be less brilliant if you do. Just chop the jalapeño and stir all the ingredients together.

COOK'S TIP on tomatillos

Choose firm tomatillos with close-fitting papery skin. Remove the brown skin and thoroughly rinse the tomatillos before cooking.

PER SERVING

CALORIES 52
TOTAL FAT 4.0 g
 Saturated Fat 0.5 g
 Trans Fat 0.0 g
 Polyunsaturated Fat 0.5 g
 Monounsaturated Fat 2.5 g
CHOLESTEROL 0 mg
SODIUM 76 mg
CARBOHYDRATES 4 g
 Fiber 1 g
 Sugars 3 g
PROTEIN 1 g
DIETARY EXCHANGES
 1 fat

PER SERVING

TOMATO-CILANTRO SALSA
CALORIES 44
TOTAL FAT 3.5 g
 Saturated Fat 0.5 g
 Trans Fat 0.0 g
 Polyunsaturated Fat 0.5 g
 Monounsaturated Fat 2.5 g
CHOLESTEROL 0 mg
SODIUM 78 mg
CARBOHYDRATES 3 g
 Fiber 1 g
 Sugars 2 g
PROTEIN 1 g
DIETARY EXCHANGES
 1 fat

dark chocolate sauce with hazelnuts

SERVES 16; 2 TABLESPOONS PER SERVING

A small amount of espresso powder intensifies the color as well as the flavor of this chocolate sauce without making it taste like mocha.

1 12-ounce can fat-free evaporated milk
1 cup packed light or dark brown sugar
½ cup unsweetened cocoa powder (dark preferred)

2 tablespoons light corn syrup
½ teaspoon instant espresso powder
¼ cup chopped hazelnuts, dry-roasted
1 teaspoon vanilla extract

In a medium saucepan, whisk together the milk, brown sugar, cocoa powder, corn syrup, and espresso powder. Bring to a boil over medium-high heat. Reduce the heat and simmer for 4 to 6 minutes, or until the desired consistency.

Stir in the hazelnuts and vanilla. The sauce is best when served warm, but it is good (and stays pourable) when cold. Refrigerate leftover sauce in an airtight container for up to one week. Reheat it in a microwave oven on 75 percent power (medium high) until warm.

PER SERVING

CALORIES 102
TOTAL FAT 1.5 g
  Saturated Fat 0.0 g
  Trans Fat 0.0 g
  Polyunsaturated Fat 0.0 g
  Monounsaturated Fat 1.0 g
CHOLESTEROL 1 mg
SODIUM 33 mg
CARBOHYDRATES 20 g
  Fiber 1 g
  Sugars 17 g
PROTEIN 3 g
DIETARY EXCHANGES
  1½ carbohydrate, ½ fat

raspberry port sauce

SERVES 4; ¼ CUP PER SERVING

For a simple yet sophisticated dessert, serve this sauce over poached fruit or fat-free vanilla frozen yogurt or ice cream.

1½ cups frozen unsweetened raspberries, blueberries, or a combination	3 tablespoons sugar
	1 tablespoon cornstarch
	½ teaspoon vanilla extract
¼ cup port	

In a small saucepan, stir together all the ingredients except the vanilla until the cornstarch is dissolved. Bring to a boil over medium-high heat. Cook for about 45 seconds, or until slightly thickened. Remove from the heat.

Stir in the vanilla. Let stand for 15 minutes so the flavors blend. Serve or cover and refrigerate to serve cold.

PER SERVING

CALORIES 99
TOTAL FAT 0.0 g
  Saturated Fat 0.0 g
  Trans Fat 0.0 g
  Polyunsaturated Fat 0.0 g
  Monounsaturated Fat 0.0 g
CHOLESTEROL 0 mg
SODIUM 2 mg
CARBOHYDRATES 21 g
  Fiber 2 g
  Sugars 14 g
PROTEIN 0 g
DIETARY EXCHANGES
  ½ fruit, 1 carbohydrate

easy jubilee sauce

SERVES 12; 2 TABLESPOONS PER SERVING

This sauce is *so* easy to put together. Keep the ingredients and some fat-free ice cream on hand for unexpected company.

1 16-ounce jar all-fruit black cherry spread	¼ cup port
	½ teaspoon almond extract

In a small bowl, stir together the ingredients. Serve or cover and refrigerate to serve cold.

COOK'S TIP

This sauce is named for the classic dessert cherries jubilee, which is flambéed and served over ice cream. This one is quicker, and there's no fire to put out.

PER SERVING

CALORIES 88
TOTAL FAT 0.0 g
  Saturated Fat 0.0 g
  Trans Fat 0.0 g
  Polyunsaturated Fat 0.0 g
  Monounsaturated Fat 0.0 g
CHOLESTEROL 0 mg
SODIUM 1 mg
CARBOHYDRATES 21 g
  Fiber 0 g
  Sugars 16 g
PROTEIN 0 g
DIETARY EXCHANGES
  1½ carbohydrate

orange sauce

SERVES 4; ¼ CUP PER SERVING

This sauce is scrumptious over Easy Apple Cake (page 573), Delicious Rice Pudding (page 613), Double-Ginger Squares (page 576), or Cinnamon-Orange Pancakes (page 553).

2 cups fresh orange juice	1 tablespoon fresh lemon juice
1 tablespoon cornstarch	2 teaspoons light tub margarine
1 tablespoon water	½ teaspoon grated orange zest
1 tablespoon sugar	

In a small saucepan, bring the orange juice to a simmer over medium heat. Simmer until reduced by half.

Put the cornstarch in a small bowl. Add the water, whisking to dissolve.

Whisk in a little orange juice. Whisk the cornstarch mixture into the juice remaining in the pan.

Whisk in the sugar. Cook for 1 to 2 minutes, or until thickened. Remove from the heat.

Whisk in the lemon juice, margarine, and orange zest.

PER SERVING

CALORIES 84
TOTAL FAT 1.0 g
  Saturated Fat 0.0 g
  Trans Fat 0.0 g
  Polyunsaturated Fat 0.0 g
  Monounsaturated Fat 0.5 g
CHOLESTEROL 0 mg
SODIUM 17 mg
CARBOHYDRATES 18 g
  Fiber 0 g
  Sugars 14 g
PROTEIN 1 g
DIETARY EXCHANGES
  1 fruit

breads and breakfast dishes

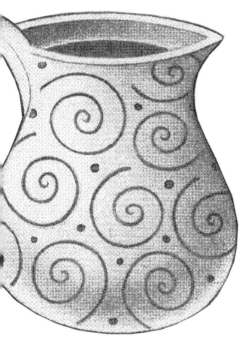

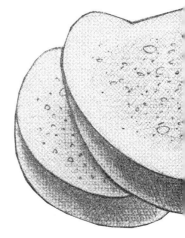

Applesauce-Raisin Bread with Streusel Topping

Apple Coffee Cake

Banana-Raisin Coffee Cake with Citrus Glaze

Quick Orange Streusel Cake

Easy Refrigerator Rolls

Southern Raised Biscuits

Parmesan-Herb Breadsticks

Muffins

Fruit Muffins

Whole-Wheat Muffins

Apricot-Cinnamon Muffins

Oat Bran Fruit Muffins

Blueberry-Banana Muffins

Eye-Opener Breakfast Cookies

Slow-Cooker Pumpkin Oatmeal

Maple and Banana Tapioca

Muesli

Apple-Berry Couscous

Baked Pear Pancake

Cinnamon-Orange Pancakes

Perfect Pumpkin Pancakes

Multigrain Apple Pancakes

Red, White, and Blueberry Waffles

Peachy Stuffed French Toast

Country-Style Breakfast Casserole

Stacked Sausage and Eggs

Breakfast Pizzas

Mexican Breakfast Pizzas

Strata with Canadian Bacon, Spinach, and Tomatoes

Mango Sunrise Breakfast Parfaits

basic bread

SERVES 32; 1 SLICE PER SERVING

Sharpen your culinary skills with this step-by-step bread recipe. You'll even get a bit of exercise from lively kneading.

¼ cup lukewarm water (105°F to 115°F)
2 ¼-ounce packages active dry yeast
1¾ cups fat-free milk
2½ tablespoons sugar
2 tablespoons canola or corn oil

4 cups all-purpose flour and 2 cups all-purpose flour, plus more as needed, divided use
1 teaspoon salt
Cooking spray

Pour the water into a large bowl. Add the yeast, stirring to dissolve. Let stand for 5 minutes, or until the mixture bubbles.

Stir in the milk, sugar, and oil.

Gradually stir in 4 cups flour and the salt. Using a sturdy spoon, beat for about 30 seconds, or until smooth.

Gradually add some of the remaining 2 cups flour, beating with the spoon after each addition, until the dough starts to pull away from the side of the bowl. Add more flour if necessary to make the dough stiff enough to handle.

Lightly flour a flat surface. Turn out the dough. Knead for 6 to 8 minutes, gradually adding enough of the remaining flour to make the dough smooth and elastic. (The dough shouldn't be dry or stick to the surface. You may not need all the flour, or you may need up to ½ cup more if the dough is too sticky.)

Lightly spray a large bowl with cooking spray. Put the dough in the bowl, turning to coat. Cover with a slightly damp dish towel. Let the dough rise in a warm, draft-free place (about 85°F) for about 1 hour, or until doubled in bulk.

Punch down the dough. Divide in half. Shape into loaves. Lightly spray two 9 x 5 x 3-inch loaf pans with cooking spray. Put the dough in the loaf pans. Cover each with a slightly damp dish towel. Let the dough rise in a warm, draft-free place (about 85°) for about 30 minutes, or until doubled in bulk.

PER SERVING

CALORIES 103
TOTAL FAT 1.0 g
  Saturated Fat 0.0 g
  Trans Fat 0.0 g
  Polyunsaturated Fat 0.5 g
  Monounsaturated Fat 0.5 g
CHOLESTEROL 1 mg
SODIUM 79 mg
CARBOHYDRATES 20 g
  Fiber 1 g
  Sugars 2 g
PROTEIN 3 g
DIETARY EXCHANGES
  1½ starch

While the dough is rising, preheat the oven to 425°F.

Bake the loaves for 15 minutes. Reduce the heat to 375°F. Bake for 30 minutes, or until the bread registers 190°F on an instant-read thermometer or sounds hollow when rapped with your knuckles. Remove the bread from the pans and let cool on cooling racks for 15 to 20 minutes before cutting.

HERB BREAD

Just before kneading, add to the dough 2 teaspoons caraway seeds; ½ teaspoon ground nutmeg; ½ teaspoon dried rosemary, crushed; and ¼ teaspoon dried thyme, crumbled. Proceed as directed.

COOK'S TIP on breadmaking

The more you practice, the easier it will be to develop a feel for when the dough has the proper consistency. If you knead in too much flour or overknead the dough, it will feel dry and stiff, and the resulting loaf can be heavy. If you use too little flour or don't knead the dough enough, your loaf won't retain its shape during baking.

Resist the urge to knead the dough completely flat against your counter or board. This can cause your dough to become sticky.

For basic kneading, fold the dough toward you. Using the heels of one or both hands, push the dough forward and slightly down in an almost rocking motion. Rotate the dough a quarter-turn and repeat. Follow this procedure until the dough is smooth and elastic. Add small amounts of flour when the dough starts to stick to the counter. Make note of the time you start, and knead for the amount of time called for in your recipe.

PER SERVING

HERB BREAD
CALORIES 103
TOTAL FAT 1.0 g
  Saturated Fat 0.0 g
  Trans Fat 0.0 g
  Polyunsaturated Fat 0.5 g
  Monounsaturated Fat 0.5 g
CHOLESTEROL 1 mg
SODIUM 79 mg
CARBOHYDRATES 20 g
  Fiber 1 g
  Sugars 2 g
PROTEIN 3 g
DIETARY EXCHANGES
  1½ starch

whole-wheat french bread

1 SLICE PER SERVING

You'll love the versatility of this nutty-flavored bread. Make a standard loaf in your bread machine, or use the dough cycle and shape the dough into baguettes to finish.

	1-pound machine (12 servings)	1½-pound machine (18 servings)	2-pound machine (24 servings)
Whole-wheat flour	1¼ cups	2 cups	2½ cups
Bread flour	1 cup	1½ cups	2 cups
Fat-free dry milk	1 tablespoon	1½ tablespoons	2 tablespoons
Salt	½ teaspoon	¾ teaspoon	1 teaspoon
Canola or corn oil	1 tablespoon	1½ tablespoons	2 tablespoons
Honey	1 tablespoon	1½ tablespoons	2 tablespoons
Water	1 cup less 1 tablespoon	1⅓ cups	1⅞ cups
Active dry yeast	1 teaspoon	1½ teaspoons	2 teaspoons

Put the ingredients in the bread machine container in the order recommended by the manufacturer. Select the basic/white bread cycle. Proceed as directed.

PER SERVING

1-POUND AND 2-POUND LOAF
CALORIES 102
TOTAL FAT 1.5 g
  Saturated Fat 0.0 g
  Trans Fat 0.0 g
  Polyunsaturated Fat 0.5 g
  Monounsaturated Fat 1.0 g
CHOLESTEROL 0 mg
SODIUM 101 mg
CARBOHYDRATES 19 g
  Fiber 2 g
  Sugars 2 g
PROTEIN 3 g
DIETARY EXCHANGES
  1½ starch

PER SERVING

1½-POUND LOAF
CALORIES 104
TOTAL FAT 1.5 g
  Saturated Fat 0.0 g
  Trans Fat 0.0 g
  Polyunsaturated Fat 0.5 g
  Monounsaturated Fat 1.0 g
CHOLESTEROL 0 mg
SODIUM 101 mg
CARBOHYDRATES 20 g
  Fiber 2 g
  Sugars 2 g
PROTEIN 4 g
DIETARY EXCHANGES
  1½ starch

honey-wheat oatmeal bread

SERVES 16; 1 SLICE PER SERVING

There's nothing like a slice of homemade oatmeal quick bread to soak up soups or sauces—or just to enjoy by itself.

Cooking spray
1½ cups all-purpose flour
½ cup whole-wheat flour
½ cup uncooked quick-cooking oatmeal and 2 tablespoons uncooked quick-cooking oatmeal, divided use
¼ cup toasted wheat germ

2 teaspoons baking powder
1 teaspoon baking soda
¼ teaspoon salt
1½ cups low-fat buttermilk
¼ cup egg substitute
2 tablespoons honey
1 tablespoon olive oil

Preheat the oven to 375°F. Lightly spray an 8½ x 4½ x 2½-inch loaf pan with cooking spray.

In a large bowl, stir together the flours, ½ cup oatmeal, wheat germ, baking powder, baking soda, and salt. Make a well in the center.

Pour the buttermilk, egg substitute, honey, and oil into the well. Stir until the flour mixture is just moistened but no flour is visible. Don't overmix; the batter may have a few lumps. Spoon into the pan, gently smoothing the top. Sprinkle with the remaining 2 tablespoons oatmeal.

Bake for 40 to 45 minutes, or until a wooden skewer inserted all the way to the bottom in the center comes out clean. Transfer the pan to a cooling rack. Let cool for 5 minutes. Turn the bread out onto the rack and let cool for 10 minutes before slicing.

PER SERVING

CALORIES 101
TOTAL FAT 1.5 g
  Saturated Fat 0.5 g
  Trans Fat 0.0 g
  Polyunsaturated Fat 0.5 g
  Monounsaturated Fat 1.0 g
CHOLESTEROL 1 mg
SODIUM 198 mg
CARBOHYDRATES 18 g
  Fiber 1 g
  Sugars 4 g
PROTEIN 4 g
DIETARY EXCHANGES
  1 starch

focaccia

SERVES 16; 1 WEDGE PER SERVING

Delicious on its own, useful for getting that last bite of spaghetti sauce, and even a replacement for pizza crust, this popular flatbread from Italy serves many purposes.

1½ cups bread flour or all-purpose flour and 1 cup bread flour or all-purpose flour, plus more as needed, divided use

¼ cup semolina flour or all-purpose flour

¼ cup all-purpose flour, plus more as needed for flouring surface, kneading, and rolling out dough, divided use

1 ¼-ounce package fast-rising yeast

1 tablespoon olive oil

2 teaspoons dried Italian seasoning, crumbled

1 teaspoon garlic powder

¼ teaspoon salt

1¼ cups warm water (120°F to 130°F)

Olive oil spray

1 tablespoon pine nuts

1 teaspoon dried rosemary, crushed

In a large bowl, stir together 1½ cups bread flour, semolina flour, ¼ cup all-purpose flour, yeast, oil, Italian seasoning, garlic powder, and salt.

Pour the water into the flour mixture. Using a sturdy spoon, beat for 30 seconds.

Gradually add some of the remaining 1 cup bread flour, beating with the spoon after each addition, until the dough starts to pull away from the side of the bowl. Add more flour if necessary to make the dough stiff enough to handle.

Lightly flour a flat surface. Turn out the dough. Knead for 6 to 8 minutes, gradually adding enough of the remaining flour to make the dough smooth and elastic. (The dough shouldn't be dry or stick to the surface. You may not need the additional flour, or you may need up to ½ cup more if the dough is too sticky. See Cook's Tip on Breadmaking, page 517.) Cover the dough with a slightly damp dish towel. Let rest for 10 minutes.

Lightly spray a 14-inch pizza pan with olive oil spray. Using your fingers, press the dough to the edge of the pan. Lightly spray with olive oil spray. Press in the pine nuts. Sprinkle with the rosemary. Cover with a slightly damp dish towel. Let the dough rise in a warm, draft-free place (about 85°F) for about 30 minutes.

While the dough is rising, preheat the oven to 375°F.

Bake for 20 to 25 minutes, or until golden brown. Remove the bread from the pan and let cool on a cooling rack for at least 10 minutes before slicing.

BREAD MACHINE INSTRUCTIONS

Follow the manufacturer's instructions for the basic/white bread cycle.

For a flat loaf, use the bread machine only to mix the dough, following the manufacturer's directions for the dough cycle. Remove the dough when it is ready. Shape it. Sprinkle with the pine nuts and rosemary. Bake as directed above. For a regular loaf, add the pine nuts and rosemary with the other ingredients.

	1-pound machine (12 servings)	1½-pound machine (18 servings)	2-pound machine (24 servings)
Water	¾ cup	1¼ cups	1½ cups
Bread flour or all-purpose flour	1⅔ cups	2½ cups	3⅓ cups
Semolina flour or all-purpose flour	3 tablespoons	¼ cup	⅓ cup
All-purpose flour	3 tablespoons	¼ cup	⅓ cup
Active dry yeast	2 teaspoons	2½ teaspoons	1 tablespoon
Olive oil	2¼ teaspoons	1 tablespoon	1½ tablespoons
Dried Italian seasoning, crumbled	1½ teaspoons	2 teaspoons	1 tablespoon
Garlic powder	¾ teaspoon	1 teaspoon	1½ teaspoons
Salt	⅛ teaspoon	¼ teaspoon	½ teaspoon

FOCACCIA SANDWICH LOAVES

SERVES 8; 1 LOAF PER SERVING

Lightly spray two baking sheets with cooking spray. After kneading, let the dough rest for 10 minutes. Divide into 8 pieces. Shape into disks. Put on the baking sheets. Cover each baking sheet with a slightly damp dish towel. Let the dough rise for 30 minutes in a warm, draft-free place (about 85°F). Bake as directed for 15 to 20 minutes, or until golden brown. Remove the bread from the sheets and let cool on a cooling rack before slicing in half horizontally.

PER SERVING

FOCACCIA SANDWICH LOAVES
CALORIES 212
TOTAL FAT 3.0 g
    Saturated Fat 0.5 g
    Trans Fat 0.0 g
    Polyunsaturated Fat 0.5 g
    Monounsaturated Fat 1.5 g
CHOLESTEROL 0 mg
SODIUM 75 mg
CARBOHYDRATES 39 g
    Fiber 2 g
    Sugars 0 g
PROTEIN 7 g
DIETARY EXCHANGES
    2½ starch

apricot-pecan bread

SERVES 16; 1 SLICE PER SERVING

A slice of this fruit-and-nut-studded bread is a treat with breakfast or as a take-along snack.

1 cup lukewarm water (105°F to 115°F)
1 ¼-ounce package active dry yeast
¼ teaspoon sugar
1½ cups whole-wheat flour
1½ cups all-purpose flour, plus more as needed for flouring surface, kneading, and rolling out dough, divided use

½ cup chopped dried apricots
¼ cup coarsely chopped pecans
2 tablespoons olive oil
1 tablespoon honey
¼ teaspoon ground nutmeg
¼ teaspoon salt
Cooking spray

Pour the water into a small bowl. Add the yeast and sugar, stirring to dissolve. Let stand for 5 minutes, or until the mixture bubbles.

Meanwhile, in a large bowl, stir together the flours. Remove 1 cup of the mixture and set aside.

Stir the apricots, pecans, oil, honey, nutmeg, and salt into the flour in the large bowl.

Pour the yeast mixture into the flour mixture, stirring for about 30 seconds.

Stir in small amounts of the reserved 1 cup flour until the dough starts to pull away from the side of the bowl.

Lightly flour a flat surface. Turn out the dough. Knead for 7 to 8 minutes, gradually adding enough of the remaining flour to make the dough smooth and elastic. You may not need all the flour. Shape into a ball.

Wipe the mixing bowl with a paper towel. Lightly spray the bowl with cooking spray. Put the dough in the bowl, turning to coat all sides. Cover the bowl with a slightly damp dish towel and put in a warm, draft-free place (about 85°F). Let the dough rise for 1 hour, or until doubled in bulk.

PER SERVING

CALORIES 125
TOTAL FAT 3.5 g
  Saturated Fat 0.5 g
  Trans Fat 0.0 g
  Polyunsaturated Fat 0.5 g
  Monounsaturated Fat 2.0 g
CHOLESTEROL 0 mg
SODIUM 38 mg
CARBOHYDRATES 22 g
  Fiber 2 g
  Sugars 3 g
PROTEIN 3 g
DIETARY EXCHANGES
  1½ starch, ½ fat

Lightly spray an 8½ x 4½ x 2½-inch loaf pan and a cutting board with cooking spray.

Punch down the dough. Transfer to the cutting board. Press or roll the dough into a 10-inch square. Roll the dough into a cylinder and press the ends to seal. Fold the ends under the dough to form a loaf. Place the bread with the folded ends down in the loaf pan. Cover with a slightly damp dish towel and let rise in a warm, draft-free place for 30 minutes, or until doubled in bulk.

While the dough is rising, preheat the oven to 375°F.

Bake the bread for 30 minutes, or until it registers 190°F on an instant-read thermometer or sounds hollow when rapped with your knuckles. Turn the bread out onto a cooling rack and let cool for 15 to 20 minutes before slicing.

jalapeño cheese bread

SERVES 20; 1 SLICE PER SERVING

Smoked paprika and beer lend an interesting touch to this easy-to-prepare quick bread.

Cooking spray
3 cups all-purpose flour, plus more as needed
1 teaspoon baking soda
½ teaspoon baking powder
1 cup shredded low-fat Cheddar cheese

2 tablespoons drained and chopped pickled jalapeños
1½ cups beer (light or nonalcoholic)
1 tablespoon olive oil
½ teaspoon smoked or regular paprika (optional)

Preheat the oven to 350°F. Lightly spray a large baking sheet with cooking spray.

In a large bowl, whisk together the flour, baking soda, and baking powder.

Stir in the Cheddar and jalapeños. Make a well in the center.

Pour the beer and oil into the well. Stir until the flour absorbs the liquids (the mixture will be slightly sticky). Spoon the dough onto the center of the baking sheet.

Using lightly floured hands, shape the dough into a 9 x 6-inch oval loaf. Sprinkle with the paprika.

Bake for 40 to 45 minutes, or until the bread is golden brown and sounds hollow when rapped with your knuckles. Remove the bread from the baking sheet and let cool on a cooling rack for at least 15 minutes before slicing.

PER SERVING

CALORIES 90
TOTAL FAT 1.5 g
  Saturated Fat 0.5 g
  Trans Fat 0.0 g
  Polyunsaturated Fat 0.0 g
  Monounsaturated Fat 0.5 g
CHOLESTEROL 1 mg
SODIUM 128 mg
CARBOHYDRATES 15 g
  Fiber 1 g
  Sugars 0 g
PROTEIN 3 g
DIETARY EXCHANGES
  1 starch

COOK'S TIP on smoked paprika

Smoked paprika, which comes from Spain, is like chipotle peppers without the heat. Use it to enhance refried beans, salsa, dips, rice dishes, marinades, and many other foods that would work well with a smoky flavor.

peppercorn-dill flatbread

SERVES 15; 4 PIECES PER SERVING

Enjoy flatbread as a snack by itself or with a heart-healthy dip or spread, such as Roasted-Pepper Hummus (page 14).

2 cups all-purpose flour, plus more as needed for flouring surface, kneading, and rolling out dough
1 cup whole-wheat flour
1 tablespoon olive oil
2 teaspoons baking powder
2 teaspoons celery seeds
2 teaspoons dried dillweed, crumbled
1 teaspoon sugar
1 teaspoon pepper (coarsely ground preferred)
½ teaspoon baking soda
¼ teaspoon salt
1¼ cups low-fat buttermilk
Cooking spray

In a large bowl, stir together the flours, oil, baking powder, celery seeds, dillweed, sugar, pepper, baking soda, and salt. Make a well in the center.

Pour the buttermilk into the well. Stir until the mixture forms a ball.

Lightly flour a flat surface. Turn out the dough. Knead for 2 minutes. Return the dough to the bowl. Cover with a slightly damp dish towel. Let the dough rest for 10 to 15 minutes.

Preheat the oven to 400°F. Lightly spray two large baking sheets with cooking spray.

Lightly flour the flat surface again if more flour is needed. Roll out the dough ⅛ inch thick. Using a pizza cutter or sharp knife, cut the dough into strips about 1½ inches wide by 4 inches long (you should get about 60). Transfer to the baking sheets. Prick each strip with a fork.

Bake for 15 minutes, or until crisp. Transfer the baking sheets to cooling racks. Let the flatbread cool for 15 to 20 minutes. Store in an airtight container for up to seven days.

PER SERVING

CALORIES 107
TOTAL FAT 1.5 g
  Saturated Fat 0.5 g
  Trans Fat 0.0 g
  Polyunsaturated Fat 0.0 g
  Monounsaturated Fat 1.0 g
CHOLESTEROL 1 mg
SODIUM 157 mg
CARBOHYDRATES 20 g
  Fiber 2 g
  Sugars 1 g
PROTEIN 4 g
DIETARY EXCHANGES
  1½ starch

walnut bread

SERVES 16; 1 SLICE PER SERVING

Here's a simple way to celebrate the robust flavor of walnuts.

Cooking spray
2 cups all-purpose flour
½ cup firmly packed light brown sugar
2 teaspoons baking powder
¼ teaspoon salt

¼ teaspoon baking soda
1 cup fat-free milk
¼ cup egg substitute
½ cup finely chopped walnuts,
 dry-roasted

Preheat the oven to 350°F. Lightly spray an 8½ x 4½ x 2½-inch loaf pan with cooking spray.

In a large bowl, sift together the flour, brown sugar, baking powder, salt, and baking soda.

In another large bowl, whisk together the milk and egg substitute.

Add the flour mixture and walnuts to the milk mixture. Stir just until the dry ingredients are moistened but no flour is visible. Don't overmix. Pour into the loaf pan, gently smoothing the top.

Bake for 40 minutes, or until a wooden toothpick inserted in the center comes out clean. Using a metal spatula, loosen the bread from the sides of the pan. Turn out onto a cooling rack and let cool.

PER SERVING

CALORIES 114
TOTAL FAT 2.5 g
 Saturated Fat 0.5 g
 Trans Fat 0.0 g
 Polyunsaturated Fat 2.0 g
 Monounsaturated Fat 0.5 g
CHOLESTEROL 1 mg
SODIUM 123 mg
CARBOHYDRATES 20 g
 Fiber 1 g
 Sugars 8 g
PROTEIN 3 g
DIETARY EXCHANGES
 1½ starch

zucchini bread with pistachios

SERVES 32; 1 SLICE PER SERVING

Some surprise ingredients—Fuji apple, extra-light olive oil, and pistachios—add a fruity nuance, color, and crunch that set this zucchini bread apart.

Cooking spray
2 cups all-purpose flour
1 cup whole-wheat flour
1 cup sugar
½ cup firmly packed light brown sugar
¼ cup chopped unsalted pistachio nuts
1 teaspoon ground cinnamon
1 teaspoon baking powder

1 teaspoon baking soda
⅛ teaspoon salt
2 cups shredded zucchini (about 12 ounces)
1 medium Fuji or Granny Smith apple, peeled and shredded (about 1 cup)
¾ cup egg substitute
½ cup unsweetened apple juice
2 tablespoons extra-light olive oil

Preheat the oven to 375°F. Lightly spray two 8½ x 4½ x 2½-inch loaf pans with cooking spray.

In a medium bowl, stir together the flours, sugars, pistachios, cinnamon, baking powder, baking soda, and salt.

Add the remaining ingredients. Stir just until the dry ingredients are moistened but no flour is visible. Don't overmix. Pour into the loaf pans, gently smoothing the tops.

Bake for 55 to 60 minutes, or until a wooden toothpick inserted in the center comes out clean. Using a metal spatula, loosen the bread from the sides of the pans. Turn out onto a cooling rack and let cool for 20 minutes before slicing.

COOK'S TIP

You can bake this bread in two 8-inch square baking pans (lightly sprayed with cooking spray) for 35 to 40 minutes, or until a wooden toothpick inserted in the center comes out clean. Cool as directed in the recipe above.

PER SERVING

CALORIES 100
TOTAL FAT 1.5 g
  Saturated Fat 0.0 g
  Trans Fat 0.0 g
  Polyunsaturated Fat 0.5 g
  Monounsaturated Fat 1.0 g
CHOLESTEROL 0 mg
SODIUM 75 mg
CARBOHYDRATES 20 g
  Fiber 1 g
  Sugars 11 g
PROTEIN 2 g
DIETARY EXCHANGES
  1 starch, ½ carbohydrate

sweet potato bread

SERVES 16; 1 SLICE PER SERVING

Incredibly moist and studded with crunchy pecans, this loaf bread is brimming with healthy ingredients—carrots, applesauce, pineapple juice, and sweet potato, one of nature's superfoods.

Cooking spray
2 cups all-purpose flour
¾ cup firmly packed light brown sugar
½ cup shredded carrot
¼ cup chopped pecans
1½ teaspoons baking powder
1 teaspoon ground cinnamon
½ teaspoon baking soda
¼ teaspoon ground nutmeg

1 cup mashed cooked sweet potatoes, fresh (about 8 ounces raw) or canned without liquid or in water, well drained if in water
⅓ cup pineapple juice
1 large egg
¼ cup unsweetened applesauce
1 tablespoon canola or corn oil

Preheat the oven to 350°F. Lightly spray an 8½ x 4½ x 2½-inch loaf pan with cooking spray.

In a large bowl, stir together the flour, brown sugar, carrot, pecans, baking powder, cinnamon, baking soda, and nutmeg. Make a well in the center.

Add the remaining ingredients to the well. Stir just until moistened but no flour is visible. Don't overmix; the batter may be slightly lumpy. Pour into the loaf pan, gently smoothing the top.

Bake for 1 hour 15 minutes, or until a wooden toothpick inserted in the center comes out clean. Transfer the pan to a cooling rack. Let the bread cool for 10 minutes, then turn out onto a cooling rack and let cool completely, about 1 hour, before slicing. Wrap any remaining bread in plastic wrap and refrigerate for up to one week.

PER SERVING

CALORIES 139
TOTAL FAT 2.5 g
  Saturated Fat 0.5 g
  Trans Fat 0.0 g
  Polyunsaturated Fat 0.5 g
  Monounsaturated Fat 1.5 g
CHOLESTEROL 13 mg
SODIUM 95 mg
CARBOHYDRATES 27 g
  Fiber 1 g
  Sugars 12 g
PROTEIN 2 g
DIETARY EXCHANGES
  2 starch

velvet pumpkin bread

SERVES 16; 1 SLICE PER SERVING

The name says it all—this bread has a wonderful texture, and just wait till you smell it baking!

Cooking spray	2 teaspoons baking powder
1 cup canned solid-pack pumpkin (not pie filling)	1 teaspoon ground cinnamon
½ cup egg substitute	½ teaspoon ground ginger
⅓ cup fat-free milk	¼ teaspoon ground nutmeg
2 tablespoons light tub margarine, melted	⅛ teaspoon salt
1 tablespoon canola or corn oil	½ cup chopped pecans, dry-roasted
2 cups all-purpose flour	½ cup sugar
	½ cup firmly packed light brown sugar

Preheat the oven to 350°F. Lightly spray a 9 x 5 x 3-inch loaf pan with cooking spray.

In a medium bowl, whisk together the pumpkin, egg substitute, milk, margarine, and oil.

In a large bowl, sift together the flour, baking powder, cinnamon, ginger, nutmeg, and salt.

Stir the pecans and sugars into the flour mixture. Make a well in the center.

Pour the pumpkin mixture into the well. Stir just until the flour mixture is moistened but no flour is visible. Don't overmix. Pour into the loaf pan, gently smoothing the top.

Bake for 1 hour, or until a wooden toothpick inserted in the center comes out clean. Using a metal spatula, loosen the bread from the sides of the pan. Turn out onto a cooling rack and let cool.

COOK'S TIP on leftover canned pumpkin

Store the leftover pumpkin in an airtight plastic container in the refrigerator for up to one week. For longer storage, put the pumpkin in ice cube trays to freeze. Transfer the frozen pumpkin cubes to a resealable plastic freezer bag. Add the cubes to soups or stews. Or freeze the remaining pumpkin in an airtight plastic container. Thaw in the refrigerator before using.

PER SERVING

CALORIES 155
TOTAL FAT 4.0 g
 Saturated Fat 0.5 g
 Trans Fat 0.0 g
 Polyunsaturated Fat 1.0 g
 Monounsaturated Fat 2.5 g
CHOLESTEROL 0 mg
SODIUM 100 mg
CARBOHYDRATES 27 g
 Fiber 2 g
 Sugars 14 g
PROTEIN 3 g
DIETARY EXCHANGES
 1 starch, 1 carbohydrate,
 ½ fat

bananas foster bread

SERVES 16; 1 SLICE PER SERVING

The taste and texture of this bread are great—and it's moist, moist, moist! You'll love how it captures the flavor of bananas Foster.

Cooking spray
1½ cups all-purpose flour
½ cup sugar
2 teaspoons baking powder
1 teaspoon baking soda
⅛ teaspoon salt
3 very ripe medium bananas, mashed (about 1½ cups)
4 large egg whites, lightly beaten with a fork

½ cup toasted wheat germ
¼ cup unsweetened applesauce
¼ cup low-fat buttermilk
1 tablespoon canola or corn oil
1 teaspoon rum extract
½ teaspoon ground cinnamon
½ teaspoon imitation butter flavoring
¼ cup firmly packed light brown sugar

Preheat the oven to 350°F. Lightly spray an 8½ x 4½ x 2½-inch loaf pan with cooking spray.

In a large bowl, sift together the flour, sugar, baking powder, baking soda, and salt.

Add the remaining ingredients except the brown sugar. Stir just until combined but no flour is visible. Don't overmix. Pour into the loaf pan, gently smoothing the top.

Sprinkle the brown sugar over the batter.

Bake for 1 hour, or until a wooden toothpick inserted in the center comes out clean. Transfer the pan to a cooling rack. Let cool for at least 10 minutes. Using a metal spatula, loosen the bread from the sides of the pan. Turn out onto a cooling rack and let cool.

PER SERVING

CALORIES 130
TOTAL FAT 1.5 g
  Saturated Fat 0.0 g
  Trans Fat 0.0 g
  Polyunsaturated Fat 0.5 g
  Monounsaturated Fat 0.5 g
CHOLESTEROL 0 mg
SODIUM 166 mg
CARBOHYDRATES 26 g
  Fiber 2 g
  Sugars 13 g
PROTEIN 4 g
DIETARY EXCHANGES
  1 starch, ½ carbohydrate

whole-wheat apricot bread

SERVES 16; 1 SLICE PER SERVING

Bits of dried apricot flavor each bite of this quick bread. You may be tempted to dunk your slice in hot tea or flavored coffee.

Cooking spray	2 teaspoons baking powder
1 cup chopped dried apricots	¼ teaspoon baking soda
1 cup whole-wheat flour	½ cup unsweetened applesauce
1 cup all-purpose flour	½ cup fat-free evaporated milk
½ cup sugar	¼ cup egg substitute
½ cup finely chopped walnuts, dry-roasted	1 tablespoon canola or corn oil

Preheat the oven to 350°F. Lightly spray a 9 x 5 x 3-inch loaf pan with cooking spray.

In a large bowl, stir together the apricots, flours, sugar, nuts, baking powder, and baking soda.

In a small bowl, whisk together the remaining ingredients. Add to the apricot mixture. Stir just until the dry ingredients are moistened but no flour is visible. Don't overmix. Pour into the loaf pan, gently smoothing the top.

Bake for 40 to 50 minutes, or until a wooden toothpick inserted in the center comes out clean. Using a metal spatula, loosen the bread from the sides of the pan. Turn out onto a cooling rack and let cool for 1 hour before slicing.

PER SERVING

CALORIES 142
TOTAL FAT 3.5 g
  Saturated Fat 0.5 g
  Trans Fat 0.0 g
  Polyunsaturated Fat 2.0 g
  Monounsaturated Fat 1.0 g
CHOLESTEROL 1 mg
SODIUM 93 mg
CARBOHYDRATES 26 g
  Fiber 2 g
  Sugars 12 g
PROTEIN 4 g
DIETARY EXCHANGES
  1 starch, ½ carbohydrate, ½ fat

orange wheat bread

SERVES 16; 1 SLICE PER SERVING

Whole-wheat flour, wheat germ, walnuts, and fruit make this quick bread nutritious as well as delicious.

Cooking spray
2 cups all-purpose flour
½ cup whole-wheat flour
½ cup toasted wheat germ
½ cup sugar
¼ cup chopped walnuts, dry-roasted
1 tablespoon baking powder

½ teaspoon baking soda
2 tablespoons grated orange zest
1 cup fresh orange juice
⅓ cup unsweetened applesauce
¼ cup egg substitute
1 tablespoon canola or corn oil

Preheat the oven to 350°F. Lightly spray a 9 x 5 x 3-inch loaf pan with cooking spray.

In a large bowl, stir together the flours, wheat germ, sugar, walnuts, baking powder, and baking soda.

Add the remaining ingredients. Stir just until the dry ingredients are moistened but no flour is visible. Don't overmix. Pour into the loaf pan, gently smoothing the top.

Bake for 55 minutes, or until a wooden toothpick inserted in the center comes out clean. Using a metal spatula, loosen the bread from the sides of the pan. Turn out onto a cooling rack and let cool.

PER SERVING

CALORIES 141
TOTAL FAT 2.5 g
  Saturated Fat 0.5 g
  Trans Fat 0.0 g
  Polyunsaturated Fat 1.5 g
  Monounsaturated Fat 1.0 g
CHOLESTEROL 0 mg
SODIUM 125 mg
CARBOHYDRATES 26 g
  Fiber 2 g
  Sugars 9 g
PROTEIN 4 g
DIETARY EXCHANGES
  1½ starch

cranberry bread

SERVES 16; 1 SLICE PER SERVING

If you froze some extra cranberries when they were plentiful, you'll be able to enjoy this bread all year long.

Cooking spray
2 cups all-purpose flour
⅔ cup firmly packed light brown sugar
2 teaspoons baking powder
½ teaspoon baking soda
¼ teaspoon ground allspice or ground nutmeg
⅛ teaspoon salt

1 cup fresh or frozen cranberries, chopped (don't thaw if frozen)
2 teaspoons grated orange zest
¾ cup fresh orange juice
¼ cup egg substitute
1 tablespoon canola or corn oil
2 teaspoons vanilla extract

Preheat the oven to 350°F. Lightly spray an 8½ x 4½ x 2½-inch loaf pan with cooking spray.

In a large bowl, stir together the flour, brown sugar, baking powder, baking soda, allspice, and salt. Make a well in the center.

In a medium bowl, stir together the remaining ingredients. Pour into the well. Stir just until the dry ingredients are moistened but no flour is visible. Don't overmix. Pour into the loaf pan, gently smoothing the top.

Bake for 50 to 60 minutes, or until a wooden toothpick inserted in the center comes out clean. Using a metal spatula, loosen the bread from the sides of the pan. Turn out onto a cooling rack and let cool.

PER SERVING

CALORIES 112
TOTAL FAT 1.0 g
    Saturated Fat 0.0 g
    Trans Fat 0.0 g
    Polyunsaturated Fat 0.5 g
    Monounsaturated Fat 0.5 g
CHOLESTEROL 0 mg
SODIUM 119 mg
CARBOHYDRATES 23 g
    Fiber 1 g
    Sugars 10 g
PROTEIN 2 g
DIETARY EXCHANGES
    1½ starch

applesauce-raisin bread with streusel topping

SERVES 16; 1 SLICE PER SERVING

Serve a warm slice of this bread with a steaming cup of orange-flavored tea and a cinnamon stick stirrer.

Cooking spray

BREAD

1 cup unsweetened applesauce
½ cup sugar
¼ cup firmly packed light brown sugar
¼ cup egg substitute
2 tablespoons fat-free milk
1 tablespoon canola or corn oil
2 cups all-purpose flour
2 teaspoons baking powder
1 teaspoon ground cinnamon
¼ teaspoon ground nutmeg

⅛ teaspoon ground cloves
⅛ teaspoon salt
½ cup raisins

TOPPING

2 tablespoons light brown sugar
2 tablespoons uncooked quick-cooking oatmeal
2 tablespoons chopped pecans, dry-roasted
1 tablespoon light tub margarine
½ teaspoon ground cinnamon

Preheat the oven to 350°F. Lightly spray a 9 x 5 x 3-inch loaf pan with cooking spray.

In a large bowl, whisk together the applesauce, sugars, egg substitute, milk, and oil.

In a medium bowl, sift together the remaining bread ingredients except the raisins.

Stir the raisins into the flour mixture. Stir the flour mixture into the applesauce mixture. Stir just until the dry ingredients are moistened but no flour is visible. Don't overmix. Pour into the loaf pan, gently smoothing the top.

In a small bowl, stir together the topping ingredients. Sprinkle over the batter.

Bake for 50 to 60 minutes, or until a wooden toothpick inserted in the center comes out clean. Using a metal spatula, loosen the bread from the sides of the pan. Turn out onto a cooling rack and let cool.

PER SERVING

CALORIES 145
TOTAL FAT 2.0 g
  Saturated Fat 0.0 g
  Trans Fat 0.0 g
  Polyunsaturated Fat 0.5 g
  Monounsaturated Fat 1.0 g
CHOLESTEROL 0 mg
SODIUM 85 mg
CARBOHYDRATES 30 g
  Fiber 1 g
  Sugars 16 g
PROTEIN 2 g
DIETARY EXCHANGES
  1 starch, 1 carbohydrate

apple coffee cake

SERVES 9

You'll love the crisp crumb topping and moist center of this coffee cake.

Cooking spray

COFFEE CAKE
1½ cups all-purpose flour
½ cup sugar
2½ teaspoons baking powder
½ teaspoon ground cinnamon
1 medium Granny Smith apple, peeled and grated
¾ cup fat-free milk
¼ cup unsweetened applesauce
1 large egg white, beaten until frothy
¼ teaspoon vanilla extract

TOPPING
⅓ cup firmly packed dark brown sugar
⅓ cup uncooked quick-cooking oatmeal
1½ tablespoons all-purpose flour
1 tablespoon light tub margarine, melted
1 teaspoon ground cinnamon

Preheat the oven to 375°F. Lightly spray a 9-inch square baking pan with cooking spray.

In a large bowl, sift together the flour, sugar, baking powder, and cinnamon.

In a small bowl, stir together the remaining coffee cake ingredients. Add to the flour mixture. Stir just until the dry ingredients are moistened but no flour is visible. Don't overmix. Pour into the baking pan, gently smoothing the top.

In a small bowl, stir together the topping ingredients. Sprinkle over the batter.

Bake for 30 to 35 minutes, or until a wooden toothpick inserted in the center comes out clean. Transfer the pan to a cooling rack. Let cool for about 30 minutes.

PER SERVING

CALORIES 193
TOTAL FAT 1.0 g
    Saturated Fat 0.0 g
    Trans Fat 0.0 g
    Polyunsaturated Fat 0.5 g
    Monounsaturated Fat 0.5 g
CHOLESTEROL 1 mg
SODIUM 139 mg
CARBOHYDRATES 43 g
    Fiber 2 g
    Sugars 23 g
PROTEIN 4 g
DIETARY EXCHANGES
    2 starch, 1 carbohydrate

banana-raisin coffee cake with citrus glaze

SERVES 12

This many-flavored coffee cake tastes best when eaten within a few hours of baking.

½ cup golden raisins
¼ cup unsweetened apple juice
½ cup low-fat buttermilk
1 large egg
3 tablespoons honey
1 tablespoon canola or corn oil
2 cups all-purpose flour
1½ teaspoons baking powder
1 teaspoon baking soda
¼ cup firmly packed light brown sugar

½ teaspoon ground ginger
½ teaspoon ground cinnamon
2 medium bananas, mashed (about 1 cup)
½ cup confectioners' sugar, sifted
1 tablespoon fresh orange juice (plus more if needed)
1 tablespoon fresh lemon juice (plus more if needed)

Preheat the oven to 350°F.

In a small bowl, stir together the raisins and apple juice. Let stand for 5 minutes.

In a large bowl, whisk together the buttermilk, egg, honey, and oil. Stir the raisin mixture into the buttermilk mixture.

In another large bowl, sift together the flour, baking powder, and baking soda.

Stir the brown sugar, ginger, and cinnamon into the flour mixture.

Stir the flour mixture and bananas into the buttermilk mixture just until the flour mixture is moistened but no flour is visible. Don't overmix. Spoon into a nonstick 10-inch Bundt pan.

Bake for 30 to 35 minutes, or until a wooden toothpick inserted in the center comes out clean. Transfer the pan to a cooling rack and let cool for 10 minutes. Turn out onto the cooling rack. Let cool completely. Transfer to a serving plate.

In a small bowl, whisk together the confectioners' sugar, 1 tablespoon orange juice, and 1 tablespoon lemon juice until smooth. Gradually whisk in additional juice if needed for consistency. Drizzle over the coffee cake.

PER SERVING

CALORIES 191
TOTAL FAT 2.0 g
  Saturated Fat 0.5 g
  Trans Fat 0.0 g
  Polyunsaturated Fat 0.5 g
  Monounsaturated Fat 1.0 g
CHOLESTEROL 18 mg
SODIUM 175 mg
CARBOHYDRATES 41 g
  Fiber 1 g
  Sugars 21 g
PROTEIN 4 g
DIETARY EXCHANGES
  1 starch, 1 fruit, 1 carbohydrate

quick orange streusel cake

SERVES 9

The orange juice and zest make this coffee cake smell wonderful as it bakes—definitely worth waking up to!

Cooking spray

CAKE

2 cups all-purpose flour
⅓ cup sugar
2 teaspoons baking powder
¼ teaspoon baking soda
⅛ teaspoon salt
2 teaspoons grated orange zest
½ cup fresh orange juice
½ cup fat-free milk
⅓ cup unsweetened applesauce

¼ cup egg substitute
1 tablespoon canola or corn oil
1 teaspoon vanilla extract

TOPPING

¼ cup chopped pecans or walnuts, dry-roasted
¼ cup firmly packed light brown sugar
2 tablespoons all-purpose flour
1 tablespoon light tub margarine, melted

Preheat the oven to 375°F. Lightly spray an 8-inch square baking pan with cooking spray.

In a large bowl, sift together 2 cups flour, sugar, baking powder, baking soda, and salt. Make a well in the center.

In a medium bowl, whisk together the remaining cake ingredients. Pour into the well. Stir just until the dry ingredients are moistened but no flour is visible. Don't overmix. Pour into the baking pan, gently smoothing the top.

In a small bowl, stir together the topping ingredients. Sprinkle over the batter.

Bake for 28 to 33 minutes, or until a wooden toothpick inserted in the center comes out clean. Transfer the pan to a cooling rack. Let cool for about 30 minutes.

PER SERVING

CALORIES 219
TOTAL FAT 4.5 g
    Saturated Fat 0.5 g
    Trans Fat 0.0 g
    Polyunsaturated Fat 1.5 g
    Monounsaturated Fat 2.5 g
CHOLESTEROL 1 mg
SODIUM 188 mg
CARBOHYDRATES 40 g
    Fiber 1 g
    Sugars 17 g
PROTEIN 5 g
DIETARY EXCHANGES
    1½ starch,
    1 carbohydrate, ½ fat

easy refrigerator rolls

SERVES 36; 1 ROLL PER SERVING

Enjoy these yeast rolls at your convenience. Mix and refrigerate the simple dough. When you want homemade rolls, shape them, let them rise, bake them, and enjoy!

¼ cup lukewarm water and 1 cup lukewarm water (105°F to 115°F), divided use
1 ¼-ounce package active dry yeast
2 large egg whites
¼ cup canola or corn oil

½ cup sugar
1 teaspoon salt
4 cups whole-wheat or all-purpose flour
Cooking spray

Pour ¼ cup water into a small bowl. Add the yeast, stirring to dissolve. Let stand for 5 minutes, or until the mixture bubbles.

In a large bowl, lightly whisk the egg whites. Add the following ingredients in order, stirring after each addition: oil, sugar, yeast mixture, salt, remaining 1 cup water, and flour. Cover and refrigerate for 12 hours to four days.

Lightly spray a baking sheet with cooking spray. Make 36 rolls in your favorite shape. Transfer to the baking sheet. Cover with a slightly damp dish towel. Let rise in a warm, draft-free place (about 85°F) for 2 hours.

Preheat the oven to 375°F.

Bake for 10 minutes, or until lightly browned.

PER SERVING

CALORIES 71
TOTAL FAT 2.0 g
  Saturated Fat 0.0 g
  Trans Fat 0.0 g
  Polyunsaturated Fat 0.5 g
  Monounsaturated Fat 1.0 g
CHOLESTEROL 0 mg
SODIUM 69 mg
CARBOHYDRATES 13 g
  Fiber 2 g
  Sugars 3 g
PROTEIN 2 g
DIETARY EXCHANGES
  1 starch

southern raised biscuits

SERVES 15; 2 BISCUITS PER SERVING

You don't need to be from the South to love these tall, flaky biscuits.

1 cup low-fat buttermilk, slightly warmed (105°F to 115°F)

1 ¼-ounce package active dry yeast

2½ cups all-purpose flour, plus more as needed for flouring surface, kneading, rolling out dough, and cutting biscuits

¼ cup sugar

½ teaspoon baking soda

½ teaspoon salt

¼ cup canola or corn oil

Cooking spray

Pour the buttermilk into a small bowl. Add the yeast, stirring to dissolve. Let stand for 5 minutes, or until the mixture bubbles.

In a large bowl, stir together 2½ cups flour, sugar, baking soda, and salt.

Add the buttermilk mixture and oil to the flour mixture. Stir just until the ingredients hold together. Don't overmix.

Lightly flour a flat surface. Turn out the dough. Knead gently 20 to 30 times. Roll out or pat to ¼-inch thickness. With a floured 1-inch biscuit cutter, cut out 60 biscuits, reflouring the biscuit cutter as needed. Lightly spray the top of each biscuit with cooking spray.

Lightly spray a baking sheet with cooking spray. Put 30 biscuits on it. Put a second biscuit on top of each. Cover with a slightly damp dish towel. Let rise in a warm, draft-free place (about 85°F) for about 2 hours.

Preheat the oven to 375°F.

Bake the biscuits for 12 to 15 minutes, or until the tops are light golden brown.

PER SERVING

CALORIES 130
TOTAL FAT 4.0 g
   Saturated Fat 0.5 g
   Trans Fat 0.0 g
   Polyunsaturated Fat 1.0 g
   Monounsaturated Fat 2.5 g
CHOLESTEROL 1 mg
SODIUM 137 mg
CARBOHYDRATES 20 g
   Fiber 1 g
   Sugars 4 g
PROTEIN 3 g
DIETARY EXCHANGES
   1½ starch, ½ fat

parmesan-herb breadsticks

SERVES 18; 1 BREADSTICK PER SERVING

Nothing soaks up the last spoonful of spaghetti sauce, such as Fresh Tomato and Roasted Red Bell Pepper Sauce (page 506), or gravy, such as Mushroom Gravy (page 494), quite like these soft homemade breadsticks.

Cooking spray
2 cups all-purpose flour, plus more as needed for shaping breadsticks
1 cup whole-wheat flour
2 tablespoons minced green onions (green part only)
1 tablespoon snipped fresh dillweed or 1 teaspoon dried, crumbled

1 teaspoon baking soda
½ teaspoon baking powder
¼ teaspoon pepper
⅛ teaspoon salt
1½ cups low-fat buttermilk
2 tablespoons olive oil
2 tablespoons shredded or grated Parmesan cheese

Preheat the oven to 350°F. Lightly spray a large baking sheet with cooking spray.

In a large bowl, whisk together the flours, green onions, dillweed, baking soda, baking powder, pepper, and salt. Make a well in the center.

Pour the buttermilk and oil into the well. Stir just until moistened. Don't overmix.

With lightly floured hands, divide the dough into 18 pieces. Shape each piece into a 4-inch-long cylinder (slightly wetting your hands with cold water will help keep the dough from sticking). Place the cylinders about 1 inch apart on the baking sheet. Sprinkle with the Parmesan.

Bake for 20 to 22 minutes, or until golden brown. For a slightly crisp outside, transfer the rolls to a cooling rack. Let cool for 5 minutes before serving. For slightly warmer and less crisp rolls, put them in a bread basket lined with a dish towel, cover, and let rest for 5 minutes.

PER SERVING

CALORIES 97
TOTAL FAT 2.0 g
  Saturated Fat 0.5 g
  Trans Fat 0.0 g
  Polyunsaturated Fat 0.5 g
  Monounsaturated Fat 1.0 g
CHOLESTEROL 1 mg
SODIUM 129 mg
CARBOHYDRATES 17 g
  Fiber 1 g
  Sugars 1 g
PROTEIN 3 g
DIETARY EXCHANGES
  1 starch

muffins

SERVES 12

Muffins aren't just for breakfast and brunch. They are so easy to make that you can enjoy them anytime.

Cooking spray	1¼ cups fat-free milk
2 cups sifted all-purpose flour	¼ cup egg substitute
2 tablespoons sugar	¼ cup unsweetened applesauce
1 tablespoon baking powder	1 tablespoon canola or corn oil
⅛ teaspoon salt	

Preheat the oven to 425°F. Lightly spray a 12-cup muffin pan with cooking spray.

In a large bowl, sift together the flour, sugar, baking powder, and salt. Make a well in the center.

In a medium bowl, whisk together the remaining ingredients. Pour into the well. Stir until the flour mixture is just blended but no flour is visible. Don't overmix. The batter should be slightly lumpy. Spoon into the muffin cups.

Bake for 20 to 25 minutes, or until a wooden toothpick inserted in the center comes out clean. Transfer the pan to a cooling rack. Let cool for about 30 minutes.

FRUIT MUFFINS
Add ½ cup fruit, such as blueberries, to the batter.

PER SERVING
CALORIES 108
TOTAL FAT 1.5 g
   Saturated Fat 0.0 g
   Trans Fat 0.0 g
   Polyunsaturated Fat 0.5 g
   Monounsaturated Fat 1.0 g
CHOLESTEROL 1 mg
SODIUM 146 mg
CARBOHYDRATES 20 g
   Fiber 1 g
   Sugars 4 g
PROTEIN 4 g
DIETARY EXCHANGES
   1½ starch

PER SERVING
MUFFINS WITH BLUEBERRIES
CALORIES 111
TOTAL FAT 1.5 g
   Saturated Fat 0.0 g
   Trans Fat 0.0 g
   Polyunsaturated Fat 0.5 g
   Monounsaturated Fat 1.0 g
CHOLESTEROL 1 mg
SODIUM 146 mg
CARBOHYDRATES 21 g
   Fiber 1 g
   Sugars 5 g
PROTEIN 4 g
DIETARY EXCHANGES
   1½ starch

whole-wheat muffins

SERVES 12

Serve these fragrant muffins fresh out of the oven with Curried Chicken Salad (page 121) and apple or pear wedges.

Cooking spray
1 cup whole-wheat flour
¾ cup all-purpose flour
¼ cup toasted wheat germ
¼ cup sugar
2½ teaspoons baking powder
½ teaspoon ground cinnamon
⅛ teaspoon ground cloves or ground nutmeg

⅛ teaspoon salt
1 cup fat-free milk
½ cup grated zucchini
⅓ cup unsweetened applesauce
¼ cup egg substitute
1 tablespoon canola or corn oil
1 teaspoon grated orange zest
3 tablespoons chopped walnuts, dry-roasted

Preheat the oven to 375°F. Lightly spray a 12-cup muffin pan with cooking spray.

In a large bowl, stir together the flours, wheat germ, sugar, baking powder, cinnamon, cloves, and salt. Make a well in the center.

In a medium bowl, whisk together the remaining ingredients except the walnuts. Pour into the well.

Add the walnuts. Stir until the flour mixture is just moistened but no flour is visible. Don't overmix; the batter should be slightly lumpy. Spoon into the muffin cups.

Bake for 20 to 25 minutes, or until a wooden toothpick inserted in the center comes out clean. Transfer the pan to a cooling rack. Let the muffins cool for a few minutes in the pan before serving.

TIME-SAVER

For dry-roasted nuts ready at a moment's notice, prepare extras and store them in an airtight container in the freezer. You don't even need to thaw them.

PER SERVING

CALORIES 124
TOTAL FAT 3.0 g
  Saturated Fat 0.5 g
  Trans Fat 0.0 g
  Polyunsaturated Fat 1.5 g
  Monounsaturated Fat 1.0 g
CHOLESTEROL 1 mg
SODIUM 128 mg
CARBOHYDRATES 21 g
  Fiber 2 g
  Sugars 6 g
PROTEIN 4 g
DIETARY EXCHANGES
  1½ starch, ½ fat

apricot-cinnamon muffins

SERVES 12

Each of these muffins contains a triple dose of apricot goodness. They are great for breakfast, snacks, and lunch boxes.

Cooking spray	⅛ teaspoon salt
¼ cup firmly packed light brown sugar	1 8-ounce can apricots in extra-light syrup, well drained, ½ cup liquid reserved, apricots cut into ¼-inch cubes
2 tablespoons chopped walnuts	
½ teaspoon ground cinnamon and 1 teaspoon ground cinnamon, divided use	
	1 cup fat-free apricot or peach yogurt
2 cups all-purpose flour	2 large egg whites
⅓ cup sugar	1 4-ounce jar pureed baby food apricots
2 teaspoons baking powder	
1 teaspoon baking soda	1 teaspoon almond extract

Preheat the oven to 375°F. Lightly spray a 12-cup muffin pan with cooking spray.

In a small bowl, stir together the brown sugar, walnuts, and ½ teaspoon cinnamon. Set aside.

In a large bowl, stir together the flour, sugar, baking powder, baking soda, salt, and remaining 1 teaspoon cinnamon. Make a well in the center.

In a medium bowl, stir together the remaining ingredients. Pour into the well. Stir until the flour mixture is just moistened but no flour is visible. Don't overmix; the batter should be slightly lumpy. Spoon into the muffin cups. Sprinkle with the brown sugar mixture.

Bake for 18 to 20 minutes, or until a wooden toothpick inserted in the center comes out clean. Transfer the pan to a cooling rack. Let cool for about 30 minutes.

PER SERVING

CALORIES 159
TOTAL FAT 1.0 g
    Saturated Fat 0.0 g
    Trans Fat 0.0 g
    Polyunsaturated Fat 0.5 g
    Monounsaturated Fat 0.0 g
CHOLESTEROL 1 mg
SODIUM 220 mg
CARBOHYDRATES 34 g
    Fiber 1 g
    Sugars 14 g
PROTEIN 4 g
DIETARY EXCHANGES
    2 starch

oat bran fruit muffins

SERVES 18

Do your heart a favor and start your day off right with a proper breakfast. One of these muffins, a cold glass of fat-free milk, and a bowl of sliced strawberries would fit the bill.

1½ cups high-fiber oat bran cereal	1 teaspoon baking soda
¾ cup all-purpose flour	1 teaspoon ground cinnamon
¾ cup whole-wheat flour	1 cup low-fat buttermilk
½ cup raisins	½ cup honey
½ cup chopped dried dates	½ cup egg substitute
½ cup chopped dried plums	¼ cup firmly packed dark brown sugar
2 teaspoons baking powder	3 tablespoons canola or corn oil

Preheat the oven to 400°F. Line a 12-cup and a 6-cup muffin pan with bake cups.

In a large bowl, stir together the cereal, flours, raisins, dates, dried plums, baking powder, baking soda, and cinnamon. Make a well in the center.

In a medium bowl, whisk together the remaining ingredients. Pour into the well. Stir until the cereal mixture is just moistened but no flour is visible. Don't overmix. The batter should be slightly lumpy. Spoon into the bake cups.

Bake for 20 to 25 minutes, or until a wooden toothpick inserted in the center comes out clean. Transfer the pan to a cooling rack. Let cool for about 30 minutes.

PER SERVING

CALORIES 152
TOTAL FAT 2.5 g
  Saturated Fat 0.5 g
  Trans Fat 0.0 g
  Polyunsaturated Fat 1.0 g
  Monounsaturated Fat 1.5 g
CHOLESTEROL 1 mg
SODIUM 168 mg
CARBOHYDRATES 31 g
  Fiber 2 g
  Sugars 19 g
PROTEIN 3 g
DIETARY EXCHANGES
  1 starch, 1 fruit, ½ fat

blueberry-banana muffins

SERVES 12

A fruit-lover's dream, these muffins combine blueberries, banana, orange juice, and applesauce.

Cooking spray	⅛ teaspoon salt
1 cup all-purpose flour	1 medium banana, mashed (about ½
½ cup whole-wheat flour	cup)
½ cup toasted wheat germ	½ cup fresh orange juice
⅓ cup firmly packed light brown sugar	¼ cup egg substitute
1 tablespoon baking powder	¼ cup unsweetened applesauce
½ teaspoon ground cinnamon	1 tablespoon canola or corn oil
⅛ teaspoon ground nutmeg	1 cup blueberries

Preheat the oven to 400°F. Lightly spray a 12-cup muffin pan with cooking spray.

In a large bowl, stir together the flours, wheat germ, brown sugar, baking powder, cinnamon, nutmeg, and salt. Make a well in the center.

In a small bowl, whisk together the remaining ingredients except the blueberries. Pour into the well. Stir until the flour mixture is just moistened but no flour is visible. Don't overmix; the batter should be slightly lumpy. With a rubber scraper, carefully fold the blueberries into the batter. Spoon into the muffin cups.

Bake for 15 minutes, or until a wooden toothpick inserted in the center comes out clean. Transfer the pan to a cooling rack. Let cool for about 30 minutes.

PER SERVING

CALORIES 132
TOTAL FAT 2.0 g
   Saturated Fat 0.0 g
   Trans Fat 0.0 g
   Polyunsaturated Fat 1.0 g
   Monounsaturated Fat 1.0 g
CHOLESTEROL 0 mg
SODIUM 138 mg
CARBOHYDRATES 26 g
   Fiber 2 g
   Sugars 10 g
PROTEIN 4 g
DIETARY EXCHANGES
   1½ starch

eye-opener breakfast cookies

SERVES 15; 2 COOKIES PER SERVING

Packed with good-for-you ingredients, these oatmeal cookies are great for breakfast or as a healthy snack later in the day.

Cooking spray
½ cup unsweetened applesauce
½ cup honey
¼ cup plus 2 tablespoons egg substitute
1 teaspoon grated orange zest
2 tablespoons fresh orange juice
2 tablespoons firmly packed light brown sugar
1 tablespoon canola or corn oil
2 teaspoons vanilla extract

¾ cup all-purpose flour
¾ cup whole-wheat flour
1½ teaspoons baking powder
½ teaspoon baking soda
1½ cups uncooked rolled oats
½ cup fat-free dry milk
½ cup toasted wheat germ
½ cup chopped sweetened dried cranberries
½ cup chopped pecans

Preheat the oven to 350°F. Lightly spray two large baking sheets with cooking spray.

In a large mixing bowl, using an electric mixer on medium speed, beat the applesauce, honey, egg substitute, orange zest, orange juice, brown sugar, oil, and vanilla for 1 to 2 minutes, or until smooth.

Meanwhile, in a small bowl, stir together the flours, baking powder, and baking soda. Add to the applesauce mixture, stirring just enough to combine. Beat on medium speed for 1 to 2 minutes, or until completely combined.

Add the remaining ingredients. Beat on low speed just until combined. (The dough will be slightly sticky.)

Using a small 1-tablespoon spring-loaded ice cream scoop or a tablespoon, drop by slightly heaping tablespoonfuls onto the baking sheets, allowing about 1 inch between cookies. You should have about 30 cookies. Using your fingertips, slightly flatten the cookies.

PER SERVING

CALORIES 188
TOTAL FAT 4.5 g
  Saturated Fat 0.5 g
  Trans Fat 0.0 g
  Polyunsaturated Fat 1.5 g
  Monounsaturated Fat 2.5 g
CHOLESTEROL 0 mg
SODIUM 110 mg
CARBOHYDRATES 34 g
  Fiber 3 g
  Sugars 17 g
PROTEIN 5 g
DIETARY EXCHANGES
  1 starch, 1 carbohydrate, ½ fat

Bake for 12 to 15 minutes, or until the cookies are lightly browned. Immediately transfer the cookies from the baking sheets to cooling racks. Let cool for about 30 minutes. Store any leftover cookies in an airtight container, such as a cookie tin, for up to four days. If you prefer softer cookies, store in a resealable plastic bag. Once the cookies are completely cooled, you can freeze them in a plastic freezer bag.

COOK'S TIP on drop cookies

Making drop cookies is a breeze when you use a small spring-loaded ice cream scoop, commonly available at supermarkets and gourmet cookware stores. The #50 scoop holds about one tablespoon and is an ideal size for most cookie recipes, including this one.

slow-cooker pumpkin oatmeal

SERVES 8; 1 CUP PER SERVING

Wake up and smell the oatmeal! The pumpkin-spiced cereal cooks as you sleep, so all you need to do is sprinkle it with brown sugar and walnuts.

Cooking spray

OATMEAL

2 cups uncooked steel-cut oats
½ cup firmly packed light brown sugar
1½ tablespoons ground cinnamon
¾ teaspoon ground nutmeg
1 cup canned solid-pack pumpkin (not pie filling)
6 cups water

1 cup fat-free half-and-half
1 cup raisins
1 teaspoon vanilla extract

TOPPING

2 tablespoons plus 2 teaspoons light brown sugar
¼ cup plus 1 tablespoon and 1 teaspoon chopped walnuts

Lightly spray a 3½- or 4-quart slow cooker with cooking spray.

In a large bowl, stir together the oats, ½ cup brown sugar, cinnamon, and nutmeg. Stir in the pumpkin. Gradually stir in the water and half-and-half. Stir in the raisins and vanilla.

Ladle the mixture into the slow cooker. Cook, covered, on low for 7½ to 8½ hours. Serve topped with the remaining brown sugar and walnuts.

COOK'S TIP

Refrigerate any leftover oatmeal for up to three days. Put the desired amount in a microwaveable bowl, cover it, and reheat it in the microwave on 100 percent power (high), adding a bit of fat-free milk as necessary for the desired consistency. (The chilled oatmeal will have thickened.)

COOK'S TIP on steel-cut oats

Steel-cut oats, also known as Irish oats or pinhead oats, are better than other oats for use in slow-cooker recipes because they can withstand the longer cooking time without getting mushy.

PER SERVING

CALORIES 360
TOTAL FAT 6.5 g
   Saturated Fat 0.5 g
   Trans Fat 0.0 g
   Polyunsaturated Fat 3.5 g
   Monounsaturated Fat 1.5 g
CHOLESTEROL 0 mg
SODIUM 44 mg
CARBOHYDRATES 70 g
   Fiber 11 g
   Sugars 33 g
PROTEIN 10 g
DIETARY EXCHANGES
   2 starch, 1½ fruit,
   1 carbohydrate, 1 fat

maple and banana tapioca

SERVES 4; ½ CUP PER SERVING

Usually enjoyed for dessert, tapioca changes roles and becomes a treat for a leisurely breakfast.

TAPIOCA
- 2 cups fat-free milk
- ¼ cup egg substitute
- 3 tablespoons uncooked quick-cooking tapioca
- ⅛ teaspoon salt
- ½ cup maple syrup
- 1 teaspoon vanilla extract
- ¼ teaspoon ground cinnamon
- 2 medium bananas, sliced

Cooking spray

TOPPING
- ¼ cup chopped pecans
- 2 tablespoons sugar
- ⅛ teaspoon ground cinnamon
- 1 tablespoon egg substitute

In a medium saucepan, whisk together the milk, ¼ cup egg substitute, tapioca, and salt. Let stand for 5 minutes. Cook over medium heat for 12 to 18 minutes (depending on the pan thickness and temperature of the ingredients), or until it comes to a full boil (doesn't stop bubbling when stirred) and begins to thicken, stirring constantly. Remove from the heat.

Stir in the maple syrup, vanilla, and ¼ teaspoon cinnamon.

Put the banana slices in 4 ramekins or custard cups. Spoon the tapioca over the bananas. Let cool for at least 30 minutes or refrigerate until cold, about 2 hours.

Meanwhile, preheat the oven to 350°F. Lightly spray a baking sheet with cooking spray.

In a small bowl, stir together the topping ingredients. Spoon onto the baking sheet. Using a rubber scraper, spread in a thin layer.

Bake the topping for 15 to 20 minutes, or until browned. Let cool on a cooling rack for about 30 minutes. Using a spatula, loosen the topping from the baking sheet. Break the topping into small pieces. Just before serving, sprinkle over the tapioca.

PER SERVING

CALORIES 313
TOTAL FAT 5.5 g
  Saturated Fat 0.5 g
  Trans Fat 0.0 g
  Polyunsaturated Fat 1.5 g
  Monounsaturated Fat 3.0 g
CHOLESTEROL 2 mg
SODIUM 168 mg
CARBOHYDRATES 62 g
  Fiber 2 g
  Sugars 44 g
PROTEIN 7 g
DIETARY EXCHANGES
  4 carbohydrate, 1 fat

muesli

SERVES 6; 1 CUP PER SERVING

For a change of pace, this no-cook, creamy dish incorporates the goodness of oatmeal, wheat germ, yogurt, and fresh and dried fruits. Prepare it the night before to save time in the morning.

1 cup uncooked quick-cooking
  oatmeal
1 cup fat-free vanilla yogurt
½ cup fat-free milk
¼ cup dried currants or raisins
¼ cup chopped dried apricots

2 tablespoons toasted wheat germ
1 tablespoon honey
2 cups sliced strawberries
2 tablespoons sliced almonds,
  dry-roasted

In a medium bowl, stir together the oatmeal, yogurt, milk, currants, apricots, wheat germ, and honey. Cover and refrigerate for 2 hours (the oats should be plump and tender) to two days.

To serve, stir in the strawberries. Sprinkle with the almonds.

PER SERVING

CALORIES 175
TOTAL FAT 2.5 g
  Saturated Fat 0.5 g
  Trans Fat 0.0 g
  Polyunsaturated Fat 1.0 g
  Monounsaturated Fat 1.0 g
CHOLESTEROL 1 mg
SODIUM 42 mg
CARBOHYDRATES 34 g
  Fiber 4 g
  Sugars 21 g
PROTEIN 7 g
DIETARY EXCHANGES
  1 starch, 1 fruit,
  ½ fat-free milk

apple-berry couscous

SERVES 6; 1¼ CUPS PER SERVING

This hot-grain combo uses fresh, dried, and bottled fruit and juice for flavor.

1 teaspoon canola or corn oil
2 medium apples, such as Fuji, McIntosh, or Rome Beauty, cut into ½-inch pieces (about 2 cups)
¼ cup unsweetened dried cherries or dried cranberries
¼ cup golden raisins
3 tablespoons dried currants

3 tablespoons light brown sugar
1 teaspoon ground cinnamon
2 cups unsweetened apple juice
½ cup water
1 teaspoon coarsely grated lime zest
3 tablespoons fresh lime juice
1⅔ cups uncooked whole-wheat couscous

In a large saucepan, heat the oil over low heat, swirling to coat the bottom. Add the apples, cherries, raisins, currants, brown sugar, and cinnamon, stirring to combine. Cook, covered, for 10 minutes, or until the apples have released some of their juices, stirring occasionally.

Stir in the remaining ingredients except the couscous. Increase the heat to high. Cover and bring to a boil.

Stir in the couscous. Remove from the heat. Let stand, covered, for 15 minutes. Fluff with a fork before serving.

COOK'S TIP on couscous

Couscous (KOOS-koos), which looks like tiny bits of pasta, is made from a coarse wheat flour called semolina. Couscous cooks quickly, making it a boon when you're in a hurry. The name "couscous" also refers to a stew made of the grain, lamb or chicken, and vegetables.

PER SERVING

CALORIES 392
TOTAL FAT 2.0 g
  Saturated Fat 0.0 g
  Trans Fat 0.0 g
  Polyunsaturated Fat 0.5 g
  Monounsaturated Fat 0.5 g
CHOLESTEROL 0 mg
SODIUM 8 mg
CARBOHYDRATES 89 g
  Fiber 11 g
  Sugars 31 g
PROTEIN 10 g
DIETARY EXCHANGES
  4 starch, 2 fruit

baked pear pancake

SERVES 6; 1 WEDGE PER SERVING

Serve this delicate Dutch-style pancake from the skillet. It will break apart if you try to transfer the whole pancake to a serving plate.

1 large ripe but firm pear, peeled and thinly sliced	¾ cup fat-free milk
	½ cup all-purpose flour
2 tablespoons sugar and ¼ cup sugar, divided use	3 large egg whites
	¼ cup egg substitute
¼ teaspoon ground cinnamon	½ teaspoon vanilla extract
⅛ teaspoon ground cloves	⅛ teaspoon salt
2 teaspoons canola or corn oil	2 teaspoons confectioners' sugar

Preheat the oven to 425°F.

Put the pear, 2 tablespoons sugar, cinnamon, and cloves in a medium bowl. Gently stir together to coat.

In a 10-inch ovenproof nonstick or cast iron skillet, heat the oil over medium-high heat, swirling to coat the bottom. Put the pear slices in a single layer in the skillet. Cook for 5 minutes, or until beginning to soften (don't stir).

Meanwhile, in a medium bowl, whisk together the milk, flour, egg whites, egg substitute, vanilla, salt, and remaining ¼ cup sugar until smooth. Pour over the pear slices.

Bake for 15 to 18 minutes, or until edge of the pancake is puffed and browned. Sprinkle with the confectioners' sugar just before cutting into wedges while still in the skillet.

PER SERVING

CALORIES 151
TOTAL FAT 2.0 g
  Saturated Fat 0.0 g
  Trans Fat 0.0 g
  Polyunsaturated Fat 0.5 g
  Monounsaturated Fat 1.0 g
CHOLESTEROL 1 mg
SODIUM 110 mg
CARBOHYDRATES 29 g
  Fiber 2 g
  Sugars 19 g
PROTEIN 5 g
DIETARY EXCHANGES
  ½ starch, ½ fruit,
  1 carbohydrate,
  ½ lean meat

cinnamon-orange pancakes

SERVES 4; 3 PANCAKES PER SERVING

Start the day off right with these yummy pancakes, topped with Orange Sauce (page 513), maple syrup, or sliced bananas or strawberries.

1 cup whole-wheat flour
¾ cup all-purpose flour
2 tablespoons toasted wheat germ
1 tablespoon sugar
2 teaspoons baking powder
1 teaspoon ground cinnamon

1 cup fat-free milk
1 teaspoon grated fresh orange zest
¾ cup fresh orange juice
¼ cup egg substitute
Cooking spray

If your griddle is not large enough to hold 12 pancakes at once, preheat the oven to 200°F. Place a cooling rack on a baking sheet. Set aside.

In a large bowl, stir together the flours, wheat germ, sugar, baking powder, and cinnamon.

In a small bowl, whisk together the remaining ingredients except the cooking spray. Pour into the flour mixture. Stir just until the flour mixture is moistened but no flour is visible. Don't overmix.

Lightly spray a griddle or large skillet with cooking spray. Heat over medium heat. For each pancake, ladle ¼ cup batter onto the griddle. Cook for 2 to 3 minutes, or until the tops are bubbly and the edges are dry. Turn over. Cook for 2 to 3 minutes. Transfer the pancakes to the cooling rack, placing them in a single layer and leaving space between. Put in the oven to keep warm. Repeat with the remaining batter (you should have a total of 12 pancakes).

PER SERVING

CALORIES 264
TOTAL FAT 1.5 g
  Saturated Fat 0.0 g
  Trans Fat 0.0 g
  Polyunsaturated Fat 0.5 g
  Monounsaturated Fat 0.0 g
CHOLESTEROL 1 mg
SODIUM 260 mg
CARBOHYDRATES 53 g
  Fiber 5 g
  Sugars 11 g
PROTEIN 12 g
DIETARY EXCHANGES
  3½ starch

perfect pumpkin pancakes

SERVES 4; 3 PANCAKES PER SERVING

With canned pumpkin available year-round, you can serve these fragrant pancakes whenever your family asks for them.

¾ cup plus 2 tablespoons whole-wheat pastry flour
⅓ cup all-purpose flour
¼ cup toasted wheat germ
1 tablespoon pumpkin pie spice
1¼ teaspoons baking powder
¾ cup canned solid-pack pumpkin (not pie filling)

¾ cup fat-free milk
½ cup fat-free sour cream
⅓ cup egg substitute
1 tablespoon plus 2 teaspoons firmly packed light brown sugar
2 teaspoons canola or corn oil
2 teaspoons vanilla extract
Cooking spray

If your griddle is not large enough to hold 12 pancakes at once, preheat the oven to 200°F. Place a cooling rack on a baking sheet. Set aside.

In a large bowl, stir together the flours, wheat germ, pumpkin pie spice, and baking powder.

In a medium bowl, whisk together the pumpkin, milk, sour cream, egg substitute, brown sugar, oil, and vanilla. Pour into the flour mixture. Stir just until moistened but no flour is visible. Don't overmix.

Lightly spray a griddle or large skillet with cooking spray. Heat over medium-high heat. For each pancake, ladle a generous ¼ cup batter onto the griddle. Cook for 3 to 4 minutes, or just until bubbles begin to form on the tops of the pancakes and the edges are a little dry. Reduce the heat to medium low. Gently turn the pancakes over. Cook for about 3 minutes, or until the second side is golden brown and the pancakes are fairly firm to the touch. Transfer the pancakes to the cooling rack, placing them in a single layer and leaving space between. Put in the oven to keep warm. Repeat with the remaining batter (you should have a total of 12 pancakes).

multigrain apple pancakes

SERVES 9; 2 PANCAKES AND HEAPING ¼ CUP TOPPING PER SERVING

Two kinds of leavening are used to keep these hearty pancakes nice and light.

APPLE TOPPING
6 cups thinly sliced peeled apples
   (6 to 7 medium)
¾ cup apple cider or apple juice
¼ cup plus 2 tablespoons packed light
   brown sugar
¾ teaspoon ground cinnamon

PANCAKES
2½ cups low-fat buttermilk
   ½ cup uncooked quick-cooking
   oatmeal

1 cup all-purpose flour
1 cup whole-wheat flour
¼ cup yellow cornmeal
1½ teaspoons baking powder
1 teaspoon baking soda
½ cup apple butter
¼ cup firmly packed light brown sugar
¼ cup egg substitute
1 large egg
1 teaspoon vanilla extract

In a large skillet, combine the apple topping ingredients. Bring to a boil over high heat, then reduce the heat to a vigorous simmer. Simmer for 18 to 20 minutes, or until the cider is reduced and slightly thickened. Set aside and keep warm.

Meanwhile, in a large bowl, combine the buttermilk and oatmeal. Let stand for 10 minutes. While the topping simmers and the oatmeal mixture stands, in a medium bowl, stir together the flours, cornmeal, baking powder, and baking soda.

In a small bowl, whisk together the remaining ingredients. After the standing time, whisk into the oatmeal mixture. Gently whisk in the flour mixture until it is just moistened but no flour is visible. Don't overmix.

Preheat a nonstick griddle or large nonstick skillet over medium heat. Using a ⅓-cup measure, pour the batter for several pancakes onto the griddle. Cook the pancakes for 2 to 3 minutes, or until the tops are bubbly and the edges are dry. Turn over and cook for 2 to 3 minutes, or until browned and cooked through. Transfer to a platter and keep warm. Repeat with the remaining batter until all is used. Serve with the apple topping spooned over the pancakes.

PER SERVING

CALORIES 296
TOTAL FAT 2.0 g
   Saturated Fat 0.5 g
   Trans Fat 0.0 g
   Polyunsaturated Fat 0.5 g
   Monounsaturated Fat 0.5 g
CHOLESTEROL 26 mg
SODIUM 308 mg
CARBOHYDRATES 63 g
   Fiber 4 g
   Sugars 33 g
PROTEIN 8 g
DIETARY EXCHANGES
   2 starch, 1 fruit,
   1 carbohydrate

red, white, and blueberry waffles

SERVES 4; 1 WAFFLE PER SERVING

In just minutes, you can create this colorful and oh-so-healthy beginning to your day. Enjoy on the Fourth of July or any other day of the year!

4 low-fat whole-grain frozen waffles	1 cup blueberries
1 cup fat-free vanilla yogurt	1 medium banana, sliced
1 cup sliced strawberries	

Using the package directions, toast the waffles.

Place one waffle on each plate. Spoon the yogurt over each. Top with the strawberries, blueberries, and banana. Serve immediately for the best texture.

PER SERVING

CALORIES 201
TOTAL FAT 2.0 g
  Saturated Fat 0.0 g
  Trans Fat 0.0 g
  Polyunsaturated Fat 0.5 g
  Monounsaturated Fat 0.5 g
CHOLESTEROL 1 mg
SODIUM 193 mg
CARBOHYDRATES 43 g
  Fiber 6 g
  Sugars 22 g
PROTEIN 8 g
DIETARY EXCHANGES
  1 starch, 1 fruit,
  1 carbohydrate

peachy stuffed french toast

SERVES 4; 1 PIECE PER SERVING

Sandwich a peach filling infused with nutmeg and lemon zest between slices of whole-grain bread and drizzle honey on top for a brunch delight.

2 tablespoons finely chopped pecans	1 teaspoon grated lemon zest
Cooking spray	⅛ teaspoon ground nutmeg
1 teaspoon light brown sugar	4 slices whole-grain bread (lowest
¼ teaspoon ground cinnamon	sodium available), halved
1 15-ounce can sliced peaches in	½ cup egg substitute
juice, well drained and diced	2 tablespoons fat-free milk
2 tablespoons light tub cream cheese	¼ cup honey

In a medium nonstick skillet, dry-roast the pecans in a single layer over medium heat for about 4 minutes, or until just fragrant, stirring frequently. Remove from the heat. Lightly spray the pecans with cooking spray. Return to the heat.

Stir in the brown sugar and cinnamon. Cook for 1 minute, or until the sugar is slightly dissolved, stirring occasionally. (Watch carefully so the mixture does not burn.) Transfer to a small plate. Set aside.

In a medium bowl, stir together the peaches, cream cheese, lemon zest, and nutmeg.

Put 4 half-slices of bread on a cutting board or other flat surface. Spoon the peach mixture onto each. Top with the remaining bread.

In a shallow dish, whisk together the egg substitute and milk. Dip the stuffed bread in the egg substitute mixture, turning to coat and letting the excess drip off.

Heat a large nonstick griddle or nonstick skillet over medium-high heat. Cook the bread for 2 to 3 minutes on each side, or until the outside is golden brown and the filling is heated through. Serve sprinkled with the pecans and drizzled with the honey.

PER SERVING

CALORIES 242
TOTAL FAT 5.0 g
 Saturated Fat 1.0 g
 Trans Fat 0.0 g
 Polyunsaturated Fat 1.0 g
 Monounsaturated Fat 2.0 g
CHOLESTEROL 5 mg
SODIUM 240 mg
CARBOHYDRATES 44 g
 Fiber 6 g
 Sugars 31 g
PROTEIN 9 g
DIETARY EXCHANGES
 1 starch, 1 fruit,
 1 carbohydrate,
 ½ lean meat, ½ fat

country-style breakfast casserole

SERVES 10

To have a special breakfast with no fuss, prepare this casserole of popular breakfast foods the night before.

Cooking spray
8 ounces low-fat smoked link sausage
2 tablespoons maple syrup
2 pounds frozen country-style hash brown potatoes (lowest sodium available)
2 cups fat-free milk
1½ cups egg substitute

2 1-ounce slices low-fat American cheese, diced
¼ cup shredded or grated Parmesan cheese
½ teaspoon dry mustard
¼ teaspoon pepper
2 tablespoons finely snipped green onions (green part only) (optional)

Preheat the oven to 350°F. Lightly spray a 13 x 9 x 2-inch baking pan with cooking spray.

In a medium skillet, cook the sausage over medium-high heat for 3 to 4 minutes, or until browned, turning occasionally. Remove from the skillet and cut into bite-size pieces. Wipe the skillet with paper towels. Return the sausage to the skillet.

Pour in the maple syrup. Cook for 1 minute, stirring to coat. Place the sausage in a single layer in the baking pan.

Top with the potatoes.

In a medium bowl, whisk together the remaining ingredients except the green onions. Pour over the potatoes.

Bake for 1 hour, or until the center is set (doesn't jiggle when the pan is gently shaken).

Sprinkle with the green onions. Let cool for at least 10 minutes before cutting.

COOK'S TIP

If you prepare this casserole ahead of time, cover it with plastic wrap and refrigerate. Put the cold casserole in a cold oven. Set the oven to 350°F and bake for 1 hour 10 minutes to 1 hour 15 minutes. Proceed as directed above.

PER SERVING

CALORIES 161
TOTAL FAT 1.0 g
 Saturated Fat 0.5 g
 Trans Fat 0.0 g
 Polyunsaturated Fat 0.0 g
 Monounsaturated Fat 0.5 g
CHOLESTEROL 14 mg
SODIUM 498 mg
CARBOHYDRATES 25 g
 Fiber 1 g
 Sugars 7 g
PROTEIN 13 g
DIETARY EXCHANGES
 1½ starch,
 1½ very lean meat

stacked sausage and eggs

SERVES 4

Try this for an easy but hearty breakfast when you have out-of-towners visiting or for a midnight breakfast when the conversation never stops! Serve with whole-grain English muffins.

4 ounces low-fat bulk sausage
2 to 3 ounces button mushrooms, sliced
½ large onion, chopped
½ medium green bell pepper, chopped
1 cup egg substitute

3 tablespoons fat-free milk
½ teaspoon Worcestershire sauce (lowest sodium available)
⅛ teaspoon cayenne
⅛ teaspoon salt
2 tablespoons snipped fresh parsley

In a large nonstick skillet, cook the sausage over medium-high heat for 2 to 3 minutes, or until no longer pink, stirring constantly to turn and break up the sausage. Transfer to a medium bowl.

In the same skillet, stir together the mushrooms, onion, and bell pepper. Cook for about 3 minutes, or until the onion is soft, stirring occasionally. Stir into the sausage. Cover to keep warm.

Meanwhile, in a small bowl, whisk together the egg substitute, milk, Worcestershire sauce, and cayenne.

Wipe the skillet with paper towels. Heat the skillet over medium heat. Cook the egg mixture for 2 minutes, stirring frequently. Transfer to plates. Top with the sausage mixture. Sprinkle with the salt and parsley.

PER SERVING

CALORIES 88
TOTAL FAT 1.0 g
   Saturated Fat 0.0 g
   Trans Fat 0.0 g
   Polyunsaturated Fat 0.0 g
   Monounsaturated Fat 0.0 g
CHOLESTEROL 14 mg
SODIUM 370 mg
CARBOHYDRATES 6 g
   Fiber 1 g
   Sugars 4 g
PROTEIN 12 g
DIETARY EXCHANGES
   1 vegetable,
   1½ very lean meat

breakfast pizzas

SERVES 4

Stack English muffins sky-high with scrambled eggs and veggies, crown them with tomato sauce and cheese, and serve them with a knife and fork.

8 ounces button mushrooms, sliced
1 large onion, chopped
1 medium green bell pepper, chopped
¾ cup egg substitute
¼ cup fat-free milk
½ cup no-salt-added tomato sauce, at room temperature

1 teaspoon dried Italian seasoning, crumbled
¼ teaspoon crushed red pepper flakes
2 whole-grain English muffins (lowest sodium available), split and toasted
2 tablespoons shredded or grated Parmesan cheese

In a large nonstick skillet, cook the mushrooms over medium-high heat for 4 minutes, or until soft, stirring occasionally.

Stir in the onion and bell pepper. Cook for 4 to 5 minutes, or until the onion is soft, stirring occasionally.

Meanwhile, in a small bowl, whisk together the egg substitute and milk.

Reduce the heat to medium. Pour the egg mixture over the mushroom mixture, stirring with a rubber scraper to combine. Cook until the eggs are set, stirring occasionally with the scraper. Remove from the heat.

In a small bowl, stir together the tomato sauce, Italian seasoning, and red pepper flakes.

Meanwhile, toast the English muffins.

Put the muffin halves on plates. Spoon the tomato mixture over the muffins. Top with the egg mixture. Sprinkle with the Parmesan.

MEXICAN BREAKFAST PIZZAS

8 ounces button mushrooms, sliced

1 medium onion, chopped

1 medium green bell pepper, chopped

¾ cup egg substitute

¼ cup fat-free milk

½ cup no-salt-added tomato sauce, at room temperature

½ teaspoon ground cumin

¼ teaspoon crushed red pepper flakes

4 6-inch corn tortillas

¼ cup fat-free sour cream

1 tablespoon snipped fresh cilantro

Prepare the egg and vegetable mixture as directed on page 560. Using the package directions, warm the tortillas. Spoon the egg substitute and vegetable mixture onto the tortillas. Stir together the tomato sauce with the cumin and red pepper flakes. Spoon over the tortillas. Top with the sour cream and cilantro.

strata with canadian bacon, spinach, and tomatoes

SERVES 4

Is this breakfast, lunch, or dinner? Whatever time of day, this savory casserole will leave no question of how good it tastes, with colorful spinach and tomatoes, smoky Canadian bacon, and the distinctive flavor of Swiss cheese.

Cooking spray	⅓ cup diced Canadian bacon
3 slices whole-grain bread (lowest sodium available), cubed	4 medium green onions, thinly sliced
	¼ cup shredded low-fat Swiss cheese
1 10-ounce package frozen chopped spinach, thawed and squeezed dry	¼ cup coarsely chopped fresh basil
	1½ cups fat-free milk
2 medium Italian plum (Roma) tomatoes, diced	1 cup egg substitute
	¼ teaspoon pepper

Preheat the oven to 350°F. (If you are preparing the strata mixture in advance, see the Cook's Tip). Lightly spray an 8-inch square baking pan with cooking spray.

In the baking pan, stir together the bread cubes, spinach, tomatoes, Canadian bacon, green onions, Swiss cheese, and basil.

In a medium bowl, whisk together the milk, egg substitute, and pepper. Pour over the bread mixture.

Bake for 55 to 60 minutes, or until the center is set (doesn't jiggle when the pan is gently shaken). Let cool for 10 minutes before cutting.

COOK'S TIP

If you prepare this casserole ahead of time, cover it with plastic wrap and refrigerate for up to 10 hours. Put the cold casserole in a cold oven. Set the oven to 350°F and bake for 1 hour 5 minutes to 1 hour 10 minutes, or until the center is set. Let cool for 10 minutes before cutting.

PER SERVING

CALORIES 178
TOTAL FAT 2.0 g
　Saturated Fat 1.0 g
　Trans Fat 0.0 g
　Polyunsaturated Fat 0.0 g
　Monounsaturated Fat 0.5 g
CHOLESTEROL 12 mg
SODIUM 530 mg
CARBOHYDRATES 21 g
　Fiber 5 g
　Sugars 9 g
PROTEIN 19 g
DIETARY EXCHANGES
　1 starch, 1 vegetable,
　2 very lean meat

mango sunrise breakfast parfaits

SERVES 4

Start the day out bright with this parfait and its brilliantly colored fruit.

1 medium mango, diced
1 teaspoon grated orange zest or
   grated peeled gingerroot
¼ cup fresh orange juice
1 tablespoon sugar
24 ounces fat-free vanilla yogurt

¾ cup low-fat granola, coarsely
   crumbled
1 cup fresh blueberries, raspberries,
   blackberries, or quartered
   strawberries

In a medium bowl, gently stir together the mango, orange zest, orange juice, and sugar.

Spoon the mango mixture into parfait glasses or wine goblets. Top, in order, with the yogurt, granola, and berries. Serve or cover and refrigerate for up to 4 hours.

PER SERVING

CALORIES 280
TOTAL FAT 1.0 g
   Saturated Fat 0.0 g
   Trans Fat 0.0 g
   Polyunsaturated Fat 0.0 g
   Monounsaturated Fat 0.5 g
CHOLESTEROL 3 mg
SODIUM 143 mg
CARBOHYDRATES 61 g
   Fiber 4 g
   Sugars 48 g
PROTEIN 11 g
DIETARY EXCHANGES
   1 starch, 1 fruit,
   1 fat-free milk,
   1 carbohydrate

desserts

Double-Shot Espresso Molten Cakes

Black Devil's Food Cake

Wacky Cake

Angelic Blueberry Delight

Angel Food Layers with Chocolate Custard and Kiwifruit

Blueberry-Almond Bundt Cake

Nutmeg Cake

Easy Apple Cake

Pineapple-Pumpkin Spice Cake

Carrot Cake

Double-Ginger Squares

Banana Spice Cupcakes with Nutmeg Cream Topping

Pumpkin Spice Cupcakes with Cinnamon-Sugar Topping

Spice Cupcakes with Vanilla Topping and Pineapple

Seven-Minute Frosting

Lemon-Flavored Seven-Minute Frosting

Seven-Minute Frosting with Fruit

Confectioners' Glaze

Lemon or Orange Confectioners' Glaze

Chocolate Confectioners' Glaze

Peach Clafouti

Delicate Lemon Ricotta Cheesecake with Blackberries

Pumpkin Cheesecake

Strawberry Cream Ice Box Pie

Frozen Mocha Yogurt Pie

Gingersnap Fruit Tart

Peach-Raspberry Crumble

Rhubarb-Cherry Oat Crumble

Apple-Raisin Crunch

Cherry Crisp

Deep-Dish Fruit Crisp

Cherry-Filled Phyllo Rollovers

Tropical Mini Phyllo Shells

Gingersnap and Graham Cracker Crust

Oatmeal Piecrust

Pistachio-Cardamom Meringues

Cookie Jar Snickerdoodles

Apple-Cherry Drops

Pumpkin Oaties

Bourbon Balls

Fudgy Buttermilk Brownies

Apricot-Almond Biscotti

Chocolate-Pecan Biscotti

Tropical Napoleons

Cannoli Cream with Strawberries and Chocolate

Cinnamon-Sugar Vanilla Flans with Blueberries

Chocolate Crème Brûlée

Honey-Almond Custards

Raisin-Walnut Rice Pudding

Delicious Rice Pudding

Guiltless Banana Pudding

Guiltless Strawberry Pudding

Vanilla Bread Pudding with Peaches

Berry-Filled Meringue Shells

Fruit with Vanilla Cream

Berries in Vanilla Sauce

Sweet and Fruity Salsa Bowl

Grapefruit-Orange Palette

Claret-Spiced Oranges

Baked Ginger Pears

Golden Poached Pears

Fall Fruit Medley

Frozen Raspberry Cream

Frozen Cocoa Cream with Dark Cherries

Spiced Skillet Bananas with Frozen Yogurt

Spiced Skillet Apples with Frozen Yogurt

Frozen Mini Key Lime Soufflés

Strawberries with Champagne Ice

Strawberry-Raspberry Ice

Strawberry-Banana Sorbet

Mango-Peach Sorbet

Cherry-Berry Chill

Tropical Breeze

Sunny Mango Sorbet

Tequila-Lime Sherbet

Cardinal Sundaes

Kiwifruit Sundaes

Raspberry Parfaits

double-shot espresso molten cakes

SERVES 8

These ultramoist cakes soak up the coffee-sauce topping like little sponges! The cakes are at their best while still warm.

Cooking spray
1 cup all-purpose flour
¾ cup sugar
⅓ cup unsweetened cocoa powder (dark preferred)
1 tablespoon instant coffee granules and 2 tablespoons instant coffee granules, divided use

2 teaspoons baking powder
½ cup fat-free evaporated milk
¼ cup egg substitute
3 tablespoons canola or corn oil
2 teaspoons vanilla extract
2 cups boiling water
1 cup fat-free frozen whipped topping, thawed in refrigerator

Preheat the oven to 350°F. Lightly spray eight 6-ounce ovenproof custard cups with cooking spray. Put on a baking sheet.

In a large bowl, whisk together the flour, sugar, cocoa powder, 1 tablespoon coffee granules, and baking powder.

In a small bowl, whisk together the milk, egg substitute, oil, and vanilla. Add to the flour mixture, stirring just until blended but no flour is visible. Don't overmix. Spoon into the custard cups.

In a small bowl, stir together the boiling water and remaining 2 tablespoons coffee granules until the granules are dissolved. Gently spoon 2 tablespoons mixture over the batter in each custard cup, reserving the remaining 1 cup coffee mixture.

Bake for 16 to 17 minutes, or until the edges are set and the centers are very soft. (The cakes will not look done at this point.) Transfer the custard cups to a cooling rack and let cool for 5 minutes. Just before serving, spoon about 2 tablespoons of the remaining coffee mixture over each cake. Top each with about 2 tablespoons whipped topping. Serve immediately.

PER SERVING

CALORIES 228
TOTAL FAT 6.0 g
  Saturated Fat 0.5 g
  Trans Fat 0.0 g
  Polyunsaturated Fat 1.5 g
  Monounsaturated Fat 3.5 g
CHOLESTEROL 1 mg
SODIUM 142 mg
CARBOHYDRATES 39 g
  Fiber 1 g
  Sugars 22 g
PROTEIN 4 g
DIETARY EXCHANGES
  2½ carbohydrate, 1 fat

black devil's food cake

SERVES 20

When the chocolate urge hits, try this rich, moist cake, which comes together as quickly as it disappears! Frost it with Seven-Minute Frosting (page 581), dress it up with a dusting of confectioners' sugar, or enjoy it without any topping at all.

Cooking spray	1¾ cups sugar
Unsweetened cocoa powder	1 tablespoon baking soda
for dusting the pan and ½ cup	1 cup low-fat buttermilk
unsweetened cocoa powder, divided	⅔ cup unsweetened applesauce
use	2 tablespoons canola or corn oil
2 cups all-purpose flour	1 cup strong coffee

Preheat the oven to 350°F. Lightly spray a 13 x 9 x 2-inch baking pan with cooking spray. Dust with cocoa powder, shaking to lightly coat. Shake off the excess.

Sift the flour, sugar, baking soda, and remaining ½ cup cocoa powder into a large mixing bowl.

Whisk in the buttermilk, applesauce, and oil.

In a small saucepan, bring the coffee to a boil over medium-high heat. Gently stir into the batter; the mixture will be soupy. Pour into the pan.

Bake for 35 to 40 minutes, or until a wooden toothpick inserted in the center comes out clean. Serve warm or let cool completely.

PER SERVING

CALORIES 143
TOTAL FAT 2.0 g
  Saturated Fat 0.0 g
  Trans Fat 0.0 g
  Polyunsaturated Fat 0.5 g
  Monounsaturated Fat 1.0 g
CHOLESTEROL 1 mg
SODIUM 202 mg
CARBOHYDRATES 30 g
  Fiber 1 g
  Sugars 19 g
PROTEIN 2 g
DIETARY EXCHANGES
  2 carbohydrate, ½ fat

wacky cake

SERVES 9

Traditional wacky cake is a chocolate cake that does not use eggs or milk. It is believed to have been created as a result of rationing during World War II when milk and eggs were scarce. Children will love to help you prepare this cake by making wells in the dry ingredients, then filling the wells with the liquids and stirring it all together.

Cooking spray
1½ cups all-purpose flour
1 cup sugar
¼ cup unsweetened cocoa powder
1 teaspoon baking soda
1 teaspoon vanilla extract

1 teaspoon cider vinegar
1½ tablespoons light tub margarine, melted
¼ cup unsweetened applesauce
1 cup water
1 tablespoon confectioners' sugar

Preheat the oven to 350°F. Lightly spray an 8-inch square baking pan with cooking spray.

Put the flour, sugar, cocoa powder, and baking soda in a sifter. Sift into the pan.

Make three wells in the flour mixture. Pour the vanilla into the first well, the vinegar into the second, and the margarine into the third.

Put the applesauce in a small bowl. Gradually stir in the water. Pour over the batter. Using a fork, stir together until all the dry ingredients are completely moistened.

Bake for 30 minutes, or until a wooden toothpick inserted in the center comes out clean. Transfer to a cooling rack and let cool completely. Sift the confectioners' sugar over the top.

PER SERVING

CALORIES 186
TOTAL FAT 1.0 g
  Saturated Fat 0.0 g
  Trans Fat 0.0 g
  Polyunsaturated Fat 0.5 g
  Monounsaturated Fat 0.5 g
CHOLESTEROL 0 mg
SODIUM 156 mg
CARBOHYDRATES 41 g
  Fiber 1 g
  Sugars 24 g
PROTEIN 3 g
DIETARY EXCHANGES
  3 carbohydrate

angelic blueberry delight

SERVES 10

Deeply colored blueberries, a source of antioxidants, taste wickedly good when combined with angel food cake in this melt-in-your-mouth creation.

1 8-ounce container fat-free frozen whipped topping and 1 cup fat-free frozen whipped topping, thawed in refrigerator, divided use
2 to 3 teaspoons grated orange zest
½ cup fresh orange juice

7 ounces fat-free sweetened condensed milk
1 8-inch angel food cake, cut into bite-size pieces
3 cups fresh blueberries

Spoon the 8-ounce container whipped topping into a medium bowl. Gradually whisk in the orange zest and juice.

Pour in the milk, whisking until well combined.

In a 3- to 3½-quart trifle dish or decorative bowl, layer half the cake pieces, 1 cup blueberries, and half the whipped topping mixture. Repeat. Spread with the remaining 1 cup whipped topping. Arrange the remaining 1 cup blueberries on top. Refrigerate for at least 1 hour before serving. Cover and refrigerate leftovers for up to one day.

PER SERVING

CALORIES 280
TOTAL FAT 0.0 g
  Saturated Fat 0.0 g
  Trans Fat 0.0 g
  Polyunsaturated Fat 0.0 g
  Monounsaturated Fat 0.0 g
CHOLESTEROL 4 mg
SODIUM 167 mg
CARBOHYDRATES 62 g
  Fiber 2 g
  Sugars 44 g
PROTEIN 5 g
DIETARY EXCHANGES
  4 carbohydrate

angel food layers with chocolate custard and kiwifruit

SERVES 8

Dark chocolate custard and jade-green kiwifruit nestle between layers of angel food cake in this decadent dessert.

CHOCOLATE CUSTARD
1 cup fat-free milk
½ cup sugar
¼ cup egg substitute
2 tablespoons cornstarch
2 tablespoons unsweetened cocoa powder
1 tablespoon all-purpose flour

½ teaspoon vanilla extract
___

½ 8-inch angel food cake
6 medium kiwifruit, peeled and each cut in 8 slices
¾ cup strawberry glaze
½ cup frozen fat-free whipped topping, thawed in refrigerator

In the top of a double boiler, whisk together all the custard ingredients except the vanilla. Set over a small amount of simmering water. Cook for 3 to 4 minutes, whisking occasionally until the mixture starts to thicken. Whisk constantly for about 1 minute, or until the custard is thick and smooth.

Whisk in the vanilla. Cook for 1 minute, whisking occasionally. Remove the top of the double boiler. Let the custard cool for 10 to 15 minutes. Place plastic wrap directly on the custard. Refrigerate for up to four days.

Cut the cake into 8 slices. Cut each slice in half crosswise. Put one half-slice of cake on each dessert plate. Arrange 3 slices of kiwifruit on each. Spread half the custard over the kiwifruit. Repeat. Drizzle with the strawberry glaze. Top each serving with a dollop of whipped topping.

COOK'S TIP on strawberry glaze

Look in the produce area of the grocery store for containers of strawberry glaze. Try it on cakes, pies, and fat-free ice cream.

PER SERVING

CALORIES 235
TOTAL FAT 1.0 g
  Saturated Fat 0.0 g
  Trans Fat 0.0 g
  Polyunsaturated Fat 0.5 g
  Monounsaturated Fat 0.5 g
CHOLESTEROL 27 mg
SODIUM 102 mg
CARBOHYDRATES 53 g
  Fiber 2 g
  Sugars 39 g
PROTEIN 5 g
DIETARY EXCHANGES
  3½ carbohydrate

blueberry-almond bundt cake

SERVES 16

Studded with berries and bursting with almond flavor, this fine-textured cake needs no adornment beyond a sprinkling of confectioners' sugar.

¾ cup sugar
4 ounces almond paste
2 cups all-purpose flour
2 teaspoons baking powder
½ teaspoon baking soda
¼ teaspoon salt
1 cup fat-free plain yogurt

¼ cup canola or corn oil
1 large egg
1 large egg white
1 cup fresh or frozen blueberries or cranberries
1 teaspoon confectioners' sugar

Preheat the oven to 350°F. Lightly spray a 9-inch Bundt pan with cooking spray.

In a food processor, process the sugar and almond paste until smooth.

Add the flour, baking powder, baking soda, and salt. Pulse to combine well.

In a large bowl, whisk together the yogurt, oil, egg, and egg white until smooth.

Add the sugar mixture to the yogurt mixture, stirring just until the batter is moist. Don't overmix.

Gently stir in the blueberries (the batter will be very thick). Spoon into the pan.

Bake for 40 to 45 minutes, or until a wooden toothpick inserted in the center comes out clean. Let cool on a cooling rack for 10 minutes. Turn out onto the rack and let cool completely. Put the confectioners' sugar in a fine-mesh sieve and dust the top of the cake.

COOK'S TIP

If your Bundt pan is 12 inches, you can use it for this recipe. The cake just won't be quite so tall.

COOK'S TIP

Be sure to use almond paste, not the sweeter, less coarse marzipan, in this recipe. Marzipan, made with almond paste and sugar, is not used in baking.

PER SERVING

CALORIES 180
TOTAL FAT 6.0 g
  Saturated Fat 0.5 g
  Trans Fat 0.0 g
  Polyunsaturated Fat 1.5 g
  Monounsaturated Fat 3.5 g
CHOLESTEROL 14 mg
SODIUM 149 mg
CARBOHYDRATES 28 g
  Fiber 1 g
  Sugars 15 g
PROTEIN 4 g
DIETARY EXCHANGES
  2 carbohydrate, 1 fat

nutmeg cake

SERVES 16

The tempting aroma of nutmeg will fill the air as this cake bakes. The topping provides a satisfying crunchiness.

Cooking spray
All-purpose flour for dusting the pan
CAKE
  2 cups all-purpose flour
  1 teaspoon baking powder
  1 teaspoon baking soda
  1 teaspoon ground nutmeg
  1 cup sugar
  ½ cup unsweetened applesauce
  1 large egg
  ¼ cup egg substitute
  1 tablespoon canola or corn oil
  1 teaspoon butter flavoring

1 cup low-fat buttermilk, at room
  temperature
½ teaspoon vanilla extract

TOPPING
  ⅔ cup uncooked quick-cooking oatmeal
  ⅓ cup firmly packed dark brown sugar
  2 tablespoons finely chopped pecans,
    dry-roasted
  ½ teaspoon ground nutmeg
  2 tablespoons light tub margarine,
    melted
  2 tablespoons (about) fat-free milk

Preheat the oven to 350°F. Lightly spray a 13 x 9 x 2-inch baking pan with cooking spray. Dust the pan with the flour, shaking to lightly coat. Shake off the excess.

In a medium bowl, sift together 2 cups flour, baking powder, baking soda, and 1 teaspoon nutmeg.

In a large mixing bowl, beat the sugar, applesauce, egg, egg substitute, oil, and butter flavoring until smooth.

Gradually add the flour mixture and buttermilk alternately, beginning and ending with the flour and beating after each addition.

Stir in the vanilla. Pour into the baking pan.

Bake for 30 to 35 minutes, or until a wooden toothpick inserted in the center comes out clean.

Meanwhile, in a small bowl, stir together the oatmeal, brown sugar, pecans, and remaining ½ teaspoon nutmeg. Stir in the margarine.

Slowly add the milk to the oatmeal mixture, stirring constantly, until the mixture is spreading consistency. Spread on the hot cake. Serve warm.

easy apple cake

SERVES 9

Double your enjoyment of apples with this moist cake made with diced apples and applesauce. Serve it with Orange Sauce (page 513) if desired.

Cooking spray
2 cups diced apples (peeled or unpeeled)
¾ cup sugar
1½ cups all-purpose flour
½ cup raisins
1½ teaspoons pumpkin pie spice or apple pie spice

1 teaspoon baking powder
1 teaspoon baking soda
⅛ teaspoon salt
⅓ cup unsweetened applesauce
1 large egg
1 tablespoon canola or corn oil
1 teaspoon vanilla extract

Preheat the oven to 350°F. Lightly spray an 8-inch square baking pan with cooking spray.

In a large bowl, stir together the apples and sugar. Set aside for about 10 minutes.

Meanwhile, in a medium bowl, stir together the flour, raisins, pie spice, baking powder, baking soda, and salt.

Stir the remaining ingredients into the apple mixture. Gradually stir the flour mixture into the apple mixture until no flour is visible. Spread the batter in the pan.

Bake for 35 to 40 minutes, or until a wooden toothpick inserted in the center comes out clean.

COOK'S TIP on pumpkin or apple pie spice

If you can't find either of these mixtures in the spice section or just prefer to make your own, start with four parts ground cinnamon, two parts each ground nutmeg and ground cloves, and one part each ground allspice and ground cardamom. Adjust the amounts to suit your taste.

PER SERVING

CALORIES 211
TOTAL FAT 2.5 g
    Saturated Fat 0.5 g
    Trans Fat 0.0 g
    Polyunsaturated Fat 0.5 g
    Monounsaturated Fat 1.0 g
CHOLESTEROL 24 mg
SODIUM 226 mg
CARBOHYDRATES 45 g
    Fiber 2 g
    Sugars 26 g
PROTEIN 3 g
DIETARY EXCHANGES
    3 carbohydrate, ½ fat

pineapple-pumpkin spice cake

SERVES 20

The pumpkin and pineapple are the key ingredients in keeping this healthy, hearty cake moist and richly flavorful.

Cooking spray
All-purpose flour for dusting the pan
¼ cup finely chopped pecans, dry-roasted
2 8-ounce cans crushed pineapple in its own juice, undrained
1 18.25-ounce box spice cake mix
1 cup canned solid-pack pumpkin (not pie filling) (about ½ 15-ounce can)

¾ cup egg substitute or 6 large egg whites
2 tablespoons canola or corn oil
2 teaspoons vanilla extract or 1 teaspoon vanilla, butter, and nut flavoring
2 teaspoons honey

Preheat the oven to 325°F.

Lightly spray a 10-inch Bundt pan or tube pan with cooking spray. Dust with the flour, shaking to lightly coat. Shake off the excess. Sprinkle the pecans in the pan.

Set a colander over a liquid measuring cup. Pour the pineapple into the colander. Using the back of a spoon, press on the pineapple to drain the juice into the cup. Spoon the pineapple over the pecans. Add enough water to the juice to equal 1⅓ cups.

Put the juice mixture and remaining ingredients except the honey in a large mixing bowl (these ingredients replace the eggs, oil, and water the package calls for). Follow the package directions for mixing speed and time. Pour the batter over the pineapple.

Bake for 55 minutes, or until a wooden toothpick inserted in the center comes out clean. Transfer the pan to a cooling rack and let the cake cool for 20 minutes. Invert onto a serving plate. Let cool completely, at least 1 hour. Drizzle the honey over the top of the cake, allowing it to dribble down the sides. Cover any leftover cake with plastic wrap and refrigerate for up to one week.

PER SERVING

CALORIES 150
TOTAL FAT 4.5 g
  Saturated Fat 1.0 g
  Trans Fat 0.5 g
  Polyunsaturated Fat 0.5 g
  Monounsaturated Fat 2.0 g
CHOLESTEROL 0 mg
SODIUM 190 mg
CARBOHYDRATES 26 g
  Fiber 1 g
  Sugars 15 g
PROTEIN 3 g
DIETARY EXCHANGES
  1½ carbohydrate, 1 fat

carrot cake

SERVES 12

Enjoy a piece of this cake with a cup of hot tea for a lunchtime treat.

Cooking spray
½ cup egg substitute
½ cup sugar
½ cup unsweetened applesauce
½ cup fat-free plain yogurt
¼ cup firmly packed light brown sugar
1 tablespoon canola or corn oil

2 cups all-purpose flour
1½ cups grated carrots
½ cup raisins (optional)
¼ cup chopped walnuts, dry-roasted
1½ teaspoons ground cinnamon
1 teaspoon baking soda

Preheat the oven to 350°F. Lightly spray an 8-inch square baking pan with cooking spray.

In a large bowl, whisk together the egg substitute, sugar, applesauce, yogurt, brown sugar, and oil.

In another large bowl, stir together the remaining ingredients. Add to the sugar mixture, stirring just until combined but no flour is visible. Don't overmix. Pour the batter into the pan.

Bake for 30 to 35 minutes, or until a wooden toothpick inserted in the center comes out clean.

PER SERVING

CALORIES 174
TOTAL FAT 3.0 g
  Saturated Fat 0.5 g
  Trans Fat 0.0 g
  Polyunsaturated Fat 1.5 g
  Monounsaturated Fat 1.0 g
CHOLESTEROL 0 mg
SODIUM 145 mg
CARBOHYDRATES 33 g
  Fiber 1 g
  Sugars 16 g
PROTEIN 4 g
DIETARY EXCHANGES
  2 carbohydrate, ½ fat

double-ginger squares

SERVES 9

We use both fresh and ground ginger—and even a bit of pepper—for a layering of flavor in this wonderfully moist cake. Whole-wheat flour, applesauce, and egg substitute make it health-friendly, too.

Cooking spray
1¼ cups white whole-wheat flour, or
    ¾ cup all-purpose flour plus ½ cup
    whole-wheat flour
1 teaspoon ground ginger
½ teaspoon ground cinnamon
¼ teaspoon ground cloves
⅛ teaspoon salt
⅛ teaspoon pepper
¼ cup plus 3 tablespoons
    unsweetened applesauce

¼ cup light molasses
¼ cup egg substitute
¼ cup canola or corn oil
1½ teaspoons grated peeled gingerroot
¼ cup firmly packed light brown sugar
⅓ cup boiling water
¾ teaspoon baking soda
Confectioners' sugar

Preheat the oven to 350°F. Lightly spray an 8-inch square baking pan with cooking spray.

In a medium bowl, stir together the flour(s), ground ginger, cinnamon, cloves, salt, and pepper.

In a separate medium bowl, stir together the applesauce, molasses, egg substitute, oil, and gingerroot. Crumble the brown sugar into the mixture, stirring to dissolve.

Pour the water into a small bowl. Stir in the baking soda. Stir into the applesauce mixture. Whisk into the flour mixture just until smooth. Pour into the pan.

Bake for 20 minutes, or until the top of the cake springs back when pressed lightly and a wooden toothpick inserted in the center comes out clean. Transfer to a cooling rack and let cool for at least 10 minutes.

Place a paper doily on the gingerbread. Sift the confectioners' sugar on top, then carefully remove the doily so the design is not disturbed. If you prefer, just sift the sugar over the gingerbread without using the doily. Cut into squares. Store any leftover cake in the pan, covered with plastic wrap, at room temperature for up to two days.

PER SERVING

CALORIES 172
TOTAL FAT 6.5 g
    Saturated Fat 0.5 g
    Trans Fat 0.0 g
    Polyunsaturated Fat 2.0 g
    Monounsaturated Fat 4.0 g
CHOLESTEROL 0 mg
SODIUM 159 mg
CARBOHYDRATES 27 g
    Fiber 2 g
    Sugars 14 g
PROTEIN 3 g
DIETARY EXCHANGES
    1 starch, 1 carbohydrate,
    1 fat

COOK'S TIP on microplanes

Using a microplane is one way to grate gingerroot. This handy tool also is perfect for grating citrus zest, fresh nutmeg, and Parmesan cheese.

COOK'S TIP on applesauce

Adding applesauce to cake batters provides moisture that traditionally comes from fats such as butter and margarine. Instead of the saturated fat those provide, you get extra fiber and vitamins.

banana spice cupcakes
with nutmeg cream topping

SERVES 24

Incredibly moist, these cupcakes are crowned with a luscious blend of creamy fat-free whipped topping and just the right amount of nutmeg.

CUPCAKES
- 1 18.25-ounce box spice cake mix
- 1 cup well-mashed very ripe bananas
- 1 cup unsweetened apple juice
- 2 large eggs
- 2 large egg whites
- 1 teaspoon vanilla, butter, and nut flavoring or vanilla extract

NUTMEG CREAM TOPPING
- 8 ounces fat-free frozen whipped topping, thawed in refrigerator
- 2 teaspoons ground nutmeg

Preheat the oven to 350°F.

In a large mixing bowl, stir together the cupcake ingredients. Using an electric mixer, beat on low for 30 seconds. Increase the speed to medium. Beat for 2 minutes. Spoon into two 12-cup nonstick muffin pans.

Bake for 20 minutes, or until a wooden toothpick inserted in the center of a cupcake comes out clean. Transfer to cooling racks and let cool for 15 minutes. Remove the cupcakes from the pans. Let cool completely.

Meanwhile, using a rubber scraper, gently fold the nutmeg into the whipped topping. Cover and refrigerate until ready to use.

Spread the chilled topping over the cupcakes up to 8 hours in advance. Cover and refrigerate.

PER SERVING

CALORIES 123
TOTAL FAT 2.5 g
 Saturated Fat 0.5 g
 Trans Fat 0.0 g
 Polyunsaturated Fat 0.0 g
 Monounsaturated Fat 0.5 g
CHOLESTEROL 18 mg
SODIUM 157 mg
CARBOHYDRATES 24 g
 Fiber 1 g
 Sugars 12 g
PROTEIN 2 g
DIETARY EXCHANGES
 1½ carbohydrate, ½ fat

PUMPKIN SPICE CUPCAKES
WITH CINNAMON-SUGAR TOPPING

Substitute 1 cup canned solid-pack pumpkin (not pumpkin pie filling) for the bananas. Before baking the cupcakes, sprinkle them with a mixture of 2 teaspoons sugar and ½ teaspoon ground cinnamon.

COOK'S TIP

The toppings for the banana cupcakes and the pumpkin cupcakes are interchangeable, so you might want to try the banana cupcakes with the cinnamon-sugar and the pumpkin cupcakes with the nutmeg topping sometime.

spice cupcakes
with vanilla topping and pineapple

SERVES 24

These piled-high goodies will bring you lots of compliments. You'll make these cupcakes over and over again.

CUPCAKES
1 18.25-ounce box spice cake mix
1⅓ cups water
6 large egg whites
¾ cup well-mashed very ripe bananas

VANILLA TOPPING
1 cup fat-free vanilla yogurt
2 tablespoons confectioners' sugar

½ teaspoon vanilla extract
2 cups fat-free frozen whipped topping, thawed in refrigerator

1 8-ounce can crushed pineapple in its own juice, well drained

Preheat the oven to 325°F.

In a medium mixing bowl, stir together the cupcake ingredients. Using an electric mixer, beat on low for 1 minute, or until moistened. Increase the speed to medium. Beat for 2 minutes. Spoon into two 12-cup nonstick muffin pans.

Bake for 18 minutes, or until a wooden toothpick inserted in the center of a cupcake comes out clean. Transfer to cooling racks and let cool for 15 minutes. Remove the cupcakes from the pans. Let cool completely.

Meanwhile, in a medium bowl, using a rubber scraper, fold together the yogurt, confectioners' sugar, and vanilla. Fold in the whipped topping. Cover with plastic wrap and refrigerate until needed.

Spread the whipped topping mixture over the cupcakes. Spoon the pineapple on top.

COOK'S TIP

You can top the cupcakes with the whipped topping mixture and pineapple, cover with plastic wrap, and refrigerate for up to 48 hours. Or refrigerate the cupcakes, topping mixture, and pineapple in separate containers for up to four days and assemble when needed.

seven-minute frosting

MAKES ENOUGH TO FROST A TWO-LAYER CAKE (12 SERVINGS)

Fluffy and rich tasting, this long-time favorite is especially impressive on chocolate cake, such as Black Devil's Food Cake (page 567).

1½ cups sugar
⅓ cup water
2 large egg whites
¼ teaspoon cream of tartar or
1 tablespoon light corn syrup

1 teaspoon vanilla, rum, or sherry extract

In the top of a double boiler, stir together all the ingredients except the vanilla. Using an electric mixer on high speed, beat for 1 minute. Put the top of the double boiler over a small amount of simmering water (don't let the water touch the top of the double boiler) and beat on high for 7 minutes, or until stiff peaks form. Remove the top of the double boiler from the heat.

Add the vanilla. Beat on high for 2 minutes, or until spreading consistency. Spread on a completely cooled cake.

LEMON-FLAVORED SEVEN-MINUTE FROSTING

Substitute 1 tablespoon fresh lemon juice for the vanilla extract. Add ¼ teaspoon grated lemon zest during the last minute of beating.

SEVEN-MINUTE FROSTING WITH FRUIT

Add 1 cup well-drained canned fruit, such as chopped mandarin oranges or crushed pineapple, to the cooked frosting, or substitute fruit flavoring, such as orange extract, for the vanilla extract.

FOR 1/12 RECIPE

SEVEN-MINUTE OR
LEMON-FLAVORED FROSTING
CALORIES 101
TOTAL FAT 0.0 g
  Saturated Fat 0.0 g
  Trans Fat 0.0 g
  Polyunsaturated Fat 0.0 g
  Monounsaturated Fat 0.0 g
CHOLESTEROL 0 mg
SODIUM 9 mg
CARBOHYDRATES 25 g
  Fiber 0 g
  Sugars 25 g
PROTEIN 1 g
DIETARY EXCHANGES
  1½ carbohydrate

FOR 1/12 RECIPE

SEVEN-MINUTE FROSTING
WITH FRUIT
CALORIES 111
TOTAL FAT 0.0 g
  Saturated Fat 0.0 g
  Trans Fat 0.0 g
  Polyunsaturated Fat 0.0 g
  Monounsaturated Fat 0.0 g
CHOLESTEROL 0 mg
SODIUM 10 mg
CARBOHYDRATES 28 g
  Fiber 0 g
  Sugars 28 g
PROTEIN 1 g
DIETARY EXCHANGES
  2 carbohydrate

confectioners' glaze

Use this versatile glaze to frost and decorate cupcakes, cakes, or cookies. You can even drizzle it on graham crackers or whole-grain toast.

1 cup confectioners' sugar, sifted	¼ cup (about) fat-free milk
½ teaspoon vanilla or rum extract	

In a small bowl, whisk together the confectioners' sugar and vanilla.

Gradually pour in the milk, whisking after each addition, until the desired consistency.

LEMON OR ORANGE CONFECTIONERS' GLAZE
Replace the milk with fresh lemon or orange juice.

CHOCOLATE CONFECTIONERS' GLAZE
Add 2 tablespoons unsweetened cocoa powder to the confectioners' sugar and proceed as directed.

PER SERVING

CALORIES 31
TOTAL FAT 0.0 g
  Saturated Fat 0.0 g
  Trans Fat 0.0 g
  Polyunsaturated Fat 0.0 g
  Monounsaturated Fat 0.0 g
CHOLESTEROL 0 mg
SODIUM 2 mg
CARBOHYDRATES 8 g
  Fiber 0 g
  Sugars 8 g
PROTEIN 0 g
DIETARY EXCHANGES
  ½ carbohydrate

peach clafouti

SERVES 8

A clafouti usually consists of a layer of batter topped with fresh fruit. Here, we've sandwiched the fruit between two layers of batter instead—a double treat.

Cooking spray
1½ teaspoons sugar
¼ teaspoon ground cinnamon and
½ teaspoon ground cinnamon, divided use
1¼ cups fat-free milk
1 cup all-purpose flour
¾ cup egg substitute
¼ cup firmly packed light brown sugar

1 tablespoon vanilla extract
1 teaspoon almond extract
¼ teaspoon ground nutmeg
¼ teaspoon salt
1½ pounds peaches, peeled and sliced (about 3½ cups)
3 tablespoons sliced almonds, dry-roasted

Preheat the oven to 350°F. Lightly spray a 9-inch square baking pan with cooking spray.

In a small bowl, stir together the sugar and ¼ teaspoon cinnamon. Set aside.

In a food processor or blender, process the milk, flour, egg substitute, brown sugar, vanilla, almond extract, nutmeg, salt, and remaining ½ teaspoon cinnamon until smooth. Spread about ¼ cup batter in the baking pan.

Bake for 5 to 10 minutes, or until set (the center doesn't jiggle when the pan is gently shaken). Arrange the peaches on the cooked batter. Pour the remaining batter on top. Bake for 20 minutes. Sprinkle with the almonds, then with the sugar mixture. Bake for 40 minutes, or until the center is set. Serve warm.

PER SERVING

CALORIES 159
TOTAL FAT 1.5 g
    Saturated Fat 0.0 g
    Trans Fat 0.0 g
    Polyunsaturated Fat 0.5 g
    Monounsaturated Fat 0.5 g
CHOLESTEROL 1 mg
SODIUM 138 mg
CARBOHYDRATES 30 g
    Fiber 2 g
    Sugars 16 g
PROTEIN 6 g
DIETARY EXCHANGES
    2 carbohydrate, ½ fat

delicate lemon ricotta cheesecake with blackberries

SERVES 12

Cheesecake can't get much easier to make than this one—just puree the filling, pour it into a pan, and bake!

Cooking spray
12 ounces fat-free lemon yogurt
8 ounces fat-free ricotta cheese
4 ounces light tub cream cheese
¾ cup sugar
6 large egg whites

2 teaspoons vanilla extract
2 teaspoons grated lemon zest
4 cups fresh or frozen blackberries
5 squares (2½ rectangles) low-fat graham crackers, crushed

Preheat the oven to 325°F. Lightly spray a springform pan with cooking spray.

In a food processor, process the yogurt, ricotta, cream cheese, sugar, egg whites, vanilla, and lemon zest until smooth. Pour into the pan.

Bake for 55 minutes, or until the center is almost set (jiggles slightly when the cheesecake is gently shaken). Transfer the pan to a cooling rack and let cool for 1 hour. Transfer to a large plate. Cover with plastic wrap and refrigerate for 8 to 24 hours.

Meanwhile, if using frozen blackberries, follow the package directions for thawing or put them in a shallow microwaveable dish, such as a glass pie pan, and microwave them on 100 percent power (high) for 20 to 30 seconds, or until thawed. Drain and pat dry with paper towels.

To serve, cut the desired number of pieces of cake and place on dessert plates. Sprinkle just those pieces with graham cracker crumbs. Spoon the berries on top. You can refrigerate leftovers for up to three days, but store the cake, graham cracker crumbs, and berries separately in airtight containers.

COOK'S TIP on cheesecake

Don't worry if the top of your cheesecake cracks during baking; that's normal. If moisture accumulates on the top after the cheesecake has cooled, dab gently with paper towels to remove.

PER SERVING

CALORIES 152
TOTAL FAT 2.0 g
  Saturated Fat 1.0 g
  Trans Fat 0.0 g
  Polyunsaturated Fat 0.0 g
  Monounsaturated Fat 0.5 g
CHOLESTEROL 8 mg
SODIUM 139 mg
CARBOHYDRATES 26 g
  Fiber 3 g
  Sugars 22 g
PROTEIN 7 g
DIETARY EXCHANGES
  1½ carbohydrate,
  1 lean meat

pumpkin cheesecake

SERVES 10

Lighter than traditional versions of cheesecake, this festive dessert is perfect for that special treat during the fall and winter holidays. You don't need a springform pan, and there's no water bath to fuss with.

Cooking spray
3 tablespoons cornflake crumbs
2 cups fat-free cottage cheese, undrained
8 ounces low-fat block cream cheese, softened
½ cup sugar
1 teaspoon cornstarch
¾ cup canned solid-pack pumpkin (not pie filling)

1 teaspoon vanilla extract
¾ teaspoon ground cinnamon
¾ cup egg substitute
½ cup plus 2 tablespoons fat-free frozen whipped topping, thawed in refrigerator
¼ cup plus 1 tablespoon finely chopped pecans, dry-roasted

Preheat the oven to 325°F. Lightly spray a 9-inch deep-dish pie pan with cooking spray.

Put the cornflake crumbs in the pie pan, gently shaking to coat the bottom and side.

In a food processor, process the cottage cheese for 1 minute, or until smooth and creamy.

Add the cream cheese and process for 15 seconds, or until well combined.

Add the sugar and cornstarch and process for 30 seconds, or until smooth, scraping down the side of the work bowl as necessary.

Add the pumpkin, vanilla, and cinnamon and process for 20 to 30 seconds, or until blended.

Add the egg substitute and process for 10 to 20 seconds, or until blended, scraping down the side of the work bowl as needed. Pour into the pie pan.

Bake for 45 to 50 minutes (don't open the oven door for at least 30 minutes), or until the center is set but not firm (doesn't jiggle when the pie pan is gently shaken). Transfer to a cooling rack and let cool for at least 1 hour. Cover and refrigerate for at least 2 hours before serving. Top each serving with 1 tablespoon whipped topping and 1½ teaspoons pecans.

PER SERVING

CALORIES 183
TOTAL FAT 7.5 g
  Saturated Fat 3.5 g
  Trans Fat 0.0 g
  Polyunsaturated Fat 1.0 g
  Monounsaturated Fat 3.0 g
CHOLESTEROL 18 mg
SODIUM 322 mg
CARBOHYDRATES 19 g
  Fiber 1 g
  Sugars 14 g
PROTEIN 10 g
DIETARY EXCHANGES
  1½ carbohydrate,
  1½ very lean meat, 1 fat

strawberry cream ice box pie

SERVES 8

You'll get a taste of summer in every bite of this creamy pie, regardless of the season.

Cooking spray
2 tablespoons light tub margarine
1 cup low-fat graham cracker crumbs
2 large egg whites, lightly beaten with a fork
½ cup all-fruit strawberry spread

4 cups strawberries, quartered and hulled
2 teaspoons grated orange zest
8 ounces fat-free frozen whipped topping, thawed in refrigerator

Preheat the oven to 375°F. Lightly spray a 9-inch glass pie pan with cooking spray.

In the pie pan, microwave the margarine on 100 percent power (high) for about 30 seconds, or until melted.

Stir in the graham cracker crumbs and egg whites. Press the mixture over the bottom of the pie pan.

Bake for 10 to 12 minutes, or until light golden. Transfer to a cooling rack. Let cool for at least 30 minutes.

Meanwhile, in a small microwaveable bowl, microwave the strawberry spread on 100 percent power (high) for 15 seconds, or until slightly melted.

In a large bowl, gently stir together the fruit spread, strawberries, and orange zest, coating the strawberries.

Fold in the whipped topping. Spoon into the pie pan. Refrigerate for 2 to 4 hours, or until firm (no need to cover).

PER SERVING

CALORIES 182
TOTAL FAT 2.0 g
  Saturated Fat 0.0 g
  Trans Fat 0.0 g
  Polyunsaturated Fat 0.5 g
  Monounsaturated Fat 1.0 g
CHOLESTEROL 0 mg
SODIUM 112 mg
CARBOHYDRATES 37 g
  Fiber 2 g
  Sugars 19 g
PROTEIN 2 g
DIETARY EXCHANGES
  2½ carbohydrate, ½ fat

COOK'S TIP

For a frozen treat, freeze the pie for about 4 hours, or until firm. Remove the pie from the freezer about 15 minutes before you plan to serve it so it will be easier to slice.

frozen mocha yogurt pie

SERVES 8

Kids will have fun using chocolate syrup to decorate the dessert plates for this rich-tasting pie.

Cooking spray
¾ cup chocolate graham cracker crumbs
2 cups fat-free vanilla frozen yogurt, slightly softened

2 cups fat-free coffee frozen yogurt, slightly softened
2 cups fat-free chocolate frozen yogurt, slightly softened
1 cup fat-free chocolate syrup

Lightly spray a 9-inch pie pan with cooking spray. Sprinkle with the graham cracker crumbs.

Put the vanilla yogurt on an 8-inch plate (such as a small dinner plate). Using a spoon or sturdy spatula, press down on the yogurt to cover the plate. (This will help when you put the yogurt in the pie pan.) Slip the vanilla yogurt layer into the pie pan. Using a spatula, carefully spread the yogurt over the bottom.

Repeat with the coffee yogurt, then with the chocolate yogurt. Cover with a double layer of plastic wrap. Freeze for at least 2 hours.

To serve, drizzle some of the chocolate syrup in a decorative pattern on each dessert plate. Cut the pie into 8 wedges. Place on the syrup. Drizzle the remaining syrup over the pie.

COOK'S TIP on cutting frozen desserts

Dipping a sharp knife into hot water makes cutting frozen desserts easier.

PER SERVING

CALORIES 263
TOTAL FAT 1.0 g
  Saturated Fat 0.0 g
  Trans Fat 0.0 g
  Polyunsaturated Fat 0.5 g
  Monounsaturated Fat 0.5 g
CHOLESTEROL 1 mg
SODIUM 133 mg
CARBOHYDRATES 59 g
  Fiber 0 g
  Sugars 45 g
PROTEIN 5 g
DIETARY EXCHANGES
  4 carbohydrate

gingersnap fruit tart

SERVE 8

Layers of pineapple, mango, banana, and blueberries make this dessert quite attractive.

Cooking spray

3 tablespoons light tub margarine

24 gingersnaps, processed to fine crumbs (about 1½ cups crumbs)

1 8-ounce can pineapple tidbits in their own juice, well drained, juice reserved

⅓ cup fresh orange juice

1½ tablespoons sugar

1 teaspoon cornstarch

1 teaspoon grated orange zest

1 medium mango, diced

1 medium banana, sliced

1 cup blueberries

Preheat the oven to 375°F. Lightly spray a 9-inch glass pie pan with cooking spray.

In the pie pan, microwave the margarine on 100 percent power (high) for about 30 seconds, or until melted.

Stir in the gingersnap crumbs. Press the mixture over the bottom of the pie pan.

Bake for 6 minutes, or until slightly firm to the touch. Let cool on a cooling rack for about 30 minutes. (The crust will continue to harden while cooling.)

Meanwhile, in a small saucepan, make a glaze by whisking together the reserved pineapple juice (set the pineapple aside), orange juice, sugar, and cornstarch until the cornstarch is dissolved. Bring to a boil over high heat. Boil for 1 minute, stirring occasionally. Remove from the heat.

Stir in the orange zest. Let cool for about 15 minutes, or until completely cool.

Make one layer each of the pineapple, mango, banana, and blueberries in the crust. Spoon the glaze over all. Refrigerate for at least 1 hour but no more than 8 hours before serving. (The crust will become soggy after about 8 hours.)

COOK'S TIP

You can bake the crust and prepare the glaze up to four days in advance. Cover the crust, put the glaze in an airtight container, and refrigerate them separately until time to assemble.

PER SERVING

CALORIES 172

TOTAL FAT 5.0 g

  Saturated Fat 1.0 g

  Trans Fat 0.0 g

  Polyunsaturated Fat 0.5 g

  Monounsaturated Fat 2.0 g

CHOLESTEROL 0 mg

SODIUM 108 mg

CARBOHYDRATES 32 g

  Fiber 2 g

  Sugars 21 g

PROTEIN 1 g

DIETARY EXCHANGES

  1 starch, 1 fruit, 1 fat

peach-raspberry crumble

SERVES 8

You can make this crumble when summer fruits are at their peak or in winter using frozen fruits. The almonds toast as the crumble bakes, making the topping extra crisp.

Cooking spray

FILLING
- 6 large peaches, peeled and sliced, or 4 cups frozen unsweetened sliced peaches, thawed and drained
- 2 cups fresh raspberries or frozen unsweetened raspberries (not thawed)
- 2 tablespoons all-purpose flour
- 2 teaspoons grated lemon zest

TOPPING
- ½ cup firmly packed light brown sugar
- ½ cup uncooked rolled oats
- 2 tablespoons all-purpose flour
- ½ teaspoon ground cinnamon
- 2 tablespoons canola or corn oil
- ¼ cup sliced almonds

Preheat the oven to 350°F. Lightly spray an 8-inch square glass baking dish with cooking spray.

In a large bowl, gently stir together the filling ingredients. Spoon into the baking dish.

In a medium bowl, stir together the brown sugar, oats, remaining 2 tablespoons flour, and cinnamon.

Drizzle the oil over the topping mixture. Stir until crumbly.

Stir the almonds into the topping mixture. Sprinkle over the filling.

Bake for 30 to 35 minutes, or until the topping is lightly browned. Transfer to a cooling rack. Let cool for a few minutes before serving.

COOK'S TIP

You can vary the fruits and make this crumble throughout the summer. Use nectarines or apricots for the peaches, and substitute blueberries or blackberries for the raspberries.

rhubarb-cherry oat crumble

SERVES 6

Tart rhubarb and tart red cherries need something sweeter for balance. Sweetened dried cherries and dark brown sugar do the trick.

Cooking spray

12 ounces fresh or frozen chopped rhubarb, thawed if frozen

1 14.5-ounce can pitted tart red cherries in water, undrained and checked for pits

⅓ cup sweetened dried cherries

⅓ cup firmly packed dark brown sugar and ⅓ cup firmly packed dark brown sugar, divided use

2 tablespoons cornstarch

2 teaspoons vanilla extract

½ cup uncooked quick-cooking oatmeal

¼ cup all-purpose flour

2 tablespoons canola or corn oil

½ teaspoon ground cinnamon

Preheat the oven to 375°F. Lightly spray a 9-inch glass deep-dish pie pan with cooking spray.

In a large saucepan, gently stir together the rhubarb, canned cherries with liquid, dried cherries, ⅓ cup brown sugar, and cornstarch until the cornstarch is dissolved. Bring to a boil over high heat, stirring occasionally. Boil for 1 minute, or until slightly thickened, stirring occasionally. Remove from the heat.

Stir in the vanilla. Pour into the pie pan.

In a small bowl, whisk together the oatmeal, flour, oil, cinnamon, and remaining ⅓ cup brown sugar. Sprinkle over the rhubarb mixture.

Bake for 30 minutes, or until the topping is golden. Transfer to a cooling rack. Let cool for at least 20 minutes. Serve warm or at room temperature.

COOK'S TIP on rhubarb

Fresh rhubarb is at the peak of its season from April to June, but you should be able to purchase frozen rhubarb year round.

PER SERVING

CALORIES 258
TOTAL FAT 5.5 g
  Saturated Fat 0.5 g
  Trans Fat 0.0 g
  Polyunsaturated Fat 1.5 g
  Monounsaturated Fat 3.0 g
CHOLESTEROL 0 mg
SODIUM 16 mg
CARBOHYDRATES 50 g
  Fiber 3 g
  Sugars 34 g
PROTEIN 3 g
DIETARY EXCHANGES
  3½ carbohydrate, 1 fat

apple-raisin crunch

SERVES 6

This dessert is delicious as is or topped with a small scoop of fat-free ice cream or frozen yogurt.

Cooking spray

FILLING

2 pounds baking apples, such as Fuji, McIntosh, or Rome Beauty, peeled and thinly sliced

½ cup golden raisins

⅓ cup sugar

¼ cup fresh orange juice

¼ teaspoon ground nutmeg

TOPPING

¾ cup uncooked quick-cooking oatmeal

¼ cup firmly packed dark brown sugar

2 tablespoons light tub margarine

½ teaspoon ground cinnamon

Preheat the oven to 350°F. Lightly spray an 8-inch square baking pan with cooking spray.

In a medium bowl, stir together the filling ingredients. Pour into the baking pan.

In a small bowl, stir together the topping ingredients. Sprinkle over the apple mixture.

Bake for 40 minutes. Let cool slightly before serving.

PER SERVING

CALORIES 240
TOTAL FAT 2.5 g
   Saturated Fat 0.0 g
   Trans Fat 0.0 g
   Polyunsaturated Fat 0.5 g
   Monounsaturated Fat 1.0 g
CHOLESTEROL 0 mg
SODIUM 35 mg
CARBOHYDRATES 56 g
   Fiber 3 g
   Sugars 43 g
PROTEIN 3 g
DIETARY EXCHANGES
   3½ carbohydrate, ½ fat

cherry crisp

SERVES 9

Sprinkle a crunchy oatmeal topping over juicy red cherries for a luscious dessert.

Cooking spray

FILLING

2 14.5-ounce cans pitted tart red cherries in water, drained, liquid reserved, and checked for pits

½ cup sugar

3 tablespoons cornstarch

1 tablespoon fresh lemon juice

¼ teaspoon ground cinnamon

¼ teaspoon ground nutmeg

TOPPING

¾ cup uncooked rolled oats

⅓ cup all-purpose flour

2 tablespoons light tub margarine

¼ cup firmly packed light brown sugar

¼ cup sugar

Preheat the oven to 350°F. Lightly spray an 8-inch square baking pan with cooking spray.

Pour the reserved liquid from the cherries into a medium saucepan. (Set the cherries aside.)

Stir in ½ cup sugar, cornstarch, lemon juice, cinnamon, and nutmeg. Cook over medium-high heat for 3 to 4 minutes, or until the sauce is thick and clear, whisking occasionally.

Stir in the cherries. Pour into the baking pan.

In a medium bowl, stir together the oats and flour. Using a fork or pastry blender, cut in the margarine until the mixture is crumbly. Stir in the brown sugar and remaining ¼ cup sugar. Sprinkle the topping over the cherry mixture.

Bake for 30 minutes, or until golden brown. Transfer to a cooling rack. Let cool for a few minutes before serving.

PER SERVING

CALORIES 184
TOTAL FAT 1.5 g
  Saturated Fat 0.0 g
  Trans Fat 0.0 g
  Polyunsaturated Fat 0.5 g
  Monounsaturated Fat 0.5 g
CHOLESTEROL 0 mg
SODIUM 29 mg
CARBOHYDRATES 42 g
  Fiber 2 g
  Sugars 30 g
PROTEIN 2 g
DIETARY EXCHANGES
  3 carbohydrate, ½ fat

deep-dish fruit crisp

SERVES 8

By varying the fruits in this basic crisp, you can take advantage of seasonal produce, supermarket specials, and family preferences.

FILLING

6 cups fresh or unsweetened frozen fruit (blueberries, blackberries, cherries, peaches, raspberries, apples, apricots, or any combination)
¼ cup all-purpose flour
¼ cup firmly packed light brown sugar
2 teaspoons grated lemon zest

TOPPING

½ cup uncooked quick-cooking oatmeal
½ cup firmly packed light brown sugar
¼ cup all-purpose flour
2 tablespoons light tub margarine
½ teaspoon ground cinnamon
¼ teaspoon ground nutmeg
¼ teaspoon ground allspice

Preheat the oven to 350°F.

In a 9-inch deep-dish pie pan, stir together the filling ingredients.

In a small bowl, stir together the topping ingredients with a fork, cutting the margarine into the other ingredients until slightly crumbly. Sprinkle over the fruit mixture.

Bake for 30 to 35 minutes, or until golden brown. Transfer to a cooling rack. Let cool for a few minutes before serving.

PER SERVING

CALORIES 187
TOTAL FAT 2.0 g
  Saturated Fat 0.0 g
  Trans Fat 0.0 g
  Polyunsaturated Fat 0.5 g
  Monounsaturated Fat 1.0 g
CHOLESTEROL 0 mg
SODIUM 29 mg
CARBOHYDRATES 43 g
  Fiber 3 g
  Sugars 30 g
PROTEIN 2 g
DIETARY EXCHANGES
  3 carbohydrate, ½ fat

cherry-filled phyllo rollovers

SERVES 4

You don't need chopsticks to enjoy these flaky dessert "egg rolls."

---

1 14.5-ounce can pitted tart red cherries in water, drained and checked for pits

¼ cup sugar and 2 teaspoons sugar, divided use

1 tablespoon cornstarch

1 teaspoon vanilla extract

½ teaspoon almond extract

4 14 x 18-inch sheets frozen phyllo dough, thawed

Butter-flavor cooking spray

⅛ teaspoon ground cinnamon

Preheat the oven to 400°F.

In a small saucepan, stir together the cherries, ¼ cup sugar, and cornstarch until the cornstarch is dissolved. Bring to a boil over medium-high heat, then stir. Boil for 1 to 2 minutes, or until thickened, stirring occasionally.

Remove from the heat. Stir in the vanilla and almond extracts.

Keeping the unused phyllo covered with a damp dish towel, lightly spray one sheet of dough with cooking spray. Working quickly, fold that sheet in half, bringing the short ends together. Spoon a quarter of the cherry mixture about 4 inches from one end; fold that end over the cherry mixture. Fold the sides over the cherry mixture and roll up (it should resemble an egg roll). Place with the seam side down on a nonstick baking sheet. Repeat with the remaining phyllo and cherry mixture. Lightly spray the tops of the rollovers with cooking spray.

Bake for 15 minutes, or until golden brown.

Meanwhile, in a small bowl, stir together the cinnamon and remaining 2 teaspoons sugar.

Place the rollovers on a cooling rack. Sprinkle with the cinnamon sugar. Let cool for 15 minutes.

PER SERVING

CALORIES 178
TOTAL FAT 0.5 g
  Saturated Fat 0.0 g
  Trans Fat 0.0 g
  Polyunsaturated Fat 0.5 g
  Monounsaturated Fat 0.5 g
CHOLESTEROL 0 mg
SODIUM 100 mg
CARBOHYDRATES 41 g
  Fiber 2 g
  Sugars 23 g
PROTEIN 2 g
DIETARY EXCHANGES
  2½ carbohydrate

tropical mini phyllo shells

SERVES 5; 3 MINI SHELLS PER SERVING

This is a fun treat for a quick dessert, appetizer, or snack. It's easy to double or triple the recipe, making it perfect for entertaining as well.

⅓ cup all-fruit apricot spread

1 1.9-ounce package frozen mini phyllo shells (15 mini shells), thawed

6 ounces fat-free vanilla yogurt

1 8-ounce can crushed pineapple in its own juice, well drained

3 tablespoons shredded sweetened coconut, lightly toasted

In a small microwaveable bowl, microwave the apricot spread, covered, on 100 percent power (high) for 30 seconds, or until melted.

Place the shells on a serving platter. In each shell, spoon, in order, about 1 teaspoon fruit spread, about 2 teaspoons yogurt, and about 2 teaspoons pineapple. Sprinkle with the coconut. Serve or cover with plastic wrap and refrigerate for up to 2 hours. (If filled for longer, the shells will become soft.)

PER SERVING

CALORIES 159
TOTAL FAT 3.5 g
  Saturated Fat 1.0 g
  Trans Fat 0.0 g
  Polyunsaturated Fat 0.0 g
  Monounsaturated Fat 0.0 g
CHOLESTEROL 1 mg
SODIUM 69 mg
CARBOHYDRATES 29 g
  Fiber 1 g
  Sugars 21 g
PROTEIN 2 g
DIETARY EXCHANGES
  1 starch, 1 fruit, ½ fat

gingersnap and graham cracker crust

SERVES 8

The pairing of gingersnaps and graham crackers makes this crust almost a dessert in itself. The corn syrup and apple juice bind the crumbs and make it easy to shape the piecrust.

¾ cup crushed low-fat graham crackers
¾ cup crushed gingersnaps

2 tablespoons light corn syrup
2 tablespoons unsweetened apple juice

In a medium bowl, stir together all the ingredients. Using your fingers, evenly press the mixture over the bottom and side of a 9-inch pie pan.

The crust is ready to fill and bake. If you need a pre-baked crust, bake it at 350°F for 10 minutes. Cool and fill.

oatmeal piecrust

SERVES 8

With its rustic texture and mildly nutty flavor, this more healthful version is a nice break from flour-based piecrust.

Cooking spray
3 tablespoons water
1 large egg white
1 cup uncooked rolled oats

⅓ cup uncooked oat bran
2 tablespoons canola or corn oil
⅛ teaspoon salt

Preheat the oven to 375°F. Lightly spray a 9-inch pie pan with cooking spray.

In a medium bowl, whisk together the water and egg white.

Stir in the remaining ingredients. Spoon into the pan. Using the back of the spoon, press gently to cover the bottom and ½ inch up the side.

Bake for 12 minutes, or until the crust is slightly golden on the edge and has pulled away from the side. Let cool on a cooling rack for 30 minutes before filling with a no-cook filling.

COOK'S TIP

For a slightly sweet taste, add 1 tablespoon sugar when you stir in the rolled oats, oat bran, oil, and salt.

PER SERVING

CALORIES 82
TOTAL FAT 4.5 g
    Saturated Fat 0.5 g
    Trans Fat 0.0 g
    Polyunsaturated Fat 1.5 g
    Monounsaturated Fat 2.5 g
CHOLESTEROL 0 mg
SODIUM 44 mg
CARBOHYDRATES 10 g
    Fiber 2 g
    Sugars 0 g
PROTEIN 3 g
DIETARY EXCHANGES
    ½ starch, 1 fat

pistachio-cardamom meringues

SERVES 9; 2 COOKIES PER SERVING

Cardamom lends an intoxicating flavor to these crisp-yet-chewy pistachio cookies. Pomegranate seeds (called "arils") nestled in the centers provide a burst of vibrant color and a pleasingly tart contrast to the sweet cookies.

¾ cup sugar
½ cup dry-roasted unsalted pistachio nuts
½ teaspoon ground cardamom
2 large egg whites, at room temperature

⅛ teaspoon cream of tartar
3 tablespoons pomegranate seeds (optional)

Preheat the oven to 300°F. Line 2 baking sheets with cooking parchment or silicone pan liners.

Put 1 tablespoon of the sugar in a small bowl and set aside. In a food processor, combine the remaining sugar, pistachios, and cardamom. Process for about 15 seconds, or until powdery. (A few tiny bumps from the nuts will remain.) Transfer to a large bowl.

Using an electric mixer, whisk the egg whites if your mixer has a whisk attachment or beat on medium speed until foamy. Add the cream of tartar. Increase the speed to high and continue whisking or beating for about 1 minute, or until soft peaks form. Slowly add the reserved sugar, whisking or beating on high for 20 to 30 seconds, or until stiff, glossy (but not dry) peaks form. Working quickly so the egg whites don't deflate, use a rubber scraper to gently fold them into the pistachio mixture until completely combined.

Using a small 2-tablespoon ice cream scoop or a tablespoon, drop the mixture by double tablespoons onto the baking sheets, 9 mounds to a sheet. Gently press the center of each mound with the back of a ½ teaspoon measuring spoon, creating an indentation, or "thumbprint."

Bake for 25 minutes, or until set, dried, and pale brown. Transfer the baking sheets to cooling racks and let the cookies cool on the baking sheets for 15 minutes. Using a thin metal spatula, carefully transfer the cookies from the baking sheets to a flat surface. Spoon ½ teaspoon pomegranate seeds into each thumbprint.

cookie jar snickerdoodles

SERVES 12; 2 COOKIES PER SERVING

Nutmeg perks up this healthier whole-wheat version of a classic cookie.

Cooking spray
1 tablespoon plus 1 teaspoon sugar and 1 cup sugar, divided use
2 teaspoons ground cinnamon
⅛ teaspoon ground nutmeg
3 tablespoons (about 1½ ounces) low-fat block cream cheese, at room temperature

2 tablespoons light tub margarine
¼ cup egg substitute
1 teaspoon vanilla extract
1¼ cups white whole-wheat flour
¾ cup all-purpose flour
½ teaspoon cream of tartar
¼ teaspoon baking soda
⅛ teaspoon salt

Preheat the oven to 400°F. Lightly spray 2 baking sheets with cooking spray.

On a small plate, stir together 1 tablespoon plus 1 teaspoon sugar, cinnamon, and nutmeg. Set aside.

In a medium mixing bowl, combine the cream cheese and margarine.

Add the remaining 1 cup sugar. Using an electric mixer on medium speed, beat for 2 minutes, or until blended and fluffy, scraping the side of the bowl as needed.

Add the egg substitute and vanilla. Beat on medium speed for 1 minute, or just until combined, scraping the side of the bowl as needed.

In a small bowl, whisk together the remaining ingredients. Gradually add to the batter, beating on low speed just to blend. The dough will not be smooth.

Roll into balls, 1 tablespoon of dough at a time (about 24 balls). Roll the balls in the sugar mixture. Place about 3 inches apart on the baking sheets. Using two fingers, slightly flatten the cookies by pressing on the tops of the balls.

Bake for 8 minutes, or until the edges are set but the centers are still soft. Transfer the baking sheets to cooling racks and let the cookies cool for 5 minutes. Transfer the cookies to the cooling racks and let cool completely, about 10 minutes.

PER SERVING

CALORIES 162
TOTAL FAT 2.0 g
  Saturated Fat 0.5 g
  Trans Fat 0.0 g
  Polyunsaturated Fat 0.5 g
  Monounsaturated Fat 0.5 g
CHOLESTEROL 3 mg
SODIUM 92 mg
CARBOHYDRATES 34 g
  Fiber 2 g
  Sugars 19 g
PROTEIN 3 g
DIETARY EXCHANGES
  2½ carbohydrate, ½ fat

apple-cherry drops

SERVES 32; 2 COOKIES PER SERVING

Keep lots of these plump, fruity delights on hand for when kids come over to play. You'll be the most popular parent in the neighborhood!

Cooking spray
2½ cups all-purpose flour
1 teaspoon baking powder
1 teaspoon baking soda
1 teaspoon ground cinnamon
¼ teaspoon ground nutmeg
¼ teaspoon salt
1 cup sugar
½ cup light tub margarine
¼ cup firmly packed light brown sugar

1 teaspoon vanilla extract
½ teaspoon almond extract
¼ cup egg substitute
¼ cup unsweetened applesauce
1 cup shredded peeled apple (about 1 large), Granny Smith, Gala, or Fuji preferred
½ cup unsweetened dried cherries, coarsely chopped

Preheat the oven to 350°F. Lightly spray 2 baking sheets with cooking spray.

In a medium bowl, whisk together the flour, baking powder, baking soda, cinnamon, nutmeg, and salt.

In a large bowl, using an electric mixer on medium speed, beat the sugar, margarine, brown sugar, and vanilla and almond extracts for 3 minutes.

Add the egg substitute and applesauce. Beat for 20 to 30 seconds, or until combined.

Gradually add the flour mixture, beating on low speed for about 1 minute, or until no flour is visible.

Stir in the apple and cherries. Using about half the dough, drop by heaping teaspoonfuls about 2 inches apart on the baking sheets.

Bake for 10 to 12 minutes, or until light brown. Transfer the baking sheets to cooling racks and let the cookies partially cool on the baking sheets, about 10 minutes. Transfer the cookies to the cooling racks. Repeat with the remaining batter.

Store any remaining cookies in an airtight container at room temperature for three or four days or refrigerated for up to seven days. For longer storage, layer between pieces of wax paper in an airtight freezer container and freeze for up to four months.

PER SERVING

CALORIES 88
TOTAL FAT 1.0 g
  Saturated Fat 0.0 g
  Trans Fat 0.0 g
  Polyunsaturated Fat 0.5 g
  Monounsaturated Fat 0.5 g
CHOLESTEROL 0 mg
SODIUM 97 mg
CARBOHYDRATES 18 g
  Fiber 1 g
  Sugars 10 g
PROTEIN 1 g
DIETARY EXCHANGES
  1 carbohydrate

pumpkin oaties

SERVES 20; 2 COOKIES PER SERVING

A cross between cookies and muffins, these rustic gems make tasty desserts, breakfasts, or anytime munchies.

Cooking spray
1¼ cups all-purpose flour
½ cup whole-wheat flour
2 teaspoons pumpkin pie spice
1 teaspoon baking powder
1 teaspoon baking soda
½ teaspoon salt
1 cup firmly packed light or dark brown sugar

¼ cup canola or corn oil
1 large egg
1 15-ounce can solid-pack pumpkin (not pie filling)
1 cup uncooked quick-cooking oatmeal
½ cup chopped pecans (optional)

Preheat the oven to 350°F. Lightly spray 2 baking sheets with cooking spray.

In a medium bowl, sift together the flours, pie spice, baking powder, baking soda, and salt.

Put the brown sugar, oil, and egg in a large mixing bowl. Using an electric mixer on medium speed, beat for 2 to 3 minutes, or until smooth and golden. Beat in the pumpkin until smooth.

Stir in the oatmeal. Gradually stir in the flour mixture, about one-third at a time, gently blending until no flour is visible. Stir in the pecans.

Using a small 1-tablespoon spring-loaded ice cream scoop or tablespoon, drop the dough by tablespoonfuls, 18 to 20 on each baking sheet. Dampen the heel of your hand and lightly press each cookie to flatten slightly. (These cookies don't spread as they bake.)

Bake for 14 to 18 minutes, or until the cookies appear dry. Transfer the cookies from the baking sheets to cooling racks and let cool.

PER SERVING

WITHOUT PECANS
CALORIES 147
TOTAL FAT 4.0 g
  Saturated Fat 0.5 g
  Trans Fat 0.0 g
  Polyunsaturated Fat 1.0 g
  Monounsaturated Fat 2.0 g
CHOLESTEROL 12 mg
SODIUM 166 mg
CARBOHYDRATES 26 g
  Fiber 2 g
  Sugars 13 g
PROTEIN 3 g
DIETARY EXCHANGES
  2 carbohydrate, 1 fat

PER SERVING

WITH PECANS
CALORIES 168
TOTAL FAT 6.0 g
  Saturated Fat 0.5 g
  Trans Fat 0.0 g
  Polyunsaturated Fat 1.5 g
  Monounsaturated Fat 3.5 g
CHOLESTEROL 12 mg
SODIUM 166 mg
CARBOHYDRATES 27 g
  Fiber 2 g
  Sugars 13 g
PROTEIN 3 g
DIETARY EXCHANGES
  2 carbohydrate, 1 fat

bourbon balls

SERVES 24; 2 COOKIES PER SERVING

These tasty morsels are a hit at holiday parties. Make them about a week in advance so the bourbon can permeate the cookies.

3 cups finely crushed low-fat vanilla wafers
1 cup confectioners' sugar, sifted, and ¼ cup sifted confectioners' sugar, divided use
½ cup chopped pecans, dry-roasted

3 tablespoons light corn syrup
1½ tablespoons unsweetened cocoa powder
¼ cup plus 2 tablespoons bourbon (plus more as needed)

In a large bowl, stir together all the ingredients except ¼ cup confectioners' sugar. Form the dough into about 48 small balls. (If the balls tend to crumble, stir in a few extra drops of bourbon.)

Put the remaining ¼ cup confectioners' sugar on a saucer. Roll each ball in the sugar. Put the cookies in an airtight container. For best results, refrigerate for about one week to mellow before serving.

PER SERVING

CALORIES 118
TOTAL FAT 3.0 g
  Saturated Fat 0.5 g
  Trans Fat 0.0 g
  Polyunsaturated Fat 1.0 g
  Monounsaturated Fat 1.5 g
CHOLESTEROL 5 mg
SODIUM 33 mg
CARBOHYDRATES 21 g
  Fiber 1 g
  Sugars 15 g
PROTEIN 1 g
DIETARY EXCHANGES
  1½ carbohydrate, ½ fat

fudgy buttermilk brownies

SERVES 16; 1 BROWNIE PER SERVING

Here's a wonderfully moist brownie to serve alone or topped with fat-free frozen yogurt.

Cooking spray

BROWNIES
1 cup all-purpose flour
1 cup firmly packed light brown sugar
⅓ cup unsweetened cocoa powder
½ teaspoon baking soda
¼ teaspoon salt
2 large egg whites or ¼ cup egg substitute

½ cup unsweetened applesauce
½ cup low-fat buttermilk
2 teaspoons vanilla extract

FROSTING
1½ cups sifted confectioners' sugar
¼ cup unsweetened cocoa powder
1 teaspoon vanilla extract
2 to 3 tablespoons fat-free milk

Preheat the oven to 350°F. Lightly spray a 9-inch square baking pan with cooking spray.

In a medium bowl, stir together the flour, brown sugar, ⅓ cup cocoa powder, baking soda, and salt.

In a small bowl, lightly whisk the egg whites.

Whisk the applesauce, buttermilk, and vanilla into the egg whites. Whisk into the flour mixture until well blended. Pour into the baking pan.

Bake for 30 minutes, or until a wooden toothpick inserted in the center comes out clean. Transfer to a cooling rack and let cool in the pan.

In a small bowl, stir together the confectioners' sugar and remaining ¼ cup cocoa powder.

Stir in the vanilla, then gradually stir in the milk until the frosting is spreading consistency. Spread over the cooled brownies. Cut into squares.

PER SERVING

CALORIES 149
TOTAL FAT 0.5 g
  Saturated Fat 0.0 g
  Trans Fat 0.0 g
  Polyunsaturated Fat 0.0 g
  Monounsaturated Fat 0.0 g
CHOLESTEROL 1 mg
SODIUM 96 mg
CARBOHYDRATES 34 g
  Fiber 1 g
  Sugars 26 g
PROTEIN 2 g
DIETARY EXCHANGES
  2½ carbohydrate

apricot-almond biscotti

SERVES 28; 1 COOKIE PER SERVING

Biscotti are typically baked, sliced, and baked again, making them quite hard to bite into. They soften up when dunked in hot tea or coffee.

Cooking spray

2 cups all-purpose flour, plus more as needed for kneading

⅔ cup sugar

2 teaspoons baking powder

¼ teaspoon salt

2 large eggs

2 tablespoons unsweetened applesauce

2 tablespoons canola or corn oil

1 teaspoon grated lemon zest

¼ teaspoon almond extract

¾ cup finely chopped dried apricots (about 4 ounces)

¼ cup chopped almonds, dry-roasted

¾ cup sifted confectioners' sugar

2 to 3 teaspoons water

Preheat the oven to 350°F. Lightly spray a baking sheet with cooking spray.

In a medium bowl, stir together 2 cups flour, sugar, baking powder, and salt.

In a small bowl, whisk together the eggs, applesauce, oil, lemon zest, and almond extract.

Stir the apricots and almonds into the egg mixture. Stir the egg mixture into the flour mixture.

Lightly flour a flat surface. Turn out the dough. Knead just until blended, 10 to 12 strokes. With slightly moistened hands, form into two 8-inch logs. Put the logs on the baking sheet. Slightly flatten to 2½ inches wide.

Bake for 25 minutes. Reduce the oven temperature to 300°F. Transfer the biscotti to a cooling rack and let cool for 10 minutes.

Meanwhile, put the confectioners' sugar in a small bowl. Gradually stir in the water until the desired consistency. Brush on the biscotti. Cut into ½-inch slices. Place the biscotti with a cut side down on the baking sheet.

Bake for 20 minutes, turning once halfway through. Transfer to a cooling rack and let cool.

PER SERVING

CALORIES 92
TOTAL FAT 2.0 g
  Saturated Fat 0.0 g
  Trans Fat 0.0 g
  Polyunsaturated Fat 0.5 g
  Monounsaturated Fat 1.0 g
CHOLESTEROL 15 mg
SODIUM 57 mg
CARBOHYDRATES 18 g
  Fiber 1 g
  Sugars 10 g
PROTEIN 2 g
DIETARY EXCHANGES
  1 carbohydrate, ½ fat

chocolate-pecan biscotti

SERVES 28; 1 COOKIE PER SERVING

Whether you use regular unsweetened cocoa powder or try the dark variety, you're going to enjoy these crunchy cookies. Like all other biscotti, they need a quick dunk in a beverage such as fat-free milk to soften them a bit.

Cooking spray
1½ cups all-purpose flour, plus more as needed for kneading
⅔ cup firmly packed light brown sugar
½ cup unsweetened cocoa powder
2 teaspoons baking powder
¼ teaspoon salt
2 large eggs

2 tablespoons unsweetened applesauce
2 tablespoons canola or corn oil
1 teaspoon vanilla extract
½ cup finely chopped pecans, dry-roasted
¾ cup sifted confectioners' sugar
2 to 3 teaspoons water

Preheat the oven to 350°F. Lightly spray a baking sheet with cooking spray.

In a medium bowl, stir together the flour, brown sugar, cocoa powder, baking powder, and salt.

In a small bowl, whisk together the eggs, applesauce, oil, and vanilla.

Whisk the pecans into the egg mixture. Whisk the egg mixture into the flour mixture.

Lightly flour a flat surface. Turn out the dough. Knead just until blended, 10 to 12 strokes. With slightly moistened hands, form into two 8-inch logs. Put the logs on the baking sheet. Slightly flatten to 2½ inches wide.

Bake for 25 minutes. Reduce the oven temperature to 300°F. Transfer the biscotti to a cooling rack and let cool for 10 minutes.

Meanwhile, put the confectioners' sugar in a small bowl. Gradually stir in the water until the desired consistency. Brush on the biscotti. Cut into ½-inch slices. Place the biscotti with a cut side down on the baking sheet.

Bake for 20 minutes, turning once halfway through. Transfer to a cooling rack and let cool.

PER SERVING

CALORIES 91
TOTAL FAT 3.0 g
  Saturated Fat 0.5 g
  Trans Fat 0.0 g
  Polyunsaturated Fat 1.0 g
  Monounsaturated Fat 1.5 g
CHOLESTEROL 15 mg
SODIUM 56 mg
CARBOHYDRATES 15 g
  Fiber 1 g
  Sugars 9 g
PROTEIN 2 g
DIETARY EXCHANGES
  1 carbohydrate, ½ fat

tropical napoleons

SERVES 4

Phyllo dough, fat-free ricotta cheese, and juicy tropical fruit give these Napoleons a decadent feel while keeping them as good for you as they are good to eat.

Butter-flavor cooking spray
2 14 x 18-inch sheets frozen phyllo dough, thawed
1 tablespoon fat-free tub cream cheese, at room temperature
½ cup fat-free ricotta cheese
3 tablespoons frozen orange juice concentrate

½ cup fat-free frozen whipped topping, thawed in refrigerator
1 cup chopped pineapple chunks (fresh preferred), drained if canned
1 cup chopped mango (fresh preferred), drained if bottled
2 teaspoons confectioners' sugar

Preheat the oven to 350°F. Lightly spray a baking sheet with cooking spray.

Place a large piece of wax paper on a flat surface. Carefully place one sheet of phyllo on the wax paper so a long side of the dough is closest to you. Keeping the unused phyllo covered with a damp cloth or damp paper towels to prevent drying, lightly spray the phyllo with cooking spray. Working quickly, place the second sheet of phyllo on the sprayed sheet. Press the top sheet firmly to make it stick to the first sheet. Spray with cooking spray.

Cut the dough in half lengthwise. Place one half on top of the other, pressing down firmly to make the layers of dough stick. Prick the top of the dough with a fork. Cut the dough lengthwise into 3 strips. Cut each strip crosswise into 4 strips. You should have 12 rectangles. Place on the baking sheet.

Bake for 11 minutes, or until golden. Transfer the baking sheet to a cooling rack and let the phyllo cool completely, 10 to 15 minutes.

Meanwhile, in a medium bowl, stir the cream cheese until it softens slightly.

In a small food processor or blender, process the ricotta for 30 seconds, or until smooth. Add to the cream cheese.

Stir the orange juice concentrate into the cream cheese mixture. Fold in the whipped topping.

Carefully spread one-third of the ricotta mixture over four of the rectangles. Place the pineapple on the ricotta. Carefully spread another one-third of the ricotta mixture over four more rectangles. Place these, with the ricotta mixture side up, on the rectangles with the pineapple. Place the mango on the ricotta mixture. Carefully spread the remaining one-third of the ricotta mixture over the last four rectangles. Place these rectangles with the ricotta mixture side down on the mango. You should have four stacks of three phyllo rectangles each, starting and ending with phyllo. Put the confectioners' sugar in a sieve. Sprinkle over the tops. Serve immediately.

COOK'S TIP

Paper-thin phyllo is the perfect way to enjoy flaky pastries without the fat of traditional puff pastry dough. Layering the dough with butter-flavor cooking spray in place of butter or oil reduces the fat in phyllo dishes even further. Be sure to follow the package directions when thawing phyllo dough.

cannoli cream with strawberries and chocolate

SERVES 6; ⅔ CUP PER SERVING

Creamy and elegant, this make-ahead dessert is just the way to end a meal for company.

¼ cup cold fat-free milk and ½ cup fat-free milk, divided use	1 teaspoon vanilla extract
1 envelope unflavored gelatin	8 to 10 fresh or unsweetened frozen strawberries, hulled if fresh, thawed if frozen
¾ cup fat-free ricotta cheese	
¾ cup fat-free cottage cheese	3 tablespoons shaved sweet chocolate
½ cup sugar	

Pour ¼ cup cold milk into a food processor or blender. Sprinkle the gelatin over the milk. Let stand for 2 minutes.

Meanwhile, in a small saucepan, bring the remaining ½ cup milk to a boil over high heat. Add to the gelatin mixture after the standing time. Process for 1 minute, or until the gelatin is completely dissolved.

Add the ricotta cheese, cottage cheese, sugar, and vanilla. Process for 2 minutes. Divide the mixture between two medium bowls. Rinse the food processor or blender container.

Process the strawberries until smooth (except for the seeds). Fold into one bowl of pudding.

Stir the chocolate into the other bowl.

Alternate layers of strawberry pudding and chocolate pudding in stemmed dessert dishes or wineglasses until all the ingredients are used. Refrigerate for 3 hours, or until set.

PER SERVING

CALORIES 165
TOTAL FAT 1.5 g
  Saturated Fat 1.0 g
  Trans Fat 0.0 g
  Polyunsaturated Fat 0.0 g
  Monounsaturated Fat 0.5 g
CHOLESTEROL 5 mg
SODIUM 188 mg
CARBOHYDRATES 27 g
  Fiber 1 g
  Sugars 26 g
PROTEIN 10 g
DIETARY EXCHANGES
  2 carbohydrate,
  1½ very lean meat

cinnamon-sugar vanilla flans with blueberries

SERVES 6; ½ CUP FLAN PLUS ¼ CUP BERRIES PER SERVING

The secret to success in making flans is to bake them in a water bath, or bain-marie. The secret with this recipe is to use boiling, not merely hot, water for the water bath; otherwise, the delicate custard will need about twice as much cooking time.

Cooking spray
2½ cups fat-free half-and-half
½ cup egg substitute
¼ cup sugar and 1 tablespoon sugar, divided use
1 teaspoon vanilla extract
2 cups boiling water
½ teaspoon ground cinnamon
1½ cups blueberries

Preheat the oven to 325°F. Lightly spray six 6-ounce ovenproof glass custard cups or porcelain ramekins with cooking spray.

In a large bowl, whisk together the half-and-half, egg substitute, ¼ cup sugar, and vanilla. Pour into the custard cups.

Place a 13 x 9 x 2-inch baking pan in the oven. Carefully pour the boiling water into the pan. Place the custard cups in the pan.

Bake for 40 minutes, or until a knife inserted near the center of a flan comes out clean. Carefully remove the custard cups from the pan and transfer to a cooling rack. Let cool completely, about 1 hour. Cover with plastic wrap and refrigerate until needed. (The flans don't need to be cold when you serve them.)

At serving time, run a knife around the edge of each flan. Place a dessert plate on each and invert.

In a small bowl, stir together the cinnamon and remaining 1 tablespoon sugar. Sprinkle over each flan. Spoon the blueberries around each. Serve immediately.

PER SERVING

CALORIES 141
TOTAL FAT 0.0 g
  Saturated Fat 0.0 g
  Trans Fat 0.0 g
  Polyunsaturated Fat 0.0 g
  Monounsaturated Fat 0.0 g
CHOLESTEROL 0 mg
SODIUM 142 mg
CARBOHYDRATES 30 g
  Fiber 1 g
  Sugars 21 g
PROTEIN 9 g
DIETARY EXCHANGES
  2 carbohydrate,
  1 lean meat

chocolate crème brûlée

SERVES 10; ½ CUP PER SERVING

If crème brûlée is your favorite restaurant dessert, you will be pleased to know how easy it is to make at home.

3 cups fat-free half-and-half
½ cup unsweetened cocoa powder, sifted
1½ cups egg substitute
⅔ cup sugar and scant ½ cup sugar, divided use

3 tablespoons plus 1 teaspoon mini chocolate chips
1 cup raspberries

Preheat the oven to 325°F.

In a medium microwaveable bowl, whisk together the half-and-half and cocoa (the mixture will be lumpy). Microwave, covered, on 100 percent power (high) for 1 minute to 1 minute 30 seconds, or until slightly warm. Whisk again to help dissolve the lumps.

Whisk in the egg substitute and ⅔ cup sugar. Pour ½ cup mixture into each of ten 6-ounce broilerproof custard cups.

Spoon 1 teaspoon chocolate chips into the middle of each custard cup. Place the custard cups in a large baking pan. Fill the baking pan to a depth of 1 inch.

Bake for 30 to 35 minutes, or until the centers are set (don't jiggle when the cups are removed from the water bath and gently shaken). Transfer the baking sheet to a cooling rack. Carefully remove the custard cups and transfer to another cooling rack. Let cool for 15 minutes. Cover and refrigerate for 2 hours to two days.

At serving time, preheat the broiler.

Sprinkle 2 teaspoons of the remaining sugar over each custard. Transfer the cups to a broilerproof pan.

Broil with the tops of the cups about 2 inches from the heat for 2 to 4 minutes, or until the sugar is caramelized (watch carefully so it doesn't burn). Serve topped with the raspberries.

PER SERVING

CALORIES 194
TOTAL FAT 1.5 g
  Saturated Fat 0.5 g
  Trans Fat 0.0 g
  Polyunsaturated Fat 0.0 g
  Monounsaturated Fat 0.5 g
CHOLESTEROL 0 mg
SODIUM 148 mg
CARBOHYDRATES 39 g
  Fiber 2 g
  Sugars 31 g
PROTEIN 10 g
DIETARY EXCHANGES
  2½ carbohydrate,
  1½ very lean meat

honey-almond custards

SERVES 6; ½ CUP PER SERVING

After a highly seasoned entrée, serve these honey-sweetened custards to balance the meal.

Cooking spray
2 cups fat-free milk
¾ cup egg substitute
¼ cup honey

2 teaspoons vanilla extract
¼ teaspoon almond extract
⅛ teaspoon salt

Preheat the oven to 350°F. Lightly spray six 6-ounce ovenproof custard cups with cooking spray.

In a small saucepan, heat the milk over medium-high heat until very hot but not boiling, whisking constantly. Remove from the heat.

In a medium bowl, gently whisk together the remaining ingredients.

Gently whisk in the milk (don't create foam). Pour the mixture into the custard cups. Place the cups in a large baking pan. Pour hot tap water into the pan to a depth of 1 inch.

Bake for 30 to 40 minutes, or until a knife inserted halfway between the cup and the center of the custard comes out clean (the center won't quite be firm). Transfer the pan to a cooling rack. Carefully remove the custard cups and transfer to another cooling rack.

MICROWAVE METHOD

Prepare the custard mixture as directed. Pour into microwaveable custard cups lightly sprayed with cooking spray. Put the cups in a microwaveable baking dish. Add the water as directed. Microwave on 100 percent power (high) for 12 to 15 minutes, or until the centers are just set (don't jiggle when the custard cups are gently shaken).

PER SERVING

CALORIES 90
TOTAL FAT 0.0 g
    Saturated Fat 0.0 g
    Trans Fat 0.0 g
    Polyunsaturated Fat 0.0 g
    Monounsaturated Fat 0.0 g
CHOLESTEROL 2 mg
SODIUM 146 mg
CARBOHYDRATES 16 g
    Fiber 0 g
    Sugars 16 g
PROTEIN 6.0 g
DIETARY EXCHANGES
    1 carbohydrate,
    1 very lean meat

raisin-walnut rice pudding

SERVES 4; ½ CUP PER SERVING

Rice pudding is an all-time family favorite. Cooking the rice in fat-free milk instead of water jump-starts the rich flavor and adds calcium without saturated fat.

Cooking spray
½ cup uncooked instant brown rice
1 teaspoon ground cinnamon
1¼ cups fat-free milk
½ cup fat-free half-and-half
⅓ cup raisins
¼ cup egg substitute
2 tablespoons firmly packed light brown sugar and 2 tablespoons firmly packed light brown sugar, divided use

1 teaspoon vanilla extract
½ teaspoon coconut extract
2 teaspoons light tub margarine
¼ teaspoon ground nutmeg
¼ teaspoon ground allspice
2 tablespoons chopped walnuts

Preheat the oven to 350°F. Lightly spray four 8-ounce ovenproof custard cups or ramekins with cooking spray. Set on a baking sheet.

In a small saucepan, stir together the rice and cinnamon. Stir in the milk. Cook the rice for the time directed on the package. Remove from the heat as soon as the liquid is absorbed. The rice will be firm.

Stir in the half-and-half, raisins, egg substitute, 2 tablespoons brown sugar, and vanilla and coconut extracts. Spoon into the custard cups.

Bake for 20 minutes, or until the edges of the pudding are just firm, but the centers are still soft. Transfer to a cooling rack.

Meanwhile, in a small bowl, stir together the remaining 2 tablespoons brown sugar, margarine, nutmeg, and allspice. Stir in the walnuts. Sprinkle over the hot puddings.

Bake for 10 minutes, or until the topping is hot and bubbly and the puddings are firm (the centers don't jiggle when the custard cups are gently shaken). Place the custard cups on heat-resistant saucers and serve warm, or let cool on a cooling rack for 15 to 20 minutes.

PER SERVING

CALORIES 228
TOTAL FAT 3.5 g
 Saturated Fat 0.5 g
 Trans Fat 0.0 g
 Polyunsaturated Fat 2.0 g
 Monounsaturated Fat 1.0 g
CHOLESTEROL 2 mg
SODIUM 117 mg
CARBOHYDRATES 43 g
 Fiber 2 g
 Sugars 28 g
PROTEIN 8 g
DIETARY EXCHANGES
 1 starch, 1 fruit,
 1 carbohydrate,
 ½ lean meat

delicious rice pudding

SERVES 6; ½ CUP PER SERVING

Enjoy this traditional comfort food unadorned, or try it with Easy Jubilee Sauce (page 512) as an interesting addition.

⅔ cup uncooked rice
   Cooking spray
2 cups fat-free milk, heated
⅓ cup sugar
1½ teaspoons vanilla extract
1½ teaspoons grated lemon zest
   (optional)

1 teaspoon lemon extract (optional)
¼ teaspoon ground nutmeg
½ teaspoon ground cinnamon
¼ cup egg substitute

Prepare the rice using the package directions, omitting the salt and margarine. Set aside.

Preheat the oven to 350°F.

Lightly spray a 1-quart casserole dish with cooking spray. Put the ingredients in the dish in the order listed. Stir well. Cover the dish and set in a large baking pan. Pour hot tap water into the pan to a depth of 1 inch.

Bake for 1 hour, or until the mixture is thick. Serve warm or cover and refrigerate to serve chilled.

COOK'S TIP on bain-marie

Using a bain-marie (bahn mah-REE), or water bath, is a technique for cooking custards and some other fragile foods. The container holding the food is placed in a larger pan (also called a bain-marie) that holds a small amount of hot, not boiling, water. (If the water starts to boil, add a little cold water.) The technique keeps the food from separating or curdling.

PER SERVING

CALORIES 150
TOTAL FAT 0.0 g
  Saturated Fat 0.0 g
  Trans Fat 0.0 g
  Polyunsaturated Fat 0.0 g
  Monounsaturated Fat 0.0 g
CHOLESTEROL 2 mg
SODIUM 56 mg
CARBOHYDRATES 31 g
  Fiber 0 g
  Sugars 16 g
PROTEIN 5 g
DIETARY EXCHANGES
  2 carbohydrate

guiltless banana pudding

SERVES 10; ¾ CUP PER SERVING

It's so rich tasting and creamy that you'll wonder how this revised favorite can be guiltless.

1 cup fat-free milk

1 1-ounce package fat-free, sugar-free vanilla instant pudding mix

8 ounces fat-free frozen whipped topping, thawed in refrigerator

⅔ cup fat-free sweetened condensed milk

2 tablespoons plus 1 teaspoon fresh lemon juice, or to taste

20 low-fat vanilla wafers, whole or crushed

2 medium bananas, thinly sliced

In a large mixing bowl, whisk or beat the fat-free milk and pudding mix until thickened.

Fold in the whipped topping, milk, and lemon juice. Layer half the vanilla wafers, half the bananas, and half the pudding mixture in an 8-inch square glass baking dish. Repeat. Place plastic wrap directly on the surface of the pudding. Refrigerate until needed.

GUILTLESS STRAWBERRY PUDDING

Replace the vanilla wafers with low-fat gingersnaps, and replace the bananas with 1 cup thinly sliced hulled strawberries.

PER SERVING

CALORIES 176
TOTAL FAT 1.5 g
  Saturated Fat 0.5 g
  Trans Fat 0.0 g
  Polyunsaturated Fat 0.5 g
  Monounsaturated Fat 0.5 g
CHOLESTEROL 7 mg
SODIUM 257 mg
CARBOHYDRATES 37 g
  Fiber 1 g
  Sugars 23 g
PROTEIN 3 g
DIETARY EXCHANGES
  2½ carbohydrate

PER SERVING

GUILTLESS STRAWBERRY
PUDDING
CALORIES 178
TOTAL FAT 1.5 g
  Saturated Fat 0.5 g
  Trans Fat 0.0 g
  Polyunsaturated Fat 0.0 g
  Monounsaturated Fat 0.5 g
CHOLESTEROL 3 mg
SODIUM 284 mg
CARBOHYDRATES 36 g
  Fiber 1 g
  Sugars 22 g
PROTEIN 3 g
DIETARY EXCHANGES
  2½ carbohydrate, ½ fat

vanilla bread pudding with peaches

SERVES 6; 2½ X 4-INCH PIECE BREAD PUDDING AND ⅓ CUP COOKED PEACHES PER SERVING

Like a soufflé, this bread pudding is puffy for only a moment. It is best when served fresh from the oven.

Cooking spray

BREAD PUDDING
1 cup fat-free milk
3 large egg whites
⅓ cup sugar
1 teaspoon vanilla, butter, and nut flavoring or vanilla extract
¾ teaspoon baking powder
¼ teaspoon ground cinnamon

⅛ teaspoon ground nutmeg
4 slices stale white bread (lowest sodium available), cut into cubes
_____
½ cup water
2 large peaches, peeled or unpeeled, thinly sliced (about 12 ounces total)
2 tablespoons sugar

Preheat the oven to 375°F. Lightly spray an 8-inch square baking pan with cooking spray.

In a large bowl, whisk together the bread pudding ingredients except the bread.

Fold in the bread cubes just until coated. Don't overmix. Spoon into the baking pan.

Bake for 25 minutes, or until a sharp knife inserted in the center comes out clean.

Meanwhile, in a medium saucepan, bring the water to a boil over high heat. Stir in the peaches and sugar. Return to a boil. Reduce the heat and simmer for 4 minutes, or until just tender. Serve over pieces of the bread pudding.

PER SERVING
CALORIES 152
TOTAL FAT 1.0 g
    Saturated Fat 0.0 g
    Trans Fat 0.0 g
    Polyunsaturated Fat 0.5 g
    Monounsaturated Fat 0.0 g
CHOLESTEROL 1 mg
SODIUM 209 mg
CARBOHYDRATES 32 g
    Fiber 1 g
    Sugars 23 g
PROTEIN 5 g
DIETARY EXCHANGES
    2 carbohydrate

berry-filled meringue shells

SERVES 6

Fresh berries with a hint of orange fill elegant-looking individual meringue shells.

MERINGUE SHELLS
- 2 large egg whites, at room temperature
- ½ teaspoon vanilla extract
- ⅛ teaspoon cream of tartar
- ½ cup sugar

FILLING
- 1 pound fresh strawberries (hulled and sliced), raspberries, blackberries, blueberries, or a combination
- 2 tablespoons frozen orange juice concentrate, thawed
- ¼ cup plus 2 tablespoons fat-free vanilla yogurt
- 2 teaspoons sugar

Preheat the oven to 300°F. Line a large baking sheet with cooking parchment. Draw six 3-inch circles on the paper; turn the paper over.

In a large mixing bowl, using an electric mixer on medium speed, beat the egg whites, vanilla, and cream of tartar for about 5 minutes, or until soft peaks form. Turn the mixer to high speed. While beating, add ½ cup sugar 1 tablespoon at a time. Beat for about 5 minutes, or until stiff peaks form, scraping down the side of the bowl once. The mixture should remain glossy and not feel grainy when rubbed between your fingers.

Using the back of a spoon, gently spread the mixture over the circles on the parchment, building up the sides to form meringue shells.

Bake for 30 minutes. Turn off the oven, leaving the meringues in the oven to dry for 1 hour. Transfer the baking sheet to a cooling rack and let cool completely, about 30 minutes. Store the meringues in an airtight container at room temperature for up to two days.

In a medium bowl, stir together the berries and orange juice concentrate. Let stand at room temperature for at least 30 minutes. Immediately before serving, spoon the berry mixture into the meringues. Top each with the yogurt and a sprinkling of the remaining 2 teaspoons sugar.

PER SERVING

CALORIES 124
TOTAL FAT 0.5 g
  Saturated Fat 0.0 g
  Trans Fat 0.0 g
  Polyunsaturated Fat 0.0 g
  Monounsaturated Fat 0.0 g
CHOLESTEROL 0 mg
SODIUM 30 mg
CARBOHYDRATES 29 g
  Fiber 2 g
  Sugars 27 g
PROTEIN 3 g
DIETARY EXCHANGES
  ½ fruit, 1½ carbohydrate

COOK'S TIP on beating egg whites

Even a single drop of egg yolk will prevent egg whites from forming peaks when beaten, so separate eggs very carefully.

COOK'S TIP on meringues

Like other meringues, these shells should not be made on a humid day. They will get a little gummy and will lose their crispness.

fruit with vanilla cream

SERVES 4

A thick, cheesecake-flavored topping covers fresh or frozen fruit.

½ cup fat-free sour cream

¼ cup sifted confectioners' sugar

2 teaspoons vanilla extract

¾ cup frozen fat-free whipped topping, thawed in refrigerator

8 ounces frozen unsweetened sliced peaches, slightly thawed, or peeled fresh peaches, hulled strawberries, blueberries, raspberries, or a combination, diced

8 slices frozen unsweetened peaches, slightly thawed, or peeled fresh peaches

In a small bowl, whisk together the sour cream, confectioners' sugar, and vanilla until smooth.

Gently fold in the whipped topping.

Put the diced fruit in a serving bowl or individual ramekins. Spoon the sour cream mixture over the fruit. Arrange the peach slices on top. Serve or cover and refrigerate for up to 2 hours.

PER SERVING

CALORIES 124
TOTAL FAT 0.5 g
  Saturated Fat 0.0 g
  Trans Fat 0.0 g
  Polyunsaturated Fat 0.0 g
  Monounsaturated Fat 0.0 g
CHOLESTEROL 5 mg
SODIUM 33 mg
CARBOHYDRATES 25 g
  Fiber 2 g
  Sugars 15 g
PROTEIN 3 g
DIETARY EXCHANGES
  1½ carbohydrate

berries in vanilla sauce

SERVES 4

Mixed berries decoratively arranged on a bed of thick, sweet vanilla cream sauce—what a beautiful way to end a meal.

---

1 cup fat-free milk and ¼ cup fat-free milk, divided use

3 tablespoons sugar

1 tablespoon plus 1 teaspoon cornstarch

1 tablespoon vanilla extract

6 ounces blueberries

8 ounces strawberries, hulled and halved

1 whole strawberry with stem (optional)

In a small saucepan, whisk together 1 cup milk and the sugar. Bring to a boil over medium-high heat, whisking occasionally.

Meanwhile, in a small bowl, whisk together the remaining ¼ cup milk and cornstarch until the cornstarch is dissolved. Whisk into the sugar mixture. Cook for 2 to 3 minutes, or until thickened, whisking constantly. Remove from the heat.

Whisk in the vanilla. Pour into a 10-inch quiche pan or onto a rimmed serving plate. Let cool for 20 minutes to set slightly.

Arrange the blueberries in a mound in the center of the sauce. Circle with the halved strawberries. Place the whole strawberry or strawberry fan (see Cook's Tip on Strawberry Fans, below) on the blueberries. Cover with plastic wrap and refrigerate for about 2 hours.

COOK'S TIP on strawberry fans

To make a strawberry fan, thinly slice the strawberry up to the stem (4 to 6 slices), but *don't* detach the stem. Gently press down with your fingertips to allow the slices to separate slightly to form a fan.

PER SERVING

CALORIES 124
TOTAL FAT 0.5 g
  Saturated Fat 0.0 g
  Trans Fat 0.0 g
  Polyunsaturated Fat 0.0 g
  Monounsaturated Fat 0.0 g
CHOLESTEROL 2 mg
SODIUM 34 mg
CARBOHYDRATES 27 g
  Fiber 2 g
  Sugars 21 g
PROTEIN 3 g
DIETARY EXCHANGES
  2 carbohydrate

sweet and fruity salsa bowl

SERVES 4

Colorful fruit tossed with fresh mint and ginger gets a tangy splash of lemon.

5 ounces strawberries, hulled and cut into ¼-inch cubes
1 medium mango, cut into ¼-inch cubes
1 medium kiwifruit, peeled and cut into ¼-inch cubes
2 tablespoons chopped fresh mint

1 tablespoon sugar
½ teaspoon grated peeled gingerroot
½ teaspoon grated lemon zest
1 tablespoon fresh lemon juice
2 cups fat-free vanilla or fruit-flavored yogurt

In a medium bowl, gently toss all the ingredients except the yogurt.

If serving right away, spoon the yogurt into bowls or wine goblets. Top with the fruit salsa. Or make the fruit salsa in advance, cover with plastic wrap, and refrigerate for up to 8 hours. Serve over the yogurt.

COOK'S TIP

If fresh mangoes aren't available, check the refrigerated section of your supermarket's produce area for bottled mango slices.

PER SERVING

CALORIES 183
TOTAL FAT 0.5 g
  Saturated Fat 0.0 g
  Trans Fat 0.0 g
  Polyunsaturated Fat 0.0 g
  Monounsaturated Fat 0.0 g
CHOLESTEROL 2 mg
SODIUM 87 mg
CARBOHYDRATES 40 g
  Fiber 2 g
  Sugars 36 g
PROTEIN 7 g
DIETARY EXCHANGES
  1 fruit, 1 fat-free milk,
  ½ carbohydrate

grapefruit-orange palette

SERVES 6

This artistic delight is excellent as dessert or as part of a weekend brunch.

---

3 medium pink or ruby red grapefruit, chilled

3 medium seedless oranges, chilled

12 ounces frozen sweetened raspberries, thawed

2 tablespoons black currant jelly or crème de cassis (black currant liqueur)

¼ cup sifted confectioners' sugar

6 fresh mint sprigs

Peel and section the grapefruit. Peel the oranges. Cut the oranges crosswise into 5 slices, then cut each slice in half. Set aside.

In a food processor or blender, process the raspberries until smooth (except for the seeds). Press through a fine-mesh strainer into a small bowl, getting as much pulp as possible. Discard the seeds.

In a small microwaveable bowl, microwave the jelly on 100 percent power (high) for 30 seconds.

Stir the jelly and sugar into the raspberry pulp.

Arrange the grapefruit sections and orange pieces alternately in a circular pattern (like flower petals) on each dessert plate. Drizzle the raspberry sauce in a circle over the fruit. Place a mint sprig in the center of each serving.

COOK'S TIP

You can prepare the fruit and sauce ahead of time. Cover and refrigerate the grapefruit sections, orange pieces, and pureed raspberries separately. Assemble just before serving.

PER SERVING

CALORIES 164
TOTAL FAT 0.0 g
   Saturated Fat 0.0 g
   Trans Fat 0.0 g
   Polyunsaturated Fat 0.0 g
   Monounsaturated Fat 0.0 g
CHOLESTEROL 0 mg
SODIUM 0 mg
CARBOHYDRATES 41 g
   Fiber 6 g
   Sugars 30 g
PROTEIN 2 g
DIETARY EXCHANGES
   2 fruit, ½ carbohydrate

claret-spiced oranges

SERVES 6

Here's a light, lovely dessert that, though simple, is elegant enough for a special occasion.

¾ cup claret or other dry red wine (regular or nonalcoholic)
½ cup water
¼ cup plus 1 tablespoon sugar
1 cinnamon stick (about 3 inches long)

1 tablespoon fresh lemon juice
2 whole cloves
4 medium oranges, peeled and sectioned

In a small saucepan, stir together all the ingredients except the oranges. Bring to a boil over medium-high heat. Reduce the heat and simmer for 5 minutes.

Put the orange sections in a medium glass bowl. Pour the sauce over the oranges. Let cool slightly. Cover and refrigerate for at least 4 hours. Discard the cinnamon stick and cloves before serving the oranges.

PER SERVING

CALORIES 107
TOTAL FAT 0.0 g
  Saturated Fat 0.0 g
  Trans Fat 0.0 g
  Polyunsaturated Fat 0.0 g
  Monounsaturated Fat 0.0 g
CHOLESTEROL 0 mg
SODIUM 1 mg
CARBOHYDRATES 22 g
  Fiber 2 g
  Sugars 20 g
PROTEIN 1 g
DIETARY EXCHANGES
  1½ carbohydrate

baked ginger pears

SERVES 8

These Asian-influenced pears go nicely with a chicken- or vegetable-based stir-fry.

8 canned pear halves in fruit juice, well drained, juice reserved
⅓ cup firmly packed light brown sugar
2 tablespoons chopped pecans, dry-roasted
1 teaspoon fresh lemon juice

¼ teaspoon ground ginger or chopped crystallized ginger to taste, plus additional crystallized ginger (optional) for garnish
8 maraschino cherries (optional)

Preheat the oven to 350°F.

Arrange the pears with the cut side up in a glass baking dish just large enough to hold them.

In a small bowl, stir together the brown sugar, pecans, lemon juice, and ginger. Spoon into the cavities of the pear halves.

Pour the reserved juice around the pears.

Bake for 15 to 20 minutes. Serve warm or cover and refrigerate to serve chilled. Garnish with bits of crystallized ginger and the cherries.

MICROWAVE METHOD

Drain the juice from the pears, reserving 1 cup. Arrange the pear halves with the cut side up in a glass pie pan. Prepare as directed. Microwave on 100 percent power (high) for 5 minutes. Let cool for at least 10 minutes before serving. Garnish with the crystallized ginger and cherries.

PER SERVING

CALORIES 86
TOTAL FAT 1.5 g
  Saturated Fat 0.0 g
  Trans Fat 0.0 g
  Polyunsaturated Fat 0.5 g
  Monounsaturated Fat 0.5 g
CHOLESTEROL 0 mg
SODIUM 6 mg
CARBOHYDRATES 19 g
  Fiber 1 g
  Sugars 17 g
PROTEIN 0 g
DIETARY EXCHANGES
  1½ carbohydrate

golden poached pears

SERVES 6

Serve these poached and chilled pears with a flute of sparkling wine or white grape juice. A great fall dessert!

6 Bartlett pears, peeled, left whole with stems intact
1 tablespoon fresh lemon juice and ¼ cup fresh lemon juice, divided use
2 12-ounce cans apricot nectar

½ cup sugar
1 teaspoon grated lemon zest
½ cup sherry (cream sherry preferred)
6 fresh mint sprigs (optional)

Sprinkle the pears with 1 tablespoon lemon juice to prevent discoloration.

In a large, deep saucepan, stir together the apricot nectar, sugar, lemon zest, and remaining ¼ cup lemon juice. Bring to a boil over medium-high heat. Reduce the heat and simmer for 5 minutes.

Stir in the sherry.

Add the pears. Simmer for 20 to 25 minutes, or until just tender, basting and turning occasionally to cook evenly. (Cooking time may vary depending on the size and firmness of the pears.) Transfer the pears to a storage container.

Continue simmering the liquid until reduced by half. Pour over the pears, cover, and refrigerate until chilled.

To serve, spoon the syrup over the pears. Garnish with the mint.

COOK'S TIP on pears

Pears are ripe when they yield to gentle pressure at the stem end. The body of the pear will still be firm. To ripen pears, put them in a paper bag and fold the top down. To speed up the process, put an apple in the bag with them. A pear's skin toughens as it cooks, so always peel before cooking.

PER SERVING

CALORIES 256
TOTAL FAT 0.5 g
  Saturated Fat 0.0 g
  Trans Fat 0.0 g
  Polyunsaturated Fat 0.0 g
  Monounsaturated Fat 0.0 g
CHOLESTEROL 0 mg
SODIUM 7 mg
CARBOHYDRATES 64 g
  Fiber 6 g
  Sugars 50 g
PROTEIN 1 g
DIETARY EXCHANGES
  3 fruit, 1 carbohydrate

fall fruit medley

SERVES 6

Although this combination of seasonal fruits is wonderful for its complementary colors, flavors, and textures, feel free to substitute whatever fruits you prefer.

2 medium apples, sliced
2 medium pears, sliced
1 Fuyu persimmon, sliced
5 ounces frozen sweetened raspberries, thawed and drained

¼ cup fresh orange juice
¼ cup kirsch (optional)

In a medium bowl, stir together the apples, pears, and persimmon.

Gently stir in the raspberries.

Pour in the orange juice and kirsch, stirring gently. Cover and refrigerate until needed.

COOK'S TIP on persimmons

A Fuyu persimmon resembles a squatty, reddish-orange tomato in shape. Firm when ripe, it can be eaten whole or sliced and will be crisp and not astringent. Hachiya persimmons, on the other hand, are very bitter until they are completely soft.

frozen raspberry cream

SERVES 8

Sweet, tart berries combine with whipped topping for a dream of a dessert.

2 large egg whites, at room temperature
2 teaspoons water
⅛ teaspoon cream of tartar
¾ cup sugar
1 10-ounce package frozen unsweetened raspberries or strawberries, thawed

1 tablespoon fresh lemon juice
1 cup fat-free frozen whipped topping, thawed in refrigerator
8 raspberries or strawberries (optional)
8 fresh mint sprigs (optional)

In the top of a double boiler, beat together the egg whites, water, and cream of tartar. Cook over simmering water for 7 to 10 minutes, or until the mixture registers 160°F. Pour into a large bowl.

Add the sugar 1 tablespoon at a time, beating constantly until smooth.

Stir in the thawed berries and lemon juice. Beat until soft peaks form.

Fold in the whipped topping. Spoon into 8 goblets. Freeze for at least 8 hours.

To serve, garnish each raspberry cream with a berry and a mint sprig.

TIME-SAVER

Skip the freezing and just refrigerate the raspberry cream for 2 hours if you're pressed for time.

PER SERVING

CALORIES 116
TOTAL FAT 0.0 g
  Saturated Fat 0.0 g
  Trans Fat 0.0 g
  Polyunsaturated Fat 0.0 g
  Monounsaturated Fat 0.0 g
CHOLESTEROL 0 mg
SODIUM 19 mg
CARBOHYDRATES 28 g
  Fiber 1 g
  Sugars 23 g
PROTEIN 1 g
DIETARY EXCHANGES
  2 carbohydrate

frozen cocoa cream with dark cherries

SERVES 4

This frozen "cream" is so smooth and, well, creamy! Make a double batch so you can have some on hand—you'll be very glad you did.

8 ounces fat-free frozen whipped topping, thawed in refrigerator	¼ cup water
	1 teaspoon cornstarch
1½ tablespoons unsweetened cocoa powder (dark preferred)	⅛ to ¼ teaspoon almond extract
8 ounces frozen dark sweet cherries, thawed	¼ cup sliced almonds, dry-roasted

Spoon the whipped topping into a medium bowl. Using a fine-mesh sieve, sift the cocoa powder over the whipped topping. Stir gently until well blended. Spoon into four 6-ounce porcelain ramekins or glass custard cups. Cover with plastic wrap. Freeze for about 2 hours, or until firm.

Meanwhile, in a medium nonstick skillet, gently stir the cherries, water, and cornstarch until the cornstarch is dissolved. Bring to boil over medium-high heat and boil for 1 minute, stirring occasionally. Remove from the heat and let cool completely, about 30 minutes.

Stir in the almond extract. Pour into a small airtight container. Cover and refrigerate until needed.

To serve, spoon the cherry mixture over the cocoa creams in the ramekins. Sprinkle with the almonds.

COOK'S TIP

Instead of making this dessert taste more "almondy," the larger amount of almond extract actually brings out the cherry flavor.

COOK'S TIP

If you made extra creams, cover them with aluminum foil and freeze them, without the cherry topping and almonds, for up to 10 days.

PER SERVING

CALORIES 175
TOTAL FAT 3.0 g
  Saturated Fat 0.0 g
  Trans Fat 0.0 g
  Polyunsaturated Fat 0.5 g
  Monounsaturated Fat 2.0 g
CHOLESTEROL 0 mg
SODIUM 32 mg
CARBOHYDRATES 31 g
  Fiber 2 g
  Sugars 14 g
PROTEIN 2 g
DIETARY EXCHANGES
  2 carbohydrate, ½ fat

spiced skillet bananas with frozen yogurt

SERVES 4

Sample a taste of the Deep South with these bananas in a brown sugar glaze.

1 tablespoon light tub margarine
2 tablespoons dark brown sugar
2 cups sliced bananas

½ teaspoon vanilla, butter, and nut flavoring or vanilla extract
2 cups fat-free vanilla frozen yogurt

In a large nonstick skillet over medium-high heat, melt the margarine, swirling to coat the bottom. Add the brown sugar, stirring until the mixture is bubbly and the sugar is dissolved.

Add the bananas, stirring gently to coat. Cook for 3 minutes, or until just softened and beginning to glaze and turn golden. Don't overcook, or the bananas will break down. Remove the skillet from the heat.

Gently stir in the flavoring. Spoon over the frozen yogurt. Serve immediately.

SPICED SKILLET APPLES WITH FROZEN YOGURT
Replace the bananas with thinly sliced peeled apples, such as Red Delicious, and replace the vanilla, butter, and nut flavoring with apple pie spice. Cook for 6 to 8 minutes, or until the apples are just tender.

PER SERVING

CALORIES 185
TOTAL FAT 1.5 g
  Saturated Fat 0.0 g
  Trans Fat 0.0 g
  Polyunsaturated Fat 0.5 g
  Monounsaturated Fat 0.5 g
CHOLESTEROL 1 mg
SODIUM 65 mg
CARBOHYDRATES 42 g
  Fiber 2 g
  Sugars 34 g
PROTEIN 4 g
DIETARY EXCHANGES
  3 carbohydrate, ½ fat

PER SERVING

SPICED SKILLET APPLES
WITH FROZEN YOGURT
CALORIES 143
TOTAL FAT 1.0 g
  Saturated Fat 0.0 g
  Trans Fat 0.0 g
  Polyunsaturated Fat 0.5 g
  Monounsaturated Fat 0.5 g
CHOLESTEROL 1 mg
SODIUM 65 mg
CARBOHYDRATES 32 g
  Fiber 1 g
  Sugars 30 g
PROTEIN 3 g
DIETARY EXCHANGES
  2 carbohydrate

frozen mini key lime soufflés

SERVES 8

No worries about these soufflés falling—they freeze in place. Make them when you have a bit of spare time, then freeze them to have on hand when you want an elegant dessert.

1 14-ounce can fat-free sweetened condensed milk

1 teaspoon grated Key lime zest or lime zest

½ cup fresh or bottled Key lime juice (fresh preferred)

2 tablespoons powdered egg whites (pasteurized dried egg whites)

¼ cup plus 2 tablespoons cold water

1 cup frozen fat-free whipped topping, thawed in refrigerator

3 Key limes or 1 large lime, cut into thin slices (optional)

To make collars for eight 2-ounce custard cups, cut aluminum foil into eight 8 x 2-inch strips. Wrap a strip around the rim of each soufflé cup to form a collar. Secure the foil with tape. This will give the illusion of a risen soufflé when the collar is removed. You can use 4-ounce custard cups without collars if you prefer.

In a medium bowl, whisk together the milk, lime zest, and lime juice until slightly thickened.

Put the powdered egg whites in a medium mixing bowl. Pour in the water. Whisk together. Let stand for 2 minutes, whisking occasionally, until the egg whites are completely dissolved and the mixture is slightly frothy. Using an electric mixer, beat on medium high for 2 to 3 minutes, or until the mixture forms stiff peaks.

Using a rubber scraper, fold the whipped topping into the milk mixture. Fold in the egg whites until just combined (the mixture will be light and fluffy).

Spoon ½ cup mixture into each custard cup. Cover individually with aluminum foil. Freeze for at least 3 hours, or until firm (will keep for up to one month, tightly covered with aluminum foil, in the freezer).

To serve, discard the foil collars. Garnish with the lime slices.

PER SERVING

CALORIES 165
TOTAL FAT 0.0 g
  Saturated Fat 0.0 g
  Trans Fat 0.0 g
  Polyunsaturated Fat 0.0 g
  Monounsaturated Fat 0.0 g
CHOLESTEROL 3 mg
SODIUM 78 mg
CARBOHYDRATES 35 g
  Fiber 0 g
  Sugars 32 g
PROTEIN 5 g
DIETARY EXCHANGES
  2½ carbohydrate

strawberries with champagne ice

SERVES 14

The flavors of strawberries and champagne marry well in this made-for-entertaining dessert.

2 medium oranges
1 medium lemon
1½ cups water
¾ cup sugar and 1 tablespoon sugar, divided use
3 tablespoons orange-flavored liqueur

2 cups champagne or other sparkling white wine and 1 cup champagne or other sparkling white wine, divided use
2 cups strawberries, hulled and halved

Using a vegetable peeler, peel the zest in strips from the oranges and lemon. Squeeze the juice from the oranges and lemon into a small bowl.

In a large saucepan, stir together the water, ¾ cup sugar, and orange and lemon zest. Bring to a boil over medium-high heat. Boil for 5 minutes. Remove from the heat. Discard the zest. Pour the liquid into a large bowl.

Stir the orange and lemon juices and liqueur into the sugar mixture. Cover and refrigerate for 2 hours.

Stir 2 cups champagne into the juice mixture. Pour into an 8-inch square baking pan. Freeze for 2 hours 30 minutes to 3 hours, or until slushy.

Beat the juice mixture in a mixing bowl or process in a food processor or blender until smooth. Pour the mixture back into the pan. Refreeze for 2 to 3 hours, stirring occasionally.

Meanwhile, put the strawberries in a medium bowl. Stir the remaining 1 cup champagne and the remaining 1 tablespoon sugar into the strawberries. Cover and refrigerate for at least 2 hours.

At serving time, using a slotted spoon, transfer the strawberries to goblets. Fill with the champagne ice.

strawberry-raspberry ice

SERVES 8

A refreshingly cool double dose of berries, this ice looks attractive in chilled wine or champagne glasses garnished with fresh mint sprigs.

6 ounces frozen white grape juice concentrate

1 cup water

1 tablespoon confectioners' sugar

8 ounces frozen unsweetened strawberries, slightly thawed

6 ounces frozen sweetened raspberries, slightly thawed

6 ice cubes (about 1 cup)

Fresh mint sprigs (optional)

In a food processor or blender, combine all the ingredients except the mint in the order listed. Process until smooth (except for the seeds), stirring occasionally. Pour into a large resealable plastic bag and seal. Put the bag on its side in the freezer and let the mixture freeze solid, at least 2 hours.

About 15 minutes before serving, remove the bag from the freezer and let the ice thaw slightly, mashing with a fork if needed. At serving time, spoon into chilled glasses. Garnish with the mint sprigs. Serve immediately.

PER SERVING

CALORIES 87
TOTAL FAT 0.0 g
  Saturated Fat 0.0 g
  Trans Fat 0.0 g
  Polyunsaturated Fat 0.0 g
  Monounsaturated Fat 0.0 g
CHOLESTEROL 0 mg
SODIUM 2 mg
CARBOHYDRATES 22 g
  Fiber 2 g
  Sugars 18 g
PROTEIN 0 g
DIETARY EXCHANGES
  1½ fruit

strawberry-banana sorbet

SERVES 5

Give your guests the star treatment—garnish this light dessert with star fruit!

1 cup peach, apricot, or strawberry nectar or fresh orange juice
¼ cup sugar
1 cup sliced hulled strawberries
1 cup sliced bananas
2 tablespoons dry white wine (regular or nonalcoholic) or fresh orange juice

1 tablespoon fresh lemon juice
1 star fruit (carambola) (optional)
Fresh mint sprigs (optional)

In a small saucepan, stir together the nectar and sugar until the sugar is dissolved. Bring to a boil over medium-high heat. Reduce the heat and simmer for 5 minutes, stirring occasionally. Pour into a medium bowl. Refrigerate for 10 to 15 minutes.

Meanwhile, in a food processor or blender, process the strawberries, bananas, wine, and lemon juice until smooth (except for the seeds). Pour into the nectar mixture, stirring well. Pour into an 8-inch square baking pan. Cover and freeze for 2 hours, stirring every 30 minutes. Freeze without stirring for 4 to 5 hours, or until completely frozen.

To serve, trim the ends off the star fruit. Cut crosswise into thin slices. Discard the seeds. Using an ice cream scoop, fill dessert dishes or wineglasses with the sorbet. Garnish with the star fruit and mint.

MANGO-PEACH SORBET

Replace the strawberries and bananas with 2 cups diced mangoes.

PER SERVING

CALORIES 108
TOTAL FAT 0.0 g
  Saturated Fat 0.0 g
  Trans Fat 0.0 g
  Polyunsaturated Fat 0.0 g
  Monounsaturated Fat 0.0 g
CHOLESTEROL 0 mg
SODIUM 4 mg
CARBOHYDRATES 27 g
  Fiber 2 g
  Sugars 21 g
PROTEIN 1 g
DIETARY EXCHANGES
  1 fruit, 1 carbohydrate

PER SERVING

MANGO-PEACH SORBET
CALORIES 114
TOTAL FAT 0.0 g
  Saturated Fat 0.0 g
  Trans Fat 0.0 g
  Polyunsaturated Fat 0.0 g
  Monounsaturated Fat 0.0 g
CHOLESTEROL 0 mg
SODIUM 5 mg
CARBOHYDRATES 29 g
  Fiber 2 g
  Sugars 26 g
PROTEIN 1 g
DIETARY EXCHANGES
  1 fruit, 1 carbohydrate

cherry-berry chill

SERVES 8

Although this dessert has the taste and texture of soft-serve ice cream, it is mostly fruit.

1 pound frozen unsweetened mixed berries	¼ cup fat-free half-and-half
¾ cup white grape juice	2 teaspoons vanilla extract
⅓ cup sugar	8 ounces frozen pitted dark (sweet) cherries, partially thawed

In a food processor or blender, process the ingredients except the cherries until smooth.

Add the cherries. Process until smooth. Serve immediately for soft serve or transfer to an airtight container and put in the freezer for at least 4 hours. If frozen, let stand at room temperature for 15 minutes before serving for peak flavor and texture.

COOK'S TIP

For easy blending, add the cherries after the other ingredients are processed. The average blender cannot hold all the ingredients for a recipe like this one without processing some of them first.

PER SERVING

CALORIES 92
TOTAL FAT 0.5 g
   Saturated Fat 0.0 g
   Trans Fat 0.0 g
   Polyunsaturated Fat 0.0 g
   Monounsaturated Fat 0.0 g
CHOLESTEROL 0 mg
SODIUM 9 mg
CARBOHYDRATES 23 g
   Fiber 2 g
   Sugars 18 g
PROTEIN 1 g
DIETARY EXCHANGES
   1½ fruit

tropical breeze

SERVES 4

You'll think you've had a quick trip to the islands when you drink this creamy blend of tropical flavors. It's best when served in glasses that have been chilled in the freezer.

½ cup pineapple juice
2 cups fat-free vanilla yogurt
¾ cup very ripe mashed bananas
¼ cup confectioners' sugar

2 teaspoons vanilla extract
½ teaspoon coconut extract
8 ice cubes (about 1⅓ cups)
4 pineapple spears (optional)

In a food processor or blender, combine all the ingredients except the pineapple spears in the order listed. Process until smooth. Pour into a large resealable plastic bag and seal. Put the bag on its side in the freezer for about 1 hour, or until the mixture is very thick.

Immediately before serving, spoon the mixture into glasses. Garnish with the pineapple spears. If the mixture is too frozen to pour or spoon into glasses, return it to the processor or blender and process until slushy.

sunny mango sorbet

SERVES 4

Thick, creamy, rich, tart, and sweet—this supersimple sorbet is all these and more. Serve it in wineglasses for that special touch.

4 cups coarsely chopped mangoes (about 5 medium)	½ cup fresh lime juice 2 tablespoons sugar

In a food processor or blender, process the ingredients until smooth. Pour into a large resealable plastic bag and seal. Put the bag on its side in the freezer for about 2 hours, or until the mixture is thick. If frozen solid, remove the bag from the freezer about 30 minutes before serving time. Stir the sorbet before serving.

COOK'S TIP

If you want a completely smooth sorbet, strain the processed mixture before freezing.

PER SERVING

CALORIES 139
TOTAL FAT 0.5 g
  Saturated Fat 0.0 g
  Trans Fat 0.0 g
  Polyunsaturated Fat 0.0 g
  Monounsaturated Fat 0.0 g
CHOLESTEROL 0 mg
SODIUM 4 mg
CARBOHYDRATES 37 g
  Fiber 3 g
  Sugars 31 g
PROTEIN 1 g
DIETARY EXCHANGES
  2½ fruit

tequila-lime sherbet

SERVES 6

Tequila and lime make a refreshing combination, as in this sherbet. Let it cool your taste buds after a spicy Tex-Mex meal.

2 tablespoons cold water and 1 cup
    water, divided use
1 envelope unflavored gelatin
¾ cup sugar

1 cup fat-free plain yogurt
1 tablespoon grated lime zest
½ cup fresh lime juice
⅓ cup tequila

In a small bowl, using a fork, stir together 2 tablespoons cold water and the gelatin. Set aside to let the gelatin soften.

In a medium saucepan, whisk together the remaining 1 cup water and the sugar. Bring to a boil over medium-high heat. Boil for 5 minutes, whisking occasionally. Remove from the heat.

Whisk in the gelatin mixture and the remaining ingredients until smooth. Pour into an 8-inch square baking pan. Freeze for 2 hours 30 minutes to 3 hours, or until slushy.

In a food processor or blender, process the mixture until smooth. Return to the pan and freeze, about 6 hours. Remove from the freezer about 15 minutes before serving.

PER SERVING

CALORIES 159
TOTAL FAT 0.0 g
  Saturated Fat 0.0 g
  Trans Fat 0.0 g
  Polyunsaturated Fat 0.0 g
  Monounsaturated Fat 0.0 g
CHOLESTEROL 1 mg
SODIUM 36 mg
CARBOHYDRATES 30 g
  Fiber 0 g
  Sugars 29 g
PROTEIN 3 g
DIETARY EXCHANGES
  2 carbohydrate

cardinal sundaes

SERVES 16

Frosty lime sherbet topped with a vibrant cardinal red berry mixture makes a delicious treat with a beautiful color contrast.

½ cup frozen unsweetened strawberries, thawed, drained, juice reserved

½ cup frozen sweetened raspberries, thawed, drained, juice reserved

1 teaspoon cornstarch

¼ teaspoon fresh lemon juice

1 tablespoon currant jelly

8 cups lime sherbet

In a small saucepan, whisk together the berry juices (set the berries aside), cornstarch, and lemon juice. Bring to a boil over medium-high heat. Cook for 1 minute, whisking constantly.

Add the jelly, whisking until melted. Remove from the heat.

Stir the berries into the sauce. Pour into a small bowl. Cover and refrigerate.

To serve, put ½ cup sherbet in each bowl. Top each serving with 1 tablespoon sauce. Cover and refrigerate any remaining topping.

kiwifruit sundaes

SERVES 4

Vibrant kiwifruit serves double duty here—it is a primary ingredient in the sauce and a tangy garnish.

4 medium kiwifruit, peeled
⅓ cup fresh orange juice and
    2 tablespoons fresh orange juice
    or orange liqueur, divided use
¼ cup honey

2 teaspoons cornstarch
1 teaspoon grated orange zest
⅛ teaspoon almond extract
2 cups fat-free frozen yogurt or
    fat-free ice cream, any flavor

In a food processor or blender, process 2 kiwifruit until smooth (except for the seeds). Slice the remaining kiwifruit. Set aside.

In a medium microwaveable bowl, whisk together the processed kiwifruit, ⅓ cup orange juice, honey, and cornstarch. Microwave, covered, on 100 percent power (high) for 3 minutes, stirring once halfway through.

Stir the orange zest, remaining 2 tablespoons orange juice, and almond extract into the kiwifruit mixture.

Spoon the frozen yogurt into dessert bowls. Spoon the sauce over the yogurt. Top with the sliced kiwifruit.

PER SERVING

CALORIES 209
TOTAL FAT 0.5 g
  Saturated Fat 0.0 g
  Trans Fat 0.0 g
  Polyunsaturated Fat 0.0 g
  Monounsaturated Fat 0.0 g
CHOLESTEROL 1 mg
SODIUM 44 mg
CARBOHYDRATES 51 g
  Fiber 2 g
  Sugars 44 g
PROTEIN 4 g
DIETARY EXCHANGES
  1 fruit, 2½ carbohydrate

raspberry parfaits

SERVES 6

These beautiful raspberry parfaits are deliciously light and refreshing.

2 cups frozen unsweetened raspberries, thawed, undrained
2 tablespoons sugar
½ teaspoon fresh lemon juice
¼ teaspoon vanilla extract
1 large peach, peeled and diced, or 1¾ cups frozen unsweetened sliced peaches, thawed and diced

1 pint fat-free vanilla ice cream or fat-free vanilla frozen yogurt
¼ cup fat-free frozen whipped topping, thawed in refrigerator
3 tablespoons sliced almonds, dry-roasted

In a food processor or blender, process the raspberries, sugar, lemon juice, and vanilla for 15 to 20 seconds, or until smooth (except for the seeds).

Spoon 1 tablespoon sauce into each parfait or small wineglass. Top with the peaches and ice cream. Spoon the remaining raspberry sauce over the ice cream. Top each serving with a dollop of whipped topping. Sprinkle with the almonds.

PER SERVING

CALORIES 143
TOTAL FAT 1.5 g
    Saturated Fat 0.0 g
    Trans Fat 0.0 g
    Polyunsaturated Fat 0.5 g
    Monounsaturated Fat 1.0 g
CHOLESTEROL 0 mg
SODIUM 45 mg
CARBOHYDRATES 31 g
    Fiber 2 g
    Sugars 20 g
PROTEIN 4 g
DIETARY EXCHANGES
    ½ fruit, 1½ carbohydrate, ½ fat

how your diet affects your heart

We know for a fact that everyday lifestyle choices such as diet have a major impact on the long-term health of your heart. Your cardiovascular system is crucial to your overall well-being, and it makes sense to do what you can to protect every component. Certain dietary choices, however, contribute to your chances of developing the conditions that increase your risk of heart disease, such as high blood pressure, high blood cholesterol, and diabetes.

HOW YOUR DIET CAN HURT YOUR HEART

Understanding how the following common dietary elements can contribute to your health risk will help you make heart-smart choices when shopping for food, cooking at home, and eating out.

Saturated Fat, Trans Fat, and Cholesterol

Many diseases of the heart, especially heart attacks in middle age and later in life, are linked to the buildup of plaque on arterial walls that is caused by long-term high blood levels of LDL ("bad") cholesterol and low levels of HDL ("good") cholesterol. Although genetic factors can affect cholesterol levels and overall heart health, in many people unhealthy cholesterol levels result from unhealthy dietary choices, such as eating a lot of foods rich in saturated fat, trans fat, and cholesterol. Although for years it was assumed that dietary cholesterol caused high blood cholesterol, we now know that a high intake of saturated and trans fats is what triggers the body's production of excess LDL cholesterol.

Sodium

A high intake of sodium increases blood pressure. In turn, the constant force of added pressure can damage arterial walls, making them thicker and less elastic. Over time, these changes reduce blood flow, forcing your heart to work harder to pump the blood that delivers oxygen to the rest of your body. Untreated high blood pressure significantly increases the likelihood of heart disease and stroke, and the higher the blood pressure, the greater the risk.

Excess Calories

When you eat more calories than you burn, you gain weight. To carry those extra pounds, your body needs to produce more energy. To provide that energy, your heart must work harder to pump blood and deliver oxygen. The increased workload gradually weakens and enlarges the heart, leaving it more vulnerable. At the same time, extra weight raises blood pressure and increases your chance of developing diabetes, both of which put you at greater risk for heart disease and stroke. Another consequence of excess calorie intake is high blood levels of triglycerides, another form of fat that is present in the blood. When calories are not used for energy, the excess calories are carried to fat cells in the form of triglycerides, which may also contribute to arterial plaque and increase risk.

Added Sugars

Sugar has no nutritional value other than to provide calories. A high intake of added sugars (as opposed to naturally occurring sugars) has been implicated in the rise in obesity and may be associated with increased risks for high blood pressure, high triglyceride levels, and other risk factors for heart disease and stroke.

HOW YOU CAN PROTECT YOUR HEART

Thanks to recent advances in our understanding of cardiovascular disease, we know more than ever about the health factors that can delay or prevent heart disease. These factors include being a non-smoker, keeping blood pressure and cholesterol levels at normal levels, having a normal body mass index, being physically active—and eating a healthy diet.

To reduce your risk of heart disease, make healthy behavior and choices part of your everyday lifestyle. You can get started by using the heart-healthy recipes in this cookbook along with the information in the following appendixes on how to shop and cook smart for your heart. For more information on diet, lifestyle, and heart disease, visit the American Heart Association's Web site at www.americanheart.org.

shopping with your heart in mind

Heart-healthy eating habits start with planning ahead and making good choices at the grocery store. Since you're more likely to eat what you have on hand, it's a smart strategy to stock your pantry, freezer, and fridge with nutritious foods. If you don't buy the foods that sabotage your efforts to eat well, you'll have fewer opportunities to be tempted by them.

MEAL PLANNING

To keep your healthy eating on course, try planning your meals—at least the entrées—for the whole week *before* you head to the grocery store. As you create your weekly meal plans, choose a variety of foods from all the food groups discussed next. In addition, use the following information to help you plan how much food to buy from each food group. The recommended numbers of servings given here are based on a daily intake of 2,000 calories; adjust accordingly if you need fewer or more calories each day. Remember that balance and variety are the keys to both good nutrition and a satisfied palate.

Next, make a grocery list of everything you'll need for preparing the healthy meals and snacks you've planned. Shopping with a detailed list will save time in the grocery store and minimize impulse buying.

At-a-Glance Shopping Guidelines

- **VEGETABLES AND FRUITS:** Choose a variety of vegetables and fruits in many colors. As a rule, the more deeply colored, the more packed with vitamins and minerals.
    - ✓ *Aim for 5 servings of vegetables and 4 of fruits* <u>each day</u>.

- **DAIRY:** Choose fat-free and low-fat (preferably 1%) dairy products, including milk, yogurt, and cheese.
    - ✓ *Aim for 2 to 3 servings of these products* <u>each day</u>.

- **WHOLE GRAINS AND HIGH-FIBER FOODS:** Try a variety of whole-grain breads, cereals, and pastas; choose whole grains such as brown and wild rice, bulgur, barley, and quinoa.
    - ✓ *Aim for 6 servings of grains* <u>each day</u>, *with at least 3 from whole grains.*

- **FISH:** Include fish, preferably fish rich in omega-3 fatty acids, such as salmon, tuna, and trout, in your weekly eating plan.
  - ✓ *Aim for at least 2 servings of fish, preferably fatty fish,* <u>each week</u>.

- **POULTRY AND MEATS:** Choose lean poultry and cuts of meats, such as skinless chicken breasts and sirloin, round steak, and flank steak.
  - ✓ *Aim for no more than 6 ounces of cooked (8 ounces raw) lean poultry and meats* <u>each day</u>.

- **LEGUMES, NUTS, AND SEEDS:** It's a good idea to include vegetarian entrées for at least two of your weekly meals. Use choices such as kidney beans, chickpeas, edamame (green soybeans), and lentils for fiber-rich protein. Round out your planning with unsalted nuts and seeds, such as almonds, walnuts, and pumpkin seeds. Because nuts and seeds are high in calories, remember that one serving is about 1½ ounces.
  - ✓ *Aim for 3 to 4 servings* <u>each week</u>.

- **FATS AND OILS:** Choose healthy unsaturated oils, such as canola, corn, and olive. Avoid unhealthy fats, such as stick butter and margarine, shortening, and most commercial baked goods.
  - ✓ *Aim for up to 2 to 3 servings of healthy fats and oils* <u>each day</u>.

- **SUGARY BEVERAGES, SNACKS, AND SWEETS:** No more than half of your daily discretionary calories should come from added sugars. Also limit snack foods and other processed and packaged foods because they often are high in sodium, saturated fat, trans fat, and cholesterol, as well as added sugar.
  - ✓ *Aim to limit added sugars from beverages and foods to 100 calories (about 6 teaspoons or 25 grams)* <u>each day</u> *for women and 150 calories (about 9 teaspoons or 38 grams)* <u>each day</u> *for men.*

SMART SHOPPING TIPS

With your grocery list in hand, it's time to go shopping. Whenever possible, avoid going to the market on an empty stomach. When you are hungry, your food choices may be driven more by your hunger than by your list. To stay focused on the core nutrient-rich foods, begin by filling your cart with fresh produce, dairy products, fish, poultry, and meats, which usually are located around the perimeter of the store. Then visit the inner aisles—where the packaged and processed foods usually are stocked—to find what's left on your list, including whole-grain foods and canned or frozen vegetables and fruits. If possible, stay clear of the aisles that stock candy, snacks, sugary sodas, and baked goods.

When you are tempted to buy a product because it's on sale, ask yourself whether it is a healthy choice. If that food is going to add unnecessary calories, saturated fat, trans fat, cholesterol, or sodium to your table, it's not a bargain. On the other hand, it's okay to be flexible when that makes sense. For example, if strawberries are on your list but blueberries are on sale, the nutrition quality is close enough to justify the switch. If you find your store is out of the salmon you want, just substitute another fish (preferably another rich in omega-3 fatty acids) rather than forgoing your meal plan.

Here are some additional tips to keep in mind when you are in the grocery store.

Vegetables and Fruits

- Look for a variety of produce in every color: spinach, broccoli, asparagus, green beans, and dark lettuces, such as arugula, for green; blueberries and eggplant for blue/purple; tomatoes, red bell peppers, strawberries, and watermelon for red; carrots, sweet potatoes, apricots, and cantaloupe for orange; summer squash and wax beans for yellow. The deeper colored choices tend to be richer in nutrients.
- Try new flavors and textures by experimenting with vegetables you haven't eaten before, and try new preparation methods to find out what you like best.
- In addition to buying fresh produce, keep on hand frozen and no-salt-added canned veggies and fruits packed in water or light syrup. There is little nutritional difference as long as you avoid foods processed with sodium, sugar, or unhealthful fats.
- Bump up your intake of vegetables and fruits by using them in unexpected places: Add spinach to meat loaf, shredded zucchini to brownies, or diced apples to soup.

Dairy Products

- Buy fat-free or low-fat (1% or ½%) milk. If at first the taste of the fat-free milk doesn't appeal to you, try drinking 2% milk for a couple of weeks, then switch to 1% for a while. Transition to ½% if available, and finally to fat free. An alternative is to buy a carton of fat-free milk and one of whole milk, then use half of each with your bowl of cereal, for example. Gradually reduce the amount of whole milk until you've become used to the taste of the fat-free milk by itself.
- Buy fat-free and low-fat versions of cheeses, such as Cheddar, mozzarella, American, and Swiss.

- Limit creamy cheeses, such as brie and processed cheese spreads, to occasional use since they tend to be high in saturated fat.
- Select fat-free and low-fat versions of other dairy products, such as yogurt, sour cream, cream cheese, and half-and-half.
- Choose from the wide selection of fat-free and low-fat dairy desserts, such as frozen yogurt and ice cream.
- Buy fat-free nondairy coffee creamers and whipped toppings to replace products loaded with coconut, palm, or palm kernel oil. Read labels carefully and avoid the products that are high in saturated fat.

Fish and Shellfish

- Try experimenting with different types of fish rich in omega-3 fatty acids, such as salmon, tuna, halibut, and trout.
- Buy both fresh and frozen fish. Keeping individually wrapped fillets in the freezer makes it convenient to have fish any night of the week. (You can quickly defrost wrapped fillets in a bowl of cool water.)
- Pick up cans of water-packed, very low sodium tuna and cans or pouches of salmon to keep on hand in your pantry.
- Include shellfish if you like; they are excellent sources of protein and very low in saturated fat. Be mindful, however, that many are also high in cholesterol.
- If you are concerned about mercury exposure, keep in mind that the risks from mercury exposure in fish depend on the amount eaten and the levels of mercury in the individual fish itself. For most people, the benefits of eating fish far outweigh the risks. You can minimize risk by choosing varieties of fish that are lower in mercury, such as salmon, catfish, and canned light tuna. In particular, women who are pregnant, planning to become pregnant, or nursing—and young children—should avoid eating the kinds of fish known to have high levels of mercury, such as shark and swordfish.

Whole Grains and High-Fiber Foods

- Read ingredient lists on products carefully because front-of-package labeling can be confusing or even misleading. Look for breads, cereals, pastas, and flours that list whole grains, such as whole wheat, first in the ingredient list.
- Try the new whole-grain products that are appearing on store shelves. Many pastas are now made from whole-grain flour, multigrain flour, or a combination.

- Buy brown rice instead of white rice. White rice is a grain, but much of the nutritive value is removed along with the husk, bran, and germ.
- Add oats, barley, bulgur, millet, quinoa, and other grains to your cart. Try preparing them in fat-free, low-sodium broth for a side dish or as part of an entrée. These foods are high in fiber, relatively low in calories, and economical, too.

Poultry and Meats

- Purchase skinless white-meat poultry because it is lower in saturated fat than the dark meat. If you buy poultry with skin, such as a roasting chicken, discard the skin before eating the meat.
- Be sure the ground chicken or turkey you buy is lean and ground without the skin. (If you can't tell whether the skin was included in packaged ground poultry, ask your butcher to grind some skinless white meat for you.)
- Look for lean beef cuts, such as round, chuck, sirloin, or flank steak.
- Avoid cuts that are heavily marbled (streaks of fat throughout the meat). These cuts are higher in saturated fat.
- Choose extra-lean ground beef, which means 95 percent lean meat with only 5 percent fat.
- Choose pork tenderloin and loin chops and, less often, lower-sodium ham and Canadian bacon for alternatives to red meat.
- Look for the cold cuts that are lowest in sodium and fat. Always check the nutrition labels, because most cold cuts are quite high in sodium even if the fat content is low.
- Buy an unbasted turkey and baste it yourself with unsalted, fat-free broth rather than buying a prebasted turkey. Most prebasted birds are injected with liquids that contain extra sodium and saturated fat.

Legumes, Nuts, and Seeds

- Stock your pantry with beans, whether canned with no salt added or dried; they are rich in fiber and complex carbohydrates that provide energy. Beans are a great alternative to meat and poultry: One cup of beans can provide between 15 and 20 grams of protein.
- Add edamame (green soybeans) to your cart as a protein source and fiber boost in salads, entrées, and snacks.
- Buy nuts and seeds without added salt. Keep them on hand to add to salads and desserts, or snack on a small handful (about 1½ ounces).

Fats and Oils

- Be sure your pantry includes nonstick cooking sprays made with vegetable oil. Use them to replace butter or margarine when possible.
- Buy heart-healthy unsaturated oils such as canola, corn, olive, safflower, soybean, and sunflower.
- Avoid buying stick margarine, which contains saturated and trans fats. Instead buy fat-free spray margarine or light tub margarine.
- Look for fat-free or low-fat salad dressings that are also low in sodium, or shop for the ingredients to make your own salad dressings. (See the recipes on pages 136–139.)

Sugary Beverages, Snacks, and Sweets

- Limit sugary sodas and syrupy fruit drinks as well as beer, wine, and other alcoholic beverages. These beverages add empty calories with no nutritional value.
- Choose beverages that are low in added sugar and sodium, such as water, fat-free milk, and unsweetened fruit juices.
- Check labels carefully when shopping for packaged snacks. Look for products with no trans fat and the smallest amounts of saturated fat and sodium.
- Watch for high levels of sodium in some sports drinks and mineral waters.
- Limit your selections of commercially baked products, including muffins, biscuits, and rolls; they contain little fiber but large amounts of saturated and trans fats as well as sugar and sodium. Instead shop for the ingredients to make your own breads and desserts. (See the recipes on pages 516–639.)

NUTRITION LABELS AND FOOD ICONS

When you buy fresh produce and other unprocessed foods, you have total control over how much fat, salt, and extra calories you add. With packaged or prepared foods, however, the only way to be sure of what you're getting is to check the nutrition facts panel on each product. The United States Department of Agriculture (USDA) regulates the information on the panel to help you compare products and understand what you are buying. Other organizations use their own icon systems to help you make decisions, and some grocery stores have introduced on-shelf labeling programs. When you see an icon or wording that signals a health claim on the front of food packaging, consider the source of the information before you make your selections.

How to Read the Nutrition Facts Panel

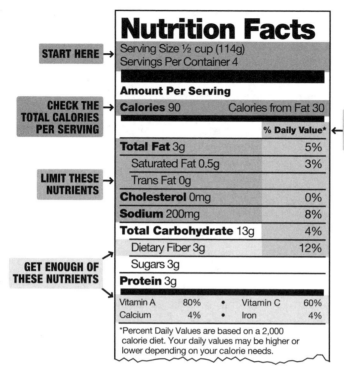

START HERE →

CHECK THE TOTAL CALORIES PER SERVING →

LIMIT THESE NUTRIENTS →

GET ENOUGH OF THESE NUTRIENTS

Nutrition Facts
Serving Size ½ cup (114g)
Servings Per Container 4

Amount Per Serving

Calories 90   Calories from Fat 30

                                    % Daily Value*

Total Fat 3g	5%
Saturated Fat 0.5g	3%
Trans Fat 0g	
Cholesterol 0mg	0%
Sodium 200mg	8%
Total Carbohydrate 13g	4%
Dietary Fiber 3g	12%
Sugars 3g	
Protein 3g	

Vitamin A	80%	Vitamin C	60%
Calcium	4%	Iron	4%

*Percent Daily Values are based on a 2,000 calorie diet. Your daily values may be higher or lower depending on your calorie needs.

Quick Guide to % DV:
5% or less is low
20% or more is high

Start at the serving size and decide how many servings you will really be consuming. If you intend to eat double the servings, you must also double the calories and nutrients. Consider how eating the food will affect your calorie balance, keeping in mind that for a 2,000-calorie diet, 40 calories per serving is considered low, 100 calories per serving is considered moderate, and 400 calories or more per serving is considered high.

The % Daily Value column tells you the percentage of each nutrient in a single serving, in terms of the daily recommended amount. As a guide, if you want to consume less of a nutrient, such as saturated fat, cholesterol, or sodium, choose foods with a lower % Daily Value (5% or less is considered low). If you want to consume more of a nutrient, such as fiber, look for foods with a higher % Daily Value (20% or more is considered high).

Be Savvy About Sodium

A few foods are naturally high in sodium, but for the most part, it is the processing that accounts for the excess sodium in commercially prepared foods. It pays to compare labels for similar products from different manufacturers, especially for sodium, because levels can vary widely. Watch for the "hidden" sodium in the common foods listed below, and look for salt-free or low-sodium versions.

- Processed or cured meats, such as bacon, bologna, hot dogs, ham, canned meat, pastrami, pepperoni, salami, and sausage
- Brined products, such as anchovies, capers, olives, and pickles
- Condiments such as barbecue sauce, ketchup, mustard, soy sauce, steak sauce, chili sauce, chutneys, pickles, relishes, and Worcestershire sauce
- Salad dressings
- Canned soups and bouillon cubes or granules
- Breads and bread products
- Cheeses
- Crackers and chips
- Frozen entrées, including pizza, and frozen vegetables with sauces
- Canned vegetables
- Salted nuts

Get to Know the Bad Fats and the Better Fats

Most foods contain a combination of fats in varying amounts. Not all fats are bad; in fact, the "better" fats, polyunsaturated and monounsaturated, provide essential nutrients and can benefit your health when eaten in moderation, especially when used to replace the "bad" fats, saturated fat and trans fat, that increase the risk for heart disease. (See Appendix A for more information on diet and heart health.) Once you know what to look for, you'll find lots of heart-healthy options when shopping for groceries.

Foods High in Bad Fats

Eating a diet high in saturated fat, trans fat, and dietary cholesterol raises LDL cholesterol, increasing your risk of heart disease. In the typical American diet, the main sources of saturated fat and cholesterol are foods from animal sources. Trans fat comes primarily from commercial foods that use hydrogenated oil, such as fried foods and baked goods. (Very small amounts of natural trans fatty acids are also found in meats and dairy products.) Although many foods that originally contained trans fat have been reformulated to reduce or eliminate it, reading labels is still a good idea. When buying a processed food, check to see what type of fat has been used. Even if a product is trans-free, remember to look at the saturated fat content, which continues to pose a real health threat. A rule of thumb is that if a fat tends to stay solid at room temperature, it is probably a saturated fat. Watch for these "bad" fats, especially if you see any of them listed as the first item in the ingredient list.

Limit your use of:

- Animal fats (lard, bacon grease, pan drippings with fat, for example)
- Full-fat dairy products (butter, cheeses, cream, for example)
- Tropical oils (coconut, palm, and palm kernel oils, for example)
- Stick margarines and products containing partially hydrogenated oil

Foods High in Better Fats

Including unsaturated fats in your diet can help protect your heart by lowering LDL and increasing HDL cholesterol. Unsaturated oils, such as canola, corn, olive, sunflower, and sesame oils, stay liquid at room temperature and are low in saturated fat and high in polyunsaturated and monounsaturated fats. Other foods that are high in unsaturated fat include most nuts and seeds, peanuts and peanut butter, and avocados.

Watch for Added Sugars

Avoid beverages and foods with added sugars, especially those with sugars listed in the first four ingredients. When reading labels, you may be surprised at how many foods are processed with added sugars. Some commonly added sugars are sucrose, dextrose, and fructose, including the high-fructose corn syrup used most often by the beverage industry. Although many people believe that high-fructose corn syrup is pure fructose, it actually contains either 42 or 55 percent fructose and is similar in composition to table sugar (sucrose). Soft drinks and other sugar-sweetened beverages are the primary source of added sugars in most Americans' diets.

AMERICAN HEART ASSOCIATION FOOD CERTIFICATION PROGRAM

Low in Saturated Fat
& Cholesterol
_____

CERTIFIED by
American Heart Association
heartcheckmark.org

The American Heart Association's heart-check mark helps you quickly and reliably find heart-healthy foods in the grocery store. When you see the heart-check mark on food packaging, you can have confidence knowing that the food has been certified by the association to meet our criteria for saturated fat and cholesterol. To learn more about how you can use the heart-check mark when you shop for groceries, visit www.heartcheckmark.org.

It can be a challenge to break lifelong habits, especially if you're not used to shopping with good health as your focus. You may not switch from buying unhealthy foods to heart-healthy foods overnight, but you *can* earn big health dividends by gradually making small changes each week. With each change in your buying habits, you and your family will move a step closer to eating better. Remember that heart-healthy grocery shopping is a good first step to heart-healthy eating—and cooking!

APPENDIX C
cooking for a healthy heart

Some cooking methods, such as deep-fat frying, are guaranteed to add calories and unhealthy fat to any food. Fortunately, many more methods help retain vitamins and minerals and create dishes that are good to eat and good for your heart.

COOKING TECHNIQUES

To keep calories and saturated fat to a minimum, avoid any cooking method that adds fat or allows food to cook in its own fat. Instead, use these tried-and-true techniques that enhance flavor and preserve nutrients.

Braising or Stewing

Braising (for pot roast, for example) and stewing (for stew and chili, for example) are great slow-cooking methods that tenderize tougher cuts of meat. Braising is also excellent for cooking root vegetables, and stewing is a good way to prepare some fresh fruits, such as apples, cherries, and plums. To braise, brown the food well on all sides in a pan sprayed with cooking spray or coated with a small amount of oil. Pour off any fat, add a small amount of liquid and whatever seasonings you wish, cover tightly, and simmer. For stewing, follow the same directions, but add enough liquid to cover the food. Because fat cooks out of meat and poultry into the liquid during the cooking process, it's a good idea to cook these dishes a day ahead, then refrigerate. The chilled fat will harden and rise to the surface, making it easy to remove before you reheat the food. The chilling step also lets the flavors of most braised and stewed dishes blend and intensify.

Grilling or Broiling

Similar in result, both grilling (cooking over direct heat) and broiling (cooking under direct heat) allow fat from meat and poultry to drip away as it cooks, producing a crisp browned exterior and a tender interior. Food that can be cooked relatively quickly using high heat is best. Steaks, seafood, poultry, and vegetables are ideal. For extra flavor and to keep food moist, marinate these foods and baste during cooking. (Remember to use food safety precautions, such as boiling the marinade before using it for basting and cleaning brushes after each basting to prevent transferring bacteria from raw food.) Trim and discard all visible fat from meats and poultry before grilling or broiling; you will cut down on saturated fat and help prevent the flare-ups that dripping fat can cause. When broiling, pay attention to the distance between the food and the heat source. If a recipe says to broil about 5 inches from the heat, that means about 5 inches between the heat element and the top of the food, not the top of the broiler pan.

Microwave Cooking

Microwaving is fast and easy, and it retains so much moisture that no added fats or oils are needed. Also, the nutrients are not drained away with the cooking liquid, as they may be with boiling. Microwaving is especially good for preparing fish, poultry, soups, vegetables, fruits, and other foods that cook well in moist heat. Many conventional recipes can be adapted for the microwave. Try to find a similar microwave recipe to use as a guide. In general, you will need to cut the microwave cooking time to one-fourth to one-third of the conventional time. If the food isn't cooked enough at that point, continue cooking it for short periods until it reaches the desired doneness. Remember that you will need to reduce the liquid used by one-third and to cut foods into equal sizes and shapes for more even cooking. Refer to your manufacturer's instructions for more guidance.

Poaching

For this method, food is immersed in a pan of almost-simmering seasoned liquid and cooked. Poaching works particularly well with chicken and seafood. Some of the liquids commonly used are water, wine, and fat-free, low-sodium broth. Once the food is cooked and removed from the pan, you can reduce the liquid (decrease the volume by boiling the liquid rapidly) to intensify the flavor. The reduction can be used as is or thickened into a sauce.

Slow Cooking

Cooking food in a slow cooker takes several hours, but because you simply fill and cover the cooker, then turn it on, this method requires very little of your time. (You may want to brown meats first to add color and deepen flavor.) When you use a slow cooker, don't fill it more than one-half to two-thirds full. Since slow cookers work by keeping heat and moisture in, don't lift the lid for a status check or to stir the ingredients unless a recipe tells you to do so. Be sure to layer ingredients according to the recipe, because foods placed at the bottom of the cooker will cook faster than those at the top. Once your meat and vegetables are cooked and you've removed them from the slow cooker, you can thicken the remaining liquid into a delicious sauce by reducing it in the cooker, uncovered, on high or in a saucepan.

Steaming

Any food that can be boiled or simmered, such as vegetables, seafood, and chicken, can be steamed. Cooking food in a steamer basket over a small amount of liquid, such as water or broth, in a tightly covered saucepan or skillet keeps in natural flavor, color, and vitamins and minerals. You can also add herbs or spices to the liquid for extra flavor. Just be sure the water doesn't touch the food as it steams.

Stir-Frying

Stir-frying, or constantly stirring food as it cooks in a small amount of hot oil over high heat, results in delicious dishes combining a variety of flavors and textures. The quick cooking preserves the color, flavor, and crispness of vegetables and seals in the natural juices of meats and seafood. The constant stirring keeps the food from sticking and burning. The sloping sides of a wok are designed especially for stir-frying, but you can also use a large skillet. Everything moves quickly once you start cooking, so the key to success is to dice or slice each food into small, preferably uniform, pieces and prepare sauces before you begin stir-frying. Because the hottest area is at the base of the wok, quickly cook ingredients in sequence there, pushing cooked ingredients up on the side of the wok while you cook the next ones.

Roasting or Baking

These slow, dry-heat methods of oven cooking are similar but not quite the same. Both use dry heat, but foods such as meat and poultry are usually roasted uncovered and at higher temperatures. Roasting works very well with vegetables, too. Baking breads, casseroles, and desserts is typically done at lower heat, and the food may be either covered or uncovered. If you're preparing a roast, discard any visible fat. Season the meat and place it on a rack in a roasting pan to keep the meat from sitting in any fat drippings. Roast uncovered to the desired doneness in a preheated oven. If basting is needed, use water, wine, fruit juice, or fat-free, low-sodium broth. (When roasting poultry, leave the skin on during cooking but discard it before serving.)

Remove a roast from the oven 15 to 20 minutes before serving to let it "rest." Use an instant-read or meat thermometer to test for doneness. (Remove food from the oven to use an instant-read thermometer, which measures temperature right away. A meat thermometer stays in the food during cooking, indicating temperature as it rises.) Insert the thermometer at the thickest part of the meat, being sure that it does not rest in fat or on bone. When the thermometer shows the desired internal temperature, push it a little deeper into the meat. If the temperature drops, continue cooking until the thermometer reaches the correct temperature. If it stays the same, the meat is done. To test doneness in most baked goods, insert a wooden toothpick in the center. If it comes out clean, the cake or bread is done.

COOKING TIPS

In addition to the basics of heart-healthy cooking, our developers use certain "tricks of the trade" to keep our recipes low in saturated fat, cholesterol, and sodium while maintaining flavor. We've compiled some useful tips you can apply in your own kitchen.

- Use nonstick cookware when possible—cleanup will be easier and you usually won't need as much fat for cooking as with regular pans.
- When using cooking spray, be careful not to spray it near an open flame. If you use nonstick cookware, check your warranty information to see whether the manufacturer advises against the use of cooking spray with its products.
- As a rule of thumb, cook fish for about 10 minutes per inch of thickness. Add 5 minutes to the total time if the fish is wrapped in foil. Frozen fish requires about 20 minutes per inch of thickness, plus 10 minutes if it's wrapped in foil. Fish is done when the flesh flakes easily when tested with a fork.
- Except when roasting, either use skinless chicken parts or skin the chicken before cooking, and remove all visible fat below the skin. Use paper towels or a clean cloth to take better hold of the skin. Be sure to scrub the cutting surface and utensils well with hot, sudsy water after preparing raw poultry. Leave the skin on for roasting to keep in moisture, then discard it before serving the poultry.
- Discard all visible fat before cooking meat.
- While meat is cooking, a rich essence drips into the roasting or broiler pan along with the fat. To keep the essence without the fat, pour the contents of the pan—fat and all—into a cup or dish, cover it, and put it in the refrigerator. The next day you can easily remove the hardened fat, leaving only the flavorful juice. Use the defatted liquid to add zest to foods ranging from soups and sauces to hash, meat pies, and meat loaf.
- Cut down on saturated fat by using more vegetables and less poultry or meat in soups, stews, and casseroles. Finely chopped vegetables are great for stretching ground poultry or ground meat, too.

- Cooking with wines and spirits adds depth to the taste of food. During cooking, most alcohol evaporates, leaving the flavor and tenderizing qualities. The wines you use for cooking don't have to be expensive, but they should be good enough to drink. Avoid using cooking wines, which contain high levels of sodium.
- Seal natural juices in foods by wrapping the foods in aluminum foil or parchment before cooking. Or try wrapping foods in edible pouches made of steamed lettuce or cabbage leaves.
- Cook vegetables just until tender-crisp. Overcooked vegetables lose flavor, texture, and important nutrients.
- Keep whole-grain flour in the refrigerator for freshness.

FLAVOR TIPS

A creative cook can make food exciting, imaginative, and crowd-pleasing—without adding salt or fat—by experimenting with seasonings. Try these ideas to spice up your dishes for everyday meals as well as special occasions.

- Use fresh herbs whenever possible.
- Use gingerroot and fresh horseradish for extra flavor. Grate peeled gingerroot with a ginger grater or a flat, sheet-type grater. Use a food processor to grate peeled fresh horseradish.
- Use flavorful citrus zest, the colored part of the peel without the bitter white pith. Grate the zest or use a rasp zester, regular zester, or vegetable peeler.
- Use vinegar or citrus juice as a wonderful flavor enhancer. Try vinegar on vegetables such as greens. Wine vinegars and herb vinegars are excellent substitutes for high-calorie dressings on salads. Citrus juice works well on fruits such as melons and in place of dressing on salads. Either vinegar or citrus juice is great with fish.
- Dry-roast seeds, nuts, and whole or ground spices to bring out their full flavor. Cook them in a dry skillet or bake them on a baking sheet.
- Roast vegetables in a hot oven to caramelize their natural sugars and bring out their full flavor.
- Use dry mustard for a zesty flavor in cooking, or mix it with water to make a very sharp condiment.
- Add fresh or dried hot peppers for a little more "bite" in your dishes. To reduce the heat somewhat, don't use the membrane or the seeds. Remember: A small amount goes a long way. Wear

disposable gloves while handling the peppers or wash your hands thoroughly afterward. Skin, especially around the eyes, is very sensitive to the oil from hot peppers.

- Some vegetables and fruits, such as mushrooms, tomatoes, chile peppers, cherries, cranberries, and currants, have a more intense flavor when dried than when fresh. Use them when you want a burst of flavor. As a bonus, keep the flavored water they soaked in and use it for cooking.

QUICK AND EASY COOKING

Sometimes the last thing you want to do on a busy day is cook. Here are some ideas for dealing with this dilemma without resorting to fast foods loaded with saturated and trans fats, sodium, and calories.

- Try cooking in quantity and freezing the extra amount. Instead of one casserole, make two. Enjoy one right away and freeze the other to enjoy later. Let the second one thaw overnight in the refrigerator or use the defrost setting on your microwave to thaw more quickly, then reheat it. Other foods that lend themselves to quantity cooking and freezing include soups, spaghetti sauce, meat and poultry dishes, and breads. Preparing a roast beef, chicken, or turkey is another way to provide several family meals, including sandwiches on whole-grain bread.
- Doing a little advance preparation can cut kitchen time way down. For example, make brown rice in large quantities. Serve it first as a side dish, then use the extra with stir-fried vegetables and meats during the week, or freeze individual portions in plastic freezer bags. When preparing salad, rinse and store extra salad greens in a plastic container with a tight-fitting lid—they'll stay fresh and crisp for about a week.
- Organize your kitchen. Arrange foods, utensils, and equipment so you can cook quickly and efficiently.
- Make sure your pantry, refrigerator, and freezer are stocked with easy-to-fix foods, such as no-salt-added canned and frozen vegetables, lean ground beef, fish fillets, and chicken breasts.
- Keep a running shopping list so you can jot down items you need to replenish. You'll be less likely to have to make an emergency trip to the supermarket so you can prepare dinner.
- Review the recipe ingredients and preparation steps and assemble the needed equipment and ingredients *before you begin cooking*. Remembering this simple hint is the best way to be sure you have everything you need for preparing the dish.

- If you're making a complex dish, prepare simple foods to go with it. For example, if your entrée needs a lot of attention, fix a simple salad or pop a frozen vegetable in the microwave. If your entrée is simple, create an interesting side dish.
- Cook vegetables in the microwave to save time, retain nutrients, and maximize flavor (see page 653 for details). Microwaving is also great for heating leftover vegetables.
- Try microwave or quick stovetop versions of dishes you usually cook in the oven.
- Use other labor-saving devices, such as a food processor, convection oven, pressure cooker, or slow cooker.
- Cut down on food-transfer and cleanup time by using cookware in which food can be cooked, served, and stored.

PLANNED-OVERS

When you prepare a dinner entrée, it's often just as easy to make extra for another meal. The pairings that follow take that idea one more step: They use the "leftovers" in specific recipes designed around them, thus the name "planned-overs." When the week gets hectic, you'll really be glad you planned ahead.

- Baked Potato Soup (page 80)—Mexican Potato Skins (page 22)
- Country-Time Baked Chicken (page 215)—Six-Layer Salad with Chicken (page 122)
- Mexican Chicken and Vegetables with Chipotle Peppers (page 216)—Chipotle Chicken Wraps (page 261)
- Sweet-Spice Glazed Chicken (page 239)—Island Chicken Salad with Fresh Mint (page 126)
- Maple-Glazed Chicken (page 240)—Sesame Chicken and Vegetable Stir-Fry (page 247)
- Triple-Pepper Chicken (page 242)—Cajun Chicken Salad (page 124)
- Grilled Lemongrass Flank Steak (page 296)—Grilled Flank Steak Salad with Sweet-and-Sour Sesame Dressing (page 127)

PLAN-AHEADS

If you want to get a jump start on your next meal, consider trying a recipe that calls for marinating or slow cooking so you can do most of the preparation ahead of time. Then, when it's time to eat later on, you'll be ready in a flash. Try these suggestions:

SLOW COOKING

Turkey and Rice Soup (page 73)

Slow-Cooker Cioppino (page 203)

Slow-Cooker Dilled Chicken with Rice, Green Beans, and Carrots (page 225)

Slow-Cooker Thyme-Garlic Chicken with Couscous (page 227)

Slow-Cooker White Chili (page 260)

Brisket Stew, Slow and Easy (page 287)

Shredded Beef Soft Tacos (page 293)

Slow-Cooker Round Steak with Mushrooms and Tomatoes (page 310)

Slow-Cooker Chili (page 320)

Slow-Cooker Pork Roast with Orange-Cranberry Sauce (page 337)

Harvest Pork Stew (page 338)

Slow-Cooker Chile Verde Pork Chops (page 341)

Slow-Cooker Chickpea Stew (page 379)

Slow-Cooker Pumpkin Oatmeal (page 548)

MARINATING

Skewered Chicken Strips with Soy-Peanut Marinade (30 minutes to 8 hours; page 27)

Dijon-Marinated Vegetable Medley (4 to 8 hours; page 98)

Caribbean Grilled Chicken Breasts (2 to 12 hours; page 209)

Chicken with One-Minute Tomato Sauce (8 hours; page 232)

Grilled Lemon-Sage Chicken (30 minutes to 8 hours; page 238)

Maple-Glazed Chicken (1 to 12 hours; page 240)

Triple-Pepper Chicken (30 minutes to 4 hours; page 242)

Tandoori Ginger Chicken Strips (4 to 8 hours; page 255)

Turkey Fillets with Fresh Herbs (1 to 12 hours; page 272)

Zesty Hot-Oven Sirloin (8 hours; page 288)

Ginger-Lime Sirloin (8 hours; page 289)

Steak Marinated in Beer and Green Onions (1 to 24 hours; page 291)

Grilled Lemongrass Flank Steak (2 to 12 hours; page 296)

Steak and Vegetable Kebabs (8 hours; page 304)

Yogurt-Marinated Grilled Round Steak (8 hours; page 308)

Philadelphia-Style Cheese Steak Wrap (10 minutes to 8 hours; page 313)

Marinated Pork Tenderloin (8 hours; page 333)

Basil Roasted Peppers (30 minutes to 8 hours; page 460)

menu planning for holidays and special occasions

F ood is an important part of most holidays and celebrations through-out the year. Unfortunately, many of the foods served for these occasions are high in saturated and trans fats, calories, and sodium. The good news is that, with the recipes in this cookbook, you can enjoy both eating well and eating healthy, even during celebratory times.

We've developed the following menus to help you get started with planning holiday and special-occasion meals. Feel free to mix and match these menus to create the healthy meals that will best suit your family's tastes.

WINTER HOLIDAY MENUS

christmas dinner

APPETIZER Roasted-Pepper Hummus *14*

SIDE SOUP Winter Squash Soup *56*

ENTRÉE Stuffed Cornish Hens with Orange-Brandy Sauce *280*

SIDE DISH Apple Dressing *486*

SIDE DISH French Peas *457*

DESSERT Blueberry-Almond Bundt Cake *571*

BEVERAGE Peppermint Coffee Chiller *38*

hanukkah dinner

ENTRÉE Brisket Stew, Slow and Easy *287*

SIDE DISH Rustic Potato Patties *464*

SIDE DISH French-Style Green Beans with Pimiento and Dill Seeds *421*

DESSERT Baked Ginger Pears *623*

kwanzaa dinner

ENTRÉE Shrimp and Okra Étouffée *198*

SIDE DISH Sautéed Red Swiss Chard *481*

BREAD Sweet Potato Bread *528*

DESSERT Deep-Dish Fruit Crisp *593*

new year's eve dinner party

APPETIZER Torta with Chèvre and Sun-Dried Tomatoes *15*

ENTRÉE Fillet of Beef with Herbes de Provence *284*

SIDE DISH Risotto with Broccoli and Leeks *470*

DESSERT Strawberries with Champagne Ice *630*

BEVERAGE Sparkling Cranberry Cooler *37*

new year's day brunch

ENTRÉE Farmstand Frittata *408*

SIDE DISH Black-Eyed Peas with Canadian Bacon *456*

BREAKFAST DISH Banana-Raisin Coffee Cake with Citrus Glaze *536*

BEVERAGE Sparkling Orange Juice Cooler *37*

super bowl party

APPETIZER Mexican Potato Skins *22*

ENTRÉE Slow-Cooker Chili *320*

BREAD Jalapeño Cheese Bread *524*

DESSERT Fudgy Buttermilk Brownies *603*

chinese new year dinner

APPETIZER Sweet-and-Sour Spring Rolls *19*

ENTRÉE Classic Chinese Beef Stir-Fry *301*

SIDE DISH Stir-Fried Bok Choy with Green Onion Sauce *428*

SIDE DISH Instant Brown Rice*

DESSERT Claret-Spiced Oranges *622*

valentine's day dinner

APPETIZER Fire-and-Ice Cream Cheese Spread *13*

SOUP Creamy Basil-Tomato Soup *61*

ENTRÉE Rosé Chicken with Artichoke Hearts and Mushrooms *234*

SIDE DISH Whole-Wheat Penne*

DESSERT Cannoli Cream with Strawberries and Chocolate *608*

SPRING HOLIDAY MENUS

st. patrick's day dinner

APPETIZER Spinach Dip *7*

ENTRÉE Shepherd's Pie *326*

SIDE DISH Cabbage with Mustard-Caraway Sauce *435*

DESSERT Bourbon Balls *602*

easter dinner

ENTRÉE Herb-Rubbed Pork Tenderloin with Dijon-Apricot Mop Sauce *334*

SIDE SOUP Creamy Asparagus Soup *47*

SIDE DISH Baked Grated Carrots with Sherry *439*

SIDE DISH Lemon-Basil Rice *468*

DESSERT Carrot Cake *575*

cinco de mayo fiesta

APPETIZER Jalapeño Poppers *20*

ENTRÉE Chile-Chicken Tortilla Soup *72*

SIDE SALAD Spinach-Chayote Salad with Orange Vinaigrette *90*

SIDE DISH Instant Brown Rice*

DESSERT Tequila-Lime Sherbet *636*

mother's day breakfast

BEVERAGE Berry Good Smoothie *36*

BREAKFAST DISH Peachy Stuffed French Toast *557*

SIDE DISH Soy Breakfast Patties*

SUMMER HOLIDAY MENUS

memorial day barbeque

ENTRÉE Grilled Salmon with Cilantro Sauce *164*

SIDE SALAD Cucumber and Mango Salad with Lime Dressing *102*

SIDE DISH Mediterranean Veggie Couscous Salad *109*

DESSERT Cherry-Berry Chill *633*

father's day dinner

ENTRÉE Grilled Stuffed Flank Steak *294*

SIDE SALAD Ginger-Infused Watermelon and Mixed Berries *104*

SIDE DISH Grilled Corn on the Cob *444*

DESSERT Frozen Mini Key Lime Soufflés *629*

fourth of july barbeque

ENTRÉE Grilled Hamburgers with Vegetables and Feta *315*

SIDE SALAD Confetti Coleslaw *100*

SIDE DISH Baked Beans *424*

BEVERAGE Summer Slush *34*

labor day barbeque

ENTRÉE Caribbean Grilled Chicken Breasts *209*

SIDE SALAD Sixteen-Bean Salad *113*

SIDE DISH Grilled Asparagus*

SIDE DISH (OR DESSERT) Grilled Pineapple *491*

*Recipe not included.

kids' halloween party

APPETIZER Ranch Dip *9*

ENTRÉE Tex-Mex Lasagna *319*

SIDE SALAD Tex-Mex Cucumber Salad *91*

DESSERT Pumpkin Spice Cupcakes with Cinnamon-Sugar Topping *579*

thanksgiving feast

SIDE SALAD Wild Rice Salad with Cranberry Vinaigrette *111*

ENTRÉE Cider-Glazed Turkey Tenderloin with Harvest Vegetables *268*

SIDE DISH Cranberry Chutney *487*

SIDE DISH Mashed Potatoes with Parmesan and Green Onions *462*

GRAVY Basic Gravy *494*

DESSERT Pumpkin Cheesecake *585*

equivalents and substitutions

INGREDIENT EQUIVALENTS

Ingredient	Measurement
ALMONDS	1 ounce = ¼ cup slivers
APPLE	1 medium = ¾ to 1 cup chopped; 1 cup sliced
BASIL LEAVES, FRESH	⅔ ounce = ½ cup, chopped
BELL PEPPER, ANY COLOR	1 medium = 1 cup chopped or sliced
CARROT	1 medium = ⅓ to ½ cup chopped or sliced; ½ cup shredded
CELERY	1 medium rib = ½ cup chopped or sliced
CHEESE, HARD, SUCH AS PARMESAN	3½ ounces = 1 cup shredded 4 ounces = 1 cup grated
CHEESE, SEMIHARD, SUCH AS CHEDDAR, MOZZARELLA, OR SWISS	4 ounces = 1 cup grated
CHEESE, SOFT, SUCH AS BLUE, FETA, OR GOAT	1 ounce crumbled = ¼ cup
CUCUMBER	1 medium = 1 cup sliced
LEMON JUICE	1 medium = 2 to 3 tablespoons
LEMON ZEST	1 medium = 2 to 3 teaspoons
LIME JUICE	1 medium = 1½ to 2 tablespoons
LIME ZEST	1 medium = 1 teaspoon
MUSHROOMS (BUTTON)	1 pound = 5 to 6 cups sliced or chopped
ONIONS, GREEN	8 to 9 medium = 1 cup sliced (green and white parts)
ONIONS, WHITE OR YELLOW	1 large = 1 cup chopped 1 medium = ½ to ⅔ cup chopped 1 small = ⅓ cup chopped
ORANGE JUICE	1 medium = ⅓ to ½ cup
ORANGE ZEST	1 medium = 1½ to 2 tablespoons

STRAWBERRIES	1 pint = 2 cups sliced or chopped
TOMATOES	2 large, 3 medium, or 4 small = 1½ to 2 cups chopped
WALNUTS	1 ounce = ¼ cup chopped

EMERGENCY SUBSTITUTIONS

When you see a recipe you'd like to prepare but don't have certain ingredients on hand, or you begin a recipe only to find you're out of something, try these in-a-pinch substitutions.

If your recipe calls for	Use
ALLSPICE, 1 teaspoon	½ teaspoon ground cinnamon + 1 teaspoon ground cloves
BAKING POWDER, 1 teaspoon	¼ teaspoon baking soda + ¾ teaspoon cream of tartar
BROWN SUGAR, 1 cup	1 cup granulated sugar + 2 tablespoons molasses
BUTTERMILK, 1 cup	1 tablespoon vinegar or lemon juice + enough fat-free milk to equal 1 cup; or 1 cup fat-free plain yogurt
CAKE FLOUR, 1 cup sifted	1 cup minus 2 tablespoons sifted all-purpose flour
CONFECTIONERS' SUGAR, 1 cup	½ cup + 1 tablespoon granulated sugar
CORNSTARCH, 1 tablespoon	2 tablespoons all-purpose flour
CRACKER CRUMBS, ¾ cup	¾ to 1 cup dry bread crumbs
FLOUR FOR THICKENING, 2 tablespoons all-purpose	1 tablespoon cornstarch
FLOUR, WHOLE-WHEAT, 1 cup (for baking)	⅞ cup all-purpose flour
FRESH HERBS, 1 tablespoon	1 teaspoon dried herbs
GINGERROOT, peeled and grated, 1 tablespoon	⅛ teaspoon ground ginger
HONEY, 1 tablespoon	4 teaspoons granulated sugar + 1½ teaspoons water
LEMON JUICE, 1 teaspoon	½ teaspoon vinegar
LEMON ZEST, 1 teaspoon	½ teaspoon lemon extract

LEMONGRASS	Grated lemon zest moistened with lemon juice
MUSTARD, dry, 1 teaspoon	1 tablespoon yellow mustard
ONION, 1 small	1 teaspoon onion powder or 1 tablespoon minced dried onion
RICOTTA CHEESE, ½ cup fat-free	½ cup fat-free cottage cheese
SHERRY, 2 tablespoons	1 to 2 teaspoons vanilla extract
SOUR CREAM, 1 cup fat-free	1 cup fat-free plain yogurt
TOMATO JUICE, 1 cup	½ cup tomato sauce + ½ cup water
TOMATO SAUCE, 2 cups	¾ cup tomato paste + 1 cup water
WINE, red, ½ cup	½ cup fat-free, no-salt-added beef broth
WINE, white, ½ cup	½ cup fat-free, low-sodium chicken broth
YEAST, active dry, 1¼-ounce package	2½ teaspoons active dry or ⅔ ounce cake yeast, crumbled

ADAPTING EXISTING RECIPES

You don't need to throw away old family recipes just because you want to eat healthy. By making a few simple ingredient substitutions, you can rework almost any recipe to be high in flavor and lower in calories, saturated fat, trans fat, cholesterol, and sodium.

If your recipe calls for	Use
REGULAR BROTH OR BOUILLON	Fat-free, low-sodium broths, either homemade or commercially prepared; salt-free or low-sodium bouillon granules or cubes, reconstituted according to package directions
BUTTER OR SHORTENING	When possible, use fat-free spray margarine or light tub margarine. However, if the type of fat is critical to the recipe, especially in baked goods, you may need to use stick margarine. Choose the product that is lowest in saturated and trans fats.
BUTTER FOR SAUTÉING	Vegetable oil, such as canola, corn, or olive; cooking spray; fat-free, low-sodium broth; wine; fruit or vegetable juice
CREAM	Fat-free half-and-half; fat-free nondairy creamer; fat-free evaporated milk

EGGS	Cholesterol-free egg substitutes; 2 egg whites for 1 whole egg
EVAPORATED MILK	Fat-free evaporated milk
FLAVORED SALTS, SUCH AS ONION SALT, GARLIC SALT, AND CELERY SALT	Onion powder, garlic powder, celery seeds or flakes; or about one-fourth the amount of flavored salt indicated in the recipe
ICE CREAM	Fat-free, low-fat, or light ice cream; fat-free or low-fat frozen yogurt; sorbet; sherbet; gelato
TABLE SALT	No-salt-added seasoning blends
TOMATO JUICE	No-salt-added tomato juice
TOMATO SAUCE	No-salt-added tomato sauce; 6-ounce can of no-salt-added tomato paste diluted with 1 can of water
UNSWEETENED BAKING CHOCOLATE	3 tablespoons cocoa powder plus 1 tablespoon unsaturated oil or light tub margarine for every 1-ounce square of chocolate
WHIPPING CREAM FOR TOPPING	Fat-free whipped topping; fat-free evaporated milk (thoroughly chilled before whipping)
WHOLE MILK	Fat-free milk

INDEX

g

j

Jalapeño Cheese Bread, 524
Jalapeño Poppers, 20
Jambalaya, Chicken, 220
jícama
    Carrot Salad with Jícama and Pineapple, 101
    cook's tip on, 101
    Fish Tacos with Pico de Gallo, 153
Jollof Rice, 345
Jubilee Sauce, Easy, 512

k

Kale Crisps, 449
Key Lime Soufflés, Frozen Mini, 629
kiwifruit
    Angel Food Layers with Chocolate Custard and Kiwifruit, 570
    Asian-Style Barbecue Pork, 342
    cook's tip on, 137
    Fruit Salsa, 12
    Island Chicken Salad with Fresh Mint, 126
    Kiwifruit Sundaes, 638
    Poppy Seed Dressing with Kiwifruit, 137
    Spinach Salad with Kiwifruit and Raspberries, 88
    Sweet and Fruity Salsa Bowl, 620

l

lasagna
    Meatless Lasagna with Zucchini and Red Wine, 402–3
    Tex-Mex Lasagna, 319
    Turkey Lasagna, 274
Layered Taco Salad with Tortilla Chips, 128
leeks
    Parmesan Parsnip Puree with Leeks and Carrots, 453
    Risotto with Broccoli and Leeks, 470
legumes
    adding to diet, xiii
    Cumin and Ginger Lentils on Quinoa, 389
    Lentil Chili Soup, 77
    Mediterranean Lentils and Rice, 377
    shopping guidelines, 643, 646
    Split Pea Soup, 79
    see also beans
Lemongrass Flank Steak, Grilled, 296
lemons
    Asparagus with Lemon and Capers, 415
    Chicken Scallops al Limone, 228
    cook's tips on, 458, 504
    Crumb-Crusted Mushrooms with Lemon, 18
    Delicate Lemon Ricotta Cheesecake with Blackberries, 584
    Dilled Orange Roughy with Lemon-Caper Sauce, 158
    Fish Fillets with Lemon and Spinach, 171
    Greek Egg and Lemon Soup, 45
    Grilled Lemon-Sage Chicken, 238
    Lemon-Basil Chicken with Mushrooms, 212–13
    Lemon-Basil Rice, 468
    Lemon-Cayenne Chicken, 243
    Lemon Dressing, 139
    Lemon-Flavored Seven-Minute Frosting, 581
    Lemon or Orange Confectioners' Glaze, 582
    Sweet Lemon Snow Peas, 458
    Thai-Style Lemon and Spinach Soup, 55
lentils
    Cumin and Ginger Lentils on Quinoa, 389
    Lentil Chili Soup, 77
    Mediterranean Lentils and Rice, 377
limes
    Cauliflower and Roasted Corn with Chili Powder and Lime, 441
    Creamy Dijon-Lime Sauce, 499
    Cucumber and Mango Salad with Lime Dressing, 102
    Frozen Mini Key Lime Soufflés, 629
    Ginger-Lime Sirloin, 289
    Grilled Pineapple-Lime Salmon, 163
    Minted Cantaloupe Soup with Fresh Lime, 65
    Oven-Fried Scallops with Cilantro and Lime, 197
    Tequila-Lime Sherbet, 636
    Tomatillo-Cilantro Salsa with Lime, 509
    Tropical Minted Cantaloupe Soup with Fresh Lime, 65
Linguine with Chicken and Artichokes, 266
Linguine with White Clam Sauce, 193
Lots of Layers Dip, 5
Louisiana Beans Oregano, 423
Louisiana Skillet Pork, 347
Luscious Berry Dip, 11

m

mangoes
    Berry Explosion Salad, 103
    cook's tip on, 126

mozzarella (*continued*)

Three-Cheese Vegetable Strudel, 404–5

Tomato, Basil, and Mozzarella Salad, 94

Turkey Lasagna, 274

Muesli, 550

muffins

Apricot-Cinnamon Muffins, 543

Blueberry-Banana Muffins, 545

Fruit Muffins, 541

Muffins, 541

Oat Bran Fruit Muffins, 544

Whole-Wheat Muffins, 542

Multigrain Apple Pancakes, 555

mushrooms

Asian Spinach and Mushrooms, 473

Barley Risotto with Mushrooms and Asparagus, 369

Beef and Pasta Skillet, 322

Breakfast Pizzas, 560

Bulgur-Mushroom Burgers, 363

Burgundy Chicken with Mushrooms, 236

Chicken and Mushroom Stir-Fry, 246

Chicken with Bell Peppers and Mushrooms, 233

cook's tip on, 316

Cream of Mushroom Soup, 48

Crumb-Crusted Mushrooms with Lemon, 18

Cube Steak with Mushroom Sauce, 312

Fish Fillets in Foil, 170–71

Fresh Mushroom Soup, 49

Ground Beef Stroganoff, 316

Italian Vegetable Bake, 482

Lemon-Basil Chicken with Mushrooms, 212–13

Mexican Breakfast Pizzas, 561

Mushroom-Stuffed Fish Roll-Ups, 169

Mushrooms with Red Wine, 450

Mushrooms with White Wine and Shallots, 451

Portobello Mushrooms and Sirloin Strips over Spinach Pasta, 300

Portobello Mushroom Wrap with Yogurt Curry Sauce, 410

Portobellos with Polenta and Tomatoes, 364–65

Roast Chicken with Artichoke Hearts and Mushrooms, 234

Salisbury Steaks with Mushroom Sauce, 314

Slow-Cooker Round Steak with Mushrooms and Tomatoes, 310–11

Stuffed Mushrooms, 25

Vegetable Stir-Fry, 484

mustard

Creamy Dijon-Lime Sauce, 499

Dijon-Marinated Vegetable Medley, 98

Fiery Shrimp Dijon, 199

Mild Mustard Sauce, 502

Mustard Potato Salad, 107

Tangy Carrots, 438

n

Nectarine-Pineapple Salsa, Grilled Tuna with, 188

Nibbles, 32

noodles

Beef and Noodle Casserole Dijon, 324

Ground Beef Stroganoff, 316

rice stick, cook's tip on, 375

Rice Sticks with Asian Vegetables (Pad Thai), 374

Two-Cheese Sour Cream Noodles, 359

Vietnamese Beef and Rice Noodle Soup, 74

nutmeg

Baked Cauliflower and Carrots with Nutmeg, 440

Banana Spice Cupcakes with Nutmeg Cream Topping, 578

cook's tip on, 46

Nutmeg Cake, 572

nutrition analyses, for recipes, xix–xx

nutrition labels, reading, 647–50

nuts

adding to diet, xiii

Apricot Bulgur with Pine Nuts, 434

cook's tip on, 87

Dark Chocolate Sauce with Hazelnuts, 510

Green Beans and Rice with Hazelnuts, 422

hazelnuts, cook's tip on, 422

Nibbles, 32

Pattypan Squash with Apple-Nut Stuffing, 478

pine nuts, cook's tips on, 356, 388

Pistachio-Cardamom Meringues, 598

shopping guidelines, 643, 646

Southwestern Nibbles, 32

Zucchini Bread with Pistachios, 527

see also almonds; pecans; walnuts

o

Oat Bran Fruit Muffins, 544

oats

Apple-Raisin Crunch, 591

Cherry Crisp, 592

cook's tip on, 548

W